Patricia A. Kreutler, Ph.D.
Dorice M. Czajka-Narins, Ph.D.

SECOND EDITION

NUTRITION
In Perspective

PRENTICE-HALL, INC., Englewood Cliffs, New Jersey 07632

Library of Congress Cataloging-in-Publication Data

Kreutler, Patricia A.
   Nutrition in perspective.

   Bibliography
   Includes index.
     1. Nutrition. I. *Czajka-Narins, Dorice M.*
II. Title.
QP141.K69 1987   613.2   86–22711
ISBN 0-13-627746-2

Editorial/production supervision: Edith Riker
Interior design: Christine Gehring-Wolf
Manufacturing buyer: Harry Baisley
Cover design: Meryl Poweski
Cover photo: Four by Five, Inc.
Photo research: Ilene Cherna

Printed in the United States of America
10 9 8 7 6 5 4 3 2 1

ISBN 0-13-627746-2 01

Prentice-Hall International (UK) Limited, *London*
Prentice-Hall of Australia Pty. Limited, *Sydney*
Prentice-Hall of Canada Inc., *Toronto*
Prentice-Hall Hispanoamericana, S.A., *Mexico*
Prentice-Hall of India Private Limited, *New Delhi*
Prentice-Hall of Japan, Inc., *Tokyo*
Prentice-Hall of Southeast Asia Pte. Ltd., *Singapore*
Editora Prentice-Hall do Brasil, Ltda., *Rio de Janeiro*

CONTENTS

iii

PART TWO   Nutrition for Everyday Living

PREFACE

Nutrition is a relatively young and rapidly growing discipline. Past its infancy and childhood, it can perhaps be likened to the everchanging adolescent period: With almost daily changes as new information is discovered, older information is reinterpreted, and new applications are identified, it is truly a dynamic science.

Like the first edition, the second edition of *Nutrition In Perspective* has been written to provide students with an understanding of the fundamentals of the science of nutrition; to acquaint students with the issues facing nutritionists, scientific and governmental leaders, and consumers in contemporary society; to prepare students to evaluate nutritional claims made in the popular media; and to enable students to translate knowledge of the science of nutrition into practices that are compatible with individual philosophies and lifestyles.

Not merely an issue-oriented text, *Nutrition In Perspective* is suitable for courses meeting science distribution requirements as well as for introductory courses for nutrition, dietetics, home economics, and nursing majors. While the scientific basis of nutrition has not been underplayed, every attempt has been made to present lucid explanations of basic biological and chemical processes central to the study of nutrition. It has been the authors' experience that most students, even those without a science background, become interested and excited as they learn how the body works. For those who enroll in an introductory nutrition course with a prior knowledge of biology and chemistry, these discussions will serve as a helpful review.

Within the framework of science, presentation of current nutritional issues is a major concern of this text. In the course of their study, students will often be reminded of the importance of diversity in food consumption patterns to nutritional, and therefore overall, health.

This text is scientifically accurate and up-to-date. Reading it, students will become aware that nutrition is a dynamic discipline in which new data and interpretations are constantly emerging; they will learn that change should be anticipated. But readers should not be discouraged; rather, as they learn to appreciate the principles of the scientific method and the intricacies of the human body, they will also appreciate the significance of change in theory and knowledge and be able to place new information in perspective.

It is hoped that this introduction to the study of nutrition will encourage further study, whether formal or informal. Readers will also recognize how many and varied are the disciplines related to nutrition. Insights and talents from many fields are needed to advance the research, interpretation, and application of this subject that so strongly influences our everyday lives.

Plan of the Book

Nutrition In Perspective is divided into two major parts. In Part One, "Scientific Principles of Nutrition," the underlying biological, chemical, and regulatory mechanisms of the internal environment are presented, using a systems approach. An understanding of the basic roles of nutrients in the body prepares students to appreciate the continuity of the life cycle with its changing nutritional needs, the implications of political and societal change, consumer concerns, and the need for a diversified diet. These topics are developed in Part Two, "Nutrition for Everyday Living."

Information and ideas presented in both parts of the text will allow students to identify the totality of nutrition and enable them to adopt good personal health practices and to be informed consumers.

Features

Topics of contemporary interest are presented as "Perspectives" within each chapter. These issues are placed in the context of current scientific knowledge to stimulate thought and discussion.

In the opening chapter a definition and discussion of the Recommended Dietary Allowances are presented. This provides the student with an understanding of some of the basic concepts and terminology to be introduced in subsequent chapters of Part One. A summary and bibliography conclude each chapter.

In-Text Learning Aids

To reinforce the concepts, facts, and principles presented, a variety of learning aids is used. Visual clarification is enhanced by diagrams, figures, photographs, and material in tabular form. Tables of nutrient composition are expressed in useful portion sizes to enable students more realistically to choose appropriate foods.

Descriptions of relevant biological processes are presented in a step-by-step manner, emphasizing regulatory systems. Although the nature of the subject matter requires technical terminology, language has been kept clear and concise. Terms are set in boldface type when they are introduced, and are defined in the glossary. Frequent use of examples to illustrate scientific principles serves to encourage learning, not by memory, but through understanding. As students gain understanding of systems through the use of examples, they are encouraged to transfer their conceptual knowledge from one system to another.

Supplements

An Instructor's Manual with a Test Item File has been prepared to accompany this text. The Instructor's Manual is designed to suggest ideas for lectures, demonstrations, creative projects, and research assignments. Many of the projects are directed toward students whose major interest is in a field other than nutrition. These projects will stimulate continued interest in nutrition within the context of another discipline—and may in turn suggest to the student a further area of intellectual and professional development. The Test Item File includes questions in a variety of formats.

Acknowledgments

The author of the first edition (P.A.K.) is delighted that Dorice M. Czajka-Narins agreed to coauthor this revision, not only for her important contribution to the text, but also because our association has renewed a personal and professional relationship that began at the Massachusetts Institute of Technology.

Nutrition In Perspective reflects the talents, dedication, and enthusiasm of innumerable people. Many of the individuals who have influenced the development of this text will remain anonymous but they include our teachers at M.I.T. who made us think about all aspects of nutrition; our colleagues, too numerous to mention, who provided the interactions necessary to formulate our ideas; and our students who asked thoughtful questions. A central figure in our professional development has been Sanford A. Miller who survived having both of us as graduate students and whose valuable insights influenced our thinking. D.C.-N. would like to thank her husband, Arthur, for his support during this project and her mother Lucille Czajka, who by her help made this and other projects possible.

The production of this text could not have been realized without the cooperation and expertise of many conscientious people. The contributions of the Prentice-Hall staff are gratefully acknowledged: Susan B. Willig, executive editor, who cheerfully coordinated this revision, a challenging and seemingly endless task; Edith Riker, production editor, whose professional expertise and gentle but persistent prodding kept the authors moving along; Susan Lesan, who guided the development of this edition; and Ilene Cherna, photo researcher.

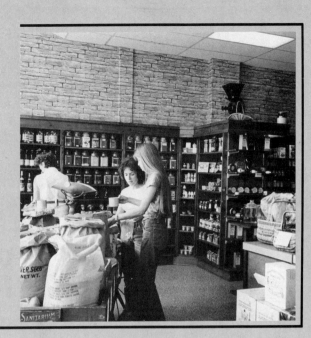

Chapter 1

INTRODUCTION
TO NUTRITION

A loaf of bread, a jug of wine, and thou said the poet long ago—and he was right. This is what it takes to keep that complex marvel called the human body going each day, day after day, for a long lifetime.

Today we call this daily fueling *nutrition*—the process of supplying our bodies with the substances needed for good health and proper functioning. But nutrition is also a science—a growing body of systematically arranged facts about the consumption and utilization of food by people. In this book we will examine nutrition as a process, using the results of nutrition as a science. But first we need to look at the background to our current knowledge and practice, the history of nutrition as a science.

A NUTRITION TIME LINE

By the nineteenth century, English sailors had become known as *Limeys* because of the practice on long voyages of supplying sailors with citrus fruit to prevent a disease known as scurvy. With the long world voyages of exploration, discovery, and trade, sailors becoming ill and dying had become a problem. They did not become ill on short voyages; why on long? By the mid-eighteenth century, one theory was diet: Only a very few kinds of food could be preserved, and the sailors were limited to them for long periods of time. In 1747 a surgeon of the English fleet, James Lind, tested this idea by varying the diets of 12 sailors. Since only those given oranges and lemons improved, Lind concluded that something in the citrus (something we now know as vitamin C) was the answer. But it took another 50 years for the British navy to make citrus juice a requirement for sailors, and another hundred after that for the discovery of vitamins and the answer to the problem of scurvy.

So like many sciences, nutrition has progressed in fits and starts, with many years passing between a discovery and an explanation of it. Some knowledge never spread beyond certain small groups in particular times. Yet other discoveries had to wait for later investigators to provide the missing links in knowledge or the development of the technology that would make facts available.

A time line showing the development of nutrition as a science might begin with the story of Daniel in the Bible. Daniel noticed that people thrive on pulse (legumes) and water, while others languish on meat and wine. But this is an anecdote, not a study that presents new ideas or understandings and influences future work.

On this basis, the nutrition time line is quite bare until the early 1600s, when the first deliberate scientific studies were made and when the physician Sanctorius, a friend of Galileo, published his studies on body weight and food consumption. Sanctorius was his own subject: He weighed himself and all the food he ate and then weighed his excretions. What he discovered was that food intake, though greater than excretory output, does not necessarily increase body weight. The answer, he thought, is that the excess is lost through perspiration.

In 1628 came William Harvey's classic publication on the circulation of the blood—which laid the foundation for the understanding of the transportation of nutrients in the body—followed by Lind's study of scurvy in 1747 and the first measurements of human energy metabolism by Lavoisier in 1789. The time line is beginning to look more crowded, but it was not until the nineteenth century that discoveries and knowledge began to grow at a fast and steady pace.

The first amino acid was discovered in 1810. In 1816, François Magendie dem-

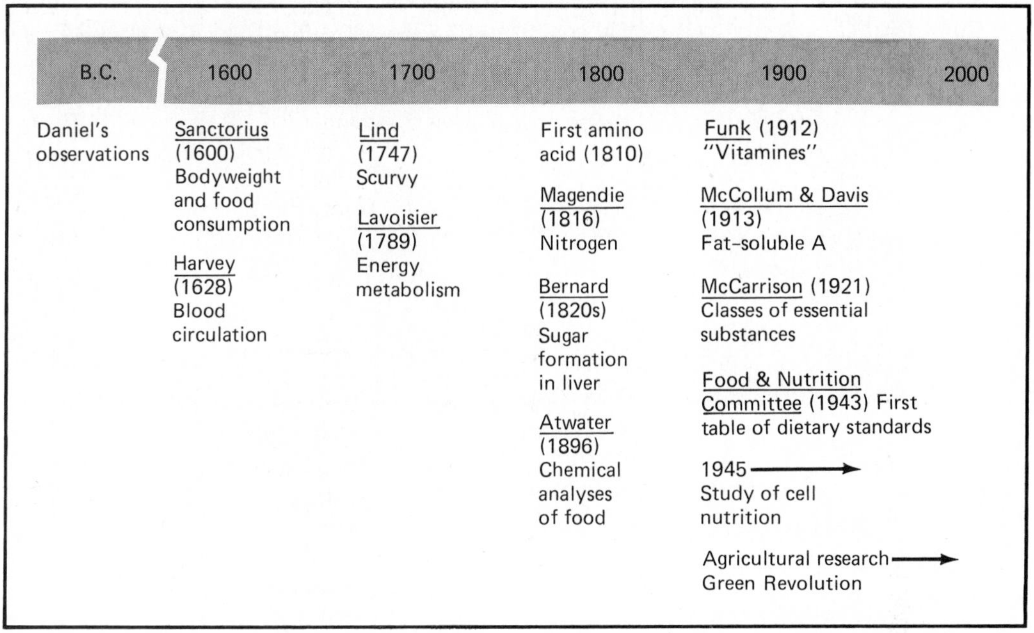

B.C.	1600	1700	1800	1900	2000

Daniel's observations

Sanctorius (1600) Bodyweight and food consumption

Harvey (1628) Blood circulation

Lind (1747) Scurvy

Lavoisier (1789) Energy metabolism

First amino acid (1810)

Magendie (1816) Nitrogen

Bernard (1820s) Sugar formation in liver

Atwater (1896) Chemical analyses of food

Funk (1912) "Vitamines"

McCollum & Davis (1913) Fat-soluble A

McCarrison (1921) Classes of essential substances

Food & Nutrition Committee (1943) First table of dietary standards

1945 ⟶ Study of cell nutrition

Agricultural research ⟶ Green Revolution

FIGURE 1-1   *Nutrition Time Line.*

onstrated that nitrogen-containing compounds were essential in the diet of dogs. His student Claude Bernard investigated sugar formation in the liver. By the 1860s, scientists in many countries were maintaining that food consisted of water, carbohydrate, fat, protein, and mineral ash. In 1896, the U.S. Department of Agriculture published its Bulletin 28, "The Chemical Composition of American Food Materials," by W. O. Atwater, who performed the first extensive analyses of food and made possible the estimation of dietary intake.

Then the mystery of the substance in citrus began to unfold. In Wisconsin in 1907, Elmer V. McCollum began to experiment with rats to try to discover what it was in food that prevented and cured such diseases as scurvy and beriberi. Joined by Marguerite Davis, who developed new techniques for using rats in research, McCollum and his colleague published a paper in 1913 describing a substance they called "fat soluble A." A year earlier, Casimir Funk coined the term *vitamine* to describe some of these substances. It soon became *vitamin* when it was found that not all vitamines are amines, or nitrogen-containing substances. By 1921 Robert McCarrison, a specialist in deficiency diseases, had realized that vitamins were only one class of the essential substances needed to maintain chemical processes in the body.

The first table of dietary standards, however, was not published until 1943, during World War II, by the Food and Nutrition Committee of the National Research Council. The explosion of technology and the development of ever more sophisticated and sensitive instruments since then has led to an equivalent explosion in new nutrition knowledge—and to worldwide efforts to improve health and life by improving both the food supply and the diet. With the electron microscope, ultracentrifuge, microchemical techniques, and radioactive isotopes, laboratory researchers can study the nutrition of the individual cell and the interaction between nutrition and proper cell growth and functioning. The surge in agricultural research

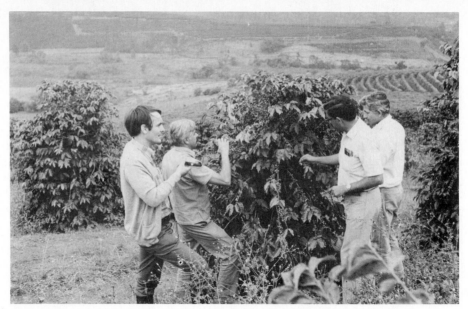

In controlled nutrition experiments, a specific food item or diet is researched. Meticulous planning, accurately recorded findings, and careful analysis are the essentials that lead to valid and logical conclusions.
United Nations

has given us the Green Revolution, as well as many new possibilities for supplying the nutritional needs of a constantly growing world population.

Armed with the results of all this research, workers in UN agencies such as WHO (World Health Organization) and FAO (Food and Agriculture Organization) are able to develop policies and programs to combat the diseases caused by deficiency and to improve overall health in many areas of the Third World. In the industrialized countries, especially our own, a steady stream of nutrition information reaches the public through the media almost on a daily basis. The time line is now jammed, as a result of what we call the scientific method.

NUTRITION AS A SCIENCE

Science deals with systematically arranged facts that demonstrate the operation of general laws that can be tested. These facts have, over many years, been arranged into laws and principles supported by controlled research studies. This controlled testing process is known as the **scientific method.** It is based on a design developed in the sixteenth century by Sir Francis Bacon, the English philosopher. The basic components of the scientific method are illustrated by what is considered to be the first controlled experiment in nutrition, Lind's scurvy study.

The experiment began with the *observation* that many English sailors became ill during long sea voyages and died. Among the explanations and theories proposed to explain this observation was the *hypothesis* that something about the sailors' diet was causing their illness. The **hypothesis** serves to limit the scope of the study. The next step in an experiment is obtaining evidence to support or refute the hypothesis. To test the hypothesis that there was a relationship between diet and illness, Lind studied 12 sailors. He gave two of them a quart of cider each day; two, 25 drops of sulfuric acid three times daily; two, vinegar; two, sea water; two, 2 oranges plus 1 lemon; and two, some nutmeg, on a daily basis. The *result* was soon apparent: Only those sailors given the citrus fruits improved. Lind drew a legitimate *conclusion* that something in the oranges and lemons cured the men.

The long-term progression of research and observation, with many years passing between a discovery and an explanation of it, has often occurred in science. Although each step, each experiment, is only a link in the chain of knowledge, much care must be taken to make it a strong link. **Controlled experiments** are the foundation on which scientific knowledge is built. In controlled nutrition experiments, a specific food item or diet is often fed to one group of subjects, while a comparable group receives a standard diet; the outcomes for both groups are then compared. Meticulous planning, accurately recorded findings, and careful analysis are the essentials of research and lead to valid and logical conclusions. Scientists are trained in these essentials, but no training can provide the qualities of vision and imagination, courage of convictions, drive, enthusiasm, patience, and persistence necessary to promote scientific discoveries.

Types of Evidence

The end product of experimentation is *evidence*, information that can be used to support the particular hypothesis being investigated. Depending on the kind of hypothesis and the methods available to test it, many different types of evidence may be obtained. In studies of nutrition, descriptive, epidemiological, and experimental evidence all have their place.

DESCRIPTIVE EVIDENCE.   A collection of facts about a situation as it exists in the environment is known as **descriptive evidence.** For example, your casual observation that about one out of ten students in your nutrition class is overweight would be considered descriptive evidence. Casual observations such as this, based on general impressions, are referred to as **anecdotal evidence.** There are obvious limitations to anecdotal reporting. This observation may be an underestimate, because students interested in nutrition may be more likely to control their weight than other students, or your sample may be biased so as to produce an overestimate, if the nutrition course is an adjunct to a weight-control workshop. Finally, such casual observations are not supported by written records, and memory may not serve correctly. Despite these limitations, anecdotal evidence can be of value by suggesting hypotheses that can then be tested by more rigorous methods, such as the *planned survey.* A survey of all the students at your college, using a specific questionnaire or work sheet on which to record weight and other data, would provide better representation of overweight and normal weight subjects and be more accurate.

EPIDEMIOLOGICAL EVIDENCE.   The survey method may suggest other questions. For example, do some factors affect overweight students but not others? You would need more than descriptive evidence to answer this question; **epidemiological evidence** would be the next step. **Epidemiology** is the study of the occurrence and distribution of factors associated with a particular phenomenon in a given population. Thus, epidemiological examination of your descriptive survey may indicate that excess weight is more prevalent in resident students than in students who commute. In scientific terms, you have found an **association** between residency and overweight. But the mere existence of an association does not necessarily indicate a cause-and-effect relationship between the variables. Just as a survey finding that heart attack victims own television sets could not be used as evidence that television causes heart disease, you could not conclude that residency causes overweight.

Despite this limitation, epidemiological evidence is important because, like descriptive evidence, it suggests hypotheses that may deserve further examination. A classic example of epidemiological evidence is the well-known Framingham study, in which several factors, such as overweight and physical inactivity, were found to be associated with the occurrence of coronary heart disease in men in a small town in Massachusetts.

EXPERIMENTAL EVIDENCE. Scientists are rarely satisfied with associations. They test hypotheses in order to establish cause-and-effect relationships. This testing process provides **experimental evidence.** In your study of overweight on campus, you may, for example, hypothesize that resident students have more opportunity than commuting students to take second and third helpings of dessert. To test this hy-

Exaggerated claims. Products and diets are described as "miraculous," "100 percent safe and effective," and "too good to believe" (this last, at least, is often true).

Hints of persecution. The "establishment" we are told, fear the acceptance of new, miraculous dietary cures of disease because it would make present knowledge obsolete and thus undermine the prestige of the medical-industrial-educational power structure. Against these groups, the faddists with a product to sell present themselves as martyred fighters for the truth.

Exploitation of insecurity. If you care about your family's health, goes this argument, you will buy my book; my blender, which somehow improves the nutritional value of your food; my pills, capsules, or tonics. To the objection that these are overpriced, there is a ready response: "Are you setting a price on health, even on life itself?" Guilt can sell products.

Impressive titles. Few legal restraints are imposed on those who choose to call themselves nutritionists, health advisors, diet specialists, or world-renowned nutrition experts. They can be distinguished from those with credentials and expertise only by careful scrutiny of their academic and professional qualifications, and few members of the public can or will do this.

So where does a person turn to get sound nutrition information? In Appendix I there is a list of organizations which provide the public with reliable nutrition information. For example, the Institute of Food Technologists, through its Expert Panel on Food Safety and Nutrition, provides accurate summary statements on topics of public interest to its regional communicators and to the membership of the organization. The regional communicators contact the science and medical media in their area and provide them with these materials. Many newspapers carry columns written by bona fide nutritionists who will answer questions. Many hospitals provide speakers from their departments of dietetics. For quick answers, there are state university cooperative extension offices in many counties. Questions about specific products can be answered by customer service representatives of the companies. There is a great deal of sound information available, but the consumer must make an effort to get it: more than simply tossing a gossip sheet on top of the groceries at the supermarket checkout.

pothesis, you might arrange to limit dessert servings in the residents' cafeteria to one per meal. If, after a long enough period of time, you found that the difference in overweight between residents and commuters had disappeared, you might conclude that extra desserts had indeed caused obesity.

Obviously, this experiment would be difficult to perform, because it would be impossible to control other important factors. Your hungry residents may substitute midnight snacks for their usual second dessert helping or not eat as often in the cafeteria. This difficulty in controlling the behavior of human subjects has produced increased reliance on experiments using nonhuman animals.

Experimental Models

Research studies in nonhuman systems are called **experimental models.** Nutritionists use **animal models.** Horses, cows, sheep, pigs, birds, cats, dogs, guinea pigs, and even microorganisms are used, but rats are by far the most popular experimental model. Each year, thousands of rats are used in diet-related studies to determine effects, if any, on health. It is very difficult, if not impossible, to perform such tests on human subjects.

Designing human experiments is difficult. To subject human beings intentionally to pain or other health hazards or to withhold possible cures is not ethical. Then, there is the problem of obtaining sufficient numbers as suitable subjects in a given place. Also, manipulation of only one test variable is difficult with human subjects. Finally, there is the problem of time. Human life is so long that young investigators would be of retirement age before they could complete an experiment in only one or two generations.

Obviously, studies of many generations are more practical in animals. Rats' small size, low maintenance cost, ease of handling, and rapid rate of reproduction have made them particularly useful. And most important to nutritionists, they are omnivorous, just as humans are, and will eat almost any kind of diet. The disadvantage of using rats is that all their internal processes are not the same as those of humans. For example, their need for certain vitamins may be different from that of humans. Rat studies may suggest applications to human nutrition, although they cannot prove beyond doubt that results in humans will be exactly the same. Nevertheless, animal models are extremely valuable because ethical, economic, and biological limitations may prohibit human testing.

Although animal models permit precise control of experimental variables, their use does not guarantee attention to other important factors. Experiments are only as good as the researchers who design them, the assumptions they make, and the testing methods they use. Is the experimental hypothesis based on accurate observation? Are the testing methods appropriate? Are important variables well controlled? Do the final conclusions follow from the observed results? Is enough information provided so that another investigator can perform the same study? These are all questions that must be asked in evaluating scientific studies.

Each year thousands of rats are used in diet-related studies to determine effects on health. It is difficult and often impossible to perform such tests on human subjects.
Hugh Rogers/Monkmeyer

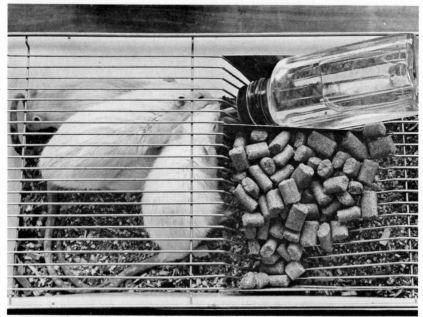

Historically, even well-controlled experiments demonstrating supportable conclusions have not always found a favorable reception in the scientific community and in the general population, especially when scientific findings differ from widely held beliefs. It often takes years before the "truth" is accepted, and many more years before long-standing theories and explanations are replaced by laws based on repeated experimentally proven facts.

But scientific research and discovery is only one aspect of nutrition; the other is the effects of different kinds of food behavior. We will look now at patterns of food consumption and use and then at what the body does with the food we do consume.

THE ECOLOGY OF FOOD AND NUTRITION

There is constant interaction between the **internal environment** inside the organism, with its precisely regulated systems, and the **external environment**, with its physical, technological, and psychosocial systems that determine the availability and choice of foods.

Food Behavior: The External Environment

Food is as much an expression of life style as choice of work, clothing, housing, and religious practices. Stylized food habits, known to sociologists as **foodways**, evolved as adaptations to the physical and social environment and are an important part of any cultural heritage.

In many societies food is not just a necessity of life but a pleasure-filled symbol of love, companionship, and achievement. Food is always a part of celebrations, the main attraction at holidays and at ritual gatherings from baptisms to funerals. An abundance of food symbolizes wealth and achievement; certain foods are exchanged as gifts; and still others, such as salt and bread, are a part of many ancient social rituals. But which foods a particular culture values, how it uses them, and which it prohibits depend on a number of factors—geography and topography, technology, economics and politics, psychology, and tradition.

GEOGRAPHY AND TOPOGRAPHY. People can eat only what is available. Dry climates foster the production of cereal grains; wet climates, the growing of rice. These environmental facts of life account for the popularity of breads and noodles in Europe and for the dependence on rice in many parts of Asia. Where soil is not fertile, the cassava and the soybean become dietary staples. Along coastlines and rivers, fish predominates in the diet. And when the food supply is uncertain, people have developed ways to preserve foods by drying or smoking for lean times. This need to have food for a time of scarcity was what gave us the sausage, the dried cod, and concentrated pastes and sauces such as the Vietnamese nuoc-mam and the Japanese miso.

Seasonal changes also have effects. Not only do they affect taste buds and appetites, but also they restrict the availability of foods. In the past, when many fresh foods were available only in season, spring was eagerly awaited because it meant the return of fresh vegetables and fruits. Where the growing season was short, ways were developed to preserve crops—canned and pickled fruits and vegetables, dried fruits and beans, jams and marmalades. And the seasons and the weather can also affect the need for certain kinds of foods. Sunlight, for example, acts on a chemical in the skin to produce vitamin D. In sunny climates where people spend a great deal of time out of doors, the need for vitamin D from food sources is reduced. Hot weather, because of excessive perspiration, may increase the need for salt and fluid. Natural disasters and unfavorable weather conditions can limit output and affect the taste, quality, and cost of agricultural products.

TECHNOLOGY. Although other animals accept the natural conditions in which they find themselves, humans have developed ways to modify their environment in order to increase the production and availability of food. In fact, the tools created by early humans and the development of animal husbandry and agriculture have provided the names—Stone Age or Iron Age—by which prehistoric periods are known.

Today, advances in irrigation, crop rotation, fertilizers, and cultivation have raised crop yields enormously even though the amount of land being farmed has decreased. Transportation methods allow us to move food products in bulk over large distances so quickly that fresh foods are available everywhere and all year round.

Refrigeration and processing techniques, large agribusiness organizations, and inventive packaging have made significant changes in our food choices and preferences. When the first settlers arrived in the New World, their diet expanded to include corn, squash, deer, wild turkey, fish, cranberries, potatoes, and nuts. By the time the United States was founded in 1776, the wealthy had a choice among local crops and imported items, although the average person was still limited to locally grown foods, simply prepared.

Today, even average Americans enjoy a wide variety of foods, and new foods, such as tofu-based frozen desserts, appear on supermarket shelves almost every day.

ECONOMICS. But despite our high technology and efficient distribution system, nutritious foods are not universally available throughout American society. Poverty sharply restricts the variety and quality of foods available and ultimately results in a vicious cycle: poor health, leading to decreased work capacity, loss of income, decreased purchasing power, decreased food intake, worsened nutritional and physical health, and further decrease in work capacity.

POLITICS. Politics has a great deal to do with socioeconomic food problems. In 1977, for example, the federal government spent about $5.7 billion on the food stamp program, which is designed to increase the availability of nourishing food to those whose incomes would not otherwise provide an adequate diet. Food supplies increase with government subsidies to farmers; incentives to improve productivity; and credit systems for purchases of seed, equipment, and fertilizers. Government stockpiling of surplus foods, price supports, and foreign commodity sales can increase prices and decrease availability. Consumers' actions can also have an effect: When meat prices rose sharply in 1973, for example, American shoppers simply boycotted meat.

PSYCHOLOGY. Advertising messages on television and radio and in newspapers and magazines tell us what is available for consumption and why we should want to consume it. These messages are directed at fulfilling not nutritional but psychosocial needs. Our physiological needs ensure that we eat, but our psychological needs

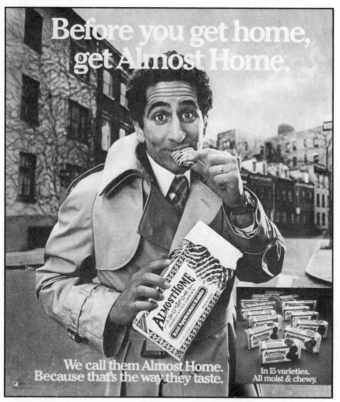

Food advertising campaigns are often based on psychological factors.
Nabisco Brands, Inc.

determine to a large extent what it is we choose to eat. Food becomes a symbol laden with social and emotional meaning.

Emotional response to food begins on the day of birth. The hungry infant learns to associate food with relief of bodily discomfort, with the warmth of a parent's body, and with the contented sleep that follows. Eating becomes associated with care, attention, and love. In adulthood, unfortunately, food can become a substitute for emotional gratification or affection. When we cannot sleep, we look for the midnight snack. When we've had a terrible day, we console ourselves with a hot fudge sundae. Food is a reward for good behavior, a punishment for bad, and a medicine (chicken soup, a cup of tea).

Food satisfies in many ways. The sensory pleasure associated with food—its appearance, aroma, and taste—does much to ensure that we eat varied dishes in sufficient quantities. Cooking and the creation of artistic dishes are excellent opportunities for self-expression. Slicing, pounding, mixing, and kneading may be good emotional outlets. Meal planning satisfies the need to care for and nurture others. Family and personal rituals at meals give order and stability to daily life.

SOCIETY AND CULTURE. These psychological and social aspects of food and nutrition are tied to a cultural heritage. A **culture** consists of the patterned sets of reactions, the ways of life learned by and characteristic of a particular group of people. A group with a distinctive culture is a **society**; it may be a nation, an ethnic group, a village, or a tribe, for societies are defined not by size or complexity but by shared traditions and ways of life. Within most large and complex societies such as ours, there are also subcultures with different customs and traditions.

Since all human behavior is influenced by the culture in which the individual is brought up, even in our fast-changing society, much of how we live and what we eat is determined by the cultural history of our families.

Many cultural traditions and habits deal with food behavior. In traditional Malaya, China, and Japan, fathers and sons receive their food first; mothers and daughters serve meals and eat separately later. In parts of Africa and the Middle East, the oldest family members are served first. Certain Latin American cultures classify red meats and eggs as "hot foods," bad for children and pregnant women. Other cultures consider certain plants and animals inedible. What American, for example, would eat a dog or a cat?

Often cultural practices and beliefs follow a kind of "folk logic" that relates attributes of foods to their effects on the human body. Warriors in Madagascar did not eat the knees of oxen because they feared their own knee joints would become weak, like those of oxen. In many traditional hunting cultures, the heart and liver of certain animals were reserved for the hunter-warriors because these organs were believed to impact strength and courage.

Religious practices often involve food. Some may in fact be based on ecological conditions, such as the prohibition against eating pork among Jews and Muslims, both residents of areas more suitable for the raising of sheep than of pigs. There may also be an ecological basis for the sacred cow of Hindu India. Indian cattle are

All human behavior is influenced by culture and even in our ever-changing modern society, how we live and what we eat is determined by the cultural history of our own family.
Hanna Schreiber/Photo Researchers, Inc.

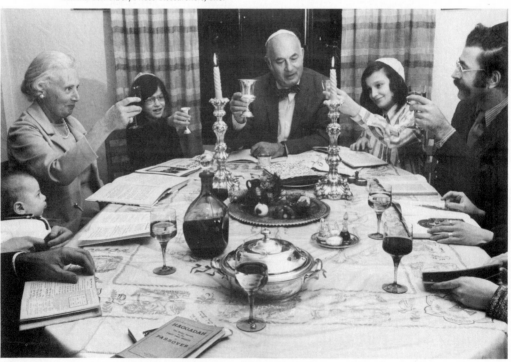

hardy; they eat waste products and can survive long periods of drought. They are useful work animals, as well as providers of dairy products and of dung, which is often the only source of fuel for cooking and heating.

Other religious food practices are based on symbolism—the egg at Easter, symbol of birth and fertility; the unleavened bread of the Jewish Passover; the salt used in Christian baptism; the food offerings at ancestral altars; the communion wafer and wine.

Social symbols associated with food also abound. In the nineteenth century, bread made with bleached white flour and white sugar was a sign of status, for these ingredients were expensive. Today, dark, whole-grain breads are status foods for "gourmet" and "health" reasons. Caviar and champagne, truffles and pheasant are symbols of both affluence and elegance. The "gourmet revolution" has changed many of our status foods, as has the growing preoccupation with health, fitness, and nutrition. Bean sprouts, raw vegetables, and traditional beans and rice are "in"; thick, juicy steak, mashed potatoes, and pie a la mode are "out."

Food Trends in the United States

Research has shown that despite, or perhaps because of, our psychosocial needs, most Americans eat a well-balanced diet. Consumers are more aware that the foods they eat may have both short and long-term effects on their health. Heart disease, weight gain, diabetes, and cancer are frequently identified as long-term health effects of the food we eat. More poultry, low-fat milk, and fresh fruits and vegetables are consumed today than 10 or 20 years ago; consumption of eggs, coffee, and whole milk is down. The use of "natural" foods has increased and more diet foods are being consumed. Many consumers base their food choices primarily on quality; an even larger number base their choices on a combination of quality and price.

Today's families eat fewer meals together and consume more foods on the run. Drive-up windows have resulted in an increase in the number of people who eat in their cars. More people eat out. Nearly three-quarters of the consumers in one survey admitted to skipping meals, primarily breakfast. More women (62.5 percent) skip meals than men (25.5 percent) or children (16.5 percent).

What about the college student? Do the habits learned at home carry over? Do the food practices of college students, for example, reflect their previous eating habits, or are students so involved with academic work and extracurricular activities that they do not make an effort to meet their nutritional needs?

According to some studies, there is good news for college students—and their concerned parents. Students, on the whole, have a firm knowledge of good nutrition and meet or exceed the recommended dietary allowances for most nutrients. When researchers compare the nutritional habits of today's college women with those of 30 years ago, they commonly find that the meal-skipping, snacking, and fad diets attributed to college students in recent years have obviously not been detrimental. What effect does the marketing of the ultra-thin, skinny, or malnourished "look" have on the eating habits of college students and other adults?

Of the 73 women in a junior/senior nutrition course, three were identified by their classmates as having either anorexia nervosa or bulimia (see Chapter 5). From data submitted as part of a project to evaluate their intake, one of the three is at the point of serious illness. From three-day food records, 93 percent and 44 percent of these students did not meet through their diet the recommended intake for iron and for calcium, respectively. Nine percent did not consume half the recommended amount of calcium each day. Fortunately many took supplements. Sup-

THE RECOMMENDED DIETARY ALLOWANCES (RDA)

The Recommended Dietary Allowances, or RDAs, are nutritional standards that will be referred to often throughout this text. To most people, the RDAs may seem authoritative. In fact, they are far from absolute, although they are indeed useful. The first version of what would become the RDAs was formulated during World War II and was intended to provide information for the development of nutrition programs in connection with national defense. Since that time, committees of the Food and Nutrition Board of the National Research Council have reevaluated the RDAs approximately every five years. The current, 9th Edition of the RDAs was published in 1980. Publication of the 1985 edition has been postponed. The RDAs can be put in perspective by keeping the following points in mind.

1. THEY ARE BASED ON ESSENTIALLY THE SAME PHILOSOPHY ALTHOUGH ACTUAL NUMBERS HAVE CHANGED. The term "allowance" was specifically chosen by the original committee to avoid implications of finality regarding the numerical values. The number of nutrients for which there are RDAs has increased from the original list of protein, vitamins A, D, and C, thiamin, riboflavin, niacin, calcium, and iron. In 1968, RDAs were established for vitamin E, folacin, pyridoxine, vitamin B_{12}, phosphorus, magnesium, and iodine as sufficient information became available on these nutrients. In 1974, the RDA for zinc was first established. No additional RDAs were established in 1980. However, for the first time, estimated safe and adequate daily dietary intakes were established for 12 additional vitamins and minerals for which there was some information, but not enough to establish RDAs. Several

changes were anticipated for the 1985 edition: changes in age categories, provision of an RDA for selenium, and revised recommendations for several vitamins and minerals. The reviewers of the committee's recommendations, however, concluded that changes in existing RDAs are warranted only for a few of these nutrients. At this point in time the revised publication schedule for the 10th edition of the RDAs has not been finalized, but it will appear eventually. Until a new report is issued, the recommendations contained in the ninth edition (1980) of the RDAs should be used.

2. THEY ARE BASED ON THE BEST INFORMATION AVAILABLE AT PRESENT ON THE ENERGY AND NUTRIENT NEEDS OF HEALTHY PEOPLE. Several sources of data have been used by various committees to determine the RDAs. These include surveys of groups of individuals to determine the relationship of nutrient intake to the presence or absence of disease; controlled feeding experiments with small numbers of individuals; and metabolic studies on laboratory animals. Although the information base upon which the recommendations rest is constantly expanding, there are still gaps in our knowledge, particularly with regard to certain age groups and for certain nutrients. For example, the most recent committee recognized formally the physiological heterogenity of the population over 50 and recommended two age categories, 51–69 years and 70 years and over. This change acknowledges that more and better data have become available on these groups since the 1980 RDAs although there is still a great need for additional knowledge and

plemented cereals were a major source of iron. The average caloric intake was 1103 kilocalories, in comparison to a recommended intake of approximate 2000 kilocalories. Many of the students do not eat meat; a few never cook a meal. On the positive side, these students met or exceeded the recommended intake for many nutrients; the nutrients mentioned above (iron and calcium) are problem nutrients for many age groups.

According to the Food and Drug Administration (FDA) 150 of the 209.2 pounds of vegetables consumed by each person in 1984 were fresh. Lettuce topped

understanding of these age groups. Another problem with setting RDAs is the vast difference in what we know about each of the nutrients. The essentiality of iron has been recognized for over 100 years and the amount of research data is enormous. However, we are still learning about iron, particularly with regard to its function as part of enzymes. Pick up the last few issues of any nutrition journal and there will be at least one article on iron. On the other hand, the essentiality of chromium was demonstrated within your lifetime and there is a lot we don't know about the role of chromium in metabolism or if everyone gets enough in their diet. A third problem is that we do not know enough about what affects the availability of a given nutrient. RDAs are based on average availability, but the availability of nutrients from an individual's self-selected diet may vary considerably from the average.

3. THEY EXCEED REQUIREMENTS BELOW WHICH AVERAGE PEOPLE WOULD BE EXPECTED TO SUFFER FROM NUTRITION DEFICIENCIES. Requirements are the smallest amount of a nutrient needed to cure or prevent a deficiency. Although average requirements can be determined, no one is "average." Human beings vary in body build, internal chemistry, age, life style, and numerous other factors that affect nutrient needs. Requirements are actual physiological needs, but they are difficult to measure, different for every individual, and in practical terms cannot be determined for each and every person. As Harper stated several years ago, "They [the RDAs] are not requirements; they are recommendations directed toward insuring the nutritional health of groups. They

must, therefore, be high enough to meet the needs of those with the highest requirements and, hence, must exceed the needs of most people."

Must we consume the amount represented by the RDA for each nutrient every day? No. Analysis of one-day food records for a large number of people may be appropriate in assessing a group. For individuals, intake data averaged over a sufficient number of days to provide an estimate of usual intake must be obtained. For most nutrients, three to seven days are adequate to obtain a time-averaged value to compare to the RDA. (Methods of dietary assessment are discussed in Chapter 10.)

Translating RDAs into needs for specific foods, rather than specific nutrients, is more difficult. The nutrient content of a sample of most foods will not be representative of all samples of that food, since nutrient content depends on such variables as climate and soil composition and nutrients may be lost in commercial or home processing and preparation. Also, interactions among nutrients affect the nutrient value of foods.

Life is not static; we will never have all the data we need to set the RDAs because of the evolving nature of our understanding of human metabolism, the epidemiology of disease, and changes in patterns of intake and interactions of nutrients with each other and other components of diet. Nutrition in general is a vigorous, complex science. The RDAs are not just simple numbers. Therefore, it should not be a surprise that the allowances are subject to differences between countries or change with the course of time.

the list. Of the 142.9 pounds of fruit each person consumed, approximately half was fresh; bananas ranked first, oranges second, and apples third. The U.S. Department of Agriculture tells us that lowfat and skim milk consumption has increased to 41 quarts per person and the amount of yogurt continues to climb, 3.18 pounds per person in 1983. Egg consumption continues to decrease while consumption of poultry and fish increases. Meat, beef, pork, veal, and lamb consumption is down to approximately 150 pounds per person for a whole year. In 1983 each of us consumed 40 gallons of soft drinks and about seven gallons of fruit juice. Many of

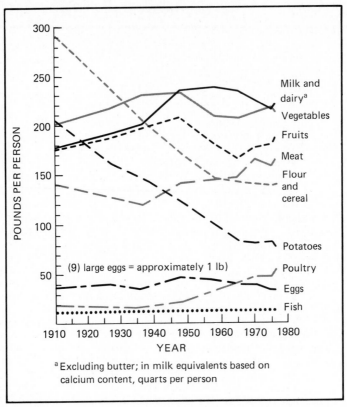

FIGURE 1-2   *Trends in Consumption in the United States in the Twentieth Century.*

these figures are based on **disappearance data** and therefore overestimate consumption, but are very useful in spotting trends. Figure 1–2 identifies several nutritional trends in this century.

The Internal Environment

"You are what you eat," or so the expression goes. But to understand the science of nutrition, we must go one step further and examine not only what is eaten but also what happens to food after it enters the internal environment of the body. The processes by which foods are utilized by the living machine can be explained in terms of basic chemistry and biology. The brief discussion which follows will therefore present some of the essentials of these sciences; additional information can be found in the appendix to this chapter.

Chemistry is the study of **matter**—anything which occupies space and has mass or weight, from a drop of water to a hamburger to you. Matter can consist of a **substance**, which contains only one kind of atom or molecule. Many of the substances in living matter contain carbon, and are therefore said to be **organic.** (Although the term *organic* is commonly believed to imply that the substance has some sort of living quality or vital force, this is not the correct meaning in science.) Four classes of nutrients—proteins, lipids, carbohydrates, and vitamins—are organic, and consequently many important materials which the body produces from nutrients are also organic. But the most abundant molecule in living things is water. Like minerals, water is an **inorganic,** or non-carbon-containing, nutrient class.

Matter can also consist of a *mixture,* which contains varying proportions of more than one kind of atom or molecule. All living things and therefore all foods, because they come from living things, are complicated mixtures of many different substances: water, proteins, minerals, vitamins, and so on. The final composition of a living thing is not, however, just a random collection of substances mixed together. Rather, substances taken in from the environment are modified under the direction of the genetic material—the DNA—in the nucleus of each cell. So if your cat eats ground beef, it turns the proteins and other materials of cow flesh into cat flesh—perhaps even into new kittens. If *you* eat ground beef, you turn the materials from a cow into human flesh, according to the orders given to the cells by the DNA within them. These remarkable transformations are brought about by the biological processes of digestion, absorption, metabolism, and excretion.

Digestion may be of two kinds. In **mechanical digestion,** pieces of food are broken down into smaller bits, but the substances present in the bits retain the same chemical identity; that is, a protein molecule remains the same protein molecule, a fat remains a fat, sucrose (table sugar) remains sucrose, and so on. In **chemical digestion,** biological catalysts or **enzymes** act on the molecules in foods to split them into smaller, different molecules: Proteins are broken down into amino acids just as the beads in a necklace separate when the string is broken, fats are broken down to their subunits (glycerol and fatty acids), and sucrose is converted to the two simple sugars of which it was composed.

Digestion occurs in the **gastrointestinal tract.** But by and large digestion occurs in the digestive tract. This is a complex tube running through the body, and food in this tract is not really inside the body proper, just as an auto in a tunnel through a mountain is not actually in the mountain. In this way, the body protects itself from direct exposure to the many foreign proteins and other substances in foods which could provoke severe allergies and other adverse reactions if they gained access to the body cells themselves.

In the **digestive system,** various types of specialized cells, which are organized into tissues and organs, each contribute their individual efforts toward accomplishing the ultimate goal of digestion: conversion of large molecules into substances small enough to pass the barrier between the digestive tract and the inner environment of the body itself.

Absorption—the passage of substances from the digestive tract into the body—may be mere passive diffusion, whereby nutrients travel from an area of high concentration (the digestive tract) to an area of lower concentration (the blood stream and lymph stream of the body). Or absorption may involve active transport, in which an organism expends energy to pump as many nutrient molecules as possible across the barrier. Although using energy simply to extract the last bit of usable material from food in the digestive tract may seem wasteful, the value to be derived later from those materials makes it worth the effort, for they would otherwise be excreted, unused, in the feces.

In general, water-soluble materials are absorbed into the blood stream, and fat-soluble ones into the lymph. The lymph bypasses the liver releasing its content into the general circulation through the thoracic duct and subclavian vein into the right atrium of the heart. Nutrients of all kinds are therefore presented to, and taken up by, each cell in the body.

Metabolism, which must occur continuously in every living cell, is then responsible for converting those substances from beef, wheat, and all the other once-living things that were eaten into substances needed by the organism that did the eating. **Metabolism**, which is simply defined as the sum total of all changes that occur after absorption and up to excretion, is far from a simple process. Thousands of different chemical reactions, many of which occur in definite sequences at dizzying speeds, are integrated into the whole known as *metabolism*. For convenience's sake, metabolism can be considered to consist of two phases: catabolism and anabolism. In **catabolism**, molecules are broken down, with the release of energy needed for functioning, or work, of the cells (muscle contraction, nerve transmission, and enzyme and hormone production, for example). In **anabolism**, substances are used to construct larger substances (hemoglobin from iron and amino acids, body fat from glycerol and fatty acids, the large glycogen molecules from many molecules of the simple sugar, glucose). Although catabolism and anabolism may be separated in order to simplify a discussion of metabolism, in the cells the two processes are intimately linked to each other; catabolism releases energy to be used in anabolism, and anabolism maintains and constantly repairs the physical structure of the cell without which neither catabolism nor any other life process could continue.

Excretion—the expelling of unused, unusable, and perhaps even detrimental materials back into the external environment—is performed by several different organs. Among the functions of the kidneys are the regulation of water and electrolyte balance and excretion of urea, a nitrogen-containing end product of protein metabolism. Excess amounts of the B vitamins are excreted in the urine. For minerals, the major route of excretion is the gut and urinary losses are negligible except in periods of stress, such as during prolonged starvation. For some minerals, for example iron, the amount present in the body is controlled by absorption; therefore if there is a defect in absorption, large concentrations of iron can accumulate in the body and the kidney is not able to excrete them.

The lungs are the organs that are primarily responsible for excreting carbon dioxide, which is formed continuously when nutrient molecules are broken down. The skin excretes certain minerals (such as the sodium and chloride which make up the salt in sweat) as well as smaller or greater quantities of water. Finally, the colon (large intestine) excretes food materials which escaped digestion, such as the various types of fiber in foods, along with a fairly large amount of water.

Each different kind of organism has its own patterns of digestion, absorption, metabolism, and excretion, based on its own particular needs. A tapeworm has no need to digest food as we do, for it lives in the digestive tract of a human or other animal which does the job of digestion for it. Excretion of salt presents such a problem for certain marine birds, with their high salt intake resulting from ingestion of sea water, that they have developed special salt-secreting glands to solve this problem. Each individual species has developed its own unique ways of incorporating part of the external environment, its food, into its internal environment. Any species that failed at this task is no longer around for us to observe, because survival is contingent upon an organism's ability to deal successfully with its nutritional needs.

Interactions Between the Internal and External Environments

This introduction to the science of nutrition has examined both the external and internal factors that influence the foods consumed and their processing in the human body. Internal and external environments clearly influence our nutritional health. In turn, nutritional health affects both these environments. What may not be so obvious is that these environments also influence each other. For example, illness, a disturbance of the internal environment, impinges on the external environment by limiting an individual's work capacity and social activities. Similarly, stressful changes in the external environment may be manifested in the internal environment as increased stomach acidity, perhaps producing ulcers, or as elevated blood pressure, perhaps causing headaches or cardiovascular problems.

Later chapters will explore the interactions between internal and external environments. They will present the basic nutrients required by the body, their functions, and their dietary sources. The watchword in the pages ahead will be *diversity*, the diversity of human needs dictating diversity in diet. Because there is no one perfect food which can supply all needed nutrients, nutritional health is closely tied to diversity.

College students, on the whole, have a knowledge of good nutrition and meet or exceed the recommended dietary allowances for most nutrients.
Laimute E. Druskis

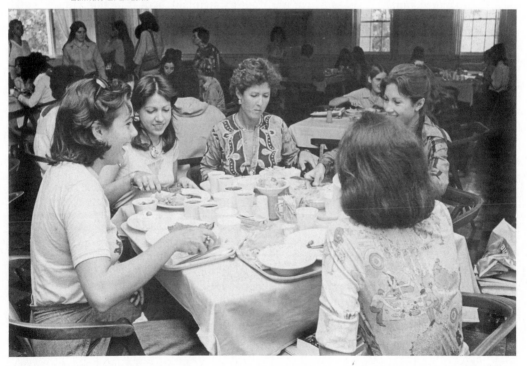

SUMMARY

Nutrition is both a science and a process. Nutritional science deals with facts and principles derived from research studies. These studies provide descriptive evidence about situations that exist in the environment, epidemiological evidence about the occurrence and distribution of factors associated with particular nutritional phenomena, and experimental evidence about proven cause-and-effect relationships. Because experimental evidence is difficult to obtain in human subjects, nutritional researchers use animal models, often rats.

Nutrition as a process is influenced by variables in the external and internal environments. External factors, such as geography, topography, technological advances, and culturally transmitted social influences, determine what foods are available to us and which ones we choose to eat. The internal environment exerts other strong pressures. The body and all the foods taken into it are made up of atoms and molecules. These atoms and molecules join together to form compounds. Organic compounds contain carbon. There are four classes of organic compounds in foods: carbohydrates, proteins, lipids, and vitamins. Inorganic molecules of water and of the minerals are also considered nutrients.

The process of nutrition involves the transformation of the atoms and molecules of food into the kinds of atoms and molecules that make up the body. This transformation occurs inside the cells. There are many specialized cells in the body, each with a particular structure suited to its particular function. Cells are organized into tissues, which in turn are organized into organs. Organs form larger organ systems.

The digestive system is of obvious importance to nutritionists. Digestive organs perform the mechanical and chemical processes by which food is digested or prepared for absorption into the blood. Specialized protein molecules, enzymes, speed the rate of these chemical reactions; each acts only on a specific substrate. Molecules of nutrients are absorbed by a variety of mechanisms into the circulatory system, from which they become available to the cells of the body.

Water-soluble nutrients are carried in the bloodstream throughout the body. Fats and fat-soluble nutrients go from the lymphatic system into the bloodstream. From the blood, nutrients enter the individual cells of the body. Here they are metabolized in one of two processes: anabolism, an energy-using process in which substances are made or synthesized; and catabolism, an energy-releasing process in which body substances are broken down into simpler substances. These processes maintain body function, renew body tissue, and produce waste products, which are excreted from the body by the lungs, skin, and kidneys. Solid wastes, representing mainly undigested components of food, accumulate in the large intestine or colon and are eliminated as feces.

Human needs for nutrients vary from one individual to the next, and during the various stages of the life cycle. The best way to provide for adequate intake of all nutrients is to eat a varied diet.

BIBLIOGRAPHY

America's Changing Diet, *FDA Consumer*, October 1985.

BEATTY, W. K. The history of nutrition: A tour of the literature. *Federation Proceedings* 36:2511, 1977.

BRIGGS, G. M. Muscle foods and human health. *Food Technology* February 1984, p. 54.

GORDON, B. M. Why we choose the foods we do. *Nutrition Today* 18:17–23, 1983.

GUTHRIE, H. A. The 1985 Recommended Dietary Allowance Committee: An Overview. *Journal of the American Dietetic Association* 85:1646–1648, 1985.

HARPER, A. E. *Recommended Dietary Allow-*

ances: *Are they what we think they are? Journal of the American Dietetic Association* 64:151–156, 1974.

HARPER, A. E. Origin of Recommended Dietary Allowances—an historic overview. *American Journal of Clinical Nutrition* 41:140–149, 1985.

HERTZLER, A. A. Children's food patterns—a review. In Food preferences and feeding problems. *Journal of the American Dietetic Association* 83:551–554, 1983.

ISSELBACHER, K. Some Comments on Future RDAs. *Journal of the American Dietetic Association* 85:1648–1649, 1985.

MONSEN, E. and A. OWEN. Awaiting the new RDAs. *Journal of the American Dietetic Association* 85:1649, 1985.

MUNRO, H. N. How well recommended are the recommended dietary allowances? *Journal of the American Dietetic Association* 71:490–497, 1977.

PRESS, F. Postponement of the 10th Edition of the RDAs. *Journal of the American Dietetic Association* 85:1644–1645, 1985.

RODIN, J. Social and immediate environmental influences on food selection. *International Journal Obesity* 4:364–370, 1980.

SANJUR, D. *Social and Cultural Perspectives In Nutrition.* Englewood Cliffs, NJ: Prentice-Hall, 1982.

SLOAN, A. E., L. C. LEONE, M. POWERS, and K. W. McNUTT. Changing consumer lifestyles. *Food Technology,* November 1984, pp. 99–103.

TODHUNTER, E. N. Some classics of nutrition and dietetics. *Journal of the American Dietetic Association* 44:100, 1964.

WAY, W. L. Food-related behaviors on prime-time television. *Journal of Nutrition Education* 15:105–109, 1983.

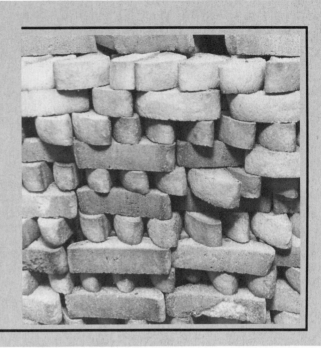

Chapter 2

CARBOHYDRATES

22

"Quick, what can I eat? I'm starved!" You've probably felt this way many times. What kind of food did you reach for? Chances are, it was a soft drink, an apple, a thick slice of bread, a ripe banana, or a chocolate bar. These foods share an important attribute; they are loaded with carbohydrates. Carbohydrate-rich foods supply quick energy to fuel the body.

Carbohydrates from grains, fruits, and vegetables account for as much as 80 percent of the energy intake of people in developing countries. In technologically advanced nations, "sweets" often replace grains, fruits, and vegetables as sources of dietary carbohydrate. What makes high-carbohydrate foods so popular? On the practical side, they are usually inexpensive and readily available. On the biological side, carbohydrates are important to many of the body's metabolic processes.

This chapter examines the biological role of carbohydrates; their composition, molecular structure, and major dietary sources; and their path from ingestion through digestion, absorption, and metabolism. Carbohydrates travel through the circulatory system in the form of simple sugars, and complex mechanisms regulate the sugar levels in the blood. Some of the problems—diabetes mellitus, hypoglycemia, and other disorders—associated with disturbances in this regulatory process will be examined. We will also look at the significance of dietary carbohydrate in supplying indigestible food remnants called *dietary fiber*, which affects the rate at which food residues move through the intestinal tract and which may have other roles as well. Against this biological background, we present trends in carbohydrate consumption in the United States and their significance in the maintenance of good health.

DEFINITION, CLASSIFICATION, SOURCES

Carbohydrates are organic compounds composed of the elements carbon (C), hydrogen (H), and oxygen (O). Generally, the hydrogen and oxygen atoms in a carbohydrate molecule are present in the ratio of 2 to 1, the same proportion in which they occur in a molecule of water. Thus, a carbohydrate molecule, with some modifications, is composed of hydrated carbon atoms.

Monosaccharides

Carbohydrates are classified according to their molecular structure and, in particular, according to the proportion of carbon atoms to the H—OH group. **Monosaccharides**, or simple sugars, contain one carbon atom for each group of two hydrogens and one oxygen. This relationship is expressed as $C_n(H_2O)_n$. (In chemical terminology, the subscript—here designated by "n"—is used to represent the number of atoms or molecules of the element or compound immediately preceding it—in this case, carbon atoms and water molecules.) Different classes of monosaccharides are distinguished by the number of carbon atoms; for example, 5-carbon sugars are called **pentoses** (from *penta-*, five, and *-ose*, carbohydrate).

The monosaccharides of most importance in nutrition are the **hexoses** or 6-carbon sugars, expressed in the general formula $C_6(H_2O)_6$, or simply $C_6H_{12}O_6$. Examples of hexoses are **glucose**, **fructose**, and **galactose**. Even though all hexoses have the same *empirical* (chemical) *formula*, they are distinguished from one another by differences in **chemical structure**, that is, by the arrangement of C, H, and

O atoms in the molecule. The differences in arrangement of the H and O atoms around the carbons in these three sugars can be seen in their structural formulas, illustrated in Figure 2–1. Although the structural differences among these three hexose molecules are slight, they are responsible for significant differences in properties. Glucose, galactose, and fructose differ in degree of sweetness and in their metabolic roles. Although other hexose molecules exist, the three shown are the most important in the study of nutrition.

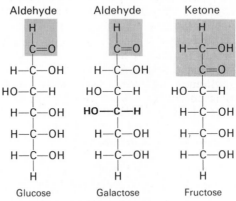

FIGURE 2-1   *Structural Formulas of Three Hexoses.*
These three hexoses differ from each other because their H and OH groups are arranged differently about the carbon atoms. Glucose and galactose both have aldehyde groups and are called *aldoses*; fructose has a ketone group and is called a *ketose*.

Two of these monosaccharides are widely found in foods. Glucose—also known as *dextrose* or *corn sugar*—is present in sweet fruits, such as berries, grapes, pears, and oranges, and in certain vegetables, notably corn and carrots. Relatively large amounts occur in honey as well. Dextrose from corn syrup is often used commercially as a sweetener in prepared foods. Fructose—sometimes called *levulose* or *fruit sugar*—is also found in most fruits and vegetables. Glucose and fructose are also contained in high fructose corn syrup (HFCS), sugar produced from starch through new technology. Galactose is not found free in foods, although it is a major constituent of the principal carbohydrate in milk, lactose.

Because the details of molecular structure are significant in organic chemistry, several ways have been devised to represent them diagrammatically. A diagram called a *ring structure* is especially convenient for illustrating large, complex molecules.

Disaccharides and Their Food Sources

Disaccharides are formed when two monosaccharides are chemically bonded together by means of a **condensation reaction**. This reaction is characterized by the release of a molecule of water, as shown by the general equation for a condensation reaction between two monosaccharides:

$$C_n(H_2O)_n + C_n(H_2O)_n \rightarrow C_{2n}(H_2O)_{2n-1} + H_2O$$

The condensation of two hexoses is written

$$2C_6(H_2O)_6 \rightarrow C_{12}(H_2O)_{11} + H_2O$$

The condensation product of glucose and fructose is sucrose—sometimes called *table sugar*—which is shown by using ring structures in Figure 2–2(a). Table sugar comes mainly from either sugar cane or sugar beets. Found in most fruits and vegetables, sucrose is also the major component of brown sugar, maple sugar, and molasses. Many processed foods are sweetened with sucrose.

The condensation product of glucose and galactose is the disaccharide **lactose** shown in Figure 2–2(b), the only significant dietary carbohydrate of animal origin. Produced solely by the mammary glands of lactating mammals, including humans, lactose—known also as *milk sugar*—is found only in milk and milk products. **Maltose**, another important disaccharide, is the result of a condensation reaction between two glucose units. See Figure 2–2(c). An intermediate product of starch breakdown during human digestion, maltose is found also in germinating seeds, in some breakfast cereals, and in fermented products such as beer.

FIGURE 2-2   *Ring Structures of Major Disaccharides.*

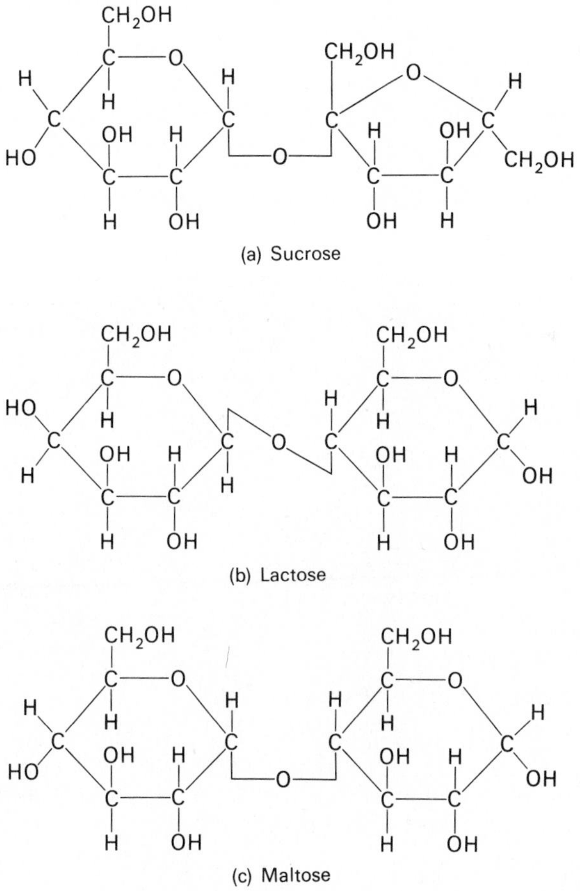

(a) Sucrose

(b) Lactose

(c) Maltose

Polysaccharides

The word **polysaccharide** means "many sugars," a logical name for a molecule in which a number of monosaccharides are combined. Polysaccharides are often referred to as **complex carbohydrates**, as contrasted with the **simple carbohydrates**—the mono- and disaccharides. A polysaccharide molecule is represented by the general empirical formula of, for example, a polyhexose: $(C_6H_{10}O_5)_n$. Monosaccharides become linked through successive condensation reactions, and one molecule of water is lost as each hexose unit is added to the molecule. The combination of from three to ten monosaccharide units in this way is sometimes known as an **oligosaccharide** (from *oligo-*, few). True polysaccharides are **polymers**, large molecules built up through the linking together of many molecular units, which may or may not be identical.

Most polysaccharides of plant origin are **starches**, of which there are several types. Different carbohydrate-containing foods—corn, wheat, and apples, for example—have different starches, each of them genetically determined. For example, amylose is a plant starch in which hundreds of glucose units are combined in a sequence of condensation reactions to form one long, straight chain. Amylopectin is another plant starch, also composed solely of glucose units, but arranged in branched chains. Various plants contain both amylose and amylopectin, although in different proportions.

The most abundant polysaccharide (and probably the most common organic molecule on earth) is cellulose, a component of plant cell walls. Cellulose resembles amylose in that it, too, is made up of glucose units arranged in a straight chain,

One facet of the biological role of carbohydrates is the significance of "dietary fiber" and how it affects the rate at which food residues move through the intestinal tract.
USDA BN-35637

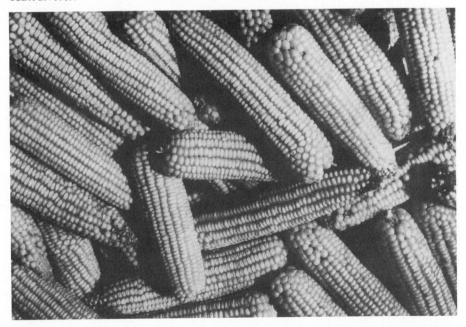

but there the resemblance stops. The key difference is in the way the glucose units are linked together. Because of the difference in linkage structure, these two polysaccharides have strikingly different chemical and physical properties and are utilized by the body in different ways. Most significant is that the human body cannot digest cellulose because the human digestive system does not have the capacity to break the cellulose linkage structure. The amylose structure, however, is readily digested. Small structural distinctions, then, make all the difference in how each molecule behaves and is utilized.

The one animal polysaccharide, **glycogen,** is not present in the food supply to an appreciable extent. Although it is stored as an energy source in some animal tissue (muscle and liver), it disappears with the death of the animal, leaving only negligible amounts in such foods as liver and fresh shellfish. The significance of glycogen for humans is its manufacture by the body during glucose metabolism.

PROPERTIES OF CARBOHYDRATES

Despite similarity in structure, the various carbohydrates differ markedly in their physical properties. The sugars—monosaccharides and disaccharides—have a sweet taste and are readily soluble in water. Polysaccharides, however, are often bland or tasteless, and are relatively insoluble. These properties make cornstarch and other such polysaccharides good thickening agents in food preparation. Their bland taste also accounts for the nearly universal practice of adding gravy and sauces to such starch-laden foods as potatoes, spaghetti, rice, and beans.

Carbohydrates in the Diet

The carbohydrate composition of some common foods is shown in Figure 2–3. These are average figures, since individual samples of any food item can vary widely. Foods are listed according to the predominant type of carbohydrate that each contains, ranging from complex (mainly polysaccharides) at the top of the graph to simple (mainly sugars) at the bottom. The main dietary carbohydrates that we obtain from cereals and potatoes, for example, are starches, whereas the main dietary carbohydrates in dried fruits and sweeteners are sugars. Baked goods and beer, with both grain and sugar components, are intermediate.

The proportion of carbohydrates in a food depends on the water content of the sample. Dried legume seeds (peas and beans) contain relatively little water until they are cooked; consequently, their carbohydrate content is concentrated and proportionately high. Milk, fresh vegetables, and fresh fruits generally have a high water content and, therefore, contain much less carbohydrate per 100-gram sample. Generally, frozen and canned fruits to which sugar has not been added have as much natural sugar as fresh fruits. However, because water has been removed, the sugar in dried fruits is more concentrated and therefore greater on a weight-for-weight basis than in fresh fruits.

Tables of food composition provide information for specific food items, usually on a per-serving basis. Data on the total carbohydrate, starch-related carbohydrates, sucrose and other sugars, and dietary fiber also appear on some package labels.

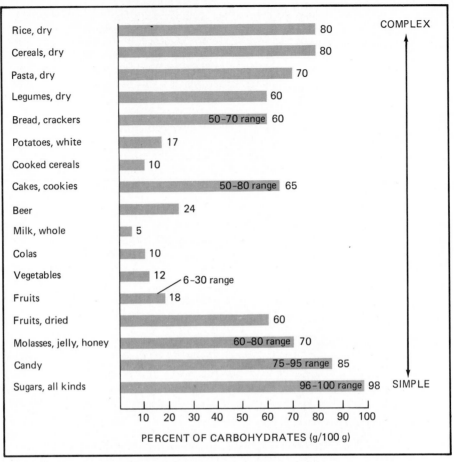

FIGURE 2-3 *Carbohydrate Composition of Selected Foods.*
Note that milk is the only food of animal origin shown; lactose, or milk sugar, is the only sugar of animal origin.

Trends in Carbohydrate Consumption

American eating habits have changed considerably during this century, especially in regard to the quantity and patterns of our use of carbohydrate-containing foods. Although total caloric intake has remained about the same, a moderate but steady decrease occurred in overall carbohydrate consumption with a corresponding increase in the proportion of calories derived from fats. There was a striking decrease in consumption of complex carbohydrates (grains and potatoes) and a corresponding increase in the consumption of simple sugars. Starch consumption decreased from 68 percent of total carbohydrate intake early in the century to 47 percent more recently; in the same period, sugar intake increased from 32 percent to 53 percent. In the last ten years, intake of sucrose has declined while use of other caloric sweeteners has almost doubled (Table 2-1). The use of "noncaloric" sweeteners has also increased particularly since the introduction of aspartame. These statistics reflect, among other things, a desire to control weight.

Table 2-1. *Amounts of various sweeteners consumed per capita in the United States since 1950. Amounts for caloric sweeteners are given in pounds. Amounts for non-caloric sweeteeners are given in "sugar equivalents."*

| | CALORIC | | | |
	Cane & Beet[1]	Corn[2]	Other[3]	Non-Caloric[4]
1950	100.6	11.5	2.7	2.9
1955	96.3	10.6	2.2	2.0
1960	97.6	11.6	2.0	2.2
1965	97.0	15.1	1.8	5.7
1970	101.8	19.3	1.5	5.8
1975	89.2	27.5	1.4	6.2
1980	83.6	40.2	1.2	7.1
1983	71.0	52.2	1.3	9.7

[1] Dry basis
[2] High fructose corn syrup, glucose, and dextrose
[3] Honey and edible syrups
[4] Negligible calories in quantities normally consumed.
Sugar Background for 1985 Farm Legislation USDA Economic Research Service, Agriculture Information Bulletin #478, 1984.

Production and distribution of foods derived from grains are less costly than are other sources of energy nutrients (proteins and fats) such as meat. Consequently, meats are status foods the world over.
Joseph P. Schuyler/Stock, Boston

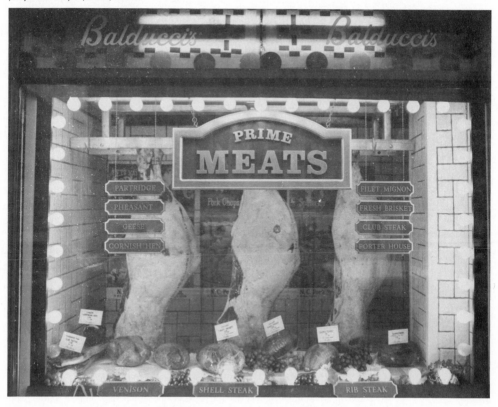

As countries throughout the world develop technologically and economically, the carbohydrate proportion of total energy intake tends to decrease. Carbohydrate consumption is, apparently, inversely proportional to economic status. The high-carbohydrate, predominantly vegetarian diet common to the poor almost everywhere is gradually replaced by a higher-fat diet containing more food items from animal sources. Production and distribution of grains and food products derived from them (cereal, pasta) are less costly than the production and distribution of foods that are better sources of other energy nutrients (proteins and fats), such as meat; consequently, meats are status foods almost everywhere.

As economic status improves there is a shift away from foods containing mainly complex carbohydrates—grains, potatoes, legumes—and toward those with more sugar. As economic status improves further and education increases, there is generally a greater interest in health and nutrition and a reintroduction of complex carbohydrates into the diet or a greater interest in slimness and consumption of limited amounts of foods high in simple sugars. Consumers who exercise and are concerned about nutrition are most likely to eat fresh fruits and vegetables. At the present time, the consumer has a choice of fruits canned in sugar syrup or in natural juices; some vegetables are canned with no added sugar or salt and cereals which emphasize fiber and vitamin content rather than "sweetness."

Another important change is the number of meals people now eat outside the home and the prepared meals brought home to eat. Because people don't cook as much as they used to years ago, more of the sugar consumed now comes from processed foods and beverages and correspondingly less is added at home (Table 2-2).

Since it is not possible to tabulate all the sugar actually measured into our cooking pots and coffee cups, and to subtract that lost when we spill a soft drink or throw away stale cake, the figures in such tables are "disappearance data;" they reflect the "disappearance" of sugar when it is distributed either through retail channels or to commercial food processors. For this reason they may not reflect actual consumption, and they should be used with this limitation in mind.

These per capita figures, moreover, represent an average, useful for comparison of overall national consumption at different periods in time, but they do not take personal differences into account. A person who eats two desserts a day, snacks on soft drinks, and drinks heavily sweetened coffee is surely consuming more than the average; someone who avoids adding sugar to food and eats only fresh fruit for dessert is consuming significantly less.

A trend difficult to quantitate is the increased consumption of those complex carbohydrates known collectively as fiber. In the United States, the average intake of dietary fiber is approximately 20 grams per day calculated from average food in-

Table 2-2. Refined sucrose usage (percent of total)				
	Household use	Processed foods	Beverages	Others[a]
1909–1913	68	21	5	6
1950	39	41	11	9
1960	34	43	14	9
1970	25	47	24	4
1980[b]	25	43	28	4

[a] Includes use by eating and drinking places, institutions, and the military.
[b] Preliminary.
Prepared by R. M. Marston, Home Economist, US Dept. Agriculture, Human Nutrition Information Service, Consumer Nutrition Center, Hyattsville, MD 20782. Personal communication. 1981.

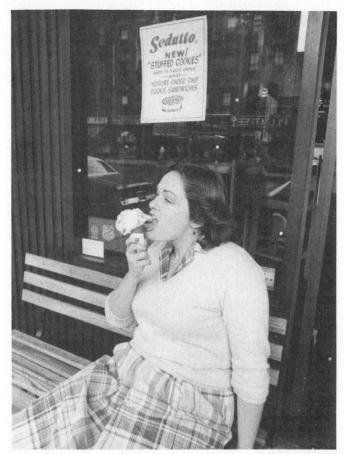

A greater amount of sugar now comes from processed foods and less is
added in the kitchen or at the table.
Teri Leigh Stratford

take and typical meal patterns. Using the amount available for consumption, the
mean intake is estimated at 25–30 grams per day, compared to 93.6 grams per day
in Mexico and 22.8 in Australia.

DIGESTION AND ABSORPTION
OF CARBOHYDRATES

Carbohydrates contained in food are not available for use by the body until after
they are changed into simple sugars and absorbed into the bloodstream. Some dietary carbohydrate is, of course, already in this form. But complex carbohydrates
must be broken down into simple sugars. Specific enzymes present in the mouth
and in certain cells of the pancreas and the small intestine play an important part in
these chemical processes.

Digestion: Enzymatic Hydrolysis

The digestive reactions of carbohydrates are hydrolytic reactions; **hydrolysis** occurs when a larger molecule is split into two smaller ones and a water molecule is added to the broken ends. By many successive repetitions of the hydrolytic reaction occurring at the oxygen bridges between two simple sugars, even very large molecules of such complex carbohydrates as starch are eventually broken down into monosaccharides.

The first chemical step in carbohydrate digestion starts as soon as food enters the mouth. Here a salivary enzyme called amylase (or **ptyalin**) is mixed with the food and begins to hydrolyze starch. The polysaccharides are progressively broken down by amylase into smaller disaccharide units. Hydrolysis of polysaccharides can take place only in the catalyzing presence of amylase.

Salivary amylase will not hydrolyze all or even very much of the starch in the bolus, because food stays in the mouth for a relatively short time. As food is swallowed, it is propelled by peristaltic action down the esophagus and into the stomach. Here the amylase mixed with the food is inactivated by gastric acid, and the hydrolysis of starch is temporarily halted.

A limited amount of carbohydrate digestion, however, does occur in the stomach. Some hydrolytic reactions, notably the one which splits sucrose into its components, glucose and fructose, occur spontaneously in an acid environment, such as that provided by gastric hydrochloric acid; such reactions need no enzyme catalysis.

Since only a small fraction of the carbohydrate is usually hydrolyzed in the stomach, the most important site of carbohydrate digestion is the small intestine, into which food passes from the stomach. At its junction with the stomach the small intestine is joined by a duct from the pancreas, which releases pancreatic amylase into the lumen of the small intestine (see Appendix J, Figure 5). This amylase, produced in certain pancreatic cells, has a slightly different structure from salivary amylase and functions under a different set of conditions, although both act to hydrolyze starches. Pancreatic amylase reduces starch to a specific disaccharide, maltose. Here the hydrolytic process catalyzed by amylase is virtually completed.

The cells of the brush border of the small intestine contain a group of enzymes—the **disaccharidases.** (Enzymes are often named by combining the name of their substrate with the suffix -*ase*.) Each member of this group—sucrase, maltase, lactase—catalyzes the hydrolysis of just one disaccharide—sucrose, maltose, or lactose—to its component simple sugars:

$$
\text{sucrose} \xrightarrow[\text{sucrase}]{\;\;H_2O\;\;} \text{glucose and fructose}
$$

$$
\text{lactose} \xrightarrow[\text{lactase}]{\;\;H_2O\;\;} \text{glucose and galactose}
$$

$$
\text{maltose} \xrightarrow[\text{maltase}]{\;\;H_2O\;\;} \text{two glucose}
$$

Although three different enzymes are involved, the chemical reaction is identical: Water is added to the bond between components of the disaccharide, and two monosaccharides are produced from each hydrolytic reaction.

Because glucose, fructose, and galactose are monosaccharides, no further digestion is needed. As shown in Figure 2–4, all the dietary carbohydrates that can be digested are hydrolyzed in the small intestine to these three monosaccharides.

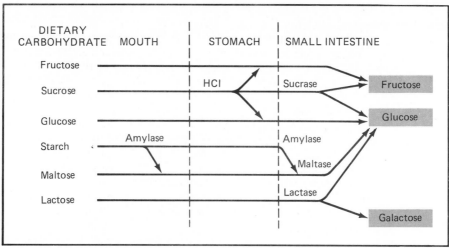

FIGURE 2-4   *Schematic Diagram of Carbohydrate Digestion.*

LACTOSE INTOLERANCE.   Many people have difficulty digesting lactose, the disaccharide in milk. Some individuals produce insufficient amounts of the enzyme **lactase**, whereas others fail to synthesize it at all. Unable to digest this sugar, they have a variety of digestive problems when they consume milk or milk products.

Lactose intolerance affects many adults and some children and infants. It is, however, only rarely present at birth, and virtually all babies are born with an adequate lactase-synthesizing capacity. In some cases, however, this capacity begins to diminish in early childhood, occasionally as early as soon after weaning.

Lactose intolerance, usually of genetic origin, may become increasingly severe with age. Individuals able to digest lactose readily are most likely to be of northern European and North African descent. An estimated 70 to 90 percent of non-Caucasians may be lactose intolerant. Temporary or even permanent intolerance can also result from gastrointestinal disease, heavy medication, surgery, or malnutrition.

The symptoms of lactose intolerance are varying degrees of abdominal distress; this may include bloating, cramps, flatulence, and/or diarrhea. Because the lactose ingested cannot be hydrolyzed, it cannot be absorbed. It remains in the small intestine and attracts water, which results in bloating. As the undigested lactose continues along the gastrointestinal tract to the large intestine, it is fermented by intestinal bacteria to organic acids and gases, causing the characteristic discomforts.

Lactose intolerance is diagnosed by a test that measures the blood glucose level after the subject has been given a measured oral dose of lactose. Lactose intolerance is present if the blood glucose level does not rise at a defined rate that indicates digestion and absorption of the test sugar into the bloodstream. The general observation has been that all non-European populations display a variable but high percentage of intolerance by this definition. This test, which requires a dose of lactose equivalent to drinking more than a liter of milk, has been criticized as being unrealistically strict, however, and some authorities even question whether it has any practical significance. According to the Committee on Nutrition of the American Pediatric Society, even children of lactose-intolerant populations should be able to drink milk in normal quantities without showing distress. In one study, for example, black American children who were diagnosed by the standard test as lactose intolerant had no difficulty digesting 1 cup (240 ml) of milk.

Most lactose-intolerant individuals are able to digest such milk products as cheese, yogurt, and ice cream. For children with a severe form of this condition, ordinary milk can be treated with a commercial lactase that will hydrolyze the lactose so that it can be absorbed. Milk can be treated with this preparation during pasteurization or drying, but the lactase is also available in powdered form to be added to milk immediately before consumption.

INDIGESTIBLE CARBOHYDRATES. Dietary fiber describes all components of food that are resistant to digestion and are eliminated in the feces. It differs from crude fiber which is the material remaining after vigorous treatment of food with alkali and acid, therefore there is more digestible fiber than crude fiber. Water insoluble fiber, such as cellulose, lignin, and most hemi-celluloses, stimulates the movement of food through the gastrointestinal tract and absorbs water to increase fecal bulk. Cellulose, the most widely occurring of all carbohydrates, is not digestible because the human body has no enzyme capable of hydrolyzing it into its component glucose units. Because it is not hydrolyzed, cellulose simply passes through the small intestine into the colon and is eventually excreted. Cellulose and amylose (starch) are very similar in structure, except that the chemical bonds connecting the glucose units are arranged differently in each of these polysaccharides. Each linkage requires its own enzyme for hydrolysis to take place, and although amylase can hydrolyze amylose, it is ineffective in dealing with the very similar cellulose. This indigestibility of cellulose in humans emphasizes the specificity of enzymes.

Enzymes that can hydrolyze cellulose are, however, produced by many microorganisms, including some normally found in the digestive tracts of various animals such as cattle and goats. Indirectly, by means of these bacterial enzymes, such animals can digest cellulose and other carbohydrates indigestible in humans. Some slight digestion of this sort is thought to be carried on by the human intestinal flora, but it is not enough to be of any practical significance. Water soluble fiber, such as pectic substances, gums and storage polysaccharides, may influence circulating glucose and insulin concentrations. Pectic substances are complex polymers originating in cell walls and fibrous parts of fruits, vegetables, and other plants. Some of them can be chemically converted to pectinic acid, a water soluble substance from which pectin, used to bind fluid in making jellies, is derived. Most commercial pectin comes from the pulp of apples and citrus fruits.

Dietary tables frequently show "crude" fiber rather than dietary fiber. Crude fiber underestimates total fiber content by as much as 80 percent of the hemicellulose, 50 to 90 percent of the lignin, and 20 to 50 percent of the cellulose.

Lack of **fiber** in the diet may be associated with cancer of the colon, diverticulosis, irritable bowel syndrome, hiatus hernia, hemorrhoids, and other diseases of the gastrointestinal system. These problems occur far less frequently among non-Westernized nonurban peoples who consume traditional diets high in fiber materials and more frequently in populations consuming a Western-style diet.

Absorption

To be utilized, the mix of monosaccharides resulting from the action of digestive enzymes must be absorbed through the cells lining the intestine. The absorptive process, occurring mostly in the jejunum (middle portion) of the small intestine, is a complex one. The simple sugars must be transported through the cells and across capillary walls into the portal vein. This movement occurs both by passive diffusion and by active transport.

Fructose is absorbed predominantly by diffusion, as are glucose and galactose when their concentrations are higher in the intestine than in the blood. When the gradient of glucose or galactose is reversed, with more of these sugars in the blood than in the intestine, active transport takes place. This process requires energy and a specific carrier system.

Several factors influence the rate of monosaccharide absorption. Concentration gradients are important, and hormones, specifically thyroxine and insulin, also appear to play a role. Studies have indicated that galactose and glucose are absorbed somewhat more rapidly than fructose; however, the efficiency of absorption of all three monosaccharides is quite high and may approach 98 percent of the digestible carbohydrate.

FUNCTION OF CARBOHYDRATES: INTERMEDIARY METABOLISM

The portal vein transports all monosaccharides directly to the liver, where fructose and galactose are converted to glucose. Thus, in studying the metabolism of carbohydrates, we are really discussing the metabolism of glucose.

The liver is the principal organ that regulates glucose metabolism, although other organs have important roles in maintaining glucose levels. **Homeostasis** is the maintenance of a constant internal environment. Glucose metabolism is in a state of dynamic equilibrium, so that cells receive an adequate supply of glucose over a period of time. Glucose metabolism ultimately produces the **ATP** (**adenosine triphosphate**) that provides energy for all cell functions. Although glucose metabolism is described as a separate process, it always occurs in conjunction with metabolism of other nutrients.

Maintenance of Blood Glucose

Tracing glucose as it leaves the liver, we can locate it in the following sources.

BLOOD GLUCOSE. Glucose circulating in the blood provides all the body cells with an energy source and with a substrate for the synthesis of other compounds. The blood glucose level is regulated by several mechanisms. In the fasting state (that is, before breakfast, or at least 12 hours after eating), glucose concentration normally ranges between 70 and 100 mg/dl. After a meal containing carbohydrates, blood glucose may rise to about 140 mg/dl, but it returns to its former level in an hour or two. Values of 70 to 110 mg/dl (fasting) are generally considered to reflect **normoglycemia** (the normal level of glucose in the blood). Abnormal functioning of the regulatory mechanisms may result in persistent **hyperglycemia** (higher than normal levels) or **hypoglycemia** (lower than normal levels). The term *dl* means "deciliter," or 100 milliliters.

MUSCLE AND LIVER GLYCOGEN. Glucose molecules are enzymatically condensed in muscle and liver cells to glycogen, the storage form of carbohydrate in animals. This process is called **glycogenesis.**

LIPIDS. By the process of **lipogenesis,** glucose can be converted to fat (see Chapter 3).

Perspective On

DIABETES AND HYPOGLYCEMIA

Regulation of blood glucose concentration results in relatively stable glucose levels in most people. The importance of this regulation can be seen by examining two abnormal conditions: diabetes mellitus, in which blood glucose level is above the normal range, and hypoglycemia, or consistently below-normal glucose levels in the blood.

DIABETES MELLITUS. Diabetes mellitus, commonly called just **diabetes,** affects as many as 12 million Americans and the incidence is increasing. Although recent improvements in diagnosis and treatment have extended the life span for people with diabetes, the disease and its complications rank third as cause of death and are responsible for the hospitalization of more than 2 million people each year, according to the American Diabetes Association.

In healthy persons, insulin, secreted by the pancreas, is the major hormone responsible for maintaining blood glucose concentration within the normal range. Patients with diabetes suffer from some abnormality of production or action of insulin—decreased synthesis of the hormone, cellular resistance to its action, or production of substances that counteract insulin's activity. As a result, the normal role of insulin in facilitating passage of glucose from the blood into the cells is impaired. Body cells are then starving in the midst of plenty; glucose can be used by cells only after it enters them and not as long as it remains outside, as it does in the diabetic. Biochemical abnormalities develop in the starved cells, which break down many of their own constituents for nourishment. The kidneys, attempting to excrete the excess blood glucose, must also excrete unusually large volumes of water (polyuria). Loss of large amounts of water causes thirst, hence increased water intake (polydipsia). These changes, plus the finding of elevated glucose levels in urine (glucosuria), suggest diabetes mellitus. The disease can be confirmed by measuring fasting glucose sometimes combined with an oral glucose tolerance test or a postprandial (literally after a meal) blood glucose. For both of the latter tests, the subject ingests a standard amount of glucose. For the glucose tolerance test, plasma glucose is measured at frequent intervals for periods up to three hours. For the postprandial measurement, a single measurement is done on the sample taken at two hours. The person with diabetes, unable to move glucose from the blood into body cells at a normal rate, will persistently have high blood glucose levels compared with those of normal people.

There are four major classifications of diabetes mellitus. Non-insulin dependent diabetes mellitus (NIDDM), formerly called adult-onset diabetes, can often be controlled by diet alone. Obesity may predispose a person to this form of diabetes. In contrast, insulin-dependent diabetes (IDDM), formerly called juvenile-onset diabetes usually develops before age 20 or 30, requires insulin injections for its control because it is characterized by a virtually total lack of insulin production by the pancreas. Impaired glucose tolerance, the third category, may carry increased risk of atherosclerotic disease. This problem is seen more frequently in the elderly than in a younger population. The exact cause of impaired glucose tolerance is not known, but certain evidence suggests chromium may play a role in some cases of intolerance. The fourth major category is gestational diabetes which has its onset or recognition during pregnancy. In most individuals there is a return to normality when pregnancy is completed. The person with gestational diabetes may or may not require insulin for management. Gestational diabetes is associated with increased perinatal complications.

Current evidence suggests that most causes of IDDM result from autoimmune destruction of the beta cells of the pancreas, initiated by a viral infection. There is evidently a genetic predisposition, but additional factors are needed before frank disease develops. Studies of twins suggest that genetic factors are predominant in the development of NIDDM. If one twin has NIDDM, the other twin will also have it in close to 100 percent of the cases; if one twin has IDDM, the other twin will have it only about 50 percent of the time.

Use of reagent strips to monitor blood glucose at home has enabled persons with diabetes mellitus to better control the concentration of glucose in their blood. Better control has the potential for reducing microvascular complications such as diabetic retinopathy, nephropathy, and possibly neuropathy. Glycosylated hemoglobin is formed by the reaction of blood glucose and hemoglobin in the red blood cells and indicates the average blood glucose concentration for the previous two to three months. A high value for glycohemoglobin indicates poor control of blood glucose and alerts the health professional to make a greater effort to educate the patient regarding diabetes.

Meal planning for patients with diabetes utilizes *exchange lists* developed by the American Diabetes Association working with the American Dietetic Association and the U.S. Public Health Service. More recently, foods have been tested for their ability to cause increased blood glucose after ingestion. The "glycemic index" is the blood glucose response during a two-hour period after the food is eaten as a percentage of the two-hour response to ingestion of an equivalent amount of glucose. Additional studies are needed to determine the usefulness of this index. The exact role of dietary fiber in management of patients with diabetes is not well defined. However, the general recommendation is that patients consume more complex carbohydate and less fat.

HYPOGLYCEMIA. Opposite from diabetes mellitus, in terms of the blood glucose scale, is the condition known as **hypoglycemia.** Hypoglycemia, due to any of several causes, is characterized by concentrations of circulating glucose sufficiently low to cause release of catecholamines and impairs central nervous system function. Diagnosis should be based on documentation of plasma glucose values in the hypoglycemic range and correction to normal with ingestion of food, not by association of non-specific symptoms with food.

Hypoglycemia, however, differs from diabetes in several important ways, in addition to the obvious difference in blood glucose levels:

1. Many of the symptoms of hypoglycemia are characteristic of anxiety or other psychological states; nervousness, weakness, sweating, and so on often occur in normal people during times of stress, such as final exam week, and do not indicate disease under these conditions.

2. Many cases of hypoglycemia are self-diagnosed and cannot be confirmed by medical examination, including laboratory tests. In recent years, hypoglycemia has become a fashionable condition. People may assume they have it merely on the basis of occasional episodes of weakness, headache, or other nonspecific complaints.

Functional hypoglycemia is overdiagnosed by the layperson and physician alike. In this condition, symptoms appear a few hours after eating and persist for less than 30 minutes. Individuals with functional hypoglycemia oversecrete insulin in response to the temporary blood glucose rise caused by eating. Oversecretion of insulin then causes a sudden and exaggerated lowering of blood glucose levels, with resulting symptoms of hypoglycemia.

Other forms of hypoglycemia occur unassociated with eating. Numerous conditions can be responsible: excess insulin taken by a diabetic, tumors of the pancreas resulting in excess insulin secretion, certain drugs, liver disease, and so on. The important point is that although all these lead to the same result, each must be treated to counteract or at least minimize the underlying abnormality.

Self-diagnosis, rare in the case of diabetes but unfortunately common in the case of hypoglycemia, is potentially dangerous; it can prevent the accurate determination and thus the effective treatment of underlying disorders responsible for symptoms of abnormal blood glucose levels.

AMINO ACIDS.   Carbohydrate derivatives can be **aminated** (by the addition of an amino, or nitrogen-containing, molecular group) to produce nonessential **amino acids**, so called because the body can synthesize them as needed. (**Essential amino acids** must be supplied in the diet; see Chapter 4.)

SPECIAL METABOLITES.   These include **nucleic acids** (the building blocks of DNA and RNA), heparin, and components of cell membranes and connective tissues, all of which contain glucose derivatives or metabolites.

CELLULAR ENERGY-PRODUCING SYSTEMS.   Body cells and tissues must have a constant supply of energy for the synthesis and catabolism (breakdown) of cell compounds, for active transport of materials across cell membranes, and for the activation of muscle and nerve cells. This energy is provided mainly by glucose.

The Maintenance Process

The interactions of these functions become clear if the entire system is viewed in terms of the regulation and utilization of blood glucose. Figure 2–5 depicts the processes that raise and lower the blood glucose level.

Maintenance of the level of glucose in the blood is the central element regulating the movement of glucose throughout the system. With very minor fluctuations, a constant level is maintained every hour of every day, despite the fact that dietary carbohydrate is ingested only at irregular intervals. Homeostasis is accomplished by

FIGURE 2-5   *Maintenance of Glucose Homeostasis.*

Levels of glucose in the blood are raised by ingestion of dietary carbohydrate, by release of fructose and galactose from storage in the liver, and by glycogenolysis and gluconeogenesis. Blood glucose levels are reduced as glucose is diverted to the energy and biochemical needs of all body tissues. After these body needs have been met, glycogenesis and lipogenesis transform glucose into glycogen and lipids, respectively, for storage. If serum levels of glucose rise higher than 160 to 180 mg/dl, the excess is excreted in the urine.

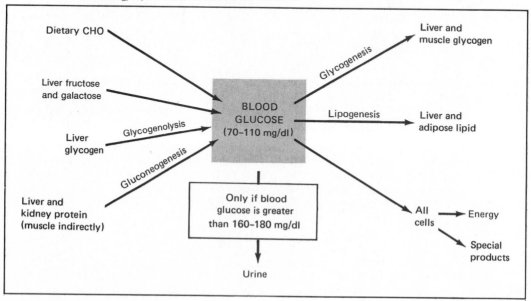

TABLE 2-3. Hormones that Influence Blood Glucose Levels

Hormone	Secreted by	Target Tissue and Effect	Net Effect on Blood Glucose
Insulin	Pancreas	Muscle: ↑ glucose uptake	↓
Thyroid hormone	Thyroid	Gastrointestinal tract: ↑ glucose absorption	↑
Glucagon	Pancreas	Liver: ↑ glycogenolysis	↑
Epinephrine	Adrenal glands	Liver and muscle: ↑ glycogenolysis	↑
Steroid hormones	Adrenal glands	Muscle; liver: ↑ gluconeogenesis	↑

Key: ↑ increase   ↓ decrease

a series of mechanisms that control the rates at which glucose is converted into glycogen or fat for storage, released from storage, reconverted into glucose, and returned to the circulation. Hormones play a key role in regulating these processes by controlling the rate and direction of the enzymatic reactions involved and by influencing the rates of active transport processes. Table 2–3 lists the sources, sites of action, and effects on blood glucose levels of several of these hormones.

When the blood glucose level falls to a "triggering" value (less than 70 mg/dl), hormonal mechanisms immediately begin functioning to restore it to normal. Glycogen stored in the liver is broken down into glucose for release to the blood. In addition, some amino acids can be **deaminated** by removal of an amino group, leaving a carbon chain, which is then converted to glucose. The glycerol part of a fat molecule can similarly be converted. These latter pathways are normally used only when dietary intake of carbohydrates is too low to replace blood glucose as it is utilized, and they become especially important during starvation or other severe stress conditions.

The precise functioning of the mechanisms for maintaining glucose homeostasis and the fact that more than one mechanism exists emphasize the great importance to health, and even to life itself, of the maintenance of a stable blood glucose level. The cells of the body must have this energy and substrate source for function and survival. Any interference with glucose supply through malfunction of these mechanisms (or simply through continued lack of food) is extremely serious and may be ultimately life-threatening.

CARBOHYDRATE STORAGE AND ENERGY PRODUCTION

Storage

Glucose, transported from the blood into the tissues, may be needed immediately, either to supply energy or as a substrate for synthesis of various products. If it is not immediately needed, however, it can be stored in the form of glycogen or converted to fat for future use. Glycogenesis occurs first, assuming that the body's capacity for glycogen storage is not yet saturated: The liver can store only about 110 grams of glycogen; muscle tissue can hold perhaps 245 grams. These figures are averages, and there may be considerable individual variation according to body size and conformation.

When the glycogen storage capacity is fully utilized, excess glucose will be converted into body fat, since the body has a much larger capacity for its storage. Lipogenesis (the synthesis of fat), like glycogen synthesis, is facilitated by insulin.

In addition to these storage mechanisms, some glucose is used for the synthesis of various important carbohydrate derivatives, such as heparin (which affects blood clotting). Because these derivatives are functioning molecules, however, they are not considered storage products in the same sense that glycogen and fat are.

Energy Production

Cells can survive only with a fairly constant and adequate supply of energy for their life processes. This energy is normally obtained from glucose, primarily by two reaction sequences or "pathways." (Although other pathways exist, the two we shall discuss here are more significant.) One of these can proceed either in the presence of adequate oxygen or under conditions of limited oxygen supply, such as might occur during vigorous exercise. This series of reactions takes place in the cytoplasm of the cell and is called the **Embden-Meyerhof pathway**, or simply **glycolysis**. The second pathway requires oxygen and functions in the mitochondria (cell organelles specialized for energy exchange). This pathway is also known as the *tricarboxylic acid (TCA) cycle*, the *citric-acid cycle*, and the **Krebs cycle**. The last name recognizes Sir Hans Krebs, an English biochemist who contributed significantly to the understanding of this metabolic cycle.

These two sequences of reactions are interrelated. Some of the reactions are also common to protein and lipid metabolism, and vitamins and minerals have their places in these reactions as well. Taken together, the interactions of substrates, enzymes, and coenzymes in these pathways are as intricate as the set of delicate parts in the mechanism of a fine watch, and as precisely controlled.

The primary function of these reaction sequences is the production of energy. There are in the body certain chemical compounds, known as high-energy compounds, that can trap and hold large amounts of energy. One of the most important of them is *adenosine triphosphate*, or ATP. High-energy compounds such as ATP can "trap" energy, much as a storage battery does, and release it as needed to power cell reactions that would not occur, or would not occur fast enough, without this energy. The ATP molecule is composed of adenine (a nitrogen compound), ribose (a pentose), and three phosphate groups. Two of these phosphates are attached to the rest of the molecule by so-called "high energy bonds." The energy in these bonds can be trapped by the cell and used to power muscle and nerve impulses for transport of materials, for heat production, and for essential biochemical reactions. Glycolysis and the Krebs cycle both result in the generation of ATP, but in markedly differing quantities.

GLYCOLYSIS. The result of this sequence is the net production of eight molecules of ATP for every glucose molecule that enters the sequence. The glucose molecule itself is converted into two 3-carbon molecules of pyruvate, which enter the Krebs cycle. Specific enzymes and coenzymes must be present to catalyze these reactions. When the cell's oxygen supply is low, some pyruvate is converted to lactic acid, utilizing the hydrogen molecules released from glucose during the reaction sequence.

KREBS CYCLE. Under aerobic conditions, pyruvate can be further oxidized with a much greater production of ATP. First, the 3-carbon pyruvate molecule crosses the mitochondrial membrane, where its initial reaction takes place. This involves the removal of a single carbon atom, in the form of a carbon dioxide (CO_2) molecule. This reaction is known as **decarboxylation.** The remaining 2-carbon fragment is a molecule of "active acetate," or **acetyl coenzyme A (acetyl CoA)**, which plays a pivotal role in intermediary metabolism.

Through a series of reactions, the two carbons in acetyl CoA become carbon dioxide. Energy is produced as the hydrogen ions released in the Krebs cycle enter and proceed through the electron transport system. This energy eventually becomes "trapped" in the high-energy compound ATP. Oxygen is important to the cell because it makes possible the oxygen-requiring energy production of the Krebs cycle. Substrates other than glucose, primarily fats and amino acids, can also be broken down via the Krebs cycle.

THE GENERATION OF HIGH-ENERGY BONDS. Much of the potential energy produced during glycolysis and the Krebs cycle becomes trapped as ATP through the electron transport system. This is a series of reactions that occurs inside the mitochondria of the cells, using vitamins and minerals as cofactors required for the reaction but not consumed in it.

If adequate oxygen is present, each set of two hydrogen atoms generated in glycolysis and the Krebs cycle passes through the electron transport system (described in Chapter 7), eventually combining with oxygen to form a molecule of water. At the same time, phosphate is joined to adenosine diphosphate (ADP) by a high-energy bond, thereby producing a molecule of ATP.

In the presence of oxygen, glycolysis yields eight molecules of ATP for each molecule of glucose. Complete oxidation through the Krebs cycle generates another 30 ATP molecules. Complete oxidation of one glucose molecule will therefore supply 38 ATP, plus a total of 6 molecules of CO_2. This CO_2 diffuses out of the cell into the blood, which carries it to the lungs, where it is released and exhaled. The overall reaction of glucose metabolism is therefore

$$C_6H_{12}O_6 + 6O_2 \rightarrow 6CO_2 + 6H_2O + 38ATP \text{ (chemical energy)}$$

Green plants, by the process of photosynthesis, use CO_2, H_2O, and the energy of sunlight to produce carbohydrate and to release oxygen:

$$6CO_2 + 6H_2O + \text{(light energy)} \rightarrow C_6H_{12}O_6 + 6O_2$$

Animals, in turn, utilize the carbohydrate in plant food sources to produce chemical energy, CO_2, and water through the processes just described. These different but interacting plant and animal energy cycles are at the heart of the food chain.

DIETARY REQUIREMENTS

Of the macronutrients, carbohydrates attracted the least interest from researchers for years. Further, the general public thought of starch as something to be avoided. More recently both researchers and the public have become more interested in the role of simple, complex, and indigestible carbohydrates. This interest has resulted from controversies surrounding the role of simple sugars and fiber in health and disease and in the role of dietary carbohydrate on metabolism and performance of skeletal muscle. The precise requirement of the human body for carbohydrate in

TABLE 2-4. Nutrient Content of Various Sweeteners (*per tbsp*)

Sweetener	kcal	(kJ)	Protein g	Fat g	CHO g	Ca mg
Corn syrup, light and dark	58	(244)	0	0	15	9.0
Honey, strained	65	(273)	0	0	17	1.0
Maple syrup, pure	53	(223)	0	0	14	21.8
Molasses, light	50	(210)	0	0	13	33.0
Molasses, blackstrap	45	(189)	0	0	11	137.0
Sugar, brown	50	(210)	0	0	13	12.0
Sugar, table	45	(189)	0	0	12	0
RDA: Males 23–50 years		—	56	—	—	800.0
Females 23–50 years		—	44	—	—	800.0

Source: C. F. Adams, *Nutritive value of American foods in common units*. Agriculture Handbook No. 456. Agricultural Research Service USDA (Washington, D.C.: U.S. Government Printing Office, 1975).

the diet is not known. The Food and Nutrition Board has recommended that a minimum of 50 to 100 grams be eaten every day. Eating fewer than 50 grams for an extended period of time could result in potentially harmful fat and protein catabolism, as we will see in later chapters. Most Americans need not worry: The average diversified diet consumed in this country provides three to four times the recommended minimum of carbohydrates. Many fad diets, however, do not. The Dietary Guidelines for Americans include one which recommends eating foods with adequate complex carbohydrate and fiber. Other countries have more specific recommendations. The Dietary Guidelines will be discussed more completely in Chapter 14.

Sugar and Disease

Sugar had been unfairly blamed for directly causing several diseases or conditions. A previously high intake of sucrose, other sugars, or carbohydrate has not been shown to be a causal factor in hypoglycemia and while sugar contributes to dental caries since it nourishes the bacteria that cause tooth decay, it is not the direct cause of dental caries.

Some lay persons attribute the development of diabetes mellitus to consumption of large amounts of sugar. However, research data does not support this for either type of diabetes mellitus. Insulin-dependent, Type I, diabetes mellitus is an autoimmune disorder which affects persons with a genetic inability to cope with viral infections that damage the pancreatic islets. A series of studies starting 50 years ago reveal that not only does occurrence of non-insulin dependent diabetes not correlate with high sucrose intake, but the intake of those who did was probably lower than average. Obesity is related to Type II diabetes mellitus, however, but obesity does not develop more readily in response to excess calories from sugar than it does from excess calories supplied by other macronutrients.

Carbohydrates, simple and complex, play another role in persons who have developed diabetes mellitus. Traditionally sugar was thought to be absorbed rapidly and cause large, fast increases in blood glucose. Complex carbohydrates were thought to be absorbed more slowly and produce a low response over a greater period of time. As a result of several recent studies we now understand that the rates of digestion of starchy foods differ. Foods are now classified by terms of glycemic

Fe mg	P mg	K mg	Thiamin mg	Riboflavin mg	Niacin mg
0.8	3.2	0.8	0	0	0
0.1	1.3	10.7	0	0.01	0.10
0.2	1.7	37.0	0	0	0
0.9	9.0	183.0	0.01	0.01	0.04
3.2	17.0	585.0	0.02	0.04	0.40
0.5	2.7	48.0	0	0	0
0	0	0.4	0	0	0
10.0	800.0	—	1.40	1.60	18.00
18.0	800.0	—	1.00	1.20	13.00

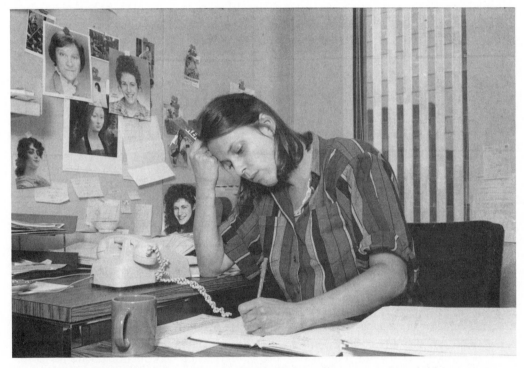

"Quick-energy" foods can be used to provide the energy boost sometimes needed for strenuous physical work but sugar taken this way is used up quickly and usually displaces other foods that have significant nutritional value in addition to energy content.
Randy Matusow

response. Glycemic response related the increase in blood glucose from a test food to the response obtained from glucose, the reference carbohydrate. Many factors including the nature of the starch, the form of the food, fiber, and such, determine the glycemic response. Initial studies suggest that having patients with either diabetes or hyperlipidemia consume low-glycemic-index foods is beneficial. Further stud-

HIGH INTENSITY SWEETENERS

Ancient humans had access to few sweet foods. Diets of meats, grains, roots, leaves, and nuts provided nutrition, but little sweetness. Except for the sugars in fruits and the honey that could be stolen from bees, sweets were in short supply. Not until the fourteenth century was sugar, as we know it, refined; even then, it was a rare and expensive delicacy. Today, sugar is readily available, inexpensive, and adds calories to the diet. For many years therefore, calorie-free nonnutritive sweeteners have been widely used by the weight conscious person, as well as by those wanting to avoid sugar for other reasons, such as diabetes mellitus. While there are no data to confirm that "diet products" produce weight loss, their availability benefits many who want to trim calories where possible.

Two sweeteners, saccharin and cyclamate, have a longer history than aspartame, the sweetener most commonly used at present. Saccharin, discovered in 1879, is about 350 times as sweet as sugar. Theodore Roosevelt loved saccharin in his chewing tobacco. Cyclamate, first marketed in 1949, was not as intensely sweet, but it masked the bitter aftertaste of saccharin.

In 1970, the FDA banned all uses of cyclamate, citing evidence that laboratory animals had developed bladder tumors as a result of ingesting a mixture of cyclamate and saccharin. The FDA's decision generated extensive scientific debate and petitions to reapprove the sweetener have been submitted. In 1984, on the basis of new evidence, a scientific committee within the FDA concluded that cyclamate is not a carcinogen. A similar decision was reached by a committee of the National Academy of Sciences in 1985. High doses of a metabolite of cyclamate produce testicular atrophy in rats (but not in mice), and this effect will be considered when the FDA makes a decision on the pending petition. Although cyclamate cannot be used in the United States at the present time, it is an approved food additive in 33 countries.

Like cyclamate, saccharin has been subjected to scientific scrutiny for many years. In fact, the safety of saccharin was questioned in the 1880s. Some years ago, 1 gram per day was considered a safe dose for humans. (In its usual commercial powdered form, saccharin is bulked with glucose. The most readily available packets contain a total of 1 gram of powder, of which 4 percent, or 40 milligrams is saccharin, equivalent in sweetening power to 2 teaspoons of sugar). A 1967 National Academy of Sciences report, undertaken at the request of the FDA, although not disagreeing with the earlier conclusion, stated that the evidence from previous studies was inadequate and called for additional research.

The first evidence that saccharin might be carcinogenic appeared in 1971. It showed that 7 of 15 rats who ingested saccharin as 5 percent of their diet for two years developed bladder cancer. Soon afterward the Canadian government began a larger-scale test of saccharin. Of 200 rats fed saccharin at the level of 5 percent of their diets, 21 developd bladder tumors, whereas only one of the control group (who received no saccharin) was so afflicted.

Citing the Delaney clause (which states that no food additive can be used if it induced cancer in man or animals) as the basis for action, the FDA proposed to ban saccharin in 1977. Because saccharin was the only low-calorie sweetener approved in the United States at that time, the public outcry against the ban was loud and clear. Opponents of the ban pointed out that the test doses were far higher in relation to body size and weight than the amounts of saccharin human users would be likely to ingest (equivalent to drinking about 1200 cans of diet soft drink every day for a lifetime). Some questioned the validity of animal, and especially nonprimate, tests.

Congress intervened, and passed the so-called "moratorium" which prohibited the FDA from banning the sweetener until more research had been done. The moratorium has been extended several times, most recently to May 1, 1987. One of the provisions of the moratorium was that foods containing saccharin must have a warning label stating that saccharin has caused cancer in laboratory animals.

Many studies have been conducted on saccharin since 1977. No other animal tested responds to saccharin in the same manner as male rats. Research is currently being done to determine the mechanism of the effect seen in male rats, which will help to evaluate whether saccharin ingestion poses a cancer risk to humans. In addition, because saccharin has been used for more than 80 years, many epidemiological studies have been conducted to determine whether saccharin use is associated with bladder cancer in humans. Most studies have been negative. Around the world, 59 countries permit the use of saccharin.

The newest "low-calorie" sweetener is aspartame. Unlike cyclamate and saccharin which contain no calories, aspartame contains 4 kcalories per gram. However, because it is about 300 times as sweet as sugar, only very small amounts are needed and its caloric contribution to food is minimal. After extensive safety testing, aspartame was approved for use in dry foods in 1981; approval for use in carbonated beverages was granted in 1983.

Aspartame is composed of two amino acids (phenylalanine and aspartic acid) and a methyl group. Individuals with phenylketonuria (PKU; see Chapter 4) must limit their intake of phenylalanine from all foods. Therefore products containing aspartame have a statement on the label informing consumers that phenylalanine is present.

Some questions have been raised about the effect of methanol which is produced by the breakdown of aspartame either in acidic beverages prior to consumption or in the gastrointestinal tract. The safety studies done to gain FDA approval for the sweetener addressed this question. Adults were given a dose of aspartame equivalent to consumption of more than fifty twelve-ounce cans of aspartame-sweetened beverage at one time. No increase in the concentration of breakdown products in the blood was detected. Infants were able to handle a somewhat lower dose adequately. Tomato juice and other foods contain methanol, often in larger amounts than that produced from the aspartame in a single can of diet soda. Boiling or temperature abuse of products containing aspartame results in a loss of sweetness intensity, not in the formation of harmful substances.

Some consumers have complained of suffering side effects after consuming aspartame. The Centers for Disease Control has analyzed more than 500 complaints and concluded that the data "do not provide evidence of the existence of serious widespread adverse health consequences." In 1985, the Council on Scientific Affairs of the American Medical Association concluded consumption of aspartame by normal persons was safe. In March 1986, the Epilepsy Institute released a statement that the organization had found aspartame to be safe for persons with epilepsy.

Since aspartame cannot be used in all foods, the search for new high intensity, low calorie sweeteners will continue. Acesulfam K has been approved for use in the United Kingdom, Germany, and Belgium, and is being considered in the United States. Other high intensity sweeteners are in various stages of development. In a society which is very conscious of weight, something that tastes like sugar without the calories is in demand. In addition, low-calorie fat substitutes are also being developed.

ies are needed to assess more foods and to better understand the factors which control rate of absorption.

Sucrose has also been implicated in heart disease, especially for the 10 percent of the population who are classified as carbohydrate-sensitive because they respond to ingestion of dietary carbohydrate (especially sucrose and fructose) with increased serum triglycerides, which have been strongly associated with the development of cardiovascular disease. As with other diseases we now understand that persons with high serum triglycerides must be classified in terms of genetic, metabolic, and environmental factors. Most researchers consider that the effect of sugar on blood lipids, however, is not well established. Again a role, if any for sugar, appears to be indirect in the development of obesity.

Modified Starches

Modified starches are used to provide texture, thicken, suspend solids, stabilize emulsions, and protect foods during processing, distribution, and storage. Animal studies using 50 percent or more of the total diet as modified starch result in diarrheae and enlargement of the cecum. Reactions do not occur if the starch is fed at 25 percent or less. From age one month, normal infants will tolerate 10 to 15 percent of the total dietary energy as starch. In one survey, the average daily intake of modified starch by 1–14 month-old infants was about 2 to 3 percent of the total intake. The American Academy of Pediatrics has recommended that use of modified or unmodified starch be as minimal as practical for infants younger than three months of age.

Exercise

Energy is derived mainly from lipids during low intesity exercise; as the level increases carbohydrate oxidation becomes the main source of energy. Well-trained athletes are better able to use lipids than untrained subjects. During high intensity exercise, lipid contributes very little and most energy for muscular work is obtained from carbohydrate metabolism. This information was incorporated into a regimen for exercise of long duration, carbohydrate loading. The regimen, carbohydrate loading, consisted of muscle glycogen depletion, carbohydrate starvation, and a supersaturation phase. The original regimen has been modified because of potential side effects. The modified program results in the same muscle glycogen concentration as the earlier one. Athletes now routinely eat 50 percent of their caloies as carbohydrate; 3 days before the event this is increased to 70 percent and training is tapered down (see Perspective On Athletes).

Alternative Sweeteners

Most of us have a "sweet tooth." Newborn infants have been shown to prefer a sweet taste. In an effort to reduce caloric intake without eliminating the pleasures of eating sweet foods, many people have been turning to alternative sweeteners. The food industry has responded by providing natural and synthetic sources of sweetness. Many of these sweeteners are not carbohydrates and are therefore discussed in Perspective On High Intensity Sweeteners (see page 44).

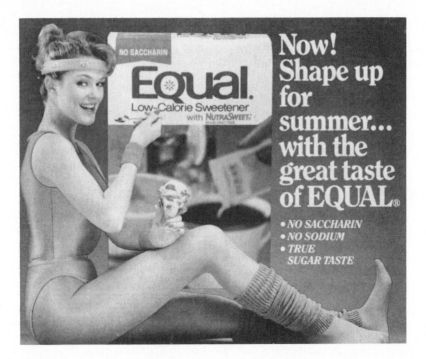

The food industry has responded to the low-calorie "sweet tooth" cravings by providing natural and synthetic sweeteners.
G. D. Searle & Company

SUMMARY

Carbohydrates, compounds of carbon, hydrogen, and oxygen in the proportions of one carbon atom to one water molecule—$C_n(H_2O)_n$—are the primary energy source in the average human diet. The two main types of carbohydrates are simple carbohydrates, or sugars, and complex carbohydrates, or starches. The names of many sugars contain the suffix *-ose* and have a prefix that defines the number of carbon atoms present in a molecule of that sugar—for example, hexoses are 6-carbon sugars, with the formula $C_6(H_2O)_6$ (or $C_6H_{12}O_6$).

Sugars may be monosaccharides (one simple sugar molecule) or disaccharides (two monosaccharides bonded together). In the bonding process, known as a condensation reaction, a molecule of water is released; therefore, the general formula for disaccharides is $C_{12}(H_2O)_{11}$. Glucose, galactose, and fructose are three different 6-carbon monosaccharides; sucrose, lactose, and maltose are three disaccharides.

Similar bonding of additional sugar units produces polysaccharide molecules (complex carbohydrates). Different arrangements of the chemical bonds within the sugar molecule (as in the monosaccharides) or between the sugar molecules (as in di- and polysaccharides) result in the formation of compounds with correspondingly different chemical and physical (for example, taste) properties.

Simple sugars are found primarily in fruits and vegetables. Sugars are commonly added to many kinds of processed foods. Complex carbohydrates are found in grains, legumes such as peas and peanuts, tubers such as potatoes, and other plant products. Lactose (milk sugar) is the only important dietary carbohydrate of animal origin.

Average consumption of sugars has been increasing, but complex carbohydrate consumption has decreased. Expansion of the food-processing industry, the widespread use of convenience foods, and other changes in food habits are among the factors involved in this shift. With increased interest in health, consumption of complex carbohydrates can be expected to rise again in the near future. Although sugar consumption has been suggested as causing several diseases, experimental evidence not only does not support these assumptions, but actually refutes them.

Disaccharides and polysaccharides in food must be converted to monosaccharides in order to be absorbed into the blood. In the process of digestion, they undergo hydrolytic reactions. The opposite of the condensation reaction, hydrolysis incorporates a water molecule to split a complex molecule into its simpler components. A specific enzyme is required to catalyze the hydrolytic reaction of each carbohydrate. If a particular enzyme is missing for any reason, its substrate cannot be digested. Lactose intolerance, for example, is a condition in which lactase, the enzyme necessary to digest lactose, is not produced in adequate quantity.

Glucose is the primary form in which digested carbohydrate enters the blood circulation. The maintenance of a constant level of glucose in the blood is of critical importance, and several body mechanisms interact to regulate that level. Diabetes and hypoglycemia are disturbances of blood glucose level regulation. From the blood, glucose enters the body cells. There it is used to produce energy by glycolysis and the Krebs cycle or to function in the synthesis of various essential compounds. Excess glucose may also be converted into glycogen or fat and stored in that form for future availability.

The Food and Nutrition Board recommends that a minimum of 50 to 100 grams of carbohydrate (about ⅛ to ¼ pound) be ingested daily, most of which should derive from grains, fruits, and vegetables. These sources contain naturally occurring simple sugars and complex carbohydrates as well as vitamins, minerals, and nonnutritive dietary fiber. The total amount of these foods should be increased in most diets. Some processed foods contain sugar accompanied by little other nutrient content. Use of such foods as a **replacement** for other foods deprives the body of the important nutrients in other foods.

Some polysaccharides cannot be digested because the human body lacks appropriate enzymes. Known as dietary fiber, undigested carbohydrates pass through the digestive tract and are excreted in the feces. Fiber content of foods is usually expressed as "crude fiber," but this is a significant underestimation of total fiber content; new methods of measuring dietary fiber accurately are being developed. Although dietary fiber contains no usable nutrients, it serves an important function in the regulation of the passage of fecal wastes. Lack of fiber in the diet may be related to such chronic ailments as diverticulosis, and also to atherosclerosis and cancer of the colon. Although questions about the role of fiber in health maintenance remain, increased consumption of high-fiber foods, especially whole-grain breads and cereals, fresh fruits, and vegetables, may be beneficial.

BIBLIOGRAPHY

Ahrens, E.H. Carbohydrates, plasma triglycerides and coronary heart disease. *Nutrition Reviews* 44:60–64, 1986.

American Diabetes Association. *What you need to know about diabetes.* New York: American Diabetes Association, 1976

———. Principles of nutrition and dietary recommendations for individuals with diabetes mellitus: 1979, *Diabetes Care* 2:520–523, 1979.

ANDERSON, T.A. Xylitol and dental caries. *Annual Review of Nutrition* 2:113–132, 1982.

BALDWIN, S.A., AND G.E. LIENHARD. Glucose transport across plasma membranes: Facilitated diffusion systems. *Trends in Biochemical Science* 6:208–211, 1981.

BEHRE, L.M. Modified starch and baby foods— the selling of fear? American Council on Science and Health, Jan/Feb, 1986.

BOLLENBACK, G.N. Sugar in health. *Cereal Foods World* 26:213–217, 1981.

BONHAM, G.S., AND D.B. BROCK. The relationship of diabetes with race, sex and obesity. *American Journal of Clinical Nutrition* 41:776–783, 1985.

BROWNLEE, M., ed. *Handbook of Diabetes Mellitus.* New York: Garland STPM Press, 1981.

BREWSTER, L. AND M. JACOBSON. *The Changing American Diet.* Washington, DC: Center for Science in the Public Interest, 1978.

CAHILL, G.F., JR. The future of carbohydrates in human nutrition. *Nutrition Reviews* 44:40–43, 1986.

CONNELL, A.M. Dietary fiber. In L.R. Johnson, ed., *Physiology of the Gastrointestinal Tract,* Vol. 2, pp. 1291–1299. Raven Press, 1981.

Council on Scientific Affairs, Division of Drugs and Technology, American Medical Association. Aspartame: Review of safety issues. *Journal of the American Medical Association* 254:400–402, 1985.

Council on Scientific Affairs, Division of Drugs and Technology, American Medical Association. Saccharin: Review of safety issues. *Journal of the American Medical Association* 254:2622–2624, 1985.

CRAPO, P.A. Theory vs. fact: The glycemic response to foods. *Nutrition Today* 19:6–11, 1984.

CZECK, M.P. Insulin action. *American Journal of Medicine* 70:142–150, 1981.

DANOWSKI, T.S., AND J.H. SUNDER. Sugar and disease in controversies in nutrition. L. Ellenbogen, ed. Vol 2, *Contemporary Issues in Clinical Nutrition.* New York: Churchill-Livingston, 1981.

DEBOGNIE, J.C., A.D. NEWCOMMER, D.B. McGILL, AND S.F. PHILLIPS. *Digest Dis. Science.* 24:225–231, 1979.

DUBRICK, M.A. Dietary supplements and health aids—a critical evaluation. Part 2— Macronutrients and fiber. *Journal of Nutrition Education* 15:88–92, 1983.

EASTWOOD, M.A. AND R. PASSMORE. A new look at dietary fiber. *Nutrition Today* 19:6–11, 1984.

Food and Nutrition Board, National Research Council. *Recommended Dietary Allowances,* 10th ed. Washington, DC: National Academy of Sciences, 1985.

GRAY, G.M. Carbohydrate absorption and malabsorption. In L.R. Johnson, ed., *Physiology of the digestive tract,* Vol. 2, pp. 1063–1072. New York: Raven Press, 1981.

HEMS, D.A. AND P.D. WHITTON. Control of hepatic glycogenolysis. *Physiological Review* 60:2–50, 1980.

HORWITZ, D.L. Advances in dietary treatment of diabetes, M. Nattrass and J.B. Santiago, eds. *Recent Advances In Diabetes I.* New York: Churchill-Livingston, 1984.

HOWE, G.R., J.D. BURCH, A.B. MILLER, et al. Artificial sweeteners and human bladder cancer. *Lancet* 2:578, 1977.

JENKINS, D.J.A., T.M.S. WOLEVER, R.H. TAYLOR, H. BARKER. Glycemic index of foods. *American Journal of Clinical Nutrition* 34:362–366, 1981.

JENKINS, D.J.A., A.L. JENKINS, T.M.S. WOLEVER, L.H. THOMPSON, AND A.V. RAO. Simple and complex carbohydrates. *Nutrition Reviews* 44:44–49, 1986.

JEQUIER, E. Carbohydrates: Energetics and performance. *Nutrition Reviews* 44:55–59, 1986.

KAY, R.M. Origin, functions, and physiological significance of dietary fiber. *Journal of Lipid Research* 23:221–242, 1982.

KRITCHEVSKY, D. Dietary fiber and disease in L. Ellenbogen, ed, *Controversies In Nutrition,* Vol. 2, *Contemporary Issues in Clinical Nutrition,* New York: Churchill-Livingstone, 1981.

LECOS, C.W. Sugar: How sweet it is—and isn't. *FDA Consumer,* February 1980, pp. 21–23.

————. Sweetness minus calories = controversy. *FDA Consumer,* February, 1985. HHS No. (FDA) 85–2205.

LENNER, R.A. Specially designed sweeteners and food for diabetics: A real need? *American Journal of Clinical Nutrition* 29:726, 1976.

LINEBACK, D.R. AND G.E. INGLETT, eds. Food Carbohydrates. Westport, CT: AVI Publishing Co., 1982.

LOESCHE, W.J. Nutrition and dental decay in infants. *American Journal of Clinical Nutrition* 41:423–435, 1985.

MAKINEN, K.K., AND A. SCHEININ. Xylitol and dental caries. *Annual Review of Nutrition* 2:133–150.

MARX, J.L. Diabetes—a possible autoimmune disease. *Science* 225:1381–1383, 1984.

NELSON, R.L. Hypoglycemia: Fact or fiction? Mayo Clinic Proceedings, 60:840–850, 1985.

OLSON, C.M. AND K.P. GEMMILL. Association of sweet preference and food selection among four to five year old children. *Ecology on Food Nutrition* 11:145–150, 1981.

PAIGE, D.M. AND T.M. BAYLESS, eds. *Lactose Digestion: Clinical and Nutritional Implications*. Baltimore, MD: Johns Hopkins University Press, 1981.

PARHAM, E.S. Comparison of responses to bans on cyclamates (1969) and saccharin (1977). *Journal of the American Dietetic Association* 72(1):59, 1978.

SELVENDRAN, R.R. The plant cell wall as a source of dietary fiber: Chemistry and structure. *American Journal of Clinical Nutrition*. 39:320–337, 1984.

SHANNON, I.L. Brand name guide to sugar: Sucrose content of over 1000 common foods and beverages. Chicago: Nelson-Hall, 1977.

SHAW, J.H. Diet and dental health. *American Journal of Clinical Nutrition*. 41:1117–1131, 1985.

SIMPSON, R.W., J. MCDONALD, M.L. WAHLQVIST, L. ATLEY, AND K. OUTCH. Macronutrients have different metabolic effects on nondiabetics and diabetics. *American Journal of Clinical Nutrition* 42:449–453, 1985.

SIPERSTEIN, M.D. Type II Diabetes: Some problems in diagnosis and treatment. *Hospital Practice*, March 15, 1985.

SPILLER, G.A. AND R.M. KAY, eds. *Medical Aspects of Dietary Fiber*. New York: Plenum, 1980.

———. Sweeteners: are any of them safe? *Consumer Reports*, November 1985, pp 690–693.

TALBOT, J.M. Role of dietary fiber in diverticular disease and colon cancer. Federation Proceedings 40:2337–2342, 1981.

ULRICH, I.H., H-Y LAI, L. VONA, R.L. REID, AND M.J. ALBRINK. Alterations of fecal steroid composition induced by changes in dietary fiber consumption. *American Journal of Clinical Nutrition*. 34:2054–2060, 1981.

USDA, Economic Research Service. Sugar: Background for 1985 farm legislation. *Agriculture Information Bulletin #478*, Washington, DC: U.S.D.A. 1984.

VAHOUNY, G.V. Dietary fiber, lipid metabolism, and atherosclerosis. Fed. Proc. 41:2801–2806, 1982.

WANG, Y.M., AND J. VAN EYS. Nutritional significance of fructose and sugar alcohols. *Annual Review of Nutrition* 1:437–475, 1981.

WOLEVER, T.M.S., AND D.J.A. JENKINS. The use of the glycemic index in predicting the blood glucose response to mixed meals. *American Journal of Clinical Nutrition* 43:167–172, 1986.

WOLRAICH, M., R. MILICH, P. STUMBO, AND F. SCHULTZ. Effects of sucrose ingestion on the behavior of hyperactive boys. *Journal of Pediatrics* 106: 675–682, 1985.

WURZBURG, O.B. Nutritional aspects and safety of modified food starches. *Nutrition Reviews* 44:74–79, 1986.

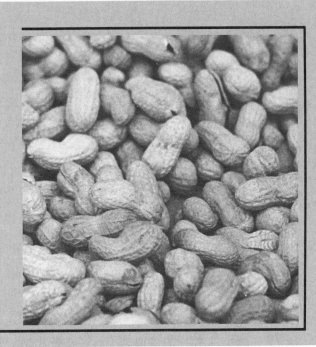

Chapter 3

LIPIDS

Long before modern knowledge of the science of nutrition existed, fats in the diet were valued as concentrated energy sources because of their ability to provide satiety—a sense of "fullness."

Early in the twentieth century, scientists observed that laboratory animals fed fat-free diets stopped growing and eventually died. Subsequently, an absence of fats was shown to cause scaly skin and other deficiency symptoms in humans. Toward the middle of the century, certain fatty substances essential for human and animal health were identified. The concept developed that two distinct aspects of dietary fats are important in nutrition:

1. A certain minimum amount of *total* fat, which can be any of numerous types such as corn oil, lard, butterfat, or many others, serves as a concentrated energy source as well as performing other functions, such as promoting absorption of certain vitamins.
2. A certain specific component of fats—an **essential fatty acid**—is required in the diet because the body cannot synthesize it as it does other fat components, and disease results from absence of this fatty acid as surely as it would from lack of a vitamin, mineral, or other essential nutrient.

For most Americans, however, fat deficiency will never be a problem; in fact, the current intake of fats far exceeds nutritional needs. Average fat consumption in the United States has risen by nearly one-third since the early years of the twentieth century. As much as 42 percent of our energy intake now comes from fats—more than is provided by either of the other two **macronutrients**, proteins and carbohydrates. Moreover, the body, as we shall see, readily synthesizes fats from other nutrient sources—as some of us know all too well.

Fat deficiency, then, is not a significant health problem in this country. Rather, it is an overabundance of dietary lipids. Excessive fat intake has been cited as a possible cause of heart disease and cancer, and the suspected relationship between fats and illness continues to generate considerable research as well as many controversial articles in both professional and popular publications. The dietary importance of fats, however, tends to be forgotten amid all the controversy.

Many body functions depend on fats. They provide an excellent source of energy, enhance transport of fat-soluble vitamins, insulate and protect internal tissues, and contribute to vital cell processes. In this chapter we shall examine these roles. We shall look also at the structures of different lipids and how they relate to their roles and functions. Finally, we shall discuss the suspected relationship between fats and disease.

WHAT ARE LIPIDS? DEFINITION

Lipid molecules differ in chemical composition, and therefore in chemical and physical properties, from the two other macronutrients. The elements found in carbohydrates—carbon, hydrogen, and oxygen—also occur in lipids, but in different proportions and with different structural arrangements. In particular, lipids contain a much lower proportion of oxygen atoms than do carbohydrates; some lipids contain nitrogen and phosphorus as well.

Because of their chemical composition, lipids do not dissolve in aqueous (water) solutions, but they do dissolve in organic solvents, such as chloroform, ether, and benzene. This can be illustrated from firsthand experience. If butter is dropped into water it will remain a glob of butter; even if the water is warmed so that the butter melts, still the butter may be seen clearly. If butter melts into your shirt, plain water will not remove it; only benzene or other solvents, such as soap, will do the job.

The composition of lipids also determines their gross, or obvious, appearance. Strictly speaking, **fats** are lipids that are solid at room temperature (butter or beef fat, for example), although as a practical matter the term *fat* is often interchangeably with *lipid*. **Oils** are lipids with melting points so low that they are liquid at room temperature (corn oil or olive oil, for example). Lipids with much higher melting points also exist but have little nutritional significance; we commonly refer to them as **waxes**. Our discussion will be concerned only with the nutrient, or edible, lipids.

LIPIDS: CLASSIFICATION

The different structures and functions of various lipids have been the basis for a number of classification systems. One such system lists lipids of nutritional interest (Table 3–1). The major lipids will be the subject of most of the discussion in this chapter. Prostaglandins, which are synthesized in the body from certain fatty acids, will be mentioned later in this chapter; **fat-soluble vitamins** will be the subject of Chapter 6.

TABLE 3–1. *Classification and functions of lipids*

Lipid	Function
1. Fatty acids	Metabolic fuel, building blocks for other lipids
Prostaglandins	Intracellular modulators
2. Glyceryl esters	
Acylglycerols	Fatty acid storage, metabolic intermediates
Phosphoglycerides	Membrane structure
3. Sphingolipids	
Sphingomyelin	Membrane structure
Glycosphingolipids	Membranes, surface antigens
4. Sterol derivatives	
Cholesterol	Membrane and lipoprotein structure
Cholesteryl esters	Storage and transport
Bile acids	Lipid digestion and absorption
Steroid hormones	Metabolic regulation
Vitamin D	Calcium and phosphorus metabolism
5. Terpenes	
Dolichols	Glycoprotein synthesis
Vitamin A	Vision, epithelial integrity
Vitamin E	Lipid antioxidant
Vitamin K	Blood coagulation

Source: R. Montgomery et al., *Biochemistry: A Case Oriented Approach*, 4th ed. (St. Louis, MO: C.V. Mosby, 1983).

CHEMICAL ORGANIZATION AND STRUCTURE

The basic structural unit of many lipid molecules is a **fatty acid**, a chain of hydrocarbons with a methyl group (CH_3) at one end and an acid or carboxyl group (COOH) attached at the other. As Table 3–1 indicates, some lipids are simple fatty acids, some are derivatives of fatty acids in combination with other substances, and others contain no fatty acid groups.

Fatty Acids

The general chemical formula for a fatty acid is

$$CH_3(CH_2)_n COOH,$$

where n is usually a multiple of two. In most fatty acids of nutritional significance, the hydrocarbon chain consists of an even number of carbon atoms ranging from 4 to 6 carbons for the so-called short-chain fatty acids, 8 to 12 carbons for medium-chain fatty acids, and 14 to 26 carbons for long-chain fatty acids. Butyric acid, for example, a 4-carbon fatty acid present in butter and other dairy products, can be written chemically either as

$$CH_3-CH_2-CH_2-COOH, \text{ or as } CH_3(CH_2)_2 COOH.$$

The value of the shorthand formula is obvious when long-chain fatty acids, such as the 14-carbon myristic acid, are considered: $CH_3(CH_2)_{12}COOH$ versus

$$CH_3-CH_2-CH_2-CH_2-CH_2-CH_2-CH_2-CH_2-CH_2-CH_2-CH_2-CH_2-CH_2-COOH.$$

Generally, each carbon in a hydrocarbon chain is attached to two hydrogen atoms and to each of two adjacent carbon atoms. Because a carbon atom has the potential for forming four such bonds, the valence requirement of carbon is 4:

$$-\overset{|}{\underset{|}{C}}-$$

A fatty acid in which the valence requirements of all carbon atoms is met in this way

$$-C-\overset{\displaystyle H}{\underset{\displaystyle H}{C}}-C-$$

is classified as a **saturated fatty acid**. That is, it is saturated with (or contains the maximum possible number of) hydrogen atoms.

Certain fatty acids are **unsaturated**; that is, some of their carbon atoms are bound to only a single hydrogen atom. To fill the remaining gaps in their valence requirement, these carbon atoms are joined by a double bond to an adjacent atom. Thus, in oleic acid, which has a total of 18 carbons, there is a double bond between the ninth and tenth carbon atoms:

$$\overset{\displaystyle H \quad H}{\underset{\displaystyle | \quad\;\; |}{CH_3(CH_2)_7C = C(CH_2)_7COOH.}}$$

(Carbon atoms are numbered from the carbon in the COOH group at the right of the chemical formula and continuing to the last carbon in the methyl group on the left.) Oleic acid, with only one double bond, is a **monounsaturated fatty acid**. A fatty acid having two or more double bonds is a **polyunsaturated fatty acid (PUFA)**.

Table 3-2 groups the naturally occurring fatty acids according to the number of carbon atoms and type of bonds between them. Note that four different fatty acids each contain 18 carbon atoms. The structural differences between these four fatty acids can most simply be expressed as 18:0, saturated stearic acid; 18:1, monounsaturated oleic acid; 18:2, polyunsaturated linoleic acid; and 18:3, polyunsaturated linolenic acid.

These numerical formulas are a convenient way to express the structures of fatty acids. The number to the left of the colon indicates the total number of carbon atoms in the molecule, and the number following the colon indicates the number of double bonds. This formula can be expanded to show the location of the double bonding as well. For examle, oleic acid can be expressed as 9-18:1, meaning that the double bond in the molecule comes after the ninth carbon atom in the chain. The chemical and numerical structural formulas for linoleic acid are

$$\overset{\displaystyle \quad\quad\quad\quad H \quad H \quad\quad\quad H \quad H}{\underset{\displaystyle \quad\quad\quad\quad | \quad\; | \quad\quad\quad\; | \quad\; |}{CH_3(CH_2)_4C = C - CH_2 - C = C(CH_2)_7COOH \text{ and } 9,12-18:2.}}$$

Linolenic acid is expressed as

$$\overset{\displaystyle \quad\quad H \quad H \quad\quad\; H \quad H \quad\quad\; H \quad H}{\underset{\displaystyle \quad\quad | \quad\; | \quad\quad\;\; | \quad\; | \quad\quad\;\; | \quad\; |}{CH_3CH_2C = C - CH_2 - C = C - CH_2 - C = C - (CH_2)_7COOH \text{ and } 9,12,15-18:3.}}$$

TABLE 3-2. *Major Naturally Occurring Fatty Acids*

NUMBER OF C ATOMS	NUMBER OF DOUBLE BONDS					
	0	1	2	3	4	5
4	Butyric					
6	Caproic					
8	Caprylic					
10	Capric					
12	Lauric					
14	Myristic					
16	Palmitic	Palmitoleic				
18	Stearic	Oleic	Linoleic*	Linolenic**		Eicosa-
20	Arachidic				Arachidonic**	Pentaenoic*

* Omega–6   ** Omega–3

Polyunsaturated fatty acids were thought for a number of years to function in a similar fashion metabolically although a structural difference was well known. This difference involves the position of the first double bond relative to the omega end of the molecule (the carbon attached to the methyl group). One class of polyunsaturated fatty acids, omega-6 fatty acids, has the first double bond on the sixth carbon from the omega end. This group includes linoleic acid. In another important class, the double bonds start at the third carbon from the omega carbon and are designated as omega-3 fatty acids. These include linolenic acid which can be slowly converted to the most common omega-3 fatty acids, eicosapentaenoic acid (EPA) and docosahexaenoic acid (DHA). Omega-3 and omega-6 fatty acids are not interconvertible metabolically and a dietary source of each may be necessary. In order to identify these two classes of polyunsaturated fatty acids, some scientists are using the designation 18:2n-6 for linoleic acid, meaning that it has an 18-carbon chain with two double bonds and the first double bond is on the sixth carbon from the omega end of the molecule. The dietary sources of these two groups of fatty acids are different.

Depending, then, on the number of hydrogen atoms in proportion to the carbon atoms, fatty acids may be saturated or unsaturated; unsaturated fatty acids may be monounsaturated or polyunsaturated; polyunsaturated fatty acids may belong to the omega-3 or omega-6 group. The differences between these forms may have dietary and health implications, as we shall see.

Although these molecules must be diagrammed in two dimensions on a page, in reality they exist in three-dimensional form. The double bonds between some carbon atoms have more flexibility than do single bonds. Consequently, the other parts of the hydrocarbon chain are able to rotate, bend, or otherwise take different positions around the double bond. Unsaturated fatty acids generally can take one of two geometric shapes. A molecule that is stretched out is known as the **trans form**, and a molecule that is folded back on itself is known as the **cis form**. (The terms are derived from Latin prefixes, *cis* meaning "on this side," and *trans* meaning "on the other side.") Each form of a molecule that exists in more than one configuration is known as an **isomer**. The *cis* and *trans* forms of oleic acid (18:1) follow along with the general structural formulas for fatty acid isomers.

$$CH_3-(CH_2)_n-\overset{\shortparallel}{C}-H$$
$$COOH-(CH_2)_n-\overset{\shortparallel}{C}-H$$

Cis form

$$CH_3-(CH_2)_n-\overset{H}{\underset{\shortparallel}{C}}$$
$$\overset{\shortparallel}{C}-(CH_2)_n COOH$$
$$H$$

Trans form

$$H\overset{\shortparallel}{C}-(CH_2)_7 COOH$$
$$H\overset{\shortparallel}{C}-(CH_2)_7 CH_3$$

Cis form

$$H\overset{\shortparallel}{C}-(CH_2)_7 COOH$$
$$H_3C(CH_2)_7-\overset{\shortparallel}{C}H$$

Trans form

Generally, the *cis* isomer is more flexible and often has a zigzag shape, important in membrane structure and function. Most naturally occurring unsaturated fatty acids are *cis* isomers. Under certain conditions, such as heat or hydrogenation (see below), these natural *cis* forms may be converted to the less flexible *trans* forms. This transformation often takes place during commercial processing of foods, as a result of which the melting points of some fats may increase. The energy value of fats, however, is not altered by such changes.

Fatty Acid Derivatives

The compound that results from the combination of one or more fatty acids with an alcohol is called an **ester**. Two categories of lipids are derived from fatty acids in this manner, *glycerol esters* and *cholesterol esters*.

GLYCEROL ESTERS. Glycerol, an important molecule derived in the body from glucose metabolism, contains three carbon atoms, each of which is attached to an alcohol group (—OH). A condensation reaction between the carboxyl group of a fatty acid and an alcohol group of glycerol results in the formation of a **glyceride**. Depending on the number of fatty acids and alcohol groups that take part in the reaction, **mono-, di-,** or **triglycerides** are formed (see Figure 3–1).

This condensation reaction is similar to the one in which a disaccharide is formed from two monosaccharides (as we saw in Chapter 2), with a molecule of water being released in the process. Remember, however, that every chemical reaction that takes place in the body must be catalyzed by a specific enzyme. Thus, each of these two reactions involves distinctive enzymes as well as different substrates.

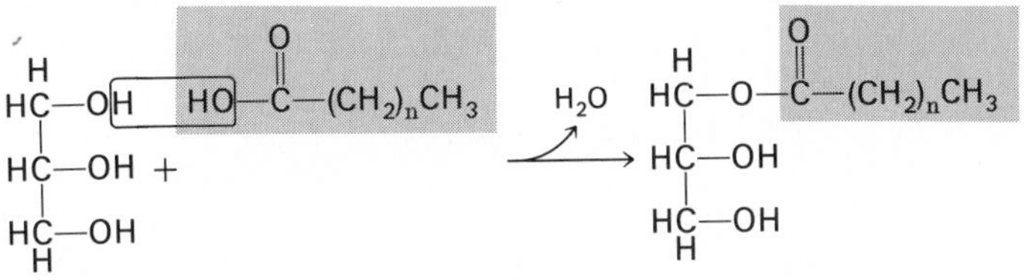

FIGURE 3-1   *Formation of a Monoglyceride.*

Successive condensation reactions incorporating the same original glycerol molecule result in the formation of diglycerides and triglycerides. Triglycerides, the most abundant type of lipid in food, result from the catalyzed reaction of glycerol and three fatty acids, a reaction which may be expressed

$$\text{glycerol} + 3 \text{ fatty acids} \longrightarrow \text{triglyceride} + 3H_2O.$$

In a simple triglyceride, all three combining fatty acids are identical. In a mixed triglyceride, however, two or three different fatty acids have condensed, or esterified, with the glycerol molecule, as shown in Figure 3–2. Most dietary triglycerides are mixed.

Phospholipids are constructed like triglycerides, except that a phosphate-containing group replaces the third fatty acid. **Lecithin** is a phospholipid.

CHOLESTEROL ESTERS. These esters are formed through condensation reactions involving the sterol cholesterol (discussed subsequently) and a fatty acid which attaches to the alcohol (—OH) group shown in Figure 3–3. Only a small quantity of dietary cholesterol is in this esterified form; most is in the form of cholesterol without a fatty acid component, that is, free cholesterol.

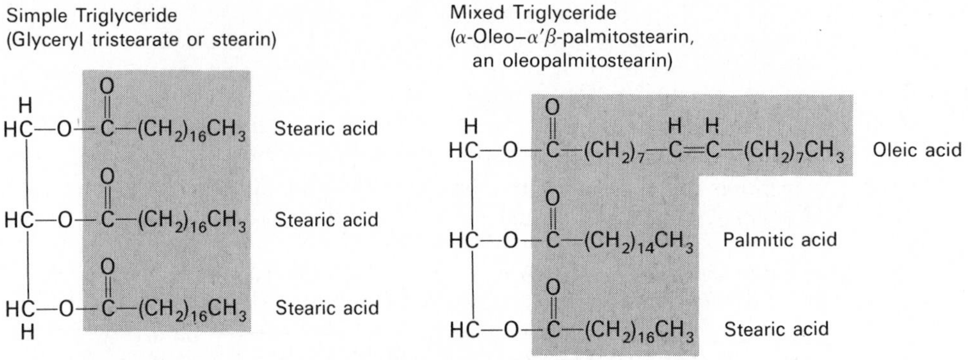
Simple Triglyceride
(Glyceryl tristearate or stearin)
Stearic acid
Stearic acid
Stearic acid
Mixed Triglyceride
(α-Oleo-α′β-palmitostearin,
an oleopalmitostearin)
Oleic acid
Palmitic acid
Stearic acid

FIGURE 3-2 *Examples of Simple and Mixed Triglycerides.*

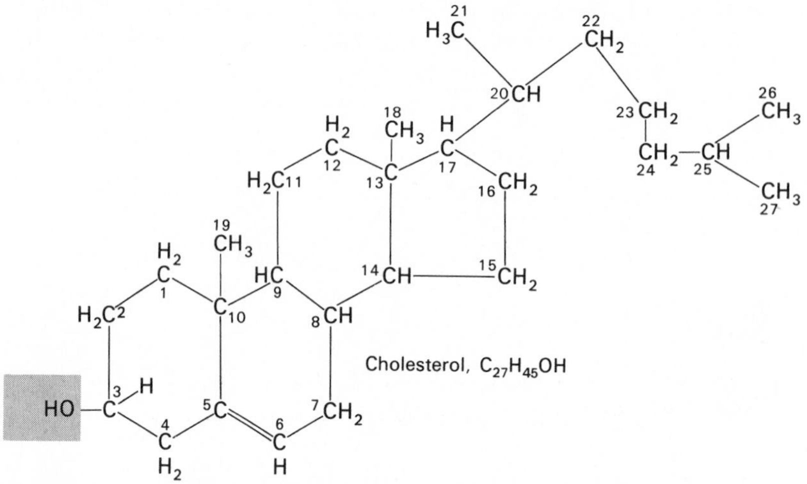
Cholesterol, C27H45OH

FIGURE 3-3 *Cholesterol Molecule.*

GLYCOLIPIDS. Compounds of one or more sugar molecules (usually glucose or galactose) with a fatty acid and nitrogen are called *glycolipids.* Cerebrosides are a group of glycolipids present in large quantities in the brain and in lesser amounts in other tissues such as the liver, spleen, and kidneys.

PROSTAGLANDINS, THROMBOXANES, AND LEUKOTRIENES. In 1962 prostaglandins (PG) were indentified as compounds capable of stimulating contraction of smooth muscle in the walls of blood vessels. Since that time PGs, thromboxanes (TXAs) and leukotrienes (LTs) have all been shown to be synthesized from 20-carbon fatty acids. EPA and arachidonic acid are both used and the types of PGs which are produced depend on the type of substrate available. The type of PG synthesized may impact on the development of diseases in humans, including heart disease.

Leukotrienes are involved in asthma, allergies, macrophage function, inflammatory responses, and immune functions. LTs are basically derived from arachidonic acid.

Sterols

Sterols, the third major dietary lipid category, are fat-soluble alcohols. The most familiar sterol is, of course, cholesterol, which has figured in extensive controversy regarding its possible contribution to atherosclerosis and coronary heart disease. A number of other important sterols are found in food as well.

Sterols differ from other lipids in having a ring structure. Typically, sterols have a nucleus of four interlocking rings, of which three contain six carbon atoms each and the fourth contains five. An alcohol (—OH) group is attached to carbon number 3 of the first ring, and a chain of eight or more carbon atoms is attached to carbon number 17 of the fourth ring. The valence requirement of all carbon atoms is met through single or double bonding to adjacent carbon atoms and through attachment to one or more hydrogen atoms. These linkages can be clearly seen in the diagrammatic representation of cholesterol in Figure 3–3. Another way of illustrating the chemical structure is depicted in Figure 3–4.

Although the role of cholesterol in disease is being debated, there is no question about the necessity for this lipid in the human body. Cholesterol is important as a precursor of several important compounds, particularly the steroid hormones (which include cortisone and the sex hormones), and for the production of vitamin D and bile salts.

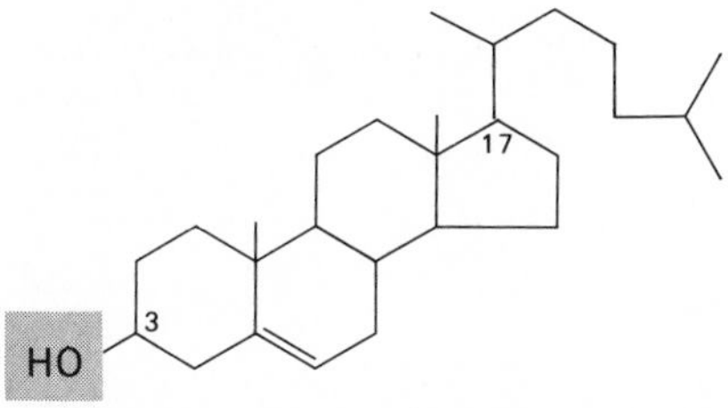

FIGURE 3-4   *Structural Diagram of a Cholesterol Molecule.*
Another way of illustrating chemical structure is depicted above. A comparison of Figures 3-3 and 3-4 will show that each angle in Figure 3-4 represents a carbon atom with the number of hydrogen atoms needed to satisfy valence requirements. Note that a single line repesents single bonding, and a double line represents double bonding. The hydroxyl group at carbon number 3 provides the attachment for a fatty acid in the ester linkage (or condensation reaction) that results in a cholesterol ester. The hydrocarbon chain is shown attached to carbon number 17 of the steroid nucleus.

LIPIDS IN FOODS

Although lipids are relatively tasteless, their structure enables them to trap pleasurable flavors. The oil in tomato sauce lets it cling not only to your spaghetti but also to your taste buds. Poultry cooked without its skin, and so without its natural blanket of fat, would be almost flavorless.

Different fats and oils have distinctive flavors because of their different chemical structures. Olive oil tastes different from peanut oil, and both taste different from sesame oil. Every region, and every ethnic group, has its characteristic cooking oil,

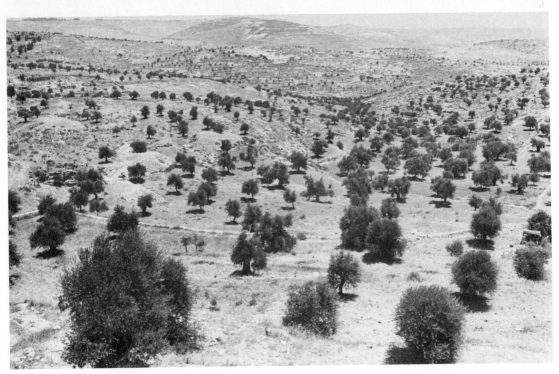

An olive grove produces the characteristic cooking oil that gives Mediterranean cuisine its distinctive flavor.

Owen Franken/Stock, Boston

which gives the cuisine its distinctive flavor. Corn oil prevails in Mexico; olive oil throughout the Mediterranean, from Greece to Italy to Spain; peanut and coconut oils in Africa; butter and lard in northern Europe; clarified butter (ghee) in India; and seal and whale oils among the Eskimo.

Functions of Fats

The palatability of fats and the greater taste appeal fats give to other foods help to ensure that our overall intake is adequate. The fat component of a meal is responsible for our feeling satisfyingly full after we have eaten. Fats and oils are digested and leave the stomach more slowly than carbohydrates or proteins, and are absorbed more slowly as well. For these reasons, the inclusion of some fatty foods in every meal will leave the eater feeling more satisfied for a longer period of time, an important consideration in the design of weight-reduction diets.

The primary function of dietary lipid is to provide a concentrated source of energy in relatively low bulk. The caloric density of fat is more than twice as great as that of either carbohydrate or protein. One gram of fat produces 9 kilocalories (37.8 kJ), whereas one gram of either carbohydrate or protein produces only 4 (16.8 kJ). Perhaps the efficiency with which fat provides the body's fuel can best be appreciated when one compares the caloric content of various food portions; one-half cup of rice (which has about 28 g carbohydrate) contains 112 kilocalories, whereas a single tablespoon of butter contains 100 kilocalories.

Another major role of dietary fats is to transport fat-soluble vitamins. Absorption of vitamins A, D, E, and K will not occur very efficiently in the absence of lipid.

Finally, dietary lipids are the source of an essential nutrient. "Essential" has a special nutritional meaning; it refers to a substance that cannot be synthesized by the body at all, or cannot be synthesized in adequate amounts, and whose lack results in specific deficiency symptoms. Linoleic acid, a PUFA, has been identified as an essential nutrient, necessary for normal growth and health maintenance. In its absence, specific deficiency symptoms develop.

When essential fatty acid (EFA) deficiency was initially described, linolenic (18:3) and arachidonic (20:4) acids were also thought to be essential. This was followed by a long period during which neither were thought to be essential. Arachidonic acid, which is about three times more effective than linoleic acid in promoting growth, is synthesized by the body from linoleic acid. One form of linolenic acid can be synthesized from linoleic acid. A second type which belongs to the omega-3 group must be obtained from the diet. Linolenic acid can be converted to EPA and DHA, but the process is very slow. Newer data suggest that omega-3 fatty acids may be essential. Monkeys whose mothers were fed diets deficient in omega-3 fatty acids during pregnancy had reduced visual acuity. Human milk contains linolenic, EPA, and DHA, and the brain contains large amounts of DHA, but at this time the answer to the question regarding the essentiality of omega-3 fatty acids cannot be answered affirmatively. Linoleic acid, be-

Certain fatty acids are essential in the nutritional sense that they cannot be synthesized by the body in adequate amounts. Therefore they must be supplied from dietary sources.
Barry L. Runk from Grant Heilman

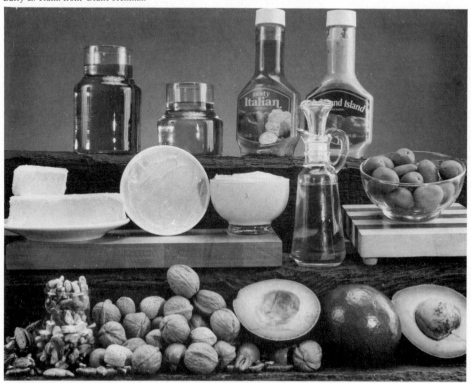

cause it cannot be synthesized by the body, is in every sense *the* essential fatty acid. Linoleic acid is present in a large number of vegetable oils, as well as in other sources. Omega-3 fatty acids are present in fish oils.

Lipid Content of Foods

Most people are aware of the "visible" fats of butter, oils, bacon, and the layer surrounding meat, but they may not realize that milk, nuts, avocados, cheese, egg yolk, pie crusts, and many other foods contain "invisible" fat in substantial quantities. In general, however, fruits, grains, and vegetables contain very little fat.

Everyone has noticed that visible fats vary from one food to another. For example, the fat of beef is whiter and firmer than that of poultry, which is in turn more solid than that found in fish. The appearance and texture of beef fat varies with the age of the animal; fat of mature beef is whiter and harder than the fat of young beef, which is soft and translucent. The difference between the lipids in butter and those in corn oil is also obvious.

TRIGLYCERIDES. Virtually all—about 90 percent—of the lipids in our food are in the form of triglycerides. The remaining tenth is primarily in the form of cholesterol and phospholipids. The length of the carbon chains and the degree of saturation of the fatty acids in the triglycerides account for the different textures, appearance, and other properties of the various dietary fats.

In general, those triglycerides containing short- and medium-chain fatty acids, as well as those containing unsaturated long-chain fatty acids, are liquid at room temperature (peanut oil). But fatty foods containing a high proportion of saturated long-chain fatty acids will be solid under the same conditions (beef fat). A single food may contain many different triglycerides, and the composite mixture of fatty acid length and degree of saturation will determine not only the physical properties but also the biological effects of a particular dietary lipid.

The fatty acid composition of various fats is listed in Table 3-3. Most food fats consist predominantly of long-chain fatty acids (16 or more carbons), with butter, milk (including human milk) and milk products, and particularly, coconut oil, containing significant amounts of short- and medium-chain fatty acids as well. Animal products generally contain significant amounts of saturated (palmitic and stearic) and monounsaturated (oleic) fatty acids, with lesser amounts of PUFA. Vegetable products, on the other hand, except for coconut oil, contain higher proportions of the long-chain unsaturated oleic and linoleic acids and lesser amounts of saturated fatty acids. Although coconut oil is largely saturated, it consists for the most part of medium- or short-chain fatty acids containing 12 or fewer carbon atoms, and is therefore liquid. People who, for health reasons or by choice, want to switch to polyunsaturated vegetable oils, should be aware that coconut oil is the exception to the vegetable oil-PUFA rule. As mentioned earlier, omega-3 fatty acids are found in fish oils. High-fat fish, such as salmon, mackerel, or trout, have more than low fat white fish such as cod or flounder.

By changing the fatty acid composition of feed, livestock with a higher PUFA content can be produced. These findings have nutritional implications for humans. Similarly, studies have shown that the fatty acid content of the adipose tissue of human infants reflects the fats received in formula or breast milk.

HYDROGENATION. We have seen that vegetable oils are liquid at room temperature because of their high proportion of polyunsaturated fatty acids. How,

TABLE 3-3. Major Fatty Acid Content of Selected Animal and Plant Origin

	SATURATED							UNSATURATED					
	4–8	Capric 10:0	Lauric 12:0	Myristic 14:0	Palmitic 16:0	Stearic 18:0	Arachidic 20:0	Palmitoleic 16:1	Oleic 18:1	Linoleic 18:2	Linolenic 18:3	Arachidonic 20:4	Other Polyenoic Acids
ANIMAL-ORIGIN FATS:													
Lard				1.5	27.0	13.5		3.0	43.5	10.5	0.5		
Chicken			2.0	7.0	25.0	6.0		8.0	36.0	14.0			
Egg					25.0	10.0			50.0	10.0	2.0	3.0	
Beef				3.0	29.0	21.0	0.5	3.0	41.0	2.0	0.5	0.5	
Butter	5.5	3.0	3.5	12.0	28.0	13.0		3.0	28.5	1.0	0.5		
Whole cow's milk[a]	6.5	2.5	3.0	11.0	28.0	12.5		2.5	26.5	2.5	1.5	trace	
Yogurt, fruit-flavored, low-fat[a]	6.0	3.0	4.0	10.5	28.0	10.0		2.0	24.0	2.0	1.0	trace	
Cheddar cheese[a]	6.0	2.0	2.0	10.5	31.0	13.0		3.0	25.0	2.0	1.0	trace	
Human milk		1.5	7.0	8.5	21.0	7.0	1.0	2.5	36.0	7.0	1.0	0.5	
Human adipose[b]			0.1–2	2–6	21–25	2–8		3–7	39–47	4–25			2–8
PLANT-ORIGIN FATS:													
Corn					12.5	2.5	0.5		29.0	55.0	0.5		
Peanut					11.5	3.0	1.5		53.0	26.0			
Cottonseed				1.0	26.0	3.0		1.0	17.5	51.5			
Soybean					11.5	4.0			24.5	53.0	7.0		
Olive					13.0	2.5		1.0	74.0	9.0	0.5		
Coconut	7.0	6.0	49.5	19.5	8.5	2.0			6.0	1.5			

a Consumer and Food Economics Institute, Composition of foods . . . dairy and egg products . . . raw, processed, prepared, USDA Agriculture Handbook No. 8-1 (Washington, D.C.: U.S. Government Printing Office, 1976).

b Adapted from E. S. West et al.: Textbook of biochemistry, 4th ed. (New York: Macmillan, 1966).

Note: Composition is given in weight percentages of the component fatty acids as determined by gas chromatography. The number of carbon atoms and the number of double bonds is indicated under the common name of the fatty acid. These data were derived from a variety of sources, and considerable variation is to be expected in individual samples.

Source: Food and Nutrition Board, Dietary fat and human health, Pub. 1147 (Washington, D.C.: National Academy of Sciences–National Research Council, 1966), p. 6.

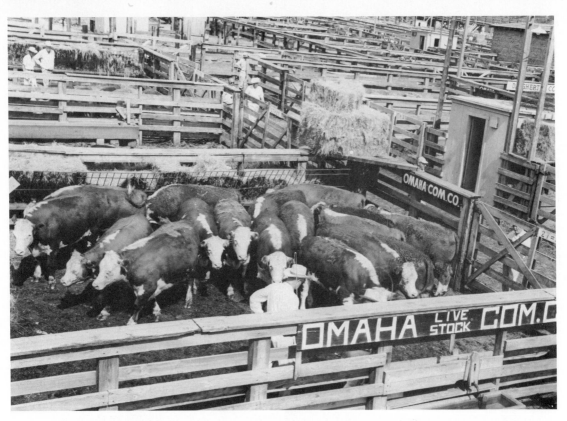

By changing the fatty acid composition of feed, livestock with a high PUFA content can be produced.
USDA

then, do we account for the fact that margarine, which consists of vegetable oils, is solid at room temperature? Food technologists found that, by the process of **hydrogenation** (chemically adding hydrogen atoms to polyunsaturated fatty acids), vegetable oils could be solidified and made spreadable. As the hydrogen atoms become attached to the carbon atoms of the molecule, the number of double bonds is reduced and the linoleic acid content is decreased. If hydrogenation is complete, the resulting fat will be saturated.

Hydrogenation may be terminated before complete saturation is achieved, resulting in a product that is only partially hydrogenated and that contains a proportionately greater quantity of monounsaturated oleic acid. Margarine, then, consists of vegetable oils that have been hydrogenated so that they have a higher proportion of saturated and monounsaturated fatty acids than the original product, and it is therefore solid at room temperature. Because the chemical nature of the lipid has been changed, its physical properties—appearance, taste, melting point—have been altered also.

When margarine was first introduced commercially as a butter substitute, consumer acceptance was poor. It did not, after all, look like butter (it was a pasty white color) nor did it taste like the "high-priced spread." Food technologists went back to their laboratories to create today's margarines, which not only have color, flavorings, and preservatives added to them but also are fortified with vitamins A and D to give them nutritive value and taste as similar as possible to those of butter. Margarine even has the same calorie count as butter, approximately 100 per tablespoon, and must, by law, contain at least 80 percent fat (as must butter). Exceptions are the "imitation" or diet margarines, which have less than 80 percent fat and contain more water than regular margarines. The fat composition of different kinds of margarine is shown in Table 3-4. Most cost less than butter, although the price differential has narrowed in recent years as consumer demand for polyunsaturated fats has grown. As one might expect, the highest-priced margarines are those with the highest PUFA content.

Hydrogenation is also used to improve the keeping qualities of liquid oils. Exposure to oxygen causes the double bonds in unsaturated fats to break down. **Oxidation** leads to undesirable odors and flavors. It is accelerated by exposure to light, air, and heat and through contact with certain metals such as iron, copper, and nickel. Partial hydrogenation, which makes oil less susceptible to oxidation, is one solution to the problem of spoilage. Other solutions include the addition of chemicals, such as BHT (butylated hydroxytoluene) and BHA (butylated hydroxyanisole), that act as **antioxidants** because they are preferentially oxidized instead of the PUFA; vitamin E is a natural antioxidant. Air-tight, dark, and cool storage conditions also retard the oxidation process.

PHOSPHOLIPIDS AND CHOLESTEROL.   Our discussion of dietary lipids has thus far concentrated on the triglycerides which account for 90 percent of our fat intake. The remaining components of dietary lipid are phospholipids and cholesterol.

Phospholipids are found in significant quantities in egg yolk and soybeans and in marginal amounts in a number of other foods. Lecithin is a major phospholipid.

Cholesterol is a natural body substance, required for several vital processes. The greater portion of the human cholesterol requirement is met by synthesis within the body. Table 3–5 shows both the fat and cholesterol content of a number of foods. Note that fat content is not an indicator of cholesterol content: Corn oil, for example, is 100 percent lipid but has no cholesterol. Cholesterol occurs only in foods of animal origin, including all meats. Organ meats such as liver and brains and egg yolks have the highest concentration. Egg yolks, in fact, contain the entire cholesterol content of the egg; there is no cholesterol in egg white. Fish and shellfish have a relatively low total lipid content and, with the exception of shrimp, have moderate amounts of cholesterol. Although low in fats, shrimp contain larger amounts of cholesterol. The concern over dietary cholesterol and its possible implication in the development of atherosclerosis will be examined later in this chapter.

Table 3-4. *Fat Composition of Margarine Types (g/tbsp)*

Margarine[a]	Total Fat	Saturated Fat	PUFA	Energy Content (kcal, rounded)
Stick (soybean oil)	11	2	1	100
Soft (soybean oil)	11	2	3	100
Soft (corn oil)	11	2	5	100
Soft diet (corn oil)	6	1	2	50

[a] Single brand, comparing various types.
Source: Adapted from *Medical Newsletter*, September 24, 1976.

Table 3-5. *Total Fat and Cholesterol Content of Selected Foods*

Food	Fat Content g/100 g	Cholesterol Content mg/100 g	Serving Size	Fat Content g/serving	Cholesterol Content mg/serving
Beef liver, raw	3.2	300	3½ oz	3.2	300
Whole eggs	11.2	548	1 large	5.6	274
Egg yolk	32.9	1602	1 large	5.6	274
Shrimp, canned, drained	1.1	150	1 c	1.4	192
Lobster, cooked, meat only	1.5	85	1 c	2.2	123
Crabmeat, canned	2.5	101	½ c	2.0	80
Beef, lean, cooked	14.7	91	3 oz	13	77
Chicken breast, cooked	7.8	84	½ breast meat and skin (98 g)	7.63	83
Haddock, flesh only	0.1	60	3½ oz	0.1	60
Oysters, meat only	2.0	50	½ c	2.4	60
Tuna, in water	0.8	63	3¼ oz	0.73	58
Clams, raw, meat only	1.6	50	½ c	1.8	57
Chicken drumstick, cooked	11.2	91	1, meat and skin (52 g)	5.8	48
Macaroni and cheese, home recipe	11.1	21	1 c	22.2	42
Hot dog, cooked	27.2	62	1 (8 per lb)	15	34
Whole milk	3.3	14	1 c	8	33
Yellow cake with chocolate frosting	13.0	44	¹⁄₁₆ of 9-in cake	10	33
Ice cream, 10% fat	10.8	45	½ c	7.1	30
Processed American cheese	31.2	94	1 oz	8.9	27
Swiss cheese	27.4	92	1 oz	7.8	26
Brownie with nuts (homemade)	31.3	83	1 (20 g)	6	17
Cream cheese	35.2	111	1 tbsp	5	16
Yogurt, plain, low-fat	1.6	6	8 oz	3.5	14
Butter	81.0	2.9	1 pat	4.1	11
Cottage cheese, 1% fat	1.0	4	1 c	2.3	10
Skim milk	0.1	2	1 c	0.4	4
Angel food cake	0.2	0	¹⁄₁₂ of 10-in cake	trace	0
Apple, raw with skin	0.4	0	1 medium	0.49	0
Banana	0.48	0	1 small	0.55	0
Bread, white	5.0	0	1 slice (22 per lb)	1	0
Corn oil	100.0	0	1 tbsp	14	0
Egg white	0	0	1 large	0	0
Margarine, vegetable	81.0	0	1 tbsp	12	0
Peanut butter	45.0	0	1 tbsp	10	0
Red kidney beans, cooked	1.7	0	1 c	1.0	0
Sweet potatoes	0.9	0	1 medium	1.0	0

Note: Generally, animal products are the food sources which contain significant amounts of cholesterol. Organ meats and eggs have the highest concentration, with the yolk containing *all* the cholesterol found in whole eggs. Fat content is not necessarily indicative of cholesterol content, as can be seen in the values for beef liver, eggs, corn oil, and margarine.

Source: Compiled from C. F. Church and H. N. Church, *Food values of portions commonly used*, 12th ed. (Philadelphia: J. B. Lippincott, 1975); and R. M. Feeley et al., Cholesterol contents of foods, *Journal of the American Dietetic Association* 61:134–149, 1972. USDA Agriculture Handbooks No. 8-1 (1976); 8-4 (1979), 8-5 (1979), 8-9 (1982), 8-11 (1982), (Washington, D.C.: U.S. Government Printing Office).

DIGESTION AND ABSORPTION

Before examining some of the specific physiological functions of lipids, we will consider the processes by which lipids in foods are transformed into lipids having structural and functional significance in the body. Although the basic principles of preparing food chemicals for entry into the blood and cells of the body are the same for lipids as they are for carbohydrates, certain important differences exist.

Because lipids are insoluble in water—which comprises the medium of cells, interstitial fluids, and the circulatory system—they must be rendered more water soluble before they can be biologically useful. This is achieved by two major mechanisms: **emulsification** and the use of specialized transport systems.

Emulsification

Lipid molecules must be emulsified in order to be able to mix with water. An emulsifier is a molecule that contains both a water-soluble and a lipid-soluble group. Emulsification takes place when the water-soluble group of such a molecule interacts with a water-based substance and the lipid-soluble group interacts with a lipid-based substance. The emulsifier acts as a bridge between two substances that would otherwise be immiscible (unblendable) (see Figure 3–5).

Bile acids and lecithin are two major biochemical emulsifiers. They disperse fat into small globules within the gastrointestinal tract, thereby increasing the surface area available to interact with digestive enzymes.

Emulsification can also be done mechanically through a process in which fat globules are broken into smaller particles so that they may be dispersed in a watery medium. The homogenization of milk is an example.

Lipid Transport

Lipids are carried through plasma in the form of **lipoproteins**. Because plasma is an aqueous medium, lipids cannot be transported without the mediation of this group

FIGURE 3-5   *Emulsification.*

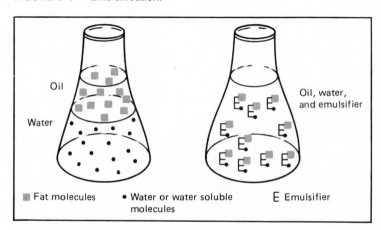

Oil

Water

Oil, water, and emulsifier

■ Fat molecules   • Water or water soluble molecules   E Emulsifier

TABLE 3-6. *Composition and Synthesis of Lipoproteins*

Lipoprotein (in order of increasing density)	Protein %	LIPID %					Carbohydrate %	Synthesized in
		Triglyceride	Cholesterol & Cholesterol esters	Phospholipid	Total			
Chylomicrons	1	90	7	2	99		trace	Intestine
VLDLs	10	60	15	14	89		1	Liver
LDLs	25	10	44	20	74		1	Liver and intestine
HDLs	50	3	16	30	49		1	Liver

of substances—proteins that tend to combine with lipids—specialized for lipid transport.

Each of the four major classes of lipoproteins performs a specific physiological function, and each differs in the proportions of its protein and lipid components. Because pure fat is lighter than water, as the proportion of lipid to protein increases, the density of the lipoprotein decreases. Thus, the lipoprotein with the greatest amount of lipid in proportion to protein will be lightest, or least dense. A comparison of the composition of these molecules is presented in Table 3–6.

Chylomicrons, the least dense type of lipoprotein, transport triglycerides and also some cholesterol. *Very low-density lipoproteins* (VLDLs), synthesized in the liver, also transport primarily triglycerides, carrying them from the liver to other tissues, especially to adipose tissue for storage. *Low-density lipoproteins* (LDLs) transport mainly cholesterol, somewhat over half of it in the form of cholesterol esters. *High-density lipoproteins* (HDLs) transport phospholipids and cholesterol esters.

Some individuals are unable to synthesize certain lipoproteins, resulting in abnormalities of lipid metabolism. These conditions are genetic in origin and are manifested by a variety of symptoms.

Lipid Digestion

No significant chemical digestion of fat occurs before dietary lipid enters the duodenum. In the stomach, however, the enzyme gastric lipase initiates hydrolysis of such highly emulsified dietary fats as those in egg yolk and milk and has some small effect on triglycerides containing short- and medium-chain fatty acids. In hydrolysis the ester bond holding the fatty acid to glycerol is broken in the presence of a facilitating enzyme, with the addition of a water molecule.

When it leaves the stomach, most fat is still in the form of large globules. Because of its low density, the fat floats on top of the chyme and is the last nutrient component to leave the stomach.

As dietary triglycerides enter the duodenum, cells of the small intestine release the hormone cholecystokinin. This substance is transported in the blood to the gall bladder, where it stimulates the release of stored bile. Bile is composed of cholesterol derivatives known as bile salts, along with water and other compounds. It is synthesized by cells in the liver and stored in the gall bladder until needed for lipid digestion. Bile, the major emulsifying agent for dietary lipids, makes it possible for digestive enzymes, which are water-soluble protein molecules, to interact with a larger surface area of the lipid particles and thus increases the effectiveness of the enzymes.

The presence of fat in the duodenum also stimulates release of *enterogastrone.* This hormone appears to regulate the rate at which fat enters the duodenum so that it will correspond with the rate of secretion of the fat-digesting enzymes from the pancreas.

Pancreatic juice, which enters the duodenum by way of the pancreatic duct, contains three enzymes that affect lipid digestion: pancreatic lipase, phospholipase, and cholesterol esterase.

Pancreatic lipase acts on long-chain triglycerides. As almost all dietary triglycerides are of this type, this enzyme is responsible for a substantial portion of lipid digestion. (Triglycerides containing medium-chain fatty acids do not usually require hydrolysis.) In the presence of pancreatic lipase, ester bonds are broken and two molecules of water are incorporated, forming a 2-monoglyceride and two fatty acids. (The 2-monoglyceride is so called because the fatty acid is attached to the second carbon of the glycerol unit.)

Similarly, *phospholipases* hydrolyze some dietary phospholipids; however, some dietary phospholipid is left intact. And *cholesterol esterase,* in the presence of bile, hydrolyzes dietary cholesterol esters, breaking them down into cholesterol and fatty acid. However, most dietary cholesterol is in the free sterol form and does not undergo digestive action at this point.

Absorption

The end products of lipid digestion are monoglycerides, fatty acids, and cholesterol; in addition, some phospholipids and short- and medium-chain triglycerides remain in essentially dietary form.

In the lumen of the small intestine, the monoglycerides, fatty acids, cholesterol, and phospholipids combine with bile to form specialized aggregates called **micelles.** Acting as an emulsifier, the bile attaches to the fatty components and enables them to become distributed through a watery medium. In this case, the digested lipids are attached to bile and suspended in the form of infinitesimal particles ready to be absorbed. In the formation of a micelle, the diameter of individual lipid particles is decreased 100 times and the surface area increased 10,000 times.

The primary site of lipid absorption is the surface of the jejunum, or middle section, of the small intestine. The intestine has an extremely large surface area because of the presence of villi or projections. Each villus contains blood vessels and a special lymph vessel called a **lacteal.**

Micellar lipids and short- and medium-chain triglycerides are absorbed directly into the mucosal cells of the jejunum by a process as yet unknown. As the lipid contents of the micelle move on their way, the bile salts are removed; they will remain in the lumen, to be reabsorbed from the ileum, or terminal portion, of the small intestine.

In the mucosal cells, several reactions take place, depending on the type of fat to be absorbed. Medium- and short-chain triglycerides are hydrolyzed by **intestinal lipase** to glycerol and short- and medium-chain fatty acids. These products, along with short- and medium-chain fatty acids that have been produced as a result of previous intestinal hydrolysis, leave the mucosal cells and enter the capillaries directly, from which they are transported by the portal vein to the liver. Fatty acids transported in the blood are bound to the protein **albumin,** which enhances their solubility.

In the meantime, long-chain fatty acids are reesterified with glycerol to produce long-chain triglycerides. Together with the cholesterol and phospholipids in the mucosa, the newly synthesized long-chain triglycerides are combined with a protein to form the lipoprotein chylomicron, a fat-rich particle which accounts for the transport of a substantial portion of dietary lipid. If a blood sample is taken a few hours after a high-fat meal has been eaten, a creamy layer will be noticed rising to the top. This layer consists of the fat-bearing chylomicrons and is a convincing demonstration indeed of their low density.

Chylomicrons enter the lymphatic system through the lacteals in the villi. Lymph vessels generally deposit their contents into the bloodstream through the thoracic duct, the pathway by which chylomicrons join the general circulation. Eventually they are carried by the hepatic artery to the liver. The liver is also the destination of the glycerol and the short- and medium-chain fatty acids which were transported directly through the capillaries and portal vein. Any excess lipid content not needed by cells in the liver will be transported to other tissues, including adipose tissue, by lipoproteins. Table 3–7 summarizes these processes.

BILE. The **enterohepatic circulation** is the mechanism by which bile becomes available for its role in lipid digestion. Bile is released from the gall bladder in response to the presence of fat at the entrance to the small intestine. Then, by means of the bile duct, it enters the duodenum, where it forms micelles with dietary lipids. As the lipid particles enter the mucosa of the jejunum, the bile salts detach from the micellar complex. Most of the bile salts are reabsorbed in the ileum, from which they enter the portal vein, which carries them back to the liver and ultimately to the gall bladder.

This enterohepatic circulation is so efficient that the relatively small total pool of bile salts, about 3 to 5 grams, is recycled many times during a day, and only a small amount (approximately 0.5 g) is lost and excreted in the feces. The lost bile salts are promptly replaced through synthesis from cholesterol, which takes place in the liver. From the liver the bile goes to the gall bladder for storage until, once again, the presence of lipid in the duodenum signals the need for its release.

DISTURBANCES OF LIPID ABSORPTION. Lipid absorption is extremely efficient, with about 95 percent of total lipid intake being absorbed. Normal adults can absorb up to as much as 300 grams of fat a day. Under certain circumstances, however, absorption is disrupted and lipids may appear in excessive amounts in the stool. This condition, known as **steatorrhea**, may be caused by any of several different factors.

In diarrhea, for example, lipids move through the intestine so rapidly that they cannot be efficiently hydrolyzed by the various enzymes. Consequently, most of the dietary fat is not absorbed and is excreted.

An obstruction of the gall bladder duct, or removal of the gall bladder itself, will decrease the amount of bile available for action in the duodenum and jejunum. After removal of the gall bladder, however, adaptive mechanisms take over. Many people who have had this operation gradually become able to tolerate normal, or nearly normal, amounts of fat in their diets. This happens because even though bile can no longer be stored, the liver synthesizes it in adequate quantity, and the bile then enters the small intestine directly from the liver.

Other causes of steatorrhea are pancreatic disease or blockage of the pancreatic duct. Decreased levels of pancreatic enzymes in the intestinal lumen will prevent adequate hydrolysis of long-chain triglycerides or cholesterol esters, and these

TABLE 3-7. *Summary of Lipid Digestion and Absorption*

Dietary Lipid	Acted on by	Digested Products	Preparation for Absorption	Absorption	In Mucosa	Product	Transport System	Destination
Long-chain triglycerides	Pancreatic lipase	2-monoglyceride + 2 fatty acids	Form micelles with bile	Absorbed into mucosa of the small intestine	Long-chain fatty acids reesterified with glycerol; all other components are unchanged	Long-chain triglycerides and other components	Combine with a protein to form chylomicrons, which first enter lymphatic system and then go into general circulation.	
Phospholipids	Pancreatic phospholipase	Fatty acids, glycerol, phosphate-containing group						
Cholesterol esters	Pancreatic cholesterol esterase	Cholesterol + fatty acid						Liver
Cholesterol								
Medium- and short-chain triglycerides				Absorbed directly into mucosa of small intestine	Hydrolyzed by intestinal lipase	Glycerol + short- and medium-chain fatty acids	Enter capillaries directly (fatty acids must first be bound to protein albumin).	

Perspective On

BODY FAT AND THE SEXES

A striking difference between the body composition of men and that of women is in the amount of fat. Whereas some 14 percent of the average man's body consists of fat, that of the average woman contains 20 to 25 percent fat. The wide range of values for normal women largely reflects variations in the fat content of certain sites, such as breasts, buttocks and hips. At birth, girls have slightly larger triceps skinfold measurements than boys. The difference increases somewhat between four and eight years of age and widens dramatically after approximately age twelve.

One hypothesis proposed to explain this sex difference is that greater fat storage in females is necessary to ensure their survival during times of severe food shortage. To achieve a high birthrate, which increases the probability of survival of the species, survival of large numbers of females is more crucial than survival of large numbers of males.

A second hypothesis holds that body fat, distributed in a certain pattern on the female body, promotes survival of the human species by sexually attracting the male. Actually, the reverse could also be the case; men may find a certain type of fat distribution attractive precisely because it is typical of the female body, and they might find any other characteristics (massive muscles, for example) attractive if women happened to possess them. This, however, is one of those hypotheses that can neither be proved nor disproved.

In the past females who stored body fat in greater quantity may have been the ones to survive periods of famine. Attainment of puberty in women may be triggered, at least in part, by a certain critical body weight. Menarche can be delayed in underfat girls. Postpubertal women may become infertile if their body fat content drops very far below the normal range. Thus models, ballet dancers, and athletes, as well as patients with anorexia nervosa, may lose their capacity to reproduce along with a large proportion of their body fat. The infertility is temporary; it is as if nature has decreed that the energy-demanding act of reproduction is best postponed in underweight women, to be resumed only after body weight increases so that fat stores are adequate to the demands of the task. As for men, the energy requirement of their role in reproduction is so slight compared with the requirements of the female's role that even the thinnest of men apparently suffer no impairment of reproductive ability because of subnormal body fat content.

lipids, which are not in a form that can be absorbed, will be excreted. For people with these and similar conditions, medium-chain triglyceride (MCT) oil with 8:0- and 10:0-chain fatty acids has been useful. Prepared by distillation from coconut oil, the short- and medium-chain fatty acids of MCT do not require hydrolysis before absorption, nor do they need to be solubilized with bile. Instead they are hydrolyzed by intestinal lipase in the mucosa and then absorbed directly into the blood vessels of the villi. Use of MCT oil, therefore, reduces the fat loss of chronic steatorrhea and the excessive energy loss that accompanies it.

Ingestion of mineral oil can also cause steatorrhea. Mineral oil is sometimes taken as a laxative or used instead of salad oil by persons on weight-loss diets. Because mineral oil does not contain any oxygen, it is not a true lipid. It cannot be digested and absorbed but merely passes through the digestive tract, accounting for its laxative action. On its way, however, it solubilizes fatty materials, including fat-soluble vitamins, and carries them along so that they cannot be absorbed. Potentially serious deficiencies of some of these substances may result from frequent ingestion of mineral oil. It is not generally advisable to use mineral oil for a laxative effect. If mineral oil is prescribed for a specific condition, it should be taken some time after eating, never during a meal.

METABOLISM OF LIPIDS

Having been digested and absorbed, lipids are now available for use by all tissues of the body, to which they are transported by lipoproteins. When the circulating lipids are needed for cell functions, an enzyme (lipoprotein lipase, which is bound to capillary and cell membranes) releases the lipid portion from its protein carrier and hydrolyzes the constituent triglyceride into glycerol and fatty acids. These molecules then enter cells for further utilization.

The metabolic needs of the organism determine the particular metabolic process that will take place. Fat breakdown, or **lipolysis**, and fat synthesis, or **lipogenesis**, are the dynamic processes of lipid metabolism. These processes are not merely the reverse of each other; each involves different pathways, reactants, and enzymes. Before examining these processes in detail, we will consider the functions of the liver and of adipose tissue, the primary regulators of lipid metabolism.

Role of the Liver

The cells of the liver constitute a complex internal biochemistry laboratory, where a number of different processes occur as they are needed. The body's requirements are signalled by hormones and enzymes that regulate the lipid metabolic processes.

Within the liver, fatty acids are synthesized by lipogenesis into new triglycerides. These are normally transported out of the liver by the lipoproteins, especially the VLDLs, which carry them to adipose tissue for storage until otherwise needed. Lipogenesis and subsequent transport are triggered by lipotropic (from Greek *tropos*, turning or changing) factors such as choline and methionine, thereby preventing excessive accumulation of fat in the liver. Carbohydrates (as well as lipids) also provide the raw materials for lipogenesis. Fatty acids and glycerol synthesized from carbohydrates follow the same pathway as the triglycerides synthesized directly from digested lipid. This process is the reason excess intake of kilocalories from carbohydrate adds to our fat reserves.

Also in the liver, long-chain fatty acids are made even longer and are desaturated, which transforms them into different fatty acids. For example, stearic acid (18:0) becomes oleic acid (18:1), and linoleic acid (18:2) becomes arachidonic acid (20:4).

But lipolysis is also occurring in the liver at the same time, as triglycerides are hydrolyzed to form fatty acids and glycerol. The triglyceride reactions are reversible and occur in response to the needs of the organism at a particular time. If there is an oversupply of lipid in the liver, lipogenesis will convert it into a form for transport and storage. If the energy needs of the organism require available lipid, on the other hand, lipolysis will occur to produce accessible lipid products for circulation. Triglycerides, then, can be hydrolyzed and resynthesized, used for energy, or used in the synthesis of other lipids, such as phospholipids and cholesterol.

In the liver, cholesterol is synthesized from 2-carbon fragments of acetyl CoA. The liver also removes cholesterol from the circulation. Cholesterol from both sources is converted to bile acids, which enter the gall bladder for storage as a component of bile.

Role of Adipose Tissue

Adipose tissue, which serves as a reservoir of stored energy, is located not only under the skin but also in the abdominal cavity and within muscle tissue. Lipids are stored primarily in the form of triglycerides. Contrary to popular belief, adipose tissue doesn't just "sit" there; it is metabolically active. Fat cells (**adipocytes**) contain both lipogenic and lipolytic enzymes. When energy intake equals energy output, enzymes and processes are in equilibrium. However, when energy intake exceeds output, lipogenesis (facilitated by the hormone insulin) predominates, and triglycerides are synthesized from fatty acids and glycerol.

When energy is in demand, the reverse process takes place. The stored triglycerides are hydrolyzed, releasing **free fatty acids (FFA)** from adipose tissue into the bloodstream. Bound to albumin, the FFA travel to other tissues to provide energy.

At any one time, the amount of FFA circulating in the plasma is normally very low, accounting for only about 5 percent of total blood lipids. The contribution of circulating FFA to energy production, however, is high. Many cells of the body, particularly muscle, preferentially use fatty acids as a source of energy, and their rapid flux throughout the circulation is vital. FFAs are a dynamic pool of potential energy and can be removed from the blood within minutes.

Several hormones influence the hydrolysis of triglycerides and the rate of release of FFA from adipose tissue—epinephrine, growth hormone, and glucagon among others. The various enzymes that catalyze lipolysis—lipases—are sensitive to these hormones and are triggered by them to catalyze the process of lipolysis in the adipocytes. Each hormone is released in response to specific metabolic conditions—stress or hypoglycemia, for example—but the net effect is to mobilize stored energy.

When there is no dietary energy source, adipose tissue is stimulated by hormones to release more fatty acids. As might be expected, blood levels of FFA will be higher during fasting than following a meal.

Biochemistry of Lipid Metabolism

We have discussed the regulatory role of the liver and of adipose tissue in fat metabolism. We will now examine these processes in greater detail from a biochemical point of view.

FATTY ACID SYNTHESIS. Fatty acids are synthesized in a complex process that requires the presence of two B vitamins, involves energy in the form of adenosine triphosphate (ATP), and uses a CO_2-containing compound, malonyl CoA. This series of reactions requires the presence of several different enzymes and several coenzymes and cannot proceed if any of these are absent. It can be thought of as a kind of molecular assembly line for the orderly building up of fatty-acid chains. Acetic acid (CH_3COOH), which is a breakdown product of nutrient metabolism, is the primary raw material, and the 16-carbon fatty acid, palmitic acid, is a major end product.

TRIGLYCERIDE SYNTHESIS. In triglyceride synthesis, fatty acids are combined or **esterified** with a glycerol molecule. The fatty acids that react with this glycerol molecule may be newly synthesized, or they may have resulted from earlier triglyceride breakdown (hydrolysis). Three fatty acids react with glycerol to form a triglyceride; two fatty acids and a phosphate-choline group react with glycerol to produce phospholipids.

β-OXIDATION. The process by which fatty acids are broken down is known as β-oxidation (beta-oxidation). Coenzyme A is a key participant in this reaction, first activating and then aiding in the oxidation of the fatty acids. A number of other enzymes and cofactors are involved as well. During each step in the process, the enzymes remove a 2-carbon fragment (acetyl CoA) from the fatty acid, leaving the fatty acid two carbons shorter. The process is repeated until complete. Thus, after seven turns of the cycle in the case of palmitic acid, eight molecules of acetyl CoA have been produced. In this manner, the complete oxidation of a fatty acid is achieved.

Acetyl CoA condenses with oxaloacetate in the Krebs cycle; ultimately, mediated by the electron transport system, the end products are CO_2, H_2O, and ATP. (The interrelationship of these several biochemical processes is shown in Figure 3–6, page 76.)

Energy production from lipids is significantly higher than that from glucose; one molecule of glucose yields 38 molecules of ATP, whereas one molecule of palmitic acid produces 129 molecules of ATP. Even 3 molecules of glucose (which contain 18 carbons, the same number as in stearic acid) yield only 114 molecules of high-energy phosphates, whereas stearic acid yields 146.

Even those fatty acids having an odd number of carbon atoms can be metabolized by β-oxidation, releasing acetyl CoA and finally a single 3-carbon molecule of propionic acid. Propionic acid can also produce energy through a reaction that depends on the presence of vitamin B_{12}. This reaction converts the 3-carbon molecule to an intermediate of the Krebs cycle, succinyl CoA. Here, then, is yet another route of energy production.

In addition to providing energy, the acetyl CoA produced by oxidation can also be utilized as the immediate source of malonyl CoA required for the synthesis of fatty acids, or it can be used for synthesis of cholesterol and other important compounds.

The entire set of interactions is extremely efficient, and no component of a compound goes to waste. The glycerol unit released during the hydrolysis of triglycerides can enter the Embden-Myerhof pathway and be metabolized to **pyruvate.**

Glycerol can also be converted to glucose. The synthesis of glucose from a precursor of noncarbohydrate origin is called **gluconeogenesis.** Glycerol, although not a major contributor to gluconeogenesis (because only a small part of the triglyceride molecule is glycerol), should not be overlooked as a contributing factor in the elevation of blood glucose levels. Fatty acids, unlike glycerol, are not gluconeogenic; that is, they cannot be converted to glucose (see caption, Figure 3–6).

The cells of adipose tissue, adipocytes, are metabolically active; within these cells, lipogenesis and lipolysis occur in dynamic equilibrium. It is also important to remember that fat can be synthesized from carbohydrates; fatty acids are synthesized from acetyl CoA, which is a product of glucose metabolism as well as of lipid metabolism. When the energy needs of the body have been met, the remaining acetyl CoA is converted to fatty acids and esterified with glycerol to produce a triglyceride. In this form, it can be stored in the adipose tissue. This set of processes occurs in a positive energy state—that is, when the supply of energy exceeds the demand for it.

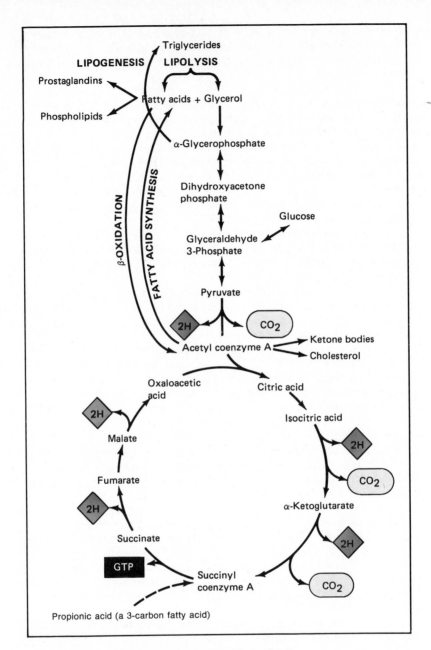

FIGURE 3-6   *Lipid Metabolism and the Krebs Cycle.*
Note that the conversion of pyruvate to acetyl CoA is irreversible; this makes it impossible to produce glucose from fatty acids, although fatty acids can be produced from glucose.

KETONE BODIES.   Most cells of the body can utilize free fatty acids for energy production. Until recently, brain cells were thought not to metabolize anything other than glucose to meet their energy needs. Now it is known that brain cells can, after a period of adaptation, convert the so-called **ketone bodies** to ATP. The ketone bodies are three derivatives of fatty acids, produced when there is an excessive rate of fatty acid breakdown in the body. In the absence of carbohydrate, as in starvation or high-protein weight-reduction diets, there will be an imbalance between lipogenesis and lipolysis in adipose tissue, with the release of excess fatty acids into the blood. Some of these fatty acids are used for energy production, but some are oxidized only partially to the ketone bodies.

The condensation of two molecules of acetyl CoA results in the formation of acetoacetate or β-hydroxybutyrate, two of the ketone bodies. The third is acetone, resulting from the decarboxylation of acetoacetate. The reasons for this incomplete oxidation are not definitely known; the diminished supply of oxaloacetate in starvation may cause a "slowdown" of the Krebs cycle.

The liver cannot utilize ketone bodies for energy because it does not have specific enzymes to do so. Normally, the body's small supply of ketones, primarily acetoacetate, is transported to skeletal and cardiac muscle. These cells produce enzymes that facilitate the oxidation of acetoacetate, providing a minor energy source for these tissues. The normal concentration of ketones in the blood is less than 2 mg/dl. When ketones are produced in excess of the capacity of the heart and skeletal muscles to oxidize them, they remain in the circulatory system, causing an increase in the level of plasma ketones.

Excessive accumulation of ketone bodies, a reflection of an imbalance between their production and utilization, is known as **ketosis**. Starvation and diabetes mellitus can produce ketosis; the lack of insulin prevents carbohydrate oxidation, and elevated ketone production is a result. Excessive levels of ketones in the blood (ketonemia) and in the urine (ketonuria) are measurable symptoms of a disturbance of carbohydrate metabolism and/or excessive lipolysis.

CHOLESTEROL METABOLISM.   Cholesterol is synthesized primarily by the cells of the liver, intestine, and adrenal glands, although all cells have the capacity to produce this sterol. Through a complicated series of reactions, the simple 2-carbon fragment, acetyl CoA, is converted to 1 or 2 grams of cholesterol daily (see Figure 3–4). In the body, endogenous (synthesized) and exogenous (dietary) cholesterol are indistinguishable.

Cholesterol is needed for the synthesis of steroid hormones, bile salts, and vitamin D—all vital substances. It is transported between tissues bound to lipoproteins, primarily the chylomicrons and LDLs. The precise requirement of the body for cholesterol is not known, but scientists agree that even the small amount produced by the body is greater than the need. Unneeded cholesterol is eliminated in the feces, about half of it in the form of bile salts and the remainder as neutral steroids. Some individuals may have substantial amounts of cholesterol in their circulation, however. Elevated levels of cholesterol in the blood have been linked with atherosclerosis and heart disease.

PHOSPHOLIPID METABOLISM.   Phospholipids are constituents of cell membranes throughout the body and play a role in cholesterol synthesis. Because of their emulsifying properties, they act as carriers of fatty acids in the blood. All cells contain phospholipids, but the cells of such metabolically active tissues as the brain, liver, and nerve tissue have particularly high concentrations. Although some phospholipids are present in the diet, the body is capable of synthesizing them in adequate amounts, and they are not considered essential in a nutritional sense. The lecithins, the most widely distributed phospholipids, are synthesized in the liver.

Phospholipids are transported primarily by HDLs. The interrelationships of the tissues involved in lipid metabolism are summarized in Figure 3–7.

ESSENTIAL FATTY ACIDS. At this time, linoleic acid is considered to be the only true essential fatty acid (EFA), since the others can be synthesized from it. Its absence from the diet produces several symptoms in both laboratory animals and humans, including skin lesions, growth retardation, liver and kidney degeneration, and increased susceptibility to infection. Adults usually have adequate stores of linoleic acid in adipose tissue. Symptoms, particularly eczema, were identified in in-

FIGURE 3-7   *Interrelationships of Body Tissues in Lipid Metabolism.*

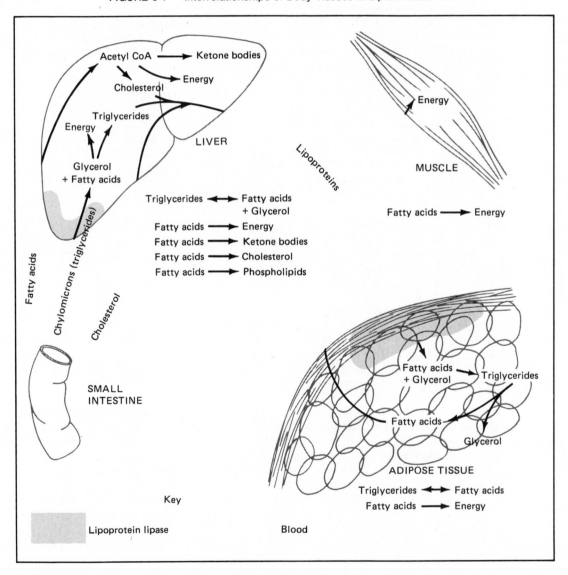

fants and in adults who received long-term, fat-free intravenous feedings at a time when lipid could not be added to the feeding for technical reasons. Infants maintained on skim milk for long periods of time have also displayed symptoms of EFA deficiency. These deficiencies are easily corrected by ingestion of small amounts of linoleic acid.

The biochemical reasons for these deficiency symptoms are still being investigated, but it is believed that EFA plays a role in the regulation of cholesterol metabolism, transport, and excretion, acting to lower blood cholesterol levels, although the fate of the removed cholesterol is unclear. In addition, as components of phospholipid molecules, EFA constitutes an important part of all cell membranes. A major role for linoleic acid is its conversion to arachidonic acid (20:4), the key molecule in the pathway leading to formation of leukotrienes, prostaglandins, and thromboxanes. LTs, PGs, and TXAs may play a role in atherogenesis by affecting platelet stickiness, blood fluidity, and endothelial growth. EPA also plays a role, apparently by determining which forms of PGs and TBAs are synthesized.

Functions of Fat in the Body

The importance of fat derives from its structural role as a component of cell membranes and its functional roles as a source of energy and a factor in the synthesis of cholesterol and its derivatives as well as of lipids, prostaglandins, and other body substances. In addition, body fat, in the form of adipose tissue, serves two other important needs. First, it acts as an insulator to help to maintain body temperature at an appropriate level by conserving heat when the external temperature is low. (The insulating effect of fat in persons with an overabundance of subcutaneous adipose tissue is well known and can present a problem in hot weather.) Second, fat deposits act as a protective cushion surrounding the kidneys, heart, and other vital organs.

Because of their important roles in the maintenance of health and well-being, dietary fats should not be avoided. They are necessary for many vital body functions, contribute energy, and add to the flavor and aroma of our foods, as well as to our feelings of satisfaction after dining.

DIETARY REQUIREMENTS

The Food and Nutrition Board has not established a Recommended Dietary Allowance for fat but suggests that adequate lipid be ingested to provide the body with essential fatty acids and carriers of fat-soluble vitamins. It has been estimated that ingesting between 15 and 25 grams of fat per day will normally meet this requirement. Studies with both animals and human subjects indicate that the requirement for EFA is fulfilled when 1 to 2 percent of the total caloric intake is provided by linoleic acid. A diet of 1,800 calories per day should provide 2 to 4 grams of linoleic acid. This is readily accomplished; many vegetable oils used in cooking and salad dressings are good sources of this essential nutrient. A single tablespoon of mayonnaise or any of several oils will more than meet the requirement of most people (see Table 3–8). In addition, foods other than oils—eggs, milk, whole grains, and many others—contain small amounts of EFA.

TABLE 3-8. *Sources of Linoleic Acid (EFA)*

	Linoleic Acid g/tbsp
Safflower oil	10
Corn, soy, and cottonseed oil	6–8
Mayonnaise	6
Peanut oil	5
Margarine	1–5
Olive oil	1

Fats in the American Diet

Since the beginning of this century, consumption of fats by Americans has been increasing (see Table 3–9). The nearly 30 percent rise in our national fat intake since 1910 is largely attributable to three categories: edible fats and oils, ice cream, and red meat. During this period, consumption of certain kinds of fats—cooking fats such as lard and shortening combined—remained about the same, while the consumption of butter and margarine combined actually declined.

Edible fats are found in almost every supermarket aisle, bottled as cooking oil and salad dressing or less obvious in such foods as "all natural" health cereals, frozen pizzas, and cake mixes. Edible fats and oils are also consumed as fast foods, most of which are deep fried. The caloric content of even low-fat meats is increased by frying. Thanks to refrigerated transport and commercial freezers, ice cream is available everywhere.

The increase in consumption of high-fat foods of animal origin such as meat results from economic prosperity. For reasons of status as well as taste, more high-fat animal foods seem to be preferred over less-expensive high-carbohydrate, plant-origin foods. Fat consumption generally increases when there is more money to be spent on food. This trend has been tempered somewhat in recent years by the increased awareness of the role of diet in health and the desire to reduce caloric intake. Consumption of beef has decreased slightly, about 10 pounds per person per year in the last 15 years. Consumption of chicken has increased rapidly and consumption of fish has increased modestly over the past ten years, reflecting the desire by many Americans to decrease fat consumption.

Cultural dietary patterns determine which fat is used within a people's cuisine and how much: Japanese foods are prepared with far less fat than are, for example, the foods of Mediterranean peoples. (National dietary patterns are, of course, directly related to the availability of certain food items as well as to cultural preferences.) Many Americans are using low-fat ethnic foods in their diets and many tra-

TABLE 3-9. *Average Fatty Acid Intake of Americans (g/day)*

	Saturated	Oleic	Linoleic
1909–13	49.8	50.3	9.0
1947–49	54.4	57.5	13.6
1967–69	57.0	63.4	19.7
1982	54.1	64.5	25.5

Adapted from R.M. Marston and S.O. Welsh. Nutrient Content of the U.S. Food Supply, 1982. *National Food Review* (USDA Economic Res Serv) Winter 25:7, 1984.

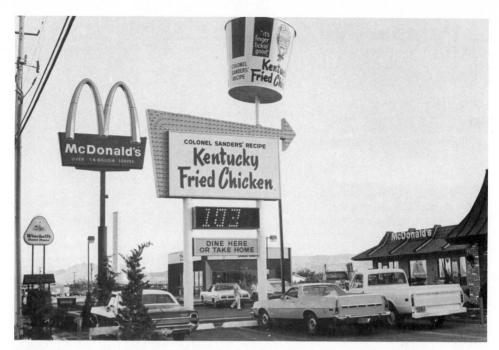

Many convenience and fast foods are notably higher in fat content than foods prepared "from scratch." Their use is generally associated with decreased consumption of whole grains and vegetables.

Van Bucher/Photo Researchers, Inc.

ditionally "rich and heavy" cuisines have now been adapted to reduce the number of calories.

Consumption of saturated fatty acids has dropped from a peak of 57.0 grams per person per day to 54.1 grams in 1982. Meanwhile, the use of vegetable fats has increased. This shift is partially related to the idea that vegetable fats are "better for you" than animal fats. Recently, fats have been assigned "good" reputations if they have a high proportion of PUFAs, and vegetable fats generally fall into this category. Exceptions are nuts and olives, which contain high levels of monounsaturated fatty acids rather than PUFAs. Also, many margarines have been partially hydrogenated for firmness and palatability, a process that lowers their PUFA content.

Diet and Health

The public has been made aware of studies linking fat consumption to heart disease, some types of cancer, and obesity. Many authoritative sources, including the American Heart Association, recommend that the current American pattern of fat consumption be altered. The 1985 Dietary Guidelines suggest "avoid too much fat, saturated fats and cholesterol." Some authorities suggest that dietary cholesterol intake should not exceed 300 milligrams daily. Many nutritionists believe, however, that this level is unrealistically and unnecessarily low for the general population.

Since the possible linkage between cholesterol and heart disease was first an-

Perspective On

DIET AND HEART DISEASE

Coronary heart disease (CHD) is a leading cause of death in affluent countries. Until menopause, women are at substantially less risk than men; in later middle age, however, women are increasingly susceptible. Epidemiological studies showing that CHD is less prevalent in some cultures than in the United States has led to considerable hypothesizing regarding the role of environmental factors such as diet. Despite extensive research, however, the subject remains controversial, with relationships suggested but not proved.

Atherosclerosis, which leads ultimately to CHD, develops from the accumulation of fatty deposits in the inner walls of the arteries. As fat deposits increase, they become surrounded by smooth muscle and connective tissue (fibrous plaques and other lesions). In this process (popularly called *hardening of the arteries*), the arterial passages become narrowed, putting great stress on the heart, which must work harder to accomplish less. In severe cases, the arterial lumen can suddenly close (occlude), resulting in a sharp decrease in blood circulation to tissues (ischemia), which causes the heart or the brain to cease functioning. The clinical names for these events are *myocardial infarction*, when heart vessels are affected, and *stroke* (or *cerebrovascular accident*), when the brain is involved.

In 1949 the U.S. Public Health Service began a large-scale study, the Epidemiologic Investigation of Cardiovascular Diseases in Framingham, Massachusetts. More than 5,000 healthy men and women aged 30 to 62 were examined every other year for evidence of CHD and other atherosclerotic conditions. Among the results was the identification of risk factors. A *risk factor* increases the probability of an event but does not predict that the event will occur. For example, it was found that men who were overweight had a higher incidence of CHD; those whose life styles included extensive physical activity had a lower incidence. Elevated levels of serum cholesterol were found consistently in association with other high-risk factors.

DIETARY FACTORS IN CHD. The Framingham study indicated that persons with serum cholesterol levels in excess of 225 mg/dl are at risk of developing CHD and that at higher levels, the risk increases markedly. Typically, Americans ingest 600 to 900 mg of cholesterol per day. It has been shown that there will be a predictable elevation of serum cholesterol levels if the intake of cholesterol is increased from 0 to 400 mg, but cholesterol intakes in larger amounts raise serum cholesterol levels higher in some individuals than in others. These studies indicate the importance of factors other than diet in determining serum cholesterol levels; for example, men's serum cholesterol increased sharply with weight gains of 7 percent or more.

Some data suggest that the high dietary cholesterol intake of westernized peoples is related both to high serum cholesterol levels and to high CHD rates. There are, however, exceptions to the high-intake high-serum level rule. Among some African groups, for example, the diet of meat and milk is as cholesterol-rich as that of any American, yet these people have virtually no CHD. Possible explanations include a high-fiber diet, more physical activity than most Americans have, and a genetic factor.

Serum cholesterol levels seem to be sensitive not only to cholesterol intake but to other components of lipid intake and metabolism as well. Saturated fat raises the level of plasma cholesterol, monounsaturated fat has no significant effect, and PUFA actually lowers blood cholesterol levels. When serum cholesterol is lowered by PUFAs, we do not know whether excess cholesterol has been excreted from the body or has shifted from the blood into tissues. The mechanisms for these observations have not yet been explained. Other nutrients may also have an effect on the development of CHD. Mineral imbalances, have also been implicated. A number of studies suggest that reductions in animal protein intake with substitution of vegetable protein result in lower serum cholesterol.

Other studies suggest that the form in which cholesterol is carried in the blood may influence the appearance of CHD. It has been observed that the level of cholesterol carried by HDLs (as opposed to other lipoproteins) is inversely related to the prevalence of CHD. Nonsmokers, people who are physically fit, and those who are not obese appear to have more HDL cholesterol than do smokers, the obese, and inactive people.

OTHER FACTORS. Nondiet factors that have been associated with CHD include genetic predisposition; hypertension; such aspects of life style as cigarette smoking, stress, and lack of exercise; the use of oral contraceptives; diabetes; obesity; and psychological factors.

Most cases of hypertension or high blood pressure have no known cause, although heredity and obesity apparently predispose people to it. Persons who are aware of being genetically predisposed and those in whom hypertension has been diagnosed should certainly decrease consumption of salt; those who are overweight would be well advised to reduce their weight and their salt intake.

It has been suggested that there is a psychological component in hypertension and CHD. In particular, persons who exhibit "type A" behavior patterns—competitive, overachieving, always-on-the-go types—are said to be more prone to heart attacks, the calmer "type B" personality being less so. The role of stress is often cited by those who claim that it characterizes Western civilization but is lacking in the lives of nonurbanized peoples. Others claim that not stress itself, but our pattern of reacting to it, is the real culprit.

Another factor often cited in CHD is the sedentary life led by most Americans in contrast to the greater physical activity of people. The Framingham results indicate that men who are least active physically have three times the risk of developing CHD as those who are most active. Exercise and physical activity may operate in a number of ways. First, those who are physically active are not likely to be obese. Second, there is evidence that the effect of exercise comes from its stimulation of the circulatory mechanism— the heart and lungs operate, it is claimed, more efficiently in a well-exercised body. There is no indication that exercise alone reduces serum cholesterol.

Cigarette smoking is clearly associated with increased risk of CHD for both men and women.

Smoking, moreover, has a synergistic effect, multiplying the influence of any other risk factor present. With only one other risk factor, smoking one pack of cigarettes per day nearly doubles the risk for men; with two or more other risk factors, cigarette smoking increases the risk by almost a third. The combinations of smoking and hypertension, or smoking and oral contraceptive use for women, are particularly dangerous; these risks can, however, be readily controlled. Coffee and moderate alcohol, both often indicted, have no significant effect.

THE DIET-CHOLESTEROL CONTROVERSY. Of all possible factors in the onset of CHD, the relationship of dietary cholesterol to serum cholesterol has most captured public attention. Sensing a sizable market, the food industry has developed cholesterol-free egg substitutes, as well as other no-cholesterol, low-saturated-fat products, such as cream and sausage substitutes. Whether or not diet can have a significant effect on serum cholesterol and whether or not a change in serum levels can affect CHD incidence and mortality are highly controversial issues.

Hundreds of studies have been done to demonstrate the effects of modifying lipid intake. Often cited are studies of vegetarians, whose levels of serum cholesterol and triglycerides are lower than those of control subjects. Reduced animal fat consumption is only one of several possible factors in the lower serum cholesterol levels. Others include total energy consumption, recent weight loss, and higher intake of vegetable protein, complex carbohydrate, and dietary fiber, which have all been advocated as cholesterol-lowering agents.

Determining the precise role of cholesterol in CHD is obviously complex. A study of the Tarahumara Indians of Mexico points up the dilemma. This population group has a low incidence of CHD, very low serum cholesterol levels, and moderate triglyceride levels. Their diet is low in cholesterol, low in total fat, and low in saturated fat. The Tarahumara also have low sugar intake, high fiber intake, and high vegetable-protein intake. They are in exceptionally good physical condition, have virtually no obesity, have low blood pressure, and are genetically fairly homogeneous. The Tarahumara, then, add little that is new to the diet-heart controversy, since no single dietary (or other) factor can be isolated to account for their low rate of CHD. In fact, this example serves to emphasize the many factors involved in atherosclerosis and heart disease.

RECOMMENDATIONS. Despite all the uncertainties, it would be advisable to reduce or eliminate as many risk factors as possible from our lives. (Factors such as age, sex, and heredity are, of course, beyond our control!) Total fat intake should be decreased to between 30 and 35 percent of total energy intake. Fat should come from a variety of sources to include omega-3 fatty acids. Overweight individuals should achieve appropriate weight. We should also, particularly if there is a family history of hypertension, reduce intake of sodium, especially table salt and increase calcium. We should try to change our patterns of reaction to stress, increase physical exercise in moderation, ingest more dietary fiber, and stop smoking. Moderation is probably the best answer.

Our expectations of results from such measures should not be unrealistic. Even a reduction in dietary cholesterol that succeeds in decreasing serum cholesterol is no guarantee against a stroke or heart attack. Because heart disease usually develops in the later years of life, it is possible that no matter how many adjustments in living and eating habits are made, the predisposition to CHD is determined by factors of earlier years.

To make such changes in eating habits, it is necessary to know the nutrient content of the foods we eat. Some manufacturers are labeling their products to indicate the amount and kinds of fat per serving; some list cholesterol, saturated fat, and PUFA content. But even where detailed labeling is absent, a consumer can be adequately informed. Because ingredients must be listed in descending order of their content in the product, labels listing liquid corn oil, for example, as a first ingredient will be relatively high in polyunsaturates, whereas "partially hydrogenated soybean oil" indicates less PUFA content, and coconut oil, of course, is largely saturated.

Other sources of information include the American Heart Association, which offers data relating to the fat content of various foods as well as specific suggestions for modifying dietary fat intake. Nutritionists in community health clinics can also provide information. Many food companies have consumer relations departments that will provide information about specific products as well.

In view of our present knowledge there is certainly no disadvantage to following the dietary recommendations, and there may be important advantages.

nounced in the 1950s, consumption of eggs, including eggs used in processed foods such as mayonnaise and cake mixes, has dropped sharply, from a high of 403 per person in 1945 to a low of 252 in 1984. Similarly, consumption of butter, implicated because of its saturated fat content, also decreased. Beef consumption, as noted above, increased until recently. Effecting the dietary changes—reducing overall lipid intake and shifting to polyunsaturates—called for by the American Heart Association and the USDA is not difficult. Use of olive and corn oils in salad dressings and cooking, substitution of margarine, especially highly unsaturated varieties, for butter; broiling or baking instead of sautéing or deep frying; more frequent servings of vegetarian, poultry, and fish as main courses; drinking skim instead of whole milk and eating ice milk in preference to ice cream—all can be easily accomplished by those who wish to modify their fat intake, either to lose or maintain weight or as part of a preventive or therapeutic program to reduce serum cholesterol.

SUMMARY

The most controversial of the major nutrients, lipids have important body functions which are often overlooked. American consumption of fats has increased by more than a third since the beginning of the century, and 42 percent of daily caloric intake, on the average, is derived from fats.

At the molecular level, lipids consist of carbon, hydrogen, and oxygen in proportions that differ from those of other nutrients. Some lipids also contain nitrogen and phosphorus. Lipid molecules are relatively insoluble in water and can be dissolved only in organic solvents. Some dietary lipids (fats) are solid at room temperatures and some are liquid (oils). A useful classification of lipids depends on their proportion in the human body. Major constituents include fatty acids, several fatty acid derivatives, and sterols and sterol derivatives. Minor constituents include the fat-soluble vitamins A, D, E, and K, the hormonelike prostaglandins, and leukotrienes.

The basic structural unit of most lipid molecules is a fatty acid, a chain of hydrocarbons with an acid (carboxyl) group at one end. In a saturated fatty acid, every carbon atom is joined by a single electrochemical bond to each of two hydrogen and two other carbon atoms. In unsaturated fatty acids, some carbon atoms are joined to only one hydrogen atom, and by a double bond, to one adjacent carbon atom. A fatty acid with one double bond is monounsaturated; with two or more, it is polyunsaturated.

Triglycerides are formed by reaction between the carboxyl groups of three fatty acids and the three alcohol (—OH) groups of glycerol. Phospholipids are formed in the same way, except that a phosphate-containing group becomes attached to one of the three alcohol groups; lecithin is an important phospholipid.

Sterols, of which cholesterol is the most important, are fat-soluble alcohols. Although high levels of cholesterol in the blood serum have been implicated in the etiology of atherosclerosis and coronary heart disease, cholesterol is an important body substance, which is created by the body daily.

The body's sources of fat are both exogenous (dietary) and endogenous (synthesized within the body), and the supply is often far in excess of need. Of all lipids, only linoleic acid cannot be synthesized; when it is not supplied in the diet, deficiency symptoms occur. For this reason linoleic acid is an essential fatty acid (EFA), necessary for growth and health. Whether omega-3 fatty acids need to be supplied in the diet has yet to be demonstrated.

Among the functions of dietary fat are its contribution to the palatability of food and to our feelings of satiety for several hours after we have eaten. The primary function of fat, however, is to provide a concentrated source of energy. In addition, fat makes possible the transport and utilization of the fat-soluble vitamins.

Virtually all lipid digestion and absorption takes place in the small intestine. Most digested lipid enters the lymphatic and subsequently the blood circulation and ultimately goes to the liver, which uses each lipid for a different process and prepares the excess for storage in adipose tissue.

The various kinds of fats are transported in the body by one or another of the four lipoproteins. Lipids become attached to emulsifiers, molecules with water-soluble and lipid-soluble components, which enable them to mix with body fluids. Bile, produced by the liver and stored in the gall bladder, is a key emulsifier, necessary for lipid digestion.

High concentrations of cholesterol in the blood have been found in association with coronary heart disease. The precise relationship between dietary fat and the development of CHD is still not clear and has generated a great deal of controversy, but there is sufficient evidence to warrant a modified dietary approach in the management and prevention of CHD processes. But diet alone is not the answer. Many risk factors have been linked to CHD. General recommendations include stopping smoking, reduction of stress, weight loss, higher fiber intake, and more exercise, in addition to lower cholesterol and higher polyunsaturated fat intake. Americans have been urged to reduce fat consumption to about 30 percent of daily energy intake.

BIBLIOGRAPHY

ADAM, O., AND G. WOLFRAM. Effect of different linoleic acid intakes on prostaglandin biosynthesis and kidney function in man. *American Journal of Clinical Nutrition* 40:763–770, 1984.

American Health Foundation. E.L. Wynder, Conference Chairman. *Plasma Lipids: Optimal Levels for Health.* New York: Academic Press, 1980.

ANDERSON, D.B., AND B.J. HOLUB. Dietary cholesterol and the synthesis of hepatic glycerides. *Lipids* 20:167–172, 1985.

BEYNEN, A.C., AND M.B. KATAN. Why do polyunsaturated fatty acids lower serum cholesterol? *American Journal of Clinical Nutrition* 42:560–563, 1985.

BRIGGS, G.M. Muscle foods and human health. *Food Technology* 39:54–57, 1985.

BROWN, M.S., P.T. KOVANEN, J.L. GOLDSTEIN. Regulation of plasma cholesterol by lipoprotein receptors. *Science* 212:628–635 1981.

BURR, G.O., AND M.M. BURR. A new deficiency disease produced by the rigid exclusion of fats from the diet. *Journal of Biological Chemistry* 82:345, 1929.

CALDWELL, M.H., T. JONSSON, AND H.B. OTHERSEN, JR. Essential fatty acid deficiency in an infant receiving prolonged parenteral alimentation. *Journal of Pediatrics* 81:894, 1972.

Consumer Reports. Cooking fats and oils. June, 1985: pp. 364–367.

CONNER, W.E., M.T. CERQUEIRA, R.W. CONNER, R.B. WALLANCE, M.R. MALINOW, AND H.R. CASDORPH. The plasma lipids, lipiproteins, and the diet of the Tarahumara Indians of Mexico. *American Journal of Clinical Nutrition* 31: 1131, 1978.

Diet for children with hyperlipidemia—A.H.A. recommendation. *Journal of the American Dietetic Association* Vol. 72:394, 1978.

DIETSCHY, J.M. Regulation of cholesterol metabolism in man and in other species. *Klinische Wochenschrift* 62:338–345, 1984.

DYERBERG, J. Dietary manipulation of prostaglandin synthesis: Beneficial or detrimental. In *Cardiovascular Pharmacology of the Prostaglandins*, A.G. Herman, P.M. Vanhoutte, H. Denolin, and A. Goossens, eds. New York: Raven Press, 1982, pp. 233–244.

DYERBERG, J. Linolenate-derived polyunsaturated fatty acids and prevention of atherosclerosis. *Nutrition Reviews* 44:125–134, 1985.

EISENBERG, S. Plasma lipoprotein conversions: the origin of low density and high density lipoproteins. *Annual N.Y. Academy of Sciences* 348:30–44 1980.

Food and Nutrition Board, National Academy of Sciences. *Recommended Dietary Alowances.*, 9 ed. Washington, DC: National Academy of Science, 1980.

GALLI, C., E. AGRADI, A. PETRONI, AND A. SOCINI. Modulation of prostaglandin production in tissues by dietary essential fatty acids. *Acta Med. Scandinavica* (Suppl.) 642:171–179, 1980.

GALTON, D.J., AND S. WALLIS. The regulation of adipose cell metabolism. *Proc. Nutr. Soc.* 41:167–173, 1982.

HENNEKENS, C.H., M.E. DROLETTE, M.J. JESSE, J.E. DAVIES, AND G.B. HUTCHINSON. Coffee drinking and death due to coronary heart disease. *New England Journal of Medicine* 294;633, 1976.

HEROLD, P.M., AND J.E. KINSELLA. Fish oil consumption and decreased risk of cardiovascular disease: A comparison of findings from animal and human feeding trails. *American Journal of Clinical Nutrition* 43:566–598, 1986.

JENKINS, C.D. Recent evidence supporting psychological and social risk factors of coronary disease. *New England Journal of Medicine* 294:987, 1033, 1976.

KEYS A. Serum cholesterol response to dietary cholesterol. *American Journal of Clinical Nutrition* 40:351–359, 1984.

KINSELLA, J.E. Food components with potential therapeutic benefits: The n-3 polyunsaturated fatty acids of fish oils. *Food Technology* 40:89, 1986.

KLEVAY, L.M. Coronary heart disease—The zinc/copper hypothesis. *American Journal of Clinical Nutrition* 28:764, 1975.

KOHRS, M.B., C. KAPICA-CYBORSKI, AND D. CZAJKA-NARINS. Iron and chromium nutriture in the elderly. *Annual Conference on Trace Substances in Environmental Health*, D. Hemphill, ed., XVIII, University of Missouri, 1984.

KROMHOUT, D., E.B. BOSSCHIETER, AND C.L. COUNLANDER. The inverse relation between fish consumption and 2-year mortality from coronary heart disease. *New England Journal of Medicine* 312:1205, 1985.

LEFEVRE, M., C.L. KEEN, B. LONNERDAL, L.S. HURLEY, AND B.O. SCHNEEMAN. Different effects of zinc and copper deficiency in composition of plasma high density lipoproteins in rats. *Journal of Nutrition* 115:359, 1985.

McCay, P.B. Physiological significance of lipid peroxidation. *Federation Proceedings* 40:173, 1981.

Mann, G.V. Coronary heart disease—doing the wrong things. *Nutrition Today,* July/August, 1985, pp. 12–14.

Mattson, F.H., and R.J. Jandacek. The effect of a non-absorbable fat on the turnover of plasma cholesterol in the rat. *Lipids* 20:273–277, 1985.

National Institutes of Health. Consensus Development Conference Statement: Lowering blood cholesterol. *Nutrition Today* 20:13–16, 1985.

Nichols, A.B., C. Rarencroft, and D.E. Lamphiear. Daily nutritional intake and serum lipid levels: The Tecumseh study. *American Journal of Clinical Nutrition* 29:1384, 1976.

Oliver, M.F. Serum cholesterol—The knave of hearts and the joker. *Lancet* 2:1090–1095, 1981.

Ostrander, J., C. Martinsen, J. McCullough, and M. Childs. Egg substitutes: use and preference—with and without nutritional information. *Journal of the American Dietetic Association* 70:267, 1977.

Patton, J.S. Gastrointestinal lipid digestion. In *Physiology of the Gastrointestinal Tract,* Vol. 2, L.R. Johnson, ed. Raven Press, New York: Raven Press, 1981, pp. 1123–1146.

Phillipson, B.E., D.W. Rothrock, W.E. Connor, W.S. Harris, and D.R. Illingworth. Reduction of plasma lipids, lipoproteins, and apoproteins by dietary fish oils in patients with hypertriglyceridemia. *New England Journal of Medicine.* 312:1210, 1985.

Sacks, F.M., W.P. Castelli, A. Donner, and E.H. Kass. Plasma lipids and lipoproteins in vegetarians and controls. *New England Journal of Medicine* 292:1148, 1975.

Shurtleff, D. Some characteristics related to the incidence of cardiovascular disease, and death: The Framingham study, 18-year followup. Washington, DC: U.S. Department of Health, Education and Welfare, National Institutes of Health, Framingham Study, Section No. 30, DHEW publication no. (NIH) 74:599, 1974.

Slover, H.T., R.H. Thompson, Jr., C.S. Davis, and G.V. Merola. *Journal of American Oil Chemists' Society* 62:775–786, 1985.

Smith, L.M., A.J. Clifford, R.K. Creveling, and C.L. Hamblin. Lipid content and fatty acid profiles of various deep-fat fried foods. *Journal of American Oil Chemists' Society* 62:996–999, 1985.

Stamler, J. Coronary heart disease: Doing the "right things." *New England Journal of Medicine* 312:1053–55, 1985.

Turjman, N., G.T. Goodman, B. Jaeger, and P.P. Nair. Metabolism of bile acids. *American Journal of Clinical Nutrition.* 40:937–941, 1984.

Vahouny, G.V. Dietary fiber, lipid metabolism, and atherosclerosis. *Federation Proceedings* 41:2801–2806, 1982.

Walker, W.J. Changing United States life-style and declining vascular mortality: Cause or coincidence? *New England Journal of Medicine* 297:163, 1977.

Wene, J.D., W.E. Conner, and L. DenBesten. The development of essential fatty acid deficiency in healthy men fed fat-free diets intravenously and orally. *Journal of Clinical Investigation* 56:127, 1975.

Willis, A.L. Essential Fatty Acids, Prostaglandins and Related Eicosanoios. In R.E. Olson, ed., *Present Knowledge in Nutrition,* 5th ed. Washington, DC: The Nutrition Foundation, Inc., 1984.

Willis, A.L. Nutritional and pharmacological factors in eicosanoid biology. *Nutrition Reviews* 39:289–301, 1981.

Chapter 4

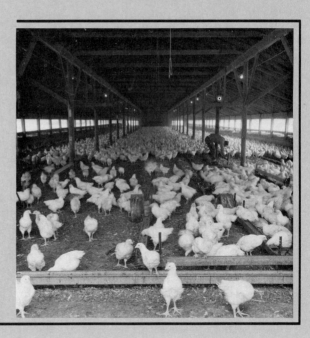

PROTEINS

Even in prehistoric times, an "animal principle" was recognized as being essential for human diets. But not until the early nineteenth century was a group of substances that acted as the "animal principle" identified. At that time, two scientists applied the word *protein* (from the Greek *proteios*, meaning "of the first rank") to this "principle." The Swedish chemist Jöns Jakob Berzelius had first proposed the word in a communication to the Dutch chemist Gerard Johannes Mulder. Mulder first used the word in published papers in 1838 to describe what he thought was a single substance that was a component of all living matter.

Although research since Mulder's time has shown that protein is not one substance but a multiplicity of substances, it has confirmed that proteins are truly "of the first rank" in importance to all life. We know now, too, that protein molecules are complex and consist of smaller entities known as *amino acids*. Some amino acids had been chemically identified as far back as 1810, even before proteins were described, but others were still being identified more than a hundred years later. Investigations of how they function are among the most exciting biochemical inquiries of our time.

Amino acids are essential for every body process, from transmission of the genetic information necessary to perpetuate every species, to the growth and maintenance of the cells of the individual organism. This is as true of one-celled microorganisms as it is of *Homo sapiens*. Body cells are able to build their own proteins from amino acids and carry out many functions by means of proteins. Although proteins can also serve as a source of energy, this is not their primary function.

Ever since proteins were identified, controversy has raged over dietary requirements. Although most Americans already consume amounts far in excess of need, numerous advertisements for protein-enriched products imply that we as a nation are a protein-deprived people. **Protein-energy malnutrition** is, however, critical in developing nations, where inadequate food supplies lead to both protein and energy undernutrition.

In this chapter we will consider the various roles of protein in the human body, sources of dietary protein, and the routes by which it supports physiological function. The interactions of protein with other nutrients, trends in protein consumption, and the nature and amount of protein necessary for health will be discussed. Finally, we will take a close look at diets that include little or no animal protein.

CLASSIFICATION, STRUCTURES, AND SOURCES: DIETARY PROTEIN

Proteins are organic compounds that always contain the elements carbon, hydrogen, oxygen, and nitrogen. Frequently, they contain sulfur and phosphorus as well, and less frequently they may contain elements such as iron, copper, and iodine.

Proteins are indeed complex molecules. The structure of each protein molecule is an assembly of amino acids, subunits whose name is derived from their chemical composition: Each has an amino (NH_2) group and a carboxyl (COOH) group, both attached to the same carbon atom. Also attached to this carbon are a hydrogen atom and a radical (R) group. The radical is different for each of the different amino acids and determines the characteristics and functions of each. The radical may be only a single hydrogen, as in glycine, or it may be a complex chemical structure, as in tryptophan. Some R groups include an additional carboxyl or amino group, a sulfur-containing group, or cyclic arrangements of carbon and other atoms. Nitrogen is the element characteristic of all amino acids and, therefore, of proteins. Most protein molecules contain from 12 to 19 percent nitrogen (usually considered 16 percent on average), a reflection of the amino acid nitrogen content.

Proline is technically an **imino acid** (having NH in a cyclic form instead of a free NH_2 group), but it is included with the amino acids because its role in protein structure is similar to theirs. Hydroxyproline and hydroxylysine contain an additional hydroxyl (—OH), added only after the parent compound (proline or lysine, respectively) has been incorporated into a protein.

Twenty-two amino acids are commonly found in foods; a few others, not present in foods, are synthesized in the body from other amino acids.

Classification of Amino Acids

Amino acids are classified in several different ways. From a functional viewpoint, those amino acids that are synthesized in the human body in adequate amounts are termed *nonessential*. Those that cannot be synthesized at all in the body, or that are synthesized in inadequate amounts, are termed *essential* because they must be supplied from food sources (see Table 4–1).

Normally, the body synthesizes all the nonessential amino acids it needs, as long as it is provided with an adequate supply of nitrogen to use for this purpose. A carbon "skeleton" around which the amino acid forms is derived from various substrates; an amino group, often transferred from other amino acids, becomes attached; the whole process is facilitated by a specific enzyme. In the case of essential amino acids, some of the enzymes required for this synthesis are either lacking or are not present in sufficient quantity.

The essential amino acids for human adults are *isoleucine, leucine, lysine, methionine, phenylalanine, threonine, tryptophan,* and *valine*. All others, with the

TABLE 4-1. *Classification of Amino Acids*

Essential			Nonessential	
NEUTRAL ALIPHATIC:				
Threonine	Thr		Glycine	Gly
Isoleucine	Ile		Alanine	Ala
Leucine	Leu		Serine	Ser
Valine	Val			
NEUTRAL CYCLIC:				
Phenylalanine	Phe		Tyrosine	Tyr
Tryptophan	Try		Proline	Pro
			Hydroxyproline	Hyp
NEUTRAL SULFUR-CONTAINING:				
Methionine	Met		Cysteine	Cys
Cysteine (infants?)	Cys			
ACIDIC:				
——			Aspartic acid	Asp
——			Glutamic acid	Glu
BASIC:				
Histidine	His		Hydroxylysine	Hyl
Lysine	Lys		Arginine	Arg

possible exceptions of *histidine* and *cysteine*, are nonessential. Until recently histidine was thought to be essential only for infants, but evidence suggests that some adults also may require exogenous histidine. Also, newborn infants may require exogenous cysteine until they mature sufficiently to produce the enzyme required for cysteine synthesis.

Under certain circumstances, cysteine and *tyrosine*, too, may have to be considered essential for humans. Normally, the body meets its requirement for cysteine by synthesizing it from methionine, and for tyrosine by converting phenylalanine. But in certain disease states, when these conversions cannot take place, cysteine and/or tyrosine must be supplied from dietary sources and are, therefore, essential amino acids.

Another classification of the amino acids is based on the chemical composition of their radicals or "side chains." Remember that all amino acids have both carboxyl and amino groups, which can be thought of as balancing each other, producing an overall neutral state of the amino acid molecule as a whole. There may, however, be additional carboxyl or amino groups present as part of the radical. If the radical contains an additional amino group, the amino acid is classified as *basic*; if it contains an additional carboxyl group, it is classified as *acidic*. And if the side chain contains no additional acidic or basic groups, the amino acid is *neutral*.

Basic and *acidic* have specific meanings in chemistry, referring to the presence of hydrogen ions (H^+). An **acid** substance will release hydrogen ions in a solution, whereas a **base** will combine with hydrogen ions. The chemical term **pH** measures relative acidity. By definition, a pH of 7 is neutral, with the number of hydrogen ions (H^+) equal to the number of hydroxyl ions (OH^-), as in water itself (H_2O). If the pH is greater than 7, the substance is basic and tends to combine with hydrogen ions; if the pH is less than 7, the substance is acidic and tends to release hydrogen ions. The pH of most physiological fluids is about 7.4.

The presence of —NH_2 or —COOH in the side chains of individual amino acids gives them their *net* basic or acidic character. For instance, in the basic amino acid lysine, the side chain NH_2 group acquires an H^+ and is ionized to NH_3^+; in aspartic acid the additional COOH gives up its hydrogen and is ionized to COO^-. These charged groups contribute to the overall structure and characteristics of the various protein molecules of which they are a part.

Neutral amino acids can be further classified according to whether they are *aliphatic*, with a straight side chain, or *aromatic* or *cyclic*, with a side chain containing a ring structure; or according to whether or not they contain sulfur.

Structure of Proteins

Protein molecules are composed of amino acids bonded together in *peptide linkage* or *peptide bond*. The central NH_2 group of one amino acid is joined to the central COOH group of another amino acid through a condensation reaction, similar to that which occurs when a monosaccharide is added to a polysaccharide, or when a fatty acid is added to a glycerol molecule: The carboxyl group gives up an —OH and the amino group an —H to release a molecule of water.

Figure 4–1 shows the formation of a dipeptide, two amino acids joined by a peptide bond. If three amino acids are joined, there will be two peptide bonds and the result is a tripeptide. Most protein molecules, however, consist of at least 50 and frequently hundreds of amino acids, and are known as **polypeptides**. But no matter how many amino acids comprise the protein molecule, they are joined together in the same peptide bonding. As a result, at one end of the protein molecule

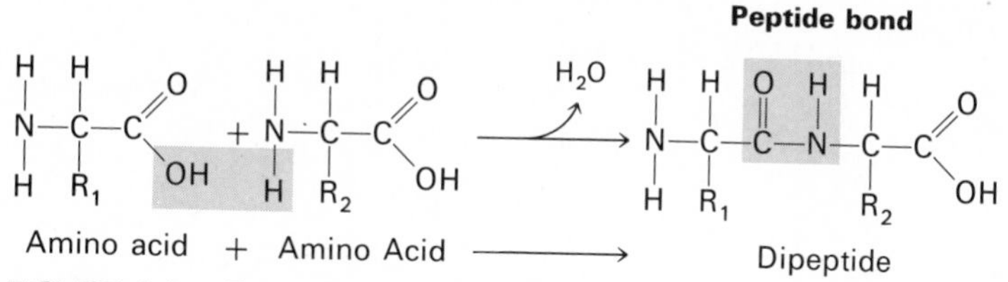

Peptide bond

Amino acid + Amino Acid ⟶ Dipeptide

FIGURE 4-1   *Formation of a Dipeptide.*

there will be a free amino group, an NH_2 that has not participated in the peptide condensation reaction. This is known as the *amino* or *N-terminal end* of the protein. Similarly, the other end of the protein chain has a free carboxyl group and is known as the *C-terminal end.*

PRIMARY STRUCTURE.   The polypeptide chain has a natural tendency to coil and become folded back on itself. This creates a complex structure, which can be described on several different levels. The primary structure of proteins depends on two factors: the sequence in which the amino acids are joined in the polypeptide chain (or chains—some proteins have more than one) and the presence of disulfide bonds.

The amino acid sequence is specific for each protein; thus, hemoglobin, collagen, the hundreds of enzymes, and all other protein molecules each consists of a specific and unique sequence. Most protein molecules contain from 15 to 20 different amino acids, and the number of possible, chemically meaningful sequences of 50 or more units that can be constructed from them is, for all practical purposes, infinite. It has been calculated that there are 10^{65} possible ways in which 20 amino acids could be arranged to form protein sequences of only 50 amino acid units, and most proteins contain more than 100 such units. Estimates indicate there are more than 100,000 distinct proteins, and therefore more than 100,000 different amino acid sequences, in the human body. (Other life forms, of course, contain other proteins.)

But primary structure also involves the presence of disulfide bonds, which are cross-links formed between the sulfur components of two cysteine units in the polypeptide chain. Cysteine has a sulfhydryl (—SH) group at one end. When two cysteine units come together to form cystine, the two sulfhydryl groups are oxidized, giving up their H atoms and leaving a strong link between the two sulfides, known as a *disulfide bond* (—S—S—). Whenever cysteines appear in a polypeptide chain they tend to form these disulfide bonds, causing the chain to fold back on itself so that sulfhydryl groups become linked. If this happens between cysteine units of two or more chains making up a single protein molecule, the bonds between those two chains are strengthened. The insulin molecule, for example, consists of two polypeptide chains linked together by two disulfide bonds; one of the chains is also linked internally by a disulfide bond (see Figure 4–2).

SECONDARY, TERTIARY, AND QUATERNARY STRUCTURE.   Secondary, tertiary, and quaternary structures refer to the three-dimensional shape of the protein molecule. *Secondary structure* results from hydrogen bonding between different amino acids within the polypeptide chain and is manifested in the characteristic coiled or helical shape of the molecule (see Figure 4–3). A hydrogen atom has a tendency to share its electron and seems to "look for" an oxygen atom to share it with. This creates a weak attraction between the hydrogen of an amino group in a peptide and

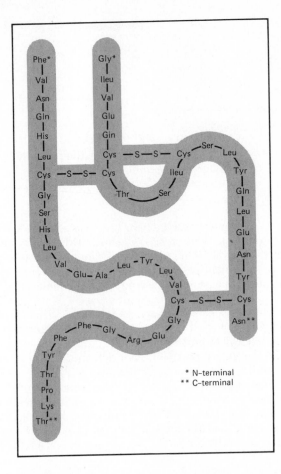

FIGURE 4-2
Polypeptide Chains of Human Insulin.

an oxygen of the carboxyl group of neighboring amino acids. Although each of these hydrogen bonds is, in itself, weak, the many hydrogen bonds between amino acids of the same chain give stability to the coiled form of the polypeptide chain. The result is a fairly regular secondary structure called the *α-helix*, which contains about 3.6 amino acids in each coil or turn. This particular helical pattern can be discerned in many protein molecules; other patterns of secondary structure have also been identified.

Tertiary structure reflects the chemical relationship of amino acids that are more distant from one another in the linear structure. Electrostatic bonding (electron

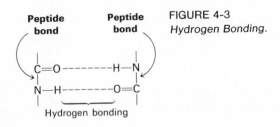

FIGURE 4-3
Hydrogen Bonding.

sharing), hydrogen bonding, and other types of bonding mechanisms link amino acids in a variety of spatial configurations.

We have been emphasizing the roles of two particular kinds of bonding—disulfide and hydrogen—in determining the architecture of the protein molecule. But it is the chemical organization of the component amino acid units, with its two reactive ends and side chain, that facilitates the different kinds of bonding (as well as the other reactions into which the resulting molecules will enter). When there is limited bonding *within* the polypeptide chain, there is a greater possibility of the formation of cross-links *between* different polypeptide chains, both within the same molecule (as in the case of insulin), or between different molecules.

Both secondary and tertiary structures allow two different basic shapes of protein molecules. *Fibrous proteins* are polypeptides that are "stretched out" so that the molecule has a somewhat linear shape. There is less internal bonding and, consequently, less coiling, leaving more side chains available to enter into cross-linkages with side chains of other similar molecules. Fibrous proteins are therefore able to provide support and structure for cells and tissues and are relatively insoluble in water. They are found, for example, in muscle (myosin), connective tissue (collagen), and hair (keratin).

Globular proteins, on the other hand, are polypeptide chains that are folded and crumpled up to form rounded or elliptical molecules. They have a substantial amount of internal bonding, along with many exposed side chains. This structure makes globular proteins relatively soluble in body fluids. Not surprisingly, enzymes, hemoglobin, and most plasma proteins are globular.

Finally, the *quaternary structure* of a protein is formed by the joining together of two or more similar protein subunits into a single large molecule, held together primarily by electrostatic forces. Hemoglobin, for example, is composed of two pairs of subunits, making four in all. Whereas all proteins have primary, secondary, and tertiary structure, only some have quaternary structure.

Under some circumstances, the structural arrangement of a protein molecule can be disrupted. Heat, acids, or mechanical action are among the forces that break the hydrogen, disulfide, or other bonds and produce this disruption, or **denaturation.** A well-known example of protein denaturation is the transformation of albumin (egg white) when it is cooked. Although in some cases denaturation is reversible, the coagulation of egg white totally alters the structure of its component polypeptide chains and cannot be reversed.

The function of proteins is a reflection of every aspect of their structure: the unique and specific amino acid composition and sequence, how the polypeptide chain is folded by internal bonding, and how subunits are combined. Even a brief introduction to the enormously complex structure of proteins leads to the conclusion that these are, in every way, complex and fascinating molecules.

Other Ways of Classifying Proteins

Another structural classification of proteins depends on whether or not a nonprotein component is present. Because of the readiness with which some polypeptides are able to react with other molecules, proteins have a notable tendency to form combinations in which they are part of a larger aggregate. In Chapter 3 we discussed lipoproteins, macromolecules with both a lipid and a protein component. Proteins that do not combine with nonprotein substances are *simple,* and those in combination are *conjugated.* Table 4–2 lists conjugated proteins according to their nonprotein components.

TABLE 4-2. *Structural Classification of Proteins*

Class of Proteins	Nonprotein Component	Example
Simple	None	Albumin
Conjugated		
Nucleoproteins	Nucleic acid (DNA, RNA)	Chromosomes
Lipoproteins	Lipids	Chylomicrons
Glycoproteins	Carbohydrate	Immunoglobulin
Metalloproteins	Metal ions (Zn, Cu, Fe)	Ferritin, carboxypeptidase
Chromoproteins	Heme, retinal	Hemoglobin, rhodopsin

Source: Adapted from R. Montgomery, R. L. Dryer, T. W. Conway, and A. A. Specter, *Biochemistry: A case-oriented approach* 4th ed. (St. Louis: C. V. Mosby, 1983), page 55.

Finally, proteins can be classified on the basis of their *physiological functions,* according to which there are six classes:

1. Enzymes, which catalyze body processes.
2. Some hormones, which regulate body processes.
3. Antibodies or immunological substances, which combat infection.
4. Structural proteins, which constitute cartilage, skin, nails, and hair.
5. Contractile proteins, which are present in skeletal muscle.
6. Blood proteins such as hemoglobin and albumin.

Proteins in Foods

You will remember that the body must obtain the essential amino acids from food for constructing its own proteins; as long as all are provided in appropriate quantity, the particular food form in which they are ingested is of no significance. Although protein can be obtained from both plant and animal foods, the latter generally contain all of the essential amino acids in amounts that will support human growth and maintain physiological functioning. These are called, somewhat incorrectly, **complete proteins.**

Incomplete proteins contain suboptimal amounts of certain essential amino acids. Except for a few in which one or more essential amino acids are totally absent, they are not literally incomplete. But they are "less" complete than most animal-derived proteins. Zein, for example, found in corn, is not capable of sustaining life if it is the sole protein being ingested. Corn, however, contains other proteins that increase the usefulness of zein.

The protein content of various foods is shown in Table 4-3. A high protein content does not, however, necessarily indicate a high **protein quality** for a given food; the essential amino acid pattern is what counts. For this reason, two foods with comparable protein content will not necessarily be of equal value to the organism. For example, 1 tablespoon of gelatin has about as much protein as 8 ounces (240 ml) of skim milk (9 g), but because gelatin is an incomplete protein, the protein quality of these two foods is not the same. Since most proteins of vegetable origin are incomplete, knowing the biological value of given foods is important especially in determining dietary protein requirements and the adequacy of vegetarian diets.

Virtually all the foods of high protein content in Table 4-3 are of animal origin: milk and milk products, meat, fish, and shellfish. The only exceptions are legumes—nuts and beans and their derivatives, such as peanut butter and tofu (soy-

TABLE 4-3. *Protein Content of Selected Foods*

Food	Serving Size	Protein Content g/Serving
Cottage cheese, uncreamed	1 c	34
Round steak, lean & fat	3½ oz	29
Swordfish, broiled	3½ oz	28
Tuna fish, in water	3½ oz	28
Scallops	3½ oz	23
Soybeans, boiled	1 c	22
Chickpeas	½ c	21
Haddock, fried	3½ oz	20
Yogurt, nonfat milk + milk solids	8 oz	13
Yogurt, low-fat + milk solids, plain	8 oz	12
Yogurt, low-fat + milk solids, fruit-flavored	8 oz	10
Milk, low-fat or skim, + solids	1 c	9–10
Almonds, roasted	⅓ c	9.5
Gelatin, dry	1 tbsp	9
Milk, whole	1 c	8
Milk, low-fat or skim	1 c	8
Yogurt, made with whole milk	8 oz	8
Cashews, roasted	⅓ c	8
Peanut butter	2 tbsp	8
Cheddar cheese	1 oz	7
Egg, whole	1 medium	6
Kidney beans	½ c	6
Broccoli, cooked	⅔ c	3
Rice, brown, cooked	⅔ c	3
Tofu (soybean curd)	1 oz	2.5
White bread, enriched	1 slice	2
Bean sprouts, raw	½ c	2
Rice, white milled, enriched	⅔ c	2
Gelatin dessert, plain	½ c	2
Carrots, cooked	½ c	1
Bouillon cube	1 cube	trace
Butter	1 tbsp	trace
Margarine; oils	1 pat	0

Sources: USDA Agricultural Handbook No. 8-1 (Washington, D.C.: U.S. Government Printing Office, 1976) 8–11 (1982); and C. F. Adams, *Nutritive value of American foods in common units*, USDA Agricultural Handbook No. 456 (Washington, D.C.: U.S. Government Printing Office, 1975).

bean curd). Note also that the protein content of milk and yogurt products varies, depending on the addition of milk solids to the low-fat varieties.

Worldwide, per capita protein availability ranges widely, from about 55 grams per day in the Far East to approximately 100 grams in the United States (see Table 4–4). In general, people in developing countries consume less protein (an average of about 58 g per capita per day) than in developed regions (almost 90 g). In developing regions, too, most protein—over 80 percent—is derived from plant food sources, compared to only about 45 percent from plant sources in developed nations.

That protein consumption is tied to availability is underscored by the figures for certain categories of protein in some places: In South and East Asia, fish consumption accounts for about 15.5 percent of all protein intake, with meat consumption

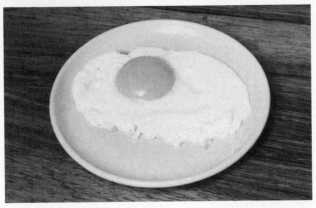

While protein can be obtained from both plant and animal food sources, the latter generally contain all of the essential amino acids in amounts that will support human growth and maintain physiological functioning.

Laimute E. Druskis

in the 6 to 7 percent range; people in West and Central Africa get a substantially greater proportion of their protein (14.8 percent) from starchy roots and tubers than do people anywhere else in the world; and Brazilians receive more than a quarter of their protein from legumes, nuts, and seeds.

The major influences on availability of plant versus animal sources of protein foods are economic and technological and have to do with such factors as methods of production (irrigation, fertilization, mechanized tilling, and slaughtering), storage facilities, transportation, and distribution (village markets versus supermarkets, for example). Traditional religious and cultural preferences (many of which also derive ultimately from technological factors) surely have some influence as well. Consumption of protein, perhaps even more than of the other major nutrients, is tied to socioeconomic factors. As a nation's or a family's socioeconomic status improves, protein, especially animal-derived protein, will form a greater proportion of the diet.

TABLE 4-4. *Protein Consumption in the United States*

Protein Type	Percent of Total Protein Consumption
ANIMAL PROTEINS, TOTAL:	68.0
Meat	42.9
Milk	20.2
Eggs	4.9
Fish	2.9
VEGETABLE PROTEINS, TOTAL:	39.6
Cereals	18.8
Fruits and vegetables	5.0
Legumes, nuts, seeds	5.5
Starchy roots, tubers	2.3

Source: Adapted from R. M. Marston and S. O. Welsh, Nutrient Content of National Food Supply in *Sourcebook on Food and Nutrition. 3rd ed.* (Chicago, IL: Marquis Academia Media, 1982).

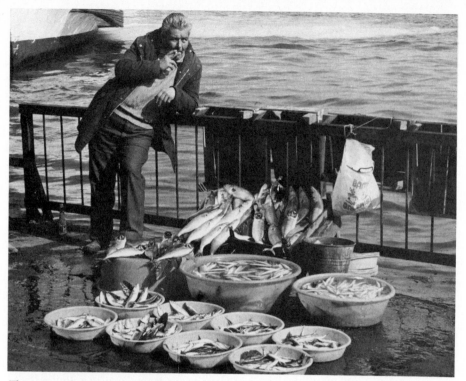

The major influences on availability of plant versus animal sources of protein foods are economic and technological and have to do with such factors as methods of production, storage facilities, transportation, and distribution. Cultural preferences have some influence as well.
Eugene Gordon

DIGESTION AND ABSORPTION

The significance of protein in foods will become clearer as we examine its functions in the body—growth, maintenance of tissues, regulation of physiological processes and, under certain conditions, a source of energy. During digestion and absorption, proteins are transformed into their constituent amino acids, which are then delivered to body cells for all these purposes.

Enzymatic Hydrolysis

In protein digestion, the peptide bonds linking amino acids in the polypeptide chain are broken down, releasing smaller peptide fragments and individual amino acids. This is a hydrolytic reaction, similar to those we have already examined for the digestion of carbohydrates and lipids, and the reverse of the condensation reaction by which the peptide bonds were formed. In hydrolysis of peptide bonds (proteolysis), which requires action by specific proteolytic enzymes, a water molecule is added at each bond (see Figure 4–4).

There is no chemical action on protein in the mouth or esophagus, although lubrication, mastication, and peristaltic action prepare protein food mechanically for

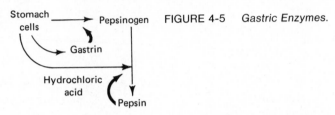

FIGURE 4-4 *Enzymatic Hydrolysis.*

Stomach cells ⟶ Pepsinogen   **FIGURE 4-5** *Gastric Enzymes.*

Gastrin

Hydrochloric acid

Pepsin

chemical attack. In the stomach, specialized cells release hydrochloric acid, which begins the denaturation of dietary protein (Figure 4–5). This loss of structure makes protein more susceptible to subsequent action by digestive enzymes. Hydrochloric acid acts also as a primer to convert the inactive precursor enzyme *pepsinogen* to **pepsin**. Pepsinogen is produced by specific cells of the stomach under the influence of the gastrointestinal hormone gastrin. Pepsin hydrolyzes large proteins into smaller polypeptides and also accelerates its own production from pepsinogen. This is, indeed, a complicated and elegantly interconnected sequence of biochemical events!

As is characteristic of the proteolytic enzymes, pepsin is selective, hydrolyzing only those bonds in which the nitrogen is provided by either phenylalanine or tyrosine. Consequently, only a small amount of protein is hydrolyzed in the stomach.

As soon as stomach contents enter the duodenum, the intestinal hormone *pancreozymin* stimulates the cells of the pancreas to release their complement of proteolytic enzymes (as well as other enzymes needed for carbohydrate and lipid digestion). These inactive precursor enzymes—*trypsinogen, chymotrypsinogen, proelastase,* and *procarboxypeptidase*—are secreted into the duodenum, where they are transformed into active participants in the digestive process. By means of *enterokinase,* an enzyme present in the duodenum, a fragment is split from the trypsinogen molecule to produce the active enzyme *trypsin.* The presence of trypsin initiates a "cascade" of further conversions, as it activates the precursor forms of *chymotrypsin, elastase,* and the *carboxypeptidases.* These enzymes are released by hydrolysis of a fragment from the polypeptide chain of their respective precursors. Now active, each of these enzymes acts on specific peptide bonds.

Trypsin selects only those bonds whose carboxyl groups are provided by arginine and lysine residues. Chymotrypsin similarly attacks only those peptide bonds where the carboxyl group is contributed by tyrosine, phenylalanine, and tryptophan. Elastase acts on a number of different amino acid residues but is the only enzyme able to hydrolyze the protein elastin, found in muscle meats. Because they attack interior peptide bonds only, and not those adjacent to the ends of the polypeptide, these three enzymes are known as **endopeptidases.** Through their action, the polypeptide chains of large protein molecules become progressively more fragmented into shorter peptide chains.

The two carboxypeptidases, on the other hand, hydrolyze the peptide bonds at the C-terminals of the peptides. Amino peptidase hydrolyzes amino acids from the N-terminal end. These *exopeptidases* release free amino acids.

The digestibility of some proteins may be affected by other substances present in particular foods, as well as by certain processing and preparation methods. Soybeans, lima beans, and peas, for example, contain a factor that has been associated with growth failure in laboratory animals. This factor, which is destroyed by heat, probably acts as an inhibitor of trypsin and perhaps chymotrypsin. The clinical and practical significance of this discovery for human nutrition is not yet clear, but it indicates these foods should probably not be eaten raw.

Excessive heating of proteins sometimes creates enzyme-resistant linkages between amino acid units (severe denaturation), which will interfere with digestion and subsequent absorption. Moderate heating, such as occurs in normal preparation and cooking, may, on the other hand, split natural cross-linkages and facilitate enzyme action.

In some instances, pancreatic deficiency or inherited diseases will interfere with efficiency of protein digestion. The result is loss of protein via the feces.

Not all the protein in the small intestine is derived from food. The digestive enzymes, for example, are themselves proteins. Moreover, protein-containing cells of the intestinal mucosa are continually being sloughed off at the outer ends of the villi as they are replaced by new cells formed at the villi bases. Together, these and other endogenous sources may provide as much as 70 grams of protein per day, in addition to the average American dietary intake of 90 to 100 grams. Since daily fecal losses of protein are only about 10 grams, total absorption in the intestine must approximate 160 grams per day.

Although most proteolysis takes place in the lumen of the small intestine, there are some enzymes in the brush borders and the intracellular fluid surrounding the mucosal cells. These dipeptidases act on the smaller peptides that are released during intestinal digestion. As soon as small peptides cross from the lumen into the mucosa (see subsequently), the brush border and intracellular peptidases begin to hydrolyze them, a process that results in the production of free amino acids.

Amino Acid Absorption

From the lumen of the small intestine, amino acids are transported to the mucosal cells by means of special carriers in an energy-dependent process. Several different carrier systems have been identified, specific for neutral, basic, or acidic amino acids or for dipeptides. Amino acids enter the general circulation through the portal vein.

Protein absorption is extremely efficient, with more than 90 percent of dietary protein absorbed as amino acids. Proteins of animal origin are digested and absorbed with even greater efficiency—97 percent—than are those in cereals, legumes, fruits, and vegetables (78 to 85 percent).

Infants are born with the ability to absorb proteins intact, without their being broken down completely. This ability, retained for a short time only, serves an important protective function. It enables antibodies, which are proteins, to be absorbed from the mother's milk and thus confers a temporary immunity against certain contagious diseases.

Except for the first month of life, however, dietary proteins cannot be absorbed in intact form but are always broken down into their component amino acids. Thus, the frequent commercial claims that certain foods contain *essential proteins* that *must* be consumed for good health cannot be reconciled with what we know of the physiology of digestion. No *protein* is essential; the individual amino acids contained in dietary proteins and released during digestion are essential to the body's physiological processes.

METABOLISM

The body's access to amino acids is regulated primarily by the liver. Following digestion of a protein-containing meal, the amino acid concentration in the portal vein increases severalfold. The liver, then, must deal with sharp fluctuations in the supply of amino acids several times a day, day after day, throughout the life of the organism. By catabolizing essential amino acids, synthesizing amino acids into proteins for use in its own processes as well as for transport through the blood to body cells, and synthesizing nonessential amino acids, the liver keeps the amino acid levels in body tissues in dynamic equilibrium.

Amino acids are thus involved in a whole range of anabolic and catabolic processes which take a number of different pathways, each influenced by many factors. We will examine the major reactions involving amino acids, beginning with protein synthesis, which is by far the primary function of amino acids in all living organisms.

Protein Synthesis

All life depends on the synthesis of new protein molecules by body cells. Of the vast number of different protein structures possible, each cell synthesizes only the ones needed for its own purposes and produces them in precisely required amounts; this is true of every cell of every living organism, be it bacterium, bat, or human being. In every individual, all cellular chemical activities are programmed by a genetic code unique to that individual. The genetic code itself is contained within the chromosomes inside every cell nucleus.

"BREAKING" THE GENETIC CODE. Chromosomes have long been recognized as being responsible for duplicating and transmitting the genetic message, and that the actual units of heredity were a component of the chromosomes known as **deoxyribonucleic acid (DNA)**. But the actual molecular structure and behavior of DNA remained a mystery until 1953, when Watson and Crick unraveled its chemical organization and proposed a model for its biochemical action. These scientists determined that the DNA molecule was an elongated double helix, whose two twisting and intertwined strands were composed of linked subunits called **nucleotides** (Figure 4–6).

Watson and Crick proposed that the two strands of a DNA molecule were held together by hydrogen bonds between specific nucleotide bases. The specificity of nucleotide bonding means that a new DNA molecule can be constructed from a single strand of the old DNA molecule: The single strand serves as a pattern to define a complementary strand. Thus, the information contained in a given pair of nucleotide chains is duplicated precisely, and hereditary information is transmitted from generation to generation. The cell-duplicating mechanism is so perfect that every cell in an individual contains identical nucleotide sequences in its DNA.

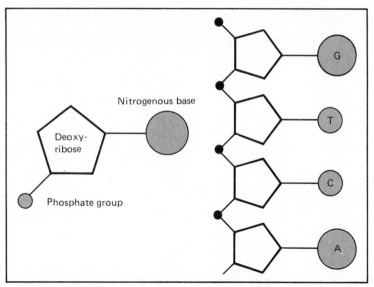

FIGURE 4-6   *Segment of a Nucleotide (DNA) Chain.*

Each nucleotide consists of deoxyribose (a 5-carbon sugar), phosphate, and a nitrogen-containing base. There are four different bases (adenine, guanine, cytosine, and thymine), and therefore four different kinds of nucleotides, usually expressed as A, G, C, and T. The sugar of one nucleotide is always attached to the phosphate group of the next, forming the "backbone" of the DNA molecule, with the different bases branching off as side chains.

The genetic code itself consists of the sequences of nucleotides within the DNA molecule, which act by programming the synthesis of the specific proteins that make up each species and individual. The actual genetic code is different for every species and for every individual within a species.

The DNA and its nucleotide sequences are located in the nucleus of the cell, however, whereas protein synthesis occurs in the cytoplasm. The genetic information, therefore, must somehow be carried from the DNA, which never leaves the cell nucleus, to the scene of the action. This is accomplished by another macromolecule, **ribonucleic acid (RNA)**, which exists in both the nucleus and the cytoplasm of the cell. RNA is very similar to DNA except that it consists of a single strand of nucleotides instead of a double strand, its 5-carbon sugar is ribose instead of deoxyribose (from which the names of the two molecules are derived), and it contains uracil (U) instead of thymine.

Actually, several kinds of RNA are required to carry out the instructions of the DNA. Messenger ribonucleic acid (mRNA) is produced in the nucleus of the cell, modeled by a single strand of DNA which partially separates from its mate for this purpose. The completed mRNA molecule then moves through the nuclear membrane and enters the cytoplasm. Here it encounters the ribosomes, the parts of the cell that actually synthesize proteins. Ribosomes are able to synthesize every protein but must be given specific "instructions" in order to "know" which proteins to produce in a given cell.

The functioning unit of protein synthesis, and thus of heredity, is a sequence of three nucleotides called a **codon.** Each codon is identified by the three letters

Perspective On

PKU, AN INBORN ERROR OF PROTEIN METABOLISM

Despite its amazing complexity, the protein synthesizing process functions to perfection in virtually every individual. But in some conditions, a key component of the mechanism fails to work. These inborn errors of metabolism are due to inherited defects that result in biochemical abnormalities, often with serious clinical symptoms. We consider here one of the most familiar of such diseases, phenylketonuria or PKU.

Usually, defects are the result of damage to a single gene, the unit by which hereditary traits are transmitted. Genes can be described as the set of nucleotide codons on a DNA molecule that direct the formation of a particular protein from its component amino acids. However, it is convenient to refer to genes in terms of their net effect, as has been traditional since Gregor Mendel first suggested their existence a century ago.

A damaged gene is known as a *mutant*. Mutations result from factors, such as exposure to radiation, that interfere with the replication of the DNA molecule. If even a single nucleotide were missing, or if an incorrect nucleotide were to replace a correct one, the mRNA strand would be transmitting the "wrong" information and keying the addition of an incorrect amino acid. If the resulting protein were a metabolic enzyme, the metabolic process for which it was necessary could not take place.

This is precisely what happens in PKU. For some reason, an incorrect nucleotide is present in the DNA strand that codes for the structure of the enzyme necessary for metabolizing phenylalanine. Since phenylalanine is an essential amino acid, a certain amount must be obtained from dietary sources. The genetic defect does not interfere with the utilization of this necessary amount. But excess phenylalanine is normally converted by the enzyme into the nonessential amino acid tyrosine, which is used for growth and other functions. If this pathway is blocked because the enzyme is missing, phenylalanine must be metabolized by alternate pathways and accumulates, along with its abnormal metabolites, in body fluids. At the same time, there is an inadequate supply of tyrosine. The combination of excessive phenylalanine and its byproducts, and inadequate tyrosine, results in the symptoms found in untreated phenylketonuric patients. The condition can be diagrammed as follows:

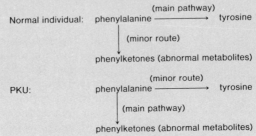

standing for its component nucleotides. There are 64 different possible codons from the combinations of the four different nucleotides (4^3). Each of 61 of them codes for only one specific amino acid; for example, AAG for lysine, AGA for arginine, GAA for glutamic acid. But there are only 22 amino acids, and so some may be called for by more than one codon: Lysine, for example, is coded by either AAG or AAA, and serine by UCU, UCC, UCA, or UCG. The remaining three codons are chain-terminating (or "nonsense") codons, which signal the end of a particular message sequence.

THE MAKING OF A POLYPEPTIDE. In the bloodstream, ready to enter the cytoplasm at an instant's notice, is a supply of amino acids that have resulted both from

The symptoms, which appear in infants between 6 and 18 months of age, include irritability, hyperactivity, convulsive seizures, lighter skin and hair color than other family members, moderate to severe mental retardation, and a general slowdown of physical growth and development. Untreated individuals have a short life expectancy, with only a 25 percent chance of surviving past the third decade.

The mutant gene that accounts for PKU exists in about 1.5 percent of the population. However, because an individual acquires chromosomes equally from each of two parents, and because a normal gene will "overrule" or be dominant over the effects of a mutant, almost all these individuals have normal or near-normal phenylalanine metabolism. They are, however, "carriers" of the recessive mutation. And if two such carriers marry, the outcome of each pregnancy can be expressed as a statistical probability. Their offspring may have two normal genes for production of the necessary enzyme (25%), may be a carrier like the parents (50%), or may have two recessive genes and therefore be afflicted with PKU.

Fortunately, PKU can now be detected by a blood test performed on newborn infants. The one individual in every 20,000 born with PKU can be identified and immediately treated through careful dietary management. PKU screening of newborns is now mandated in most states.

Dietary management consists of a carefully controlled food plan containing only enough phenylalanine for essential purposes and an adequate intake of energy, other amino acids, and all other nutrients. Phenylalanine is present in many foods of both animal and vegetable origin and is especially plentiful in milk, the basic food in the first months of life. Infants with PKU receive a special formula (Lofenelac, from which phenylalanine has been removed) supplemented by small amounts of cow's milk. As the child grows older, other foods containing some phenylalanine, mainly fruits and vegetables, are introduced. Animal foods contain excessive amounts and must generally be avoided. Near-normal growth and intellectual development can be expected if such a regime is begun in the earliest weeks of life. Treatment begun after the first year will eliminate behavioral problems but will be too late to correct mental retardation.

With our present knowledge we can only hope to alleviate the effects of genetically determined metabolic diseases such as PKU. Extensive investigations have been conducted to understand the etiology of such diseases; but much remains to be done to develop screening tests, methods of treatment, and a means of prevention.

digestion of dietary protein and from breakdown of cellular protein. Waiting in the cytoplasm are molecules of transfer ribonucleic acid (tRNA). Each tRNA molecule contains a 3-nucleotide sequence that "fits" a similar sequence on the mRNA strand, and each tRNA molecule is also able to attach to a particular amino acid from the cellular amino acid pool.

Once the mRNA enters the cytoplasm, ribosomes cluster along its length. The mRNA and its attached ribosomes are known as a polyribosome complex. Each ribosome moves along the strand of mRNA, touching two codons at a time. Codon by codon, a tRNA molecule and its amino acid arrive on the scene. Enzymes in the ribosome form a peptide bond which attaches the new amino acid to the growing peptide chain. The tRNA molecule is released, and the ribosome moves along the mRNA to the next codon, where instructions for the next amino acid in the sequence are received. As each appropriate tRNA molecule carrying its amino acid responds, the polypeptide chain grows longer.

Actually, many ribosomes move at the same time along a single strand of mRNA, each producing a protein molecule in the course of its journey. Thus, a single molecule of mRNA can direct the synthesis of many identical protein molecules. The whole process occurs very quickly, within seconds. This amazingly complex set of reactions is still being actively studied.

Some of the most intriguing questions related to protein synthesis deal with the regulation of the process: How is it initiated? How is it limited to specific proteins? All cells in the body have the same DNA information, but they obviously don't all do the same thing. Somehow, in all cells, part of the total coded information is "turned off" so that only those parts specific to the functioning of each type of cell are operative. How this "turning off" is effected is not yet clearly understood. But in every cell, the necessary combination of appropriate amino acids is "strung together" in a particular sequence, as programmed by the genetic code unique to that individual, via a series of elegant enzymatic reactions.

Several factors are involved in keeping this vital and intricate mechanism functioning smoothly. The first requirement is an adequate supply in every cell of all amino acids. This is truly an "all-or-nothing" situation: If even one of the amino acids called for by an mRNA codon is missing, synthesis of the whole polypeptide chain comes to a halt. This, then, is the reason why the "essential" amino acids must be provided by dietary protein; there is no other way for them to be available within the cell.

Energy, in the form of ATP, is the second requirement; it is needed both to initiate and to continue the process of protein synthesis. ATP activates the amino acids in the cytoplasm so that they become attached to their tRNA molecules; it moves the mRNA, tRNA, and ribosomes in their appointed courses; and it is necessary at several other stages. If there is insufficient energy, the process cannot proceed.

Protein synthesis is regulated by a number of other factors as well—so many other factors, and with functions so intricate, that description of their interactions is beyond the scope of this book.

FUNCTIONS OF SYNTHESIZED PROTEINS. All cells synthesize protein by the mechanism that has just been described but the liver and muscle are particularly important in protein metabolisms. These proteins are used as constituents of a number of important body substances for growth and maintenance of all tissues. The growth of the body depends on incorporation of newly synthesized protein into bone, muscle, skin, hair, nails, and other tissues. Most growth, of course, takes place during the earlier years of the individual's life; however, skin, nails, and hair continue to grow throughout life.

Throughout life, too, the protein in body tissues is continually being broken down into amino acids, which become part of the amino acid pool in the cells. When tissue proteins are broken down, they must be replaced by new proteins. This tissue maintenance requires a constant supply of amino acids. The amino acids that result from tissue breakdown, along with amino acids from dietary protein, are used for synthesis of new proteins and special molecules and for energy. This breakdown and replacement is known as **protein turnover**. Without an adequate supply of amino acids from both dietary and endogenous sources, protein turnover could not be accomplished.

Proteins are also important for regulation of the body's water balance. This role will be discussed more fully in Chapter 9, but here we should note that plasma proteins, such as albumin, serve the important function of maintaining **osmotic pressure** in the blood. Thus, they help to effect a proper distribution of fluid between blood and body tissues. If plasma protein levels decrease, as in protein deficiency, fluid accumulates in the tissues, a condition known as edema.

Proteins also regulate the acid-base balance (pH) of body fluids. The acidic and basic side groups of the various amino acids constituting protein molecules enable them to act as buffers and to neutralize acids and bases in the body so that the generally neutral pH level is maintained. Maintenance of pH neutrality is vital; several different regulatory mechanisms exist to preserve it.

Finally, some functional proteins are antibodies, which destroy infectious organisms and thereby fight disease.

As much as 300 grams of protein per day may be synthesized in the body of an average adult male weighing 70 kilograms. The quantity of protein synthesized is related to growth and therefore age (see Table 4–5), as well as to overall energy expenditure. A single gram of dietary protein may support the synthesis of 4 to 5 grams of tissue, regardless of age. Differences in protein needs, expressed in grams per kilogram of body weight per day, result from differences in the rate of protein synthesis (that is, the amount of protein synthesized in a given period of time).

Synthesis of Nonessential Amino Acids

About half of the more than 20 amino acids found in the human body can be synthesized in the liver from other compounds. Formation of an amino acid requires the attachment of an amino or nitrogen group to a "carbon skeleton," which contains the distinctive radical or side chain that will characterize the resulting amino acid. The carbon skeleton is a keto acid, such as pyruvate or α-ketoglutarate, which is a product of carbohydrate or fat metabolism. The nitrogen group is provided by other amino acids present in larger quantity, through the processes of transamination or deamination.

Keto and amino acids exist in pairs, related by similar structure of the carbon chain; several pairs exist. In **transamination**, an amino group is transferred from an amino acid of one pair (alanine-pyruvate) to the keto acid of another pair (α-ketoglutarate-glutamic acid). Transamination requires the assistance of specific enzymes known as transaminases and must be accompanied by pyridoxine (vitamin B_6), which serves as a coenzyme (Figure 4–7).

In **deamination**, nitrogen is released from glutamine, a basic amino acid, in the

Age Group	Body Weight (BW) kg	TOTAL BODY PROTEIN SYNTHESIS		Protein Synthesis g/g Protein Intake
		g/kg BW/day	g/day[a]	
Newborn (premature)	1.95 ± .59	17.4 ± 7.9	33.8	5.4
Infants (10–20 mos.)	9.0 ± .5	6.9 ± 1.1	62.1	5.3
Young adults (20–23 yrs.)	71 ± 15	3.0 ± 0.2	213.0	5.2
Elderly (69–91 yrs.)	56 ±	1.9 ± 0.2	106.4	4.5

TABLE 4-5. *Amount of Protein Synthesis*

[a] Calculated from Young's data.
Source: V. R. Young, W. P. Steffee, R. B. Pencharz, J. C. Winterer, and N. S. Scrimshaw, Total human body protein synthesis in relation to protein requirements at various ages, *Nature* 253:192, 1975.

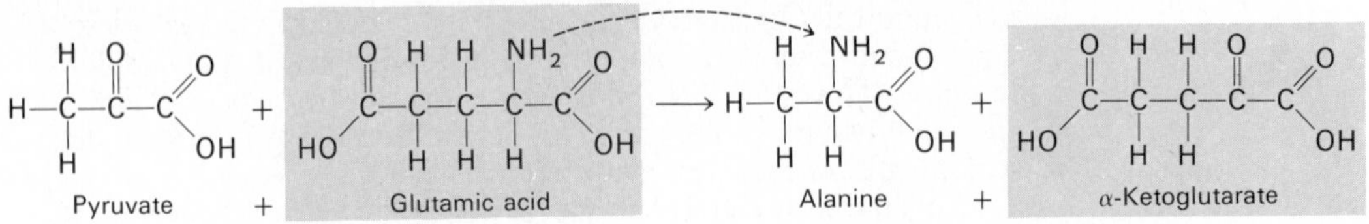

FIGURE 4-7   Transamination.

form of ammonia. A new amino acid is produced by the addition of the ammonia to a keto acid (Figure 4–8).

A steady supply of nonessential amino acids for use in protein synthesis depends on the efficient functioning of these conversion reactions. Remember that these reactions are reversible. Although nonessential amino acids can be synthesized in the body, diet is still the usual source. If, however, the diet fails to provide them in adequate amounts, this process of endogenous synthesis must take up the slack. This fail-safe mechanism ensures that the nonessential amino acids needed for protein synthesis will always be available to the cells.

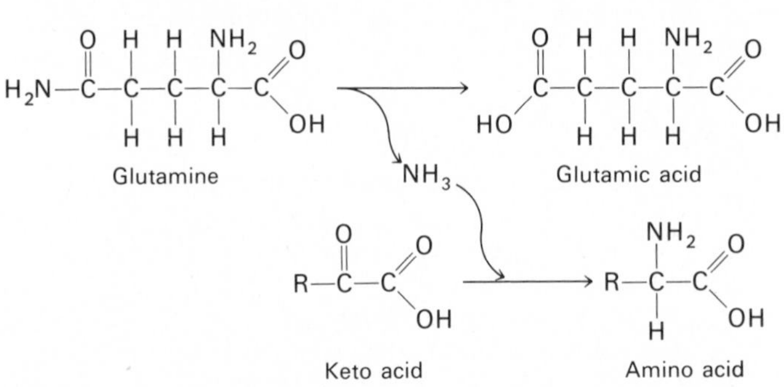

FIGURE 4-8   Deamination.

Gluconeogenesis and Energy Metabolism

When carbohydrate and lipid intake or reserves are insufficient, body proteins and amino acids can be utilized for energy needs. The same amount of energy can be obtained from protein as from carbohydrates—1 gram yields 4 kilocalories. Some amino acids can be converted to glucose by the process of gluconeogenesis. Amino acids that cannot be used immediately are generally metabolized to fat for storage. In all these processes, the participating amino acids are deaminated to provide the carbon skeleton that takes part in the particular metabolic pathway, releasing ammonia which will be disposed of by the body in the form of urea. These processes are interrelated; we will discuss first the pathways by which excess protein is converted to glucose, then the circumstances which result in nitrogen loss, and finally the synthesis of lipids from protein.

DISPOSAL OF THE CARBON SKELETON.   Once amino acids have lost their nitrogen groups, the remaining carbon skeletons enter the Krebs cycle at various points. Most amino acids are glycogenic; that is, their carbon skeletons are degraded to pyruvate or other intermediates (oxaloacetic acid, fumaric acid, succinyl CoA, α-ketoglutarate) that can be transformed into glucose. A few amino acids cannot be converted to glucose; tryptophan and leucine are purely **ketogenic**, being metabolized only to acetoacetyl CoA and acetyl CoA, which enter the Krebs cycle for the production of ATP, CO_2, and water. A few amino acids are both ketogenic and glucogenic and can be converted to acetyl CoA or to glucose.

The process of gluconeogenesis is virtually a reversal of the Embden-Meyerhof pathway (by which glucose is converted to pyruvate). The direction followed along this pathway depends on the metabolic needs of the body at a given time. Amino acids may thus be used to raise blood glucose levels, which subsequently are oxidized for energy.

DISPOSAL OF NITROGEN: THE UREA CYCLE.   Humans and other terrestrial vertebrates excrete their nitrogenous wastes (ammonia, NH_3) in the form of urea. Ammonia is highly toxic and must be removed from the blood before it can build up to dangerous concentrations. (Note: transamination alone does not release nitrogen; deamination does.) The liver removes ammonia from circulation and converts it to urea in the urea cycle. In the form of urea, the nitrogenous wastes return to the kidney, which dilutes the urea with water and adds other substances prior to excretion.

In the urea cycle, the amino acid ornithine receives ammonia from amino acid deamination and an additional amount from the amino acid aspartic acid. Adding these two nitrogenous components to its amine group, the ornithine is converted to arginine. The enzyme arginase then splits off urea from the arginine, regenerating ornithine (Figure 4–9). The urea cycle requires, in addition to specific enzymes, energy in the now-familiar form of ATP, along with CO_2. Figure 4–10 illustrates the production of urea and energy from one specific amino acid, alanine.

LIPID SYNTHESIS.   After the body's amino acid needs for protein synthesis have been met, any amino acid surplus is metabolized to fat and stored in that form.

FIGURE 4-9   *The Urea Cycle.*

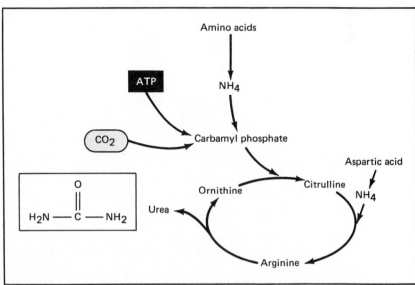

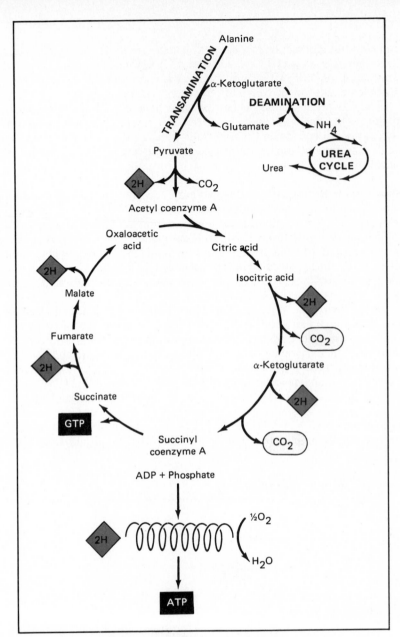

FIGURE 4-10   Summary of Amino Acid Catabolism.

This is accomplished by conversion of the amino acids to pyruvate and acetyl CoA, which are in turn converted to fatty acids. These then combine with glycerol to form a triglyceride.

SUMMARY OF PROTEIN METABOLISM.   Because of the intricate interactions between protein anabolism and catabolism, we say that these processes are in dynamic equilibrium; that is, the balance between them tips one way or the other depending on the immediate need of the individual. Figure 4–11 summarizes pro-

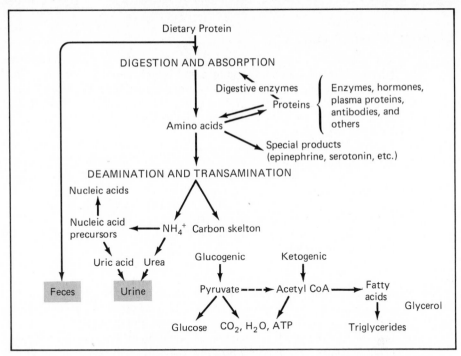

FIGURE 4-11   *Summary of Protein Metabolism.*

tein metabolism. The interaction between and regulation of these pathways depend on various factors that together determine body needs at a given time. These factors include the organism's stage in the life cycle, hormonal balance, energy status, presence of disease, and the availability of appropriate substrate (the specific amino acids needed for a given process). The continuous turnover of body protein, by normal degradation processes, provides much of the supply in the amino acid pool.

PROTEIN REQUIREMENTS

Most of the protein molecules in the body perform one or more vital roles, so very little protein is present merely as a storage form. Because protein is constantly being depleted, the supply must be replenished through diet every day. Estimates of the amount of protein that must be provided in the diet have varied widely. In the late nineteenth century, the German physiologist Carl Voit concluded, after a statistical analysis of the diets of his countrymen, that an average adult man doing moderate physical work needed 118 grams of dietary protein per day, or 1.5 grams per kilogram of body weight. In the early twentieth century, however, in a series of meticulous experiments, the American Russell H. Chittenden showed that 40 to 60 grams per day, from a varied food selection, were enough to maintain health and nitrogen balance. Later, work pioneered by William Rose demonstrated that there were requirements for individual essential amino acids as well as for overall protein intake.

Nitrogen Balance Studies

Traditionally, protein requirements have been determined through nitrogen balance studies, which compare intake and excretion of that element. Significant discoveries have been made in this way, despite the fact that precise measurements of nitrogen content of dietary protein and excretory products (urine, feces, and wastes from the skin) are time-consuming, subject to error, and especially with human subjects, expensive.

Nitrogen balance data are conveniently expressed as actual protein gained or lost over a period of time. Because approximately 16 percent of protein consists of nitrogen, it is possible to obtain a valid estimate of total protein by multiplying grams of nitrogen by 6.25. Thus, 2 grams of nitrogen would be roughly equivalent to 12.5 grams of protein. However, protein requirements can be validly estimated by the nitrogen balance method only when energy intake is adequate. Otherwise, dietary protein will be diverted to make up any energy deficit, and protein requirements will be overestimated.

COMPONENTS OF NITROGEN LOSS. As we have seen, the predominant nitrogen compound excreted in urine is urea. Certain other compounds containing nitrogen, such as creatinine and uric acid, make smaller contributions. Whenever protein intake exceeds the amount the body can use immediately, the nitrogen content of the urine increases. As protein intake decreases, the nitrogen content of the urine correspondingly decreases. However, even with very low protein intake (or none at all), a small amount of nitrogen continues to be excreted. This is known as the obligatory urinary nitrogen loss.

Nitrogen from undigested protein, both dietary and endogenous, is also excreted in the feces. On average, fecal nitrogen excretion of an adult is about 1 gram per day, but the actual amount for any individual depends on the efficiency of digestion and absorption, and possibly also on the specific dietary proteins consumed. Persons with malabsorptive disorders will have increased levels of nitrogen in the feces.

Nitrogen is also lost from the skin, principally in sloughed-off epidermal cells, in lost hair and nails, and in perspiration. Small as these contributions to overall nitrogen losses may be, they are not insignificant. In fact, profuse sweating can increase nitrogen loss substantially. However, with acclimatization to a warm environment, such losses are reduced. Loss of blood through hemorrhage will also add to nitrogen loss and may even be heavy enough to place an individual in negative nitrogen balance, in which nitrogen loss exceeds intake.

Protein Quality

Early in the twentieth century, a series of classic experiments led to the development of the concept of *protein quality*, which is an important factor in determining protein requirements. Studies with growing rats showed that growth, as measured in weight gain, was supported by the milk protein casein but not by wheat protein, and that an actual loss of weight resulted when the corn protein zein was the sole dietary protein. Further investigations made it clear that the differences in ability of these proteins to support growth were due to differences in their amino acid composition. A number of indices have since been developed for measuring protein quality, several of which are based on the nitrogen balance principle.

BIOLOGICAL VALUE.   Biological value is an index of protein quality that reflects the percentage of absorbed nitrogen from dietary protein actually utilized (retained) by the body, measured under standard conditions. The derived figure is an estimate of the adequacy of a given protein to meet body needs. The basic formula for biological value is

$$BV = \frac{N_{retained}}{N_{absorbed}} \times 100.$$

To determine the biological value of a given protein food source, that food must be fed (usually to rats) exclusively during the test period. Nitrogen content of diet, urine, and feces is measured, and numerical values are derived for use with the following equivalent formula:

$$BV = \frac{Dietary\ N - (Urinary\ N + Fecal\ N)}{Dietary\ N - Fecal\ N} \times 100$$

The greater the proportion of nitrogen retained, the higher the biological value (BV), or quality, of the protein being tested. Protein foods containing optimal quantities and proportions of all the essential amino acids, as well as adequate supplies of nonessential amino acids, will have the highest biological values. Eggs, for example, top the list with a biological value ranging from 87 to 97, a near-perfect score; cow's milk, at 85 to 90, is a close second. Note that these are animal protein sources; no plant protein even approaches these values, although rice and tofu, a soybean product, have biological values of 75. But with the exception of gelatin, no animal protein has a BV lower than 72. Generally speaking, and provided that caloric intake is adequate to meet energy needs, proteins with a biological value of 70 or more are capable of supporting growth.

When a diet consisting of mixed proteins is analyzed, the biological value of the mixture is usually greater than the average of the biological values of its component proteins. This complementary effect is due to the fact that particular amino acid deficiencies in one protein source are often made up by another source, thus increasing the usefulness of the otherwise "incomplete" proteins to the body.

The timing of ingestion is crucial to this synergistic effect of mixed proteins. Because tissues must have all the necessary amino acids present at the same time for protein synthesis to occur, complementary proteins should be eaten in the same meal for optimal effect. Otherwise, some dietary amino acids will be wasted, since an excess of one kind absorbed at a given time cannot be held over for use at a later time.

NET PROTEIN UTILIZATION.   Even the best mix of amino acids will be less available for use if it is packaged in a protein that is only partially digested. **Net protein utilization (NPU)** is an index that takes into account the relative digestibility of proteins. It is, simply, biological value multiplied by digestibility, expressed as a percent; NPU is determined by the following formulas:

$$NPU = \frac{N_{retained}}{Dietary\ N} \times 100$$

$$= \frac{Dietary\ N - (Urinary\ N + Fecal\ N)}{Dietary\ N} \times 100$$

Proteins are generally easy to digest, however, most being 90 percent or more digestible. Thus, in most cases, NPU approximates the BV.

PROTEIN EFFICIENCY RATIO. Unlike the indices previously discussed, the protein efficiency ratio (PER) is not based on nitrogen balance studies. For this reason, it is somewhat less precise than BV and NPU, but it is technically easier to derive and use. The protein efficiency ratio is defined as the change in body weight (growth) relative to the amount of protein eaten. It is usually measured in laboratory rats kept under standardized conditions. If a rat receives 2 grams of casein per day as the sole dietary protein in an otherwise standard diet, and gains 5 grams of weight per day, the PER of casein would be determined as 2.5:

$$\text{PER} = \frac{\text{Weight gain in grams}}{\text{Dietary protein in grams}}$$

Whole egg has a PER of 3.8, whereas at the other extreme, gelatin has a PER of 0. PER values are used in labeling foods to show the nutritional value of the protein they contain.

AMINO ACID SCORE. Another index of protein quality, the **chemical score,** is based on chemical analysis, not on a biological test. It compares the content of essential amino acids in a protein or protein mixture with that found in a standard reference protein, defined by the FAO/WHO (Table 4–6). The amino acid score is determined by the following formula:

$$\frac{\text{Amino acid}}{\text{score}} = \frac{\text{Milligrams of amino acid per gram of test protein}}{\text{Milligrams of amino acid per gram of reference protein}} \times 100$$

The score of the test protein is determined by the amino acid that is lowest in proportion to its amount in the reference protein. In soybeans, for example, the sulfur-containing amino acids methionine and cystine are the essential amino acids present in the smallest proportion to their level in the reference protein. Since soybean protein has only 74 percent as much of these amino acids as the reference protein, the amino acid score of soybean protein is 74. The sulfur-containing amino acids are then the limiting amino acids in soybean protein. Generally, lysine, threonine, and the sulfur-containing amino acids are the limiting amino acids in most foods. Measurement of protein quality by this method corresponds quite well to biological testing methods, emphasizing the accuracy and usefulness of all these indices.

TABLE 4-6. *Provisional Amino Acid Scoring Pattern*

Amino Acid	Suggested Level mg 1 gr Protein
Isoleucine	40
Leucine	70
Lysine	55
Methionine + cystine	35
Phenylalanine + tyrosine	60
Threonine	40
Tryptophan	10
Valine	50
Total	360

Source: FAO Nutrition Report Series No. 52, *Energy and protein requirements*, WHO Technical Report Series No. 522 (Rome: Food and Agricultural Organization, 1973), p. 63.

The significance of this concept of limiting amino acids was demonstrated when rats, whose growth had halted when they were fed on wheat protein, resumed growing when they were given supplementary lysine. Lysine is the limiting amino acid in wheat protein; supplementary amounts enabled the rats to make greater use of the other amino acids in the wheat protein. Similar results were observed when rats fed on corn protein were provided with a lysine and tryptophan supplement. Here, then, is experimental evidence for the "all-or-none" amino acid requirement previously discussed at the molecular level. (Remember, if even one of the amino acids required for synthesis of a specific protein molecule is not available in the amino acid pool when it is summoned to the ribosomes by RNA, synthesis of that protein is halted.)

This concept of limiting molecules has a number of practical applications. It is, for example, important in the dietary planning of informed vegetarians. Since every plant-origin food is low in one or more essential amino acids, vegetarians must try at every meal to include foods providing complementary proteins (Figure 4–12). In another application, food engineers are developing special products, such as mixtures of plant proteins in which the limiting amino acid of one protein component is provided by an amino acid found in greater amounts in another. Incaparina is an example of a plant protein food developed especially for child-feeding programs in Guatemala. Such foods provide a high-quality protein mix in a relatively inexpensive and easily stored form, making them as nutritious but less expensive and more readily available than animal food sources.

There have been other attempts to increase the chemical scores of foods, especially plant foods. Agricultural research has, for example, already produced new strains of wheat with increased levels of lysine and tryptophan (the limiting amino acids in traditional varieties). Direct fortification of wheat flour with lysine has also been practiced in some developing countries.

Protein-enriched products are also appearing on supermarket shelves in the United States. One recent addition is a wheat-and-soy-flour spaghetti, which also contains corn germ and added lysine. It contains 13 grams of protein per 2-ounce serving (compared to 8 grams in ordinary spaghetti), and the quality of the protein, moreover, is improved by the additional complementary amino acids. It is also more expensive than ordinary spaghetti; in a recent supermarket check, 12 ounces

FIGURE 4-12   *Food Combinations Providing Complementary Proteins.*
Combinations of foods represented in groups connected by arrows should be eaten together.

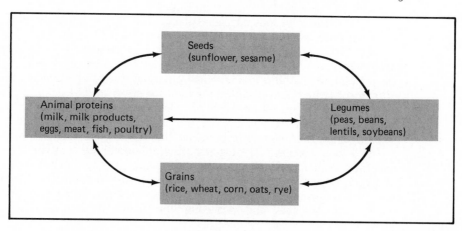

of this product cost as much as 16 ounces of the standard version. However, the new product is being marketed as a meat alternative, and it is notably less expensive per serving than most animal protein sources.

Fortified foods used in conjunction with a generally low protein diet can, however, result in an amino acid imbalance. Experiments with laboratory animals have shown that excesses of certain amino acids can create an increased need for the next most limiting amino acid, leading to diminished appetite, growth failure, and other metabolic abnormalities. That overfortification may have similar effects in humans, while not yet ascertained, should be considered a possibility.

Protein and Amino Acid Requirements

The body's needs for essential amino acids and nitrogen require dietary protein of optimal quality and adequate quantity. Obviously, the bodies of different individuals will have different needs, which are governed by a variety of factors including genetic variation, sex, age, overall health status, and perhaps climate and occupation.

In the first month of life, a stage of rapid growth, infants require at least 2 grams of protein per kilogram of body weight per day. This amount is, of course, provided in milk. Protein requirements fall gradually as the child's growth rate slows, dropping to 1.5 grams per kilogram at six months, and continue falling even more gradually as growth rate slows further.

Pregnancy substantially increases the protein requirement for women, to provide for the growth of the fetus and additional tissues in the mother. Some evidence suggests, furthermore, that efficiency of protein utilization is lowered during pregnancy, thereby increasing the need for dietary sources. During lactation, also, protein needs are markedly increased, since the milk produced by the mother must supply the protein for the infant's growth needs.

Illness and other physiological, and perhaps psychological, stresses lead to increased nitrogen loss and thus increased protein requirements. Profuse sweating increases nitrogen loss and therefore protein requirement and data now suggest that moderate and heavy exercise may result in an increase in the physiological requirement either for specific essential amino acids or for total protein. Since Americans typically consume more protein than required, there is probably no need for a further increase. Any period of nutritional inadequacy, whether from dieting or disaster, will also increase needs for protein, since available supplies will be diverted to energy needs, leaving less for protein functions.

On the basis of various nitrogen balance studies, the basal protein requirement for an average adult male has been estimated at 0.47 grams per kilogram body weight. This figure, however, is not the same as a recommendation or dietary allowance, which must take into account the greater-than-average needs of about half the population. To allow for individual variations, the basal estimate is increased by 30 percent (which also provides a margin for error) to 0.61 g/kg. A correction is also made for 75 percent efficiency of utilization, on the assumption that the average American diet contains protein with average biological values of 75. This results in an adjusted protein recommendation of 0.8 g/kg body weight per day.

For a man weighing 70 kilograms, the protein allowance is thus 56 grams per day; for a woman of 55 kilograms, it is 44 grams per day. Protein allowances have also been issued by the Food and Nutrition Board to cover the special needs of pregnant and lactating women, to distinguish between the needs of males and females at various ages, and to account for greater requirements in the years of

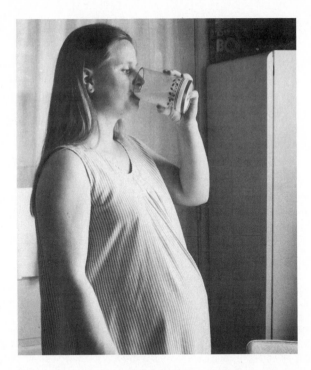

Pregnancy substantially increases the protein requirement for women.
Teri Leigh Stratford

growth (see Appendix, Table A). Generally, these allowances will meet all amino acid needs if at least half the daily intake is high-quality protein which provides all the essential amino acids in optimal balance.

EXCESS AND DEFICIENCY

Excessive intake of proteins, unlike that of other major nutrients, is not a significant dietary hazard for healthy people. A few problems have been noticed, but normal individuals can apparently tolerate large amounts of amino acids as long as all essential amino acids are included in a well-balanced pattern. In an early study, human subjects subsisted exclusively on meat, with intakes of 100 to 140 grams of protein per day, for a year without showing evidence of adverse effects.

High Intake and the Arctic Eskimo

The Eskimo people constitute a particularly interesting natural laboratory for studying the effects of a predominantly protein diet. Traditionally, approximately 82 percent of the protein intake of Eskimos in Alaska was provided by meat and fish alone, with the remainder derived from all other sources; just under a third of total calories were provided by protein. (Lipids accounted for nearly all the remaining energy intake, with carbohydrate making a negligible contribution.) Although these levels were considerably higher than those found in other populations, no adverse effects are associated with this diet pattern.

VEGETARIANISM

There is nothing new about vegetarianism; most of the world's peoples have always derived most of their nourishment from plants. This practice is, however, usually not from choice. Meat has been unobtainable for many people in most of the world throughout history. Even the cave dwellers, often pictured as clubbing mammoths and other beasts, probably ate plants more often than meat, as most primates do.

In the United States, however, some people have turned to a vegetarian diet by choice. A few have been influenced by an interest in Eastern religions such as Hinduism and Buddhism, which emphasize reverence for all life and consequently prohibit the eating of flesh. Others are following the example of certain Western religions; for Trappist monks, for example, vegetarianism is part of their vow of poverty, and for Seventh Day Adventists it is recommended although not required. Other reasons stated by American vegetarians include concern at the wastefulness of feeding grain to animals in order to produce meat; abhorrence at the slaughter of animals; and concern over health issues such as cholesterol and saturated fat intake.

The types of vegetarians are as diverse as their motivations. Some abstain only from red meat, or from red meat and poultry, and continue to eat fish; these people are not really vegetarians at all. Lacto-ovo-vegetarians eat no flesh but consume eggs and dairy products; lacto-vege-tarians consume dairy products but not eggs, and ovo-vegetarians consume eggs but not dairy products. Vegans—strict vegetarians—consume no foods of animal origin at all. Obviously, then, the quality of a vegetarian diet depends heavily on the answer to the question; Which vegetarian diet?

One of the most peculiar (and fortunately least accepted) vegetarian diets ever practiced in the United States is the Zen macrobiotic diet. This program actually consists of ten dietary plans, ranging from fairly well balanced to extremely restricted. At the most restricted level, the foods allowed consist almost solely of brown rice and tea. Even fluid intake is restricted, so that resulting health problems include kidney disease.

Historically, the main nutritional concern about vegetarian diets has been their protein content. People who include animal products of some kind (eggs, dairy products) need not be concerned about protein intake. Strict vegetarians, however, must plan carefully to obtain adequate supplies of proteins—or of essential amino acids, to be precise. Foods of plant origin should be eaten in combinations that provide a balance among lysine, tryptophan, and the sulfur-containing amino acids; these are generally the ones most lacking in foods of plant origin. Legumes, for example, are low in tryptophan and in sulfur-containing amino acids although they are good sources of lysine; nuts, seeds, and

A predominantly meat and fish diet, however, raises concern about calcium, which most populations derive from milk and other dairy products, and which is needed for bone development and maintenance. Apparently Eskimos ingest just enough soft bone and cartilage, especially of fish and sea mammals, to prevent noticeable calcium deficiencies. However, additional concern has been raised about the Eskimo diet because high protein intakes increase urinary calcium loss (see Chapter 8). High rates of bone loss have indeed been observed among older Eskimos in northern Alaska, and there is a good possibility that this condition may be associated with their high protein and relatively low calcium intake.

Surprisingly, the Eskimo have been found, despite their high-protein, high-fat diet, to have normal cholesterol levels. This is attributed to the high levels of polyunsaturated fats in the fish and lean mammals they consume. High excretion levels

most cereal gains are low in lysine but are good sources of tryptophan and sulfur-containing amino acids. Therefore, combinations of foods, such as beans and rice or corn and beans, can provide all the essential amino acids because the different foods complement each other: The shortcomings of each food are offset by the particular amino acid contributions of the other.

Although amino acid intake may not be a problem for most vegetarians, other considerations are often overlooked. Deficiencies of vitamin D, riboflavin, and calcium (especially for children) and iron for women of childbearing age are potential problems. Zinc and iodine deficiencies are possible as well. A particularly serious problem for pure vegetarians is deficiency of vitamin B_{12}, which is found only in animal-origin foods.

Adequate riboflavin, iron, and calcium can be provided by generous servings of most green, leafy vegetables. Zinc can be obtained from nuts, legumes, and wheat germ, and iodine from iodized salt and seaweed. Those vegetarians who use soy sauce and sea salt instead of commercial iodized salt face a potential iodine problem. Fortified soy milk or exposure to sunlight can provide vitamin D. Nuts and seeds, whole grains, dried fruits, and dried beans contribute iron; however women, especially during pregnancy and lactation, should have a supplemental source of this mineral.

On most vegetarian diets, and especially the more strict versions, energy consumption is low. For most adults this is not unhealthful, and may even be an advantage. However, infants and children raised on vegetarian diets may not reach their growth potential. The foods they eat provide a great deal of bulk in proportion to energy and nutrients; with relatively small stomach capacity, infants and children cannot consume the sheer quantity of plant-origin foods they need.

A serious concern for children is vitamin B_{12} deficiency, which can result from a strict vegetarian diet for the child or from breast-feeding by a strict vegetarian mother. In either case, severe anemia, growth retardation, and other major symptoms can develop in the offspring unless supplementation is provided for the pregnant and lactating vegan woman, the infant, or preferably both.

With careful planning to provide adequate amino acids, calcium, riboflavin, iron, and vitamin B_{12} in particular, a vegetarian diet can be safe and may even confer some health benefits by reducing obesity and high cholesterol levels. As with any diet, but especially those limited to plant food sources, diversity is the key to success. When any group of foods is eliminated from the diet, special care must be taken to ensure that nutrient requirements are met from alternate foods.

of nitrogenous wastes from amino acid metabolism are associated with consumption of a great deal of water and are apparently tolerated without difficulty.

Eskimos have been genetically adapted to their traditional diet. However, those who have moved to towns and cities are being exposed to, and are acquiring, some of the food habits of other Americans. Dietary acculturation is accompanied by obesity, cardiovascular diseases, hypertension, and tooth decay—problems all too familiar in the "lower forty-eight" but seldom encountered with the traditional diet.

Most humans are not quite as well adapted to high protein intakes as are Eskimos, and liver and kidney damage can result from prolonged and markedly excessive intakes. This indicates that regulation of a variety of metabolic processes is undermined when those organs must process excessive quantities of amino acids and remove large amounts of nitrogenous wastes. For this reason, too, kidney damage may result from high protein weight-loss diets. Because kidney function is not fully developed in infants, excessive protein intake is not recommended in the early months of life, and high protein foods should be introduced gradually.

Protein Deficiency

Kwashiorkor, the disease resulting from a deficit of protein relative to energy intake, was first noted in Africa and described by Williams and has subsequently been noted in Latin American and Asian populations as well. It was considered of sufficient importance that at its first meeting in 1949, the FAO/WHO Expert Committee on Nutrition called for a study of kwashiorkor etiology in Africa.

Kwashiorkor (the name of the disease is derived from a West African word which means "sickness of the child when a second baby is born") generally appears shortly after weaning. In traditional societies this usually occurs between one and four years of age and is precipitated by the arrival of a new baby who must receive the mother's milk. The young child is suddenly put on a traditional diet, consisting almost exclusively of grains and other high carbohydrate foods. Such a diet provides adequate energy but very little vegetable protein and no animal protein. Kwashiorkor is sometimes found in adults, but children are more frequently afflicted because of their higher protein and energy requirements in proportion to body weight. Adults can generally consume enough rice or other grains to meet their protein needs, but the sheer bulk of such foods necessary to approach the protein needs of children would be simply too much for them to eat.

The first symptoms may well go unnoticed. The child seems listless and loses appetite and may develop a sudden attack of diarrhea or other infection due to lowered resistance. Edema, the accumulation of interstitial fluid, especially in the legs and abdomen, follows shortly, and is often misinterpreted, since the puffiness and apparent weight gain due to fluid retention give the child a healthy and well-fed appearance for a while. Often, the first symptoms noted by the family are the loss of pigmentation in the hair and skin; the loss of some hair itself; and the development of patchy, discolored, and/or sore areas on the body. Clinical symptoms also include decreased amino acid levels in blood plasma, decreased serum albumin, fat accumulation in the liver, decreased production of pancreatic enzymes (which results in malabsorption of what little nourishment is available), and marked retardation of physical and mental growth, along with increased susceptibility to infection.

The interaction of malnutrition and infection is synergistic. Even a moderate protein shortage weakens the body's resistance. Infection, in turn, increases the need for protein and thus sets up a vicious cycle in which the protein deficit is even greater and malnutrition more severe, causing the individual to deteriorate more rapidly. In many cultures, this interaction is aggravated by the belief that food should be withheld when a person, and particularly a child, is ill. Usually infection, and not specific symptoms of kwashiorkor, leads to the child being brought for treatment.

If recognized at an early stage, kwashiorkor responds readily to feedings of skim milk and other animal protein sources, with vegetables and fat added gradually. At the beginning of treatment, only 2 to 3 grams of protein and 61 kilocalories per kilogram body weight are given, increasing to 6 or 7 grams protein and 100 to 120 kilocalories per kilogram of body weight within 10 days to 2 weeks. In advanced

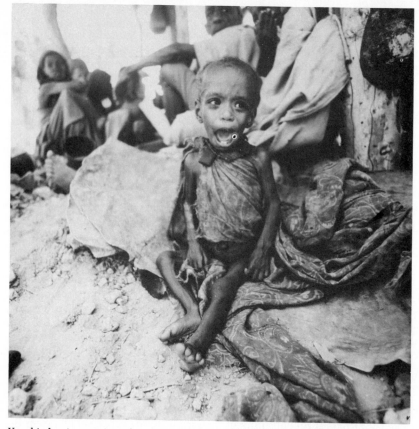

Kwashiorkor is sometimes found in adults, but children are more frequently afflicted because of their higher protein and energy requirements in proportion to body weight.
United Nations

cases, however, irreversible damage, especially to growth and the digestive system, may have already occurred. Even when treatment has been successful, the child is most likely to return home to the same inadequate diet that caused the condition in the first place, so that relapse within a matter of months is common. Mortality following repeated episodes of kwashiorkor is high.

Kwashiorkor is now being considered as only one form of protein-energy malnutrition (PEM). Another form is marasmus, the disease condition reflecting deficits of energy and caused by a generally inadequate food supply; it will be discussed in Chapter 14.

Recently, the incidence of kwashiorkor has increased in populations that have accepted bottled formula instead of mother's milk for infant feeding. Because of poverty, inadequate amounts of formula are extended with plain water (which is often unsanitary as well), and the infant receives fewer, rather than more, nutrients.

In the United States and other developed countries, kwashiorkor is rare. Occasional instances, however, have been reported. When milk was removed from the diets of two infants in Cleveland, typical symptoms of kwashiorkor developed. In both cases, misconceptions on the part of the mothers were the cause. Both infants responded to appropriate therapy, and the mothers were instructed in the importance of milk. Because American physicians are generally unfamiliar with this syndrome, and are unlikely, because of its rarity, to suspect the absence of milk from an infant's diet, diagnosis is likely to be delayed.

Although protein deficiency is rare in the United States, certain subgroups— pregnant and lactating women of low socioeconomic levels and their children, elderly persons on limited budgets, the chronically ill—may have subclinical protein deficiencies and serum levels may be low because of suboptimal intakes. Certainly the social, economic, educational, and other factors responsible for such instances should be corrected. But American protein intake is typically higher, not lower, than allowances.

TRENDS IN U.S. PROTEIN CONSUMPTION

The protein content of the American diet has remained essentially the same for most of this century, but the sources of that protein have changed considerably. The most striking changes over time are the increase in meat consumption and the decrease in the consumption of flour and cereal grains which formerly provided fully half of our protein intake. In recent years, vegetarianism has become increasingly popular. Further, many individuals concerned about their health are changing their dietary habits to include more fruits, vegetables, grains, and smaller servings of meat. This trend should be reflected soon in consumption figures. Overall, protein consumption has not varied much over the years, with little difference between the 1910 and 1980 figures of 102 and 105 grams per person per day. Meat, eggs, and dairy foods account for almost 70 percent of the protein we consume.

Exact figures on consumption of various foods vary depending on the source of information. Most information is based on consumption statistics which are derived from "disappearance data" (discussed in Chapter 2) which tally the sources available in the marketplace, but may not accurately reflect actual consumption. Consumption of beef, pork, veal, lamb, and game meats increased to a high of 163.6 pounds per person per year in 1970 (see Table 4–7). Since that time, the trend is downward so that in 1984 the figure was 153.6 pounds per person per year. In contrast, the consumption of poultry has risen steadily from 25.1 pounds per

TABLE 4-7. *Changes in consumption of the major sources of protein in the U.S. diet. Values are given as pounds per person per year for meat, poultry, fish, and yogurt; quarts per person per year for milks; and number per person per year for eggs.*

	1950	1960	1970	1980	1984
Meat*	138	147	164	158	154
Poultry	25	35	49	61	68
Fish	14	13	15	15	16
Whole milk	—	117	99	67	61
Lowfat and skim milk	—	6	20	39	41
Yogurt	—	.26	.86	2.67	3.18
Eggs	378	324	300	264	252

* Includes beef, pork, veal, lamb/mutton, and game meat.
Source: A Special Report: America's Changing Diet. *FDA Consumer*, October, 1985.

person per year in 1950 to 67.5 in 1984. After decreasing somewhat in the mid-fifties to mid-sixties, fish consumption reached a high of 15.5 pounds per person per year in 1984.

Reasons for this strong trend are not hard to find. Meat in general, and beef in particular, have always been viewed as "status" foods, and increased protein, meat, and beef consumption have been observed to accompany increased prosperity in virtually all times and places. Americans are not alone in this trend; meat consumption in Taiwan and South Korea has doubled in the past 20 years, and in Japan it has increased ninefold. Increased meat consumption is everywhere associated with improved economic conditions, suggesting that any people able to afford a high-meat diet will eat one.

But in some ways the American emphasis on beef is unique. From the time the continent was opened up for settlement, cattle raising has been a dominant force both in folklore (with its songs and stories concerning cowboys and life "on the lone prairie") and as big business. Increased industrialization of every aspect of meat production, from cattle breeding to chicken plucking, along with improved marketing practices, greatly increased availability. The more recent "fast-food"

FIGURE 4-13   *Consumption Trends for Primary Sources of Protein in the American Diet.*

Source: Adapted from L. Brewster and M. Jacobson, *The Changing American Diet* (Washington, D.C.: Center for Science in the Public Interest, 1978).

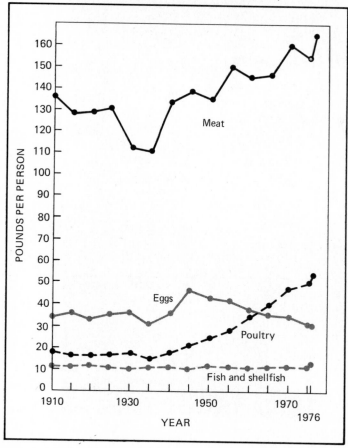

phenomenon, with its emphasis on burgers and fried chicken, has made ever more animal protein available on every street and superhighway. To these influences must be added those which at the same time decreased our consumption of plant sources of protein: disappearance of the small farm and home vegetable garden, the decline in home baking and other time-consuming methods of food preparation. With the increased availability of frozen vegetables, consumption began to increase modestly and now with the emphasis on nutrition and health there is increased consumption of fresh vegetables. Potatoes are now frequently part of our diet as fries or chips (3.9 billion pounds of potatoes ended up as frozen french fries in 1984). Fresh potato use may be boosted with increased use of microwave ovens which turn out a baked potato in minutes instead of an hour.

Meat is a nutrient dense food. One 3 ounce serving will supply nearly half the protein, 60 percent of the vitamin B_{12}, 30 percent of the zinc, 20 percent of the iron, and 20 percent of the niacin needed by a 23 to 50-year-old man. As well as being a source of iron, meat will improve the absorption of nonheme iron from

American emphasis on beef is unique, as evidenced by the popularity of the backyard barbecue.

Peter Menzel/Stock, Boston

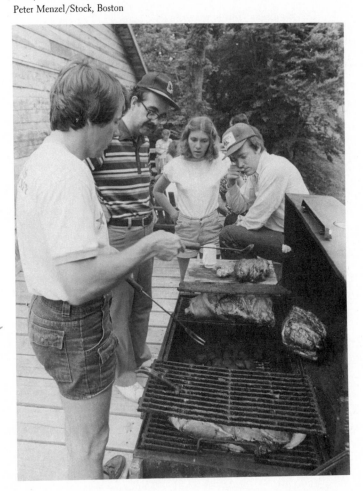

other sources. While not the only way to supply all needed nutrients, a serving of meat goes a long way toward meeting our needs.

Although the cost of beef and most other meats and fish is high, top quality proteins are available. We in the United States are far from being a protein-malnourished nation. In several studies it has been shown that even most low-income individuals consume well over the RDAs for protein. Among the few exceptions are some low-income teenage girls, pregnant and lactating women, and elderly men and women, in all of whom moderate (not major) protein deficits are related to suboptimal food intake generally. Although all such individuals would benefit from increasing their total food consumption, hardly anyone in the United States would benefit from protein supplements. Misconceptions are at the root of what has been called the "protein mystique" that would make everything, from baby food to snack food, "high protein."

Although the cost of beef and most other meats and fish is high and going higher, top-quality proteins are available at reasonable prices for most people. Eggs, beef liver, beans, peanut butter, American cheese, chicken, and dry milk are all protein "bargains." Since four servings of such foods would meet daily protein requirements for just about everyone, a good supply of dietary protein can be had for less than a dollar a day.

SUMMARY

Proteins, the largest and most complex molecules known, are organic compounds that always contain carbon, hydrogen, oxygen, and nitrogen; frequently they contain sulfur, phosphorus, and/or other elements as well.

Proteins are catalysts (enzymes) and regulators (hormones) of body processes; they are antibodies; they are components of the body's structure itself (cartilage, skin, nails, hair), of skeletal muscle, and of substances in the blood. Proteins are required for growth and for maintenance of all tissues.

Protein molecules consist of subunits, the amino acids, which are linked together by peptide bonds. All amino acids have an amino (NH_2) group; a radical (R) group, which differs for each and gives each its distinctive properties; and a carboxyl (COOH) group. Twenty-two amino acids are found in foods; a few others, not present in foods, are synthesized in the body from other amino acids. Many of those found in foods can be synthesized as well. These are the nonessential amino acids. Essential amino acids are those that cannot be synthesized in the body, or cannot be synthesized in adequate amounts, and so must be supplied in adequate amounts from dietary sources.

Complete proteins provide all the essential amino acids in optimal amounts; incomplete proteins generally contain a smaller amount of some of these. Most foods of animal origin contain complete proteins, but foods of plant origin have incomplete proteins and should be consumed in combinations that will make up for the amino acid deficiencies.

During digestion and absorption, the peptide bonds joining amino acids are hydrolyzed by various enzymes from the stomach, pancreas, and small intestine.

Amino acids are used in construction of the protein molecules needed by the body. This process of protein synthesis is programmed by hereditary material in DNA, a component of all cell nuclei. Actual protein synthesis takes place outside the cell nucleus, in bodies known as ribosomes. Protein synthesis is exceedingly complex and is regulated at several stages by various hormones. It also requires energy. As much as 300 grams of protein may be synthesized, as well as degraded, daily in the body of an adult.

When carbohydrate and fat intake or reserves are inadequate for energy needs, proteins can be utilized instead. Amino acids not needed for body processes are generally metabolized to fat for storage. Some amino acids can be converted to glucose by the process of gluconeogenesis. Carbon skeletons for these conversions are derived from deamination of amino acids, which produces nitrogenous waste in the form of ammonia.

The liver removes ammonia, which is highly toxic, from circulation and converts it to urea, which is ultimately excreted in the urine. Protein synthesis and protein breakdown are always in dynamic equilibrium or balance, depending on the needs of the individual at any given time.

Protein requirements are greatest in infancy, a period of rapid growth, at 2 grams per kilogram of body weight per day. Requirements fall gradually as growth slows and then ceases in adulthood; for average adult males it is estimated at 0.47 g/kg body weight per day. Intake recommendations, set higher to allow for individual variation and inefficiency of utilization, are 0.8 g/kg, or 56 grams per day for the reference adult man, 44 grams per day for the reference adult woman.

Kwashiorkor is a protein deficiency disease, first described in Africa in 1935, that may occur despite adequate energy intake. It typically occurs in very young children who have been suddenly weaned and placed on a predominantly starchy diet.

Protein consumption in the United States has not changed significantly in this century, averaging in the neighborhood of 100 grams per person per day. There has been a marked increase in the amount of protein derived from animal sources, especially beef, and a corresponding decrease in the amount from grains and cereals. Increased meat consumption is apparently correlated with increased affluence, since it occurs in other developed nations as well.

Vegetarianism has become increasingly popular in recent years. Those vegetarians who consume no foods of animal origin at all should choose from vegetable foods providing complementary amino acids and eat a variety of foods. Supplementation, particularly of vitamin B_{12}, soy milk fortified with vitamin D for children, and supplemental iron for pregnant and lactating women are advisable for strict vegetarians. Vegetarians who consume some animal protein in the form of fish, eggs, and/or dairy products are probably not at nutritional risk.

BIBLIOGRAPHY

BALLARD, F.J. and J.M. GUNN. Nutritional and hormonal effects on intracellular protein catabolism. *Nutritional Reviews* 40:33–42, 1982.

BARNES, L.A. Nutritional aspects of vegetarianism, health foods, and fad diets. *Nutrition Reviews*, 35:153, 1977.

BRIGGS, G.M. Muscle foods and human health. *Food Technology*, February, 1985, 54–57.

BROCK, J.F., and M. AUTRET. Kwashiorkor in Africa. *Bulletin of the World Health Organization* 5:1, 1952.

BROWN, P.T., and J.G. BERGAN. The dietary status of "new" vegetarians. *Journal of the American Dietetic Association* 67:455, 1975.

CARPENTER, K.J. Individual amino acid levels and bioavailability. In C.E. Bodwell, J.S. Adkins, and D.T. Hopkins, eds., *Protein Quality In Humans: Assessment and In Vitro Estimation.* Westport, CT: AVI Publishing, 1981, pp. 239–259.

CHOPRA, J.G., A.L. FORBES, and J.P. HABICHT. Protein the U.S. diet. *Journal of the American Dietetic Association* 72:253, 1978.

CHUNG, Y.C., Y.S. KIM, A. SHADCHEHR, A. GARRIDO, I.L. MACGREGOR, AND M.H. SLEISENGER. Protein digestion and absorption in human small intestine. *Gastroenterol.* 76:1415–1421, 1979.

CLARK, H.E., M.A. KOLLENLARK, and J.D. HALVORSON. Ability of 6 grams of nitrogen from a combination of rice, wheat, and milk to meet protein requirements of young men for 4 weeks. *American Journal of Clinical Nutrition* 31:585, 1978.

CROSBY, W.H. Can a vegetarian be well nourished? *Journal of the American Medical Association* 233:898, 1975.

DRAPER, H.H. The aboriginal Eskimo diet in modern perspective. *American Anthropologist* 79:309, 1977.

DUBRICK, M.A. Dietary supplements and health aids—a critical evaluation. Part 2—Macronutrients and fiber. *Journal of Nutritional Education* 15:88–92, 1983.

DWYER, J.T., R. PALUMBO, H. THORNE, I. VALADIAN, and R.B. REED. Preschoolers on alternate life-style diets. *Journal of the American Dietetic Association* 72:264, 1978.

Food and Agricultural Organization/World Health Organization. *Energy and protein requirements.* Rome: FAO, 1983.

FORD, J.E. Microbiological methods for protein quality assessment. In C.E. Bodwell, J.S. Adkins, and D.T. Hopkins, eds., Westport, CT: AVI Publishing, 1981.

FREEMAN, H.J. and Y.S. KIM. Digestion and absorption of protein. *Annual Review of Medicine* 29:99–116, 1978.

GAULL, G.J., J.A. STURMAN, and N.C.R. RAIHA. Development of mammalian sulphur metabolism: Absence of cystathionase in human fetal tissues. *Pediatric Research* 6:538, 1972.

GERSOVITZ, M., D. BIER, D. MATTHEWS, J. UDALL, H.N. MUNRO, and V.R. YOUNG. Dynamic aspects of whole body glycine metabolism: influence of protein intake in young adult and elderly males. *Metabolism* 29:1087–1094, 1980.

HARPER, A.E. Amino acids of nutritional importance. In Committee on Food Protection, Food and Nutritional Board, National Research Council, eds. *Toxicants Occurring Naturally In Foods*, 2nd ed. Washington, DC: National Research Council, 1973.

HELLER C.A., and E.M. SCOTT. The Alaska dietary survey (1956–1961). *Public Health Service Publication No. 999-AH-2.* Anchorage: U.S. Department of Health, Education, and Welfare, Arctic Health Research Center, 1967.

HIGGINBOTTOM, C.C., L. SEETMAN, and W.I. NYHAN. A syndrome of methylmalonic aciduria, homocystinuria, megaloblastic anemia and neurologic abnormalities in a vitamin B_{12} deficient breast-fed infant of a strict vegetarian. *New England Journal of Medicine* 299:317, 1978.

HOLTZMAN, N.A., D.W. WELCHER, and E.E. MELLITS. Termination of restricted diet in children with PKU: A randomized controlled study. *New England Journal of Medicine* 293:1121, 1975.

HOPKINS, L.L., and G.W. THOMAS. The nutritional aspects of animal protein consumption. *Nutrition Today* 19:6–14, 1984.

KOPPLE, J.D., and M.E. SWENDSEID. Evidence that histidine is an essential amino acid in normal and chronically uremic men. *Journal of Clinical Investigation* 55:881, 1975.

KREIL, G. Transfer of proteins across membranes. *Annual Review of Biochemistry.* 50:317–348, 1981.

LAPPE, F.M. *Diet For a Small Planet,* rev. ed. New York: Ballantine, 1975.

LECOS, C. FISH and fowl lure consumers from red meat. *FDA Consumer*, October, 1985, pp. 19–21.

LEWIS, H.B. Fifty years of study of the role of protein in nutrition. *Journal of the American Dietetic Association* 28:701, 1952.

LOZY, E., and D.M. HEGSTED. Calculations of the amino acid requirements of children at different ages by a factorial method. *American Journal of Clinical Nutrition* 28:1052, 1975.

LUNN, P.G. and A. AUSTIN. Dietary manipulation of plasma albumin concentration. *Journal of Nutrition* 113;1791–1802, 1983.

MILLWARD, D.J., J.C. BATES, J.G. BROWN, S.R. ROSOCHACKI, and M.J. RENNIE. Anabolic stimulation of protein breakdown related to remodeling. In *Protein Degradation in Health and Disease.* (Ciba Foundation 75), Excerpta Medica, Amsterdam, 1980, pp. 307–329.

MITCH, W.E. The influence of diet on the progression of renal insufficiency. *Annual Review of Medicine* 35:249–264, 1984.

MUNCK, B.G. Intestinal absorption of amino acids. In L.R. Johnson, ed., *Physiology of the Gastrointestinal Tract*, Vol. 2. New York: Raven Press 1981, pp. 1097–1122.

Munro, H.N. and V.R. Young. Protein metabolism and requirements. In A.N. Exton-Smith and F.I. Caird, eds, *Metabolic and Nutritional Disorders in the Elderly.* 1980.

National Academy of Sciences, Food and Nutrition Board. Recommended dietary allowances, 9th ed. Washington, DC: National Academy of Sciences, 1985.

Nutrition Reviews. Human protein deficiency—Biological changes and functional implications. Vol. 35:294, 1977.

PELLET, P.L., and V.R. YOUNG, eds. *Nutritional Evaluation of Protein Foods.* (WHTR-3/UNUP 129). Tokyo: United Nations University, 1981.

PLANTE, R.I., and M.E. HOUSTON. Exercise and protein catabolism in women. *American Nutrition Metabolism.* 28:123–129, 1984.

RADOS, B. Eggs and dairy foods: Dietary mainstays in decline. *FDA Consumer* October, 1985, pp. 11–17.

RAND, W.M., N.S. SCRIMSHAW, and V.R. YOUNG. Determination of protein allowances in human adults from nitrogen balance data. *American Journal of Clinical Nutrition* 30:1129, 1977.

RAND, W.M., N.S. SCRIMSHAW, and V.R.

YOUNG. Retrospective analysis of data from five long-term, metabolic balance studies: Implications for understanding dietary nitrogen and energy utilization. *American Journal of Clinical Nutrition* 42:1339–1350, 1985.

ROSE, W.C. Amino Acid requirements of man. Federation Proceedings 8:546, 1949.

SATTERLEE, L.D., H.F. MARSHALL, and J.M. TENNYSON. Measuring protein quality. *Journal of American Oil Chemistry Society*, 56:103–109, 1979.

SCRIMSHAW, N.S. Through a glass darkly: Discerning the practical implications of human protein-energy interrelationships. *Nutrition Reviews* 35:321, 1977.

SILK, D.B.A., Digestion and absorption of dietary protein in man. Proc. Nutr. Soc. 39:61–70, 1980.

STANBURY, J.B., D. FREDRICKSON, and J.F. WYNGAARDEN, eds. *Metabolic Basis of Inherited Disease*, 4th ed. New York: McGraw-Hill, 1978.

STERN, T.P., M.D. SCHLUTER, and C.E. DIAMOND. Nutrition, protein turnover, and physical activity in young women. *American Journal of Clinical Nutrition* 38:223–228, 1983.

VYHMEISTER, I.B., U.D. REGISTER, and L.M. SONNENBERG, Safe vegetarian diets for children. *Pediatric Clinics of North America* 24(1):203, 1977.

WIEBE, S.L., V.M. BRUCE, and B.E. McDONALD. A comparison of the effect of diets containing beef protein and plant proteins on blood lipids of healthy young men. *American Journal of Clinical Nutrition* 40:982–989, 1984.

WILLIAMS, C.D. KWASHIORKOR: A nutritional disease of children associated with a maize diet. *Lancet* 2:1151, 1935.

YOUNG, V.R. Protein metabolism and nutritional state in man. Proc. Nutr. Soc. 30:343–359, 1981.

YOUNG, V.R., W.P. STEFFEE, P.B. PENCHARZ, J.C. WINTERER, and N.S. SCRIMSHAW. Total human body protein synthesis in relation to protein requirements at various ages. *Nature* 253;192, 1975.

YOUNG, V.R. and B. TORUN. Physical activity: Impact on protein and amino acid metabolism and implications for nutritional requirements. In *Nutrition in Health and Disease and International Development*. New York: Alan R. Liss, 1981. pp. 57–85.

YU, Y.M., R.D. YANG, D.E. MATTHEWS, Z.M. WEN, J.F. BURKE, D.M. BIER and V.R. Young. Quantitative aspects of glycine and alanine nitrogen metabolism in postabsorptive young men: Effects of level of nitrogen and dispensable amino acid intake. *Journal of Nutrition* 115:399–410, 1985.

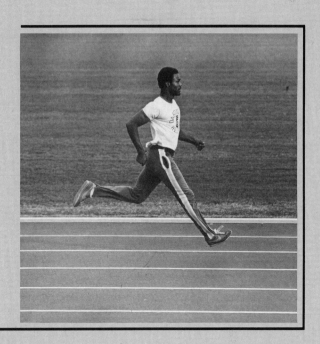

Chapter 5

ENERGY BALANCE

We need energy from nutrients for running or pulling ourselves up from a chair or making any other movement, just as a car needs gasoline to move. Similarly, we need energy while we are sitting, sleeping, or flopping on the sofa watching television, just as the car uses gasoline even while idling. But there the similarity of the body to a machine ends: If a machine is turned off completely it can be started again later, but if we stop using energy for long, we die or are irreparably damaged.

Our energy needs differ from the needs of a machine for several reasons. First, we are homeothermic (warm-blooded) animals and must, therefore constantly transform the chemical energy of nutrient molecules to heat energy to maintain our bodies at optimal temperature for the biochemical reactions occurring in our internal environments.

Second, our parts—the atoms and molecules of which our cells are made—must continuously be replaced to keep pace with the rates of their breakdown and excretion. We accomplish this replenishment only through the energy-requiring process of converting nutrients from the environment into our own cellular materials.

Third, to become adults and perpetuate our species, we must synthesize enough new material to grow to adulthood and then to support growth of the fetus and infant during pregnancy and lactation.

Compared to us, then, the car has an easy time of it. It needs energy only to move and to idle, not to keep itself warm, build and repair its own parts, or produce new little cars.

ENERGY: FORMS AND MEASUREMENT

Energy is defined as the capacity to do work. Although different aspects of this capacity are emphasized in the study of physics, chemistry, and nutrition, the essential meaning of the term is the same in all sciences.

In common usage, however, the term *energy* generally, and incorrectly, refers to enthusiasm, an inclination to be active, high spirits, and similar psychological phenomena. Thus we read of diets that are supposed to be "low in calories but high in energy," and people sometimes complain that they just "have no energy." In view of the facts that calories *are* units of energy and that absence of energy produces almost immediate death, we can see the error of equating energy with "feeling energetic."

Energy Transformations

The concept of energy as a capacity may seem somewhat abstract. However, although we can't actually see a capacity, we can see work being done, the result of energy being expended. In the work process, energy doesn't get used up and then vanish; it is transformed. Electrical energy, for example, can be changed into light and heat; just look at and touch a light bulb. The first law of thermodynamics states this well-known fact succinctly: Energy can neither be created nor destroyed. Thus, energy can be thought of as constituting a vast, eternal cycle.

The central point of the energy cycle on our planet is the sun. The sun shines on growing plants, which by the process of photosynthesis, use solar energy to convert carbon dioxide from the air and water from the soil to glucose. Carbohydrate is stored by the plants, along with other substances synthesized by the plant or taken up from the soil and air. Animals, including humans, consume the plants and thus obtain nutrients that will provide the energy required for their own life processes.

The energy provided by plant and animal foodstuffs is called *potential* energy; until it is actually used for work, it exists in storage form. Potential energy must be transformed by metabolic reactions before it can do work in the body. It is changed into several different kinds of working energy: electrical for conduction of nerve impulses, mechanical for muscle contraction and movement, chemical for anabolism and catabolism, and heat for maintenance of normal body temperature.

Energy released from the body in these various forms must be replaced. We rely, therefore, on the potential energy supplied by food for the continual replacement of energy utilized by our cells and tissues. When the amount of energy supplied is equal to the amount of energy expended in physiological processes, *equilibrium* is achieved; the organism is in a state of energy balance. If the energy supplied by foods exceeds that which is utilized, however, potential energy is stored by the body, primarily as fat; this is a *positive* energy state. Conversely, when utilization exceeds supply, potential energy is released from storage sites and transformed into the energy forms required by the body; this is a *negative* energy state.

Units of Measurement

Nutritional scientists measure energy as heat, a concept that reflects energy oxidation within the body. The traditional unit of heat measurement is the kilocalorie (Calorie, kcal). A **kilocalorie** is defined as the amount of heat required to raise the temperature of 1 kilogram (kg) of water by 1°C (generally measured from 15°C to 16°C).

The preeminence of the kilocalorie was challenged by the Seventh International Congress of Nutrition in 1969 and by the American Institute of Nutrition in 1970. These groups recommended the adoption of a different standard, the *joule*, the nonheat unit of energy measurement in the metric system. This change would bring nutritional terminology into accord with the measurements used in physics, chemistry, and the other disciplines on which the basic principles of nutrition are founded.

The metric system, which is the international measurement terminology of science, includes several similar units for specific kinds of energy: the ampere (A) for electric current, the kelvin (K) for thermodynamic temperature, and the candela (cd) for light intensity. These, along with the more familiar meter (m) for length, kilogram (kg) for mass, and second (s) for time, serve as the bases from which all other metric units are derived. By definition, a **joule** is the amount of energy expended when 1 kilogram is moved a distance of 1 meter by a force of 1 newton. By this definition, energy is a force, quite different from the concept of the kilocalorie, which expresses energy only in terms of one of its forms, heat. In metric terms, the joule is the *mechanical* (that is, work-producing) equivalent of heat.

Even though converting traditional caloric measurements into their metric equivalents may be cumbersome, nutritionists recognize that failure to follow universally accepted scientific terminology would isolate the nutritional sciences from advances in related fields. In fact, the mathematical conversion of kilocalories to kilojoules is not complex. One kilocalorie is equivalent to 4,184 joules (J), or 4.184 kilojoules (kJ), where 1,000 J = 1 kJ. Thus, the conversion of kilocalories to kJ involves multiplication of the value of kilocalories by 4.184 or, more speedily but a little less precisely, by 4.2.

Despite the ease of mathematical conversion, practical and psychological problems remain. Tables of food composition listing energy content of various foods and tables of energy requirements, now expressed in kilocalories, must be revised. To make the transition easier, journals and other publications for the specialist use the familiar nonmetric units, with their metric equivalents in parentheses; for example, "55 kcal (230 kJ)." In the future, the sequence will be reversed: "230 kJ (55 kcal)," and eventually the values will be given only in kilojoules.

Energy Value of Foods

The change from kilocalories to kilojoules will not change the methods by which food energy values are determined. The most common method involves the use of a **bomb calorimeter**, a device that determines the amount of heat produced after a dried, weighed sample of food is oxidized. The food sample is placed within the well-insulated bomb, which is then filled with pure oxygen and placed in a measured quantity of water. The sample is ignited by an electrical spark, and the temperature increase in the surrounding water is measured. Because the quantity of heat needed to raise the temperature of a given volume of water is known, the energy value of the food (its heat of combustion) can be calculated. The energy values determined by burning 1 gram of pure protein, carbohydrate, and fat are shown in the first column of Table 5–1.

Values for ethanol, commonly known as grain alcohol, are also included in this table. Ethanol, the "active" ingredient in alcoholic beverages, is metabolized primarily in the liver by the enzymes ethanol dehydrogenase and acetaldehyde dehydrogenase, both of which require a cofactor containing the vitamin niacin (Figure 5–1). Further oxidation of acetaldehyde via acetyl CoA proceeds through the Krebs cycle. Ethanol, although consumed primarily for its effect as a drug, contributes significantly to total energy intake in many individuals.

Ethanol does not require digestion and is very efficiently absorbed from the stomach and the rest of the gastrointestinal tract. This fact is reflected in the 100 percent coefficient digestibility of ethanol, listed in the second column of Table 5–1. The coefficient of digestibility is used to correct for the less than 100 percent efficiency of digestion and absorption of most nutrients, which is ultimately reflected as production of less energy in the body than in the bomb calorimeter.

The energy value of dietary protein must be corrected for a factor in addition to digestibility. Pure protein is completely oxidized in the calorimeter. In the human body, however, the urea and other nitrogenous wastes produced by amino acid ca-

TABLE 5-1. *Estimation of Physiological Fuel Value*

	Heat of Combustion kcal/g	Coefficient of Digestibility %	Urinary Loss kcal/g	PHYSIOLOGICAL FUEL VALUE	
				kcal/g[a]	kJ/g[b]
Protein	5.6	92	1.25	4	17
Carbohydrate	4.1	99	—	4	17
Fat	9.4	95	—	9	38
Ethanol	7.1	100	negligible	7	29

Note: The use of the physiological fuel value (also known as the Atwater coefficient) tends to overestimate the number of Calories that can be obtained from foods containing large amounts of undigestible carbohydrate (dietary fiber). Newer tables of food composition also consider the fact that different proteins contain different percentages of nitrogen, rather than the 16 percent that was generally assumed in the past. Appropriate correction factors have been applied in recent tables.
[a] Heat of Combustion × Coefficient of Digestibility − Urinary Loss
[b] Calculated as kcal/g × 4.2 = kJ/g

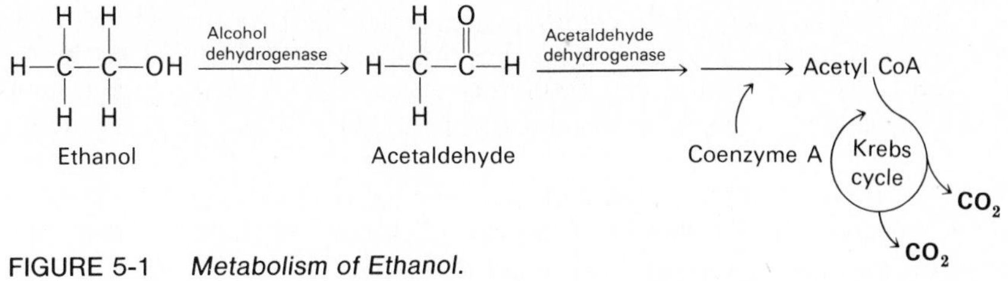

FIGURE 5-1   *Metabolism of Ethanol.*

tabolism are not converted to energy; thus, they represent a loss of part of the total energy value of consumed protein-containing food. This appears in Table 5–1 as a urinary loss of 1.25 kcal per gram of protein. The *actual* physiological fuel values (Atwater coefficients) of the energy-producing nutrients are the familiar 4 kcal/g of carbohydrate and protein, 9 kcal/g of fat, and 7 kcal/g of ethanol.

To calculate the approximate energy value of each of the foods we eat, nutritionists determine its percentage composition of carbohydrate, protein, fat, and ethanol and then multiply by the appropriate Atwater coefficients. Since different samples of the same food may differ slightly in their proportions of carbohydrate, protein, and fat, and since individuals differ in their efficiency of digestion, the energy provided by any single serving of a particular food can never be known precisely. Recognizing this, laboratories analyze many samples of each food and calculate an average, to ensure a reasonably accurate estimate of energy value.

ENERGY REQUIREMENTS

Methods of Determination

Determination of energy requirements is time-consuming and expensive. In order to know how much energy-producing food an individual requires each day, that person's daily energy expenditure must be calculated. This is the amount of energy that must be replaced to keep the body at equilibrium.

Obviously, different individuals have different energy requirements, and total energy expenditure varies from day to day even for the same individual. But by averaging the requirements of many individuals in a given group—growing children, pregnant women, adult males—the energy requirements of a typical member of that population can be estimated.

Energy expenditure is measured as heat released. The body "combusts" foodstuffs in the same way, essentially, as the bomb calorimeter does—although no electric spark is needed to initiate the process, and it doesn't happen quite as rapidly!

Several methods of measuring energy expenditure have been developed. One technique, **direct calorimetry**, utilizes the principle that heat released by the body is a product of energy expended. Measurements of the heat given off by an individual can therefore be used to calculate that individual's energy expenditure. This technique involves placing the person in a *respiratory calorimeter*, a large, ventilated, and well-insulated chamber whose exterior surface is lined with water-filled coils. Heat given off by the individual raises the temperature of the water in the coils, providing a measurement that can be converted to kilocalories or kilojoules. As you may recognize, the respiratory calorimeter is quite similar in principle to the bomb calorimeter; it can also be used to measure carbon dioxide production as well as oxygen consumption.

The ratio of the volume of CO_2 produced to the volume of O_2 consumed is known as the **Respiratory Quotient (R.Q.)**. Studies have shown that the R.Q. varies with the type of food ingested. Foods that contain greater relative proportions of oxygen require less molecular oxygen for biochemical oxidation; these foods have a higher R.Q. Glucose, the nutrient with the highest proportion of oxygen, has an R.Q. of 1. A fatty acid, such as stearic acid, with a lower proportion of oxygen, therefore requiring more molecular oxygen for metabolism, has a lower R.Q. Protein, with an oxygen content intermediate between glucose and fatty acids, has an R.Q. of approximately 0.8.

The R.Q. of a diet of mixed nutrients is approximately 0.85. In fasting and uncontrolled diabetes, where lipolysis and subsequent fatty acid oxidation is greatly accelerated, the measured R.Q. approaches 0.70. Administration of insulin, which accelerates glucose metabolism, produces an R.Q. greater than 0.85.

Because respiratory calorimeters are expensive and complicated to operate, they are not practical for routine use. Methods of **indirect calorimetry** have been devised and are both more convenient and lower in initial and operating costs. These methods depend on the fact that the amount of oxygen consumed during any activity is in direct proportion to the amount of energy liberated as heat. Calorimetric studies on many different subjects have shown that 1 liter of oxygen is required when approximately 4.8 kilocalories are liberated under basal (resting) conditions. Many experiments have confirmed this relationship.

From these figures, energy expenditures under a variety of experimental conditions can be readily calculated. All that is required is a respirometer, a lightweight apparatus that measures oxygen used and carbon dioxide exhaled. The resulting data are used to determine equivalents in kilocalories.

Factors Related to Energy Requirements

Several factors contribute to the amount of energy required by an individual at a given time: **basal metabolic rate** (BMR), physical activity, and to a lesser extent, dietary induced thermogenesis (DIT) of foods.

BASAL METABOLIC RATE. Energy is needed just to keep body systems working. Nerves firing, blood circulating, involuntary movements of muscles in the heart and diaphragm—these and other activities go on continuously in each individual, even when the body is at rest.

Researchers have studied the involuntary work of the brain, heart, muscles, and other vital organs to determine the amount of energy required for these collective processes. This energy requirement is known as the *basal metabolic rate* (BMR). BMR measurements are obtained under carefully controlled conditions. Subjects are instructed not to eat for 12 to 16 hours before testing to ensure that they are in a postabsorptive state. They must be relaxed, calm, and fully rested. Thus, testing is most frequently scheduled for early morning. The test consists of measuring oxygen consumption for six minutes with the subject at rest but awake. Standard calculations are then used to estimate the daily at-rest or basal energy requirement. Resting metabolic rate (RMR) is the energy expenditure under similar conditions except the interval since the last meal is not as long. A person's RMR will therefore be greater than their BMR. RMR is measured more frequently since testing conditions are not as strict.

Through testing of many healthy men and women, nutritionists have defined a useful rule of thumb: The BMR for adults is approximately 22 to 24 kilocalories per kilogram body weight per day (101 kJ/kg/day). Alternatively, for women of average body build, an approximation of BMR is 0.9 kcal (3.8 kJ) per kg per hour; for men, it is 1.0 kcal (4.2 kJ) per kg per hour.

To estimate your BMR, convert your body weight to kilograms (pounds ÷ 2.2); then multiply by 22 (women) or 24 (men). This gives some idea of the energy required for minimal metabolic functioning.

Basal metabolic rate is influenced by many factors, including age, sex, hormonal status, body size, and nutritional state. Infants and adolescents have the highest BMR; elderly people, the lowest. Women have a 6 to 10 percent lower metabolic rate than men. This sex difference has been attributed to women's higher proportion of adipose tissue and to hormonal differences. Hormones, the secretions of the endocrine glands, affect metabolism in many ways. Oversecretion of thyroxine by the thyroid gland (hyperthyroidism), for example, may speed up metabolism by as much as 100 percent. Conversely, undersecretion (hypothyroidism) may reduce metabolism by 30 to 40 percent. Thus, the pituitary gland, which stimulates thyroxine secretion by the thyroid, obviously exerts strong control on metabolism. Thyroxine acts slowly but maintains its effectiveness over long periods. Another important hormone, epinephrine (adrenalin), secreted by the adrenal glands, has a quick but transitory effect on metabolism. The sudden rush of energy you feel during excitement, fear, or emotional stress is the result of epinephrine secretion.

Body size and body composition also affect BMR. Bodies composed of a greater percentage of fatty tissue have a lower basal metabolism than bodies with a greater percentage of muscle tissue. This difference is due to the active oxidative processes that take place in muscle tissue, which continuously expend more energy than the processes occurring in fatty tissue. As mentioned before, men, who typically have a larger amount of lean body tissue than women, also have a higher BMR.

Most of the body's energy is lost through the skin as heat. Thus, a tall thin person, having a greater surface area than a short person of the same weight (who would obviously be fatter), would also have a higher basal metabolism. The greater the skin surface area, the greater the loss of heat, and the greater the amount of heat that must be produced to equal the heat lost.

What effect does body temperature have on the BMR? Temperature elevation increases the BMR by 7 percent for each degree Fahrenheit (0.55°C) above 98.6° (37°C). Thus, a fever of 103.6°F, which is 5°F (2.8°C) above normal, would increase basal metabolism by 35 percent. This effect applies to internal temperature changes only. Although climate influences basal metabolism somewhat, the significance of this factor has been reduced primarily because clothing and climate-control systems moderate the effects of temperature extremes.

Nutritional status also affects BMR. The more severe the state of undernutrition, the lower the BMR. This decrease is due to the loss of muscle tissue, which begins to be metabolized as fat stores are depleted, and also to a general decrease in the metabolic rate per unit of body weight. Underweight individuals who are not malnourished, however, often have a *higher* BMR per unit of body weight; this has been attributed to their relatively greater proportion of muscle mass to adipose tissue.

Obviously, so many factors influence BMR that predictions of energy requirements based on standardized tables are merely approximations. For most people, however, no matter what their actual BMR may be, more than half of their daily energy needs are devoted to continuing the vital processes of growth, regulation, and maintenance of physiological function.

PHYSICAL ACTIVITY.   Any kind of physical activity will increase the body's energy requirement above the basal level. Of course, some activities require more energy than others. Interestingly, a heavy individual will require more energy than a slim one engaged in the same activity because more energy is needed to move the greater mass of the heavier body.

The average individual spends about one-third of a normal day in sleep, an activity that doesn't greatly increase energy expenditure. Nevertheless, sleep may account for as much as one-fourth of the total daily energy requirement. Obviously, this figure varies from individual to individual. Some people enjoy relatively long periods of absolute rest during sleep, whereas others toss, turn, and move about for much of the night.

Walking, climbing, and running are necessary functions in our daily lives, and so are recreational activities. The energy cost of these activities varies according to the speed involved, the gradient and surface of the ground covered, and the weight of the individual. Predictably, the greater the speed, the steeper the level walked or the stairs climbed, the rougher the surface, or the heavier the individual, the greater the energy expenditure. Similar relationships hold for more strenuous activities, such as bicycling, skiing, and playing tennis.

For some of us, recreational time is far exceeded by work time. Obviously, strenuous physical work carries with it energy demands just as great as those required for strenuous recreation. But what of mental labor? Students are surprised to learn that their exhaustion after studying or concentrating during an examination is all psychological. Research conclusively demonstrates that mental work requires insignificant increases in energy expenditure. The energy you use in studying comes from muscle tension, opening and shutting books, or writing notes—but not from thinking!

Most adults engage in an activity mixture that is largely determined by their occupations, which have been classified according to the level of physical activity they involve. Most office and professional work is listed as "light" activity, in contrast to the "moderate" activity of light industry and the "exceptional" activity of construction work. Because people in industrialized nations are engaged primarily in light or moderate occupational activity and in spectator, rather than active, sports, the Food and Nutrition Board has issued energy guidelines tailored to the lower activity level of today's population. Tables for men indicate an average energy expenditure (in kilocalories per kilogram per hour) for very light work (seated and standing activities) of 1.5, increasing to 8.4 for heavy activities (tree felling or working with pick and shovel). The average range of energy expenditure for women is listed as 1.3 (light activity) to 8.0 (heavy activity).

DIETARY INDUCED THERMOGENESIS.   Food ingestion itself is known to increase energy expenditure. Several explanations for this increase have been advanced. It was originally attributed to the "work" involved in digestion and absorption. However, nutrients administered intravenously (bypassing the digestive system) or provided orally in the form of glucose and amino acids still produce an increase in the metabolic rate.

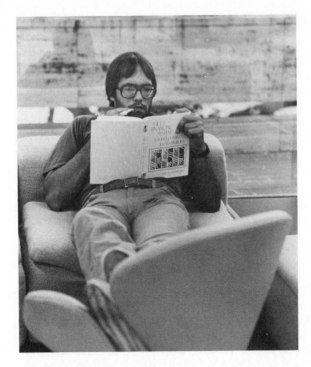

Obviously, physical work and strenuous recreation require high energy demands. But mental work requires insignificant increases in energy expenditure. Energy used in studying comes from muscle tension, opening and closing books, or writing notes—but not from thinking!

The University of Texas at Austin
News and Information Service

This thermogenic effect, known as the *specific dynamic effect* or dietary induced thermogenesis (DIT) of food, is particularly noticeable following protein ingestion. Protein increases metabolic rate by as much as 30 percent, compared with an increase for carbohydrate and fat of only 5 or 6 percent. Protein ingestion increases the body's energy requirements by stimulating urea synthesis, or alternatively, it is protein *synthesis* that increases the metabolic rate. DIT may alternatively result from "wasted energy" generated at the cellular level when the potential energy in food is converted to the free energy (usually ATP) required by the organism. The metabolic efficiency of this conversion process is 40 percent at maximum, varying with different metabolic pathways and with the nutritional status of the organism. Food ingestion may further decrease the efficiency of energy transformation, resulting in the heat loss known as the specific dynamic effect.

Whichever of the many explanations is correct, DIT is recognized as a relevant variable in any *precise* calculation of energy requirements. It has been estimated to represent approximately 6 percent of the body's total energy needs, a minor contribution compared to the energy required for basal metabolism and physical activity.

Recommendations for Energy Allowances

Precise energy requirements are difficult to establish for any one individual. Although the basal metabolic rate remains relatively stable in each person, activity patterns may vary, often on a daily basis. Tables of suggested energy allowances obviously cannot consider each of these variables as they affect every individual. As a practical compromise, the Food and Nutrition Board has made several assumptions in devising its RDA tables:

1. The average activity level of an adult (age 23 to 50) engaged in a light-activity occupation, in an environment with a mean temperature of 20°C (68°F), consists of 8 hours of sleep, 12 hours of very light activity, 3 hours of light activity, and 1 hour of moderate activity.
2. The energy expenditure during sleep is approximately 90 percent of an individual's resting basal metabolic rate. In contrast to the rigid experimental requirements of morning testing after 14 hours without eating in determining strict basal metabolism, the RMR is taken in the course of a day, with the subject at rest. Because it is not a fasting BMR, the calculation includes a correction for DIT. The RMR thus represents an average metabolic rate during a pause in the day's occupation.
3. In contrast to allowances for *nutrients*, which are set at a level above the estimated average requirement (see Chapter 1), the recommended allowance for *energy* is set at the average value thought to be consonant with good health.

Note that the energy/weight/day calculation figures in Table 5–2 compare reasonably well with the quick rule of thumb for adult BMR (22 or 24 kcal/kg body weight/day) plus 40 to 50 percent for activity.

For those who are not appreciably over or under appropriate body weight, individual energy requirements can be determined with more precision from the energy-activity guidelines of the Food and Nutrition Board. After determining how much time is spent at light, moderate, and heavier work, in other activities, and in sleep, it is possible to approximate more closely just how much energy an individual usually expends per day. Table 5–3 illustrates the method of estimating energy needs from total daily activities.

Those individuals whose weight is more than about 10 percent above or below the suggested range should calculate their energy *needs* based on their recommended, not actual, weights. For overweight people, these estimations will usually dictate a decrease in food consumption, though still within the energy level required for efficient growth and body maintenance.

But what of the overweight individual who is consuming an energy level appropriate for his or her ideal body weight, sex, and age? The Food and Nutrition Board does not recommend starvation, which would be necessary to achieve energy intakes *below* minimal need. They suggest, instead, increased *activity* to achieve the desired weight balance and to avoid degenerative arterial diseases that have been associated with a sedentary life style and obesity.

TABLE 5-2. *RDA for Energy for Adults*[a]

	BODY WEIGHT (BW)		ENERGY ALLOWANCE			
	kg	lb	kcal/day	kJ/day	kcal/kg BW/day	kJ/kg BW/day
Males						
19–22 yrs	70	154	2,900	12,200	41	174
23–50 yrs	70	154	2,700	11,340	39	162
Females						
19–22 yrs	55	120	2,100	8,820	38	160
23–50 yrs	55	120	2,000	8,400	36	153

[a] For energy recommendations for all ages see Appendix, Table A.
Source: Food and Nutrition Board, National Research Council, *Recommended dietary allowances*, 9th rev. ed. (Washington, D.C.: National Academy of Sciences, 1979).

TABLE 5-3. *Estimation of Energy Needs for a 23-Year-Old Female, 65 Inches (165 cm) Tall, 120 Pounds (54 kg)*

A. Calculation of BMR:

$$22 \text{ kcal/kg BW/day} = 22 \times 54 = 1{,}188 \text{ kcal/day}$$

B. Adjustment for physical activity:

| | TIME | ENERGY EXPENDITURE | |
ACTIVITY	hrs	kcal/kg/hr	kcal
Sleeping	8	—	—
Dressing	0.5	0.7	18.9
Driving car	1	0.9	48.6
Eating	1.5	0.4	32.4
Typing (electric typewriter)	5	0.5	135.0
Bicycling	1	2.5	135.0
Housework (making bed, 10 mins.; washing dishes, 20 mins.; vacuum cleaning, 30 mins.)	1	1–3	113.4
Sitting	5.5	0.4	118.8
Sewing by hand	0.5	0.4	10.8
Walking upstairs (2 flights)		0.036[a]	3.9
Walking downstairs (2 flights)		0.012[a]	1.3
Total			618.0

C. Subtotal for basal metabolism plus physical activity:

$$1{,}188 + 618 = 1{,}806$$

D. Dietary induced thermogenesis (+6%):

$$1806 \times .06 = 108.36$$

E. Total Energy Requirement:

$$1{,}806 + 108 = 1{,}914 \text{ kcal/day}$$

[a] Allowance per kg for 15-step staircase, disregarding time.

Most individuals do not need to rely on extensive calculations of energy requirements. The most practical way to monitor your own energy balance state is to watch the scale. It will tell you whether you are matching your intake to your daily needs! Energy allowances for persons at different stages of the life cycle, and during pregnancy and lactation, will be discussed in later chapters.

OBESITY: POSITIVE ENERGY BALANCE

A certain amount of body fat is desirable and necessary to protect against starvation and, as mentioned in Chapter 3, to protect the internal organs and provide insulation for the body. Normal energy intake and energy expenditure maintain this necessary level of body fat. At birth human infants have about 12% body fat, a greater proportion than most other animals. By one year of age the amount of fat has reached 25% of the total body weight; in the next ten years it decreases to about 15%. At puberty the amount of fat decreases in males and increases in females so that at age 18, males have about 15% body fat and females about 25%. For both sexes the percentage of fat tends to increase with age.

Definition and Diagnosis

Obesity and overweight are terms frequently used as if they are interchangeable, but they are not. Overweight signifies an increase in body weight above a reference standard usually related to height. Weight is the sum of the weight of *lean body mass*, bone, muscle, and nonfat issues, and the weight of fat. Increased weight can result from an increase in either. Athletes may be 10 percent or more above the average weight for their height and yet not be fat. Precise ways of determining lean body mass are used primarily in experiments in which body composition is determined. These methods are, however, too cumbersome and expensive for routine clinical use. Fortunately there are simpler ways to determine body fat.

Obesity is more correctly defined as a condition in which the relative proportion of body fat is abnormally high. A working definition of obesity is a little more difficult. There are three basic methods of defining obesity: social, physiological, and statistical. The social definition of obesity is culturally determined and has changed over the years. While the medical importance of obesity has been recognized since Hippocrates, "ideal weight"in times past was heavier than at the present time. The attitude of "You can't be too thin or too rich" and "Thin is in" has contributed to the dramatic increase in the incidence of anorexia nervosa and bulimia which will be discussed more completely later. The social definition of "too fat"should be replaced by one based on health concerns with an understanding that there is a strong genetic component to body size. While physical appearance may be a reasonable indicator for many people, health not fashion should be the ultimate criterion. The ramifications of the social definition of obesity will be discussed more completely in the section on underweight.

Ideally, a physiological definition of obesity is more desirable, that is, that weight at which there is least mortality (death) and morbidity (illness). Unfortunately we are not yet at the stage of understanding the best amount of fatness at each age to achieve this goal.

Using the statistical method to diagnose obesity, a certain percentage of the population, say the upper 20 percent, are defined as obese. There are two basic problems with this method. First, what reference standard or table should you use. For years, weight tables categorizing adults by sex and frame size and compiled from life insurance company statistics have been used. Although determinations of body frame size are inexact, the validity of categorizing weight by body build is supported by mortality statistics. Through the years the tables were variously labeled "ideal body weight" or "desirable body weight" or most recently, just "weight." Using data from the Build Study by the Society of Actuaries, the Metropolitan Life Insurance Company recently issued the latest version of these tables. In these tables the weight ranges for women under 5'7" are increased by 10 pounds; for those over 5'7" the increase is 15 pounds. For men 15 pounds has been added for those under 5'10" and 20 pounds for men over this height. The higher weights have created some controversy; some health professionals recommend using the old version of the tables while other suggest the newer, more liberal version. A way to avoid the controversy would be to use the Fogerty tables, developed by experts in the study of obesity which give the average weight for a given height and an acceptable range which encompasses the three body frame sizes. See Appendix D for weight tables.

The degree of "overweight" can be expressed in several ways. Relative weight is the comparison to a standard weight. Weight and height can also be related using ratios. The most frequently used ratio, the Quetelet or **body mass index (BMI)** is most highly correlated with the degree of body fat. BMI is calculated as the weight in kilograms divided by the square of the height in meters. Values above 25 for men and 27 for women are considered to indicate obesity. Values below 20 are considered to indicate underweight; those below 17 are suggestive of anorexia nervosa.

The National Center for Health Statistics has published growth charts for children and adolescents. Children throughout the country were measured to provide data for calculating the growth curves showing percentile values by sex and age from early infancy through 18 years of age. Growth charts do not correct for body build and body composition, but they are a means of comparing a given child's development in terms of height and weight with that of other children. The pattern of growth of a single child over a period of time can also be checked against the standards. An overfat infant, for example, might be in the 50th percentile for height, but the 99th percentile for weight. A large-boned child who falls at the 85th percentile for height may well be at the 85th percentile for weight with no sign of obesity. A consistent pattern of increasing percentile measures for weight with increased age may signal obesity in a growing child.

Estimation of **skinfold thickness** is another way to identify excess adiposity. Can you "pinch an inch?" If the fold of skin and underlying subcutaneous fat at your waist or the back of your arm is greater than an inch in thickness, you are probably somewhat overfat. This "pinch test" may be performed more scientifically with a measuring instrument known as skinfold calipers. Both the Health and Nutrition Examination Survey and the Ten State Nutrition Survey conducted by the U.S. Public Health Service used triceps skinfold thickness to estimate "obesity." Obesity in adults was defined as a value greater than the 85th percentile of measurements of young white adults (18 mm for males and 25 mm for females). The subscapular skinfold thickness is suggested by many as a better indicator of fatness than is the triceps skinfold thickness. Upper limits for the subscapular skinfold thickness are 19 mm for males and 25 mm for females. Tables of values for triceps and subscapular skinfold measurements are given in Appendix E. From birth girls and women have greater skinfold thickness than boys and men and young people have lower values than older people. Calipers may never replace the tape measure, however. Some researchers find significant variability in caliper measurements both from day to day and from observer to observer. They recommend a return to circumference measurements of chest, waist, hips, and biceps. These are easy to obtain and more reliable than skinfold measurements. Waist circumference, particularly for men, may be a better index of obesity than either of the two skinfolds mentioned.

Prevalence

The prevalence of overweight or obesity depends on the criteria used to define these conditions. By percent of population deviating from mean weight for 20 to 29-year-olds, 12.6 percent of women aged 20 to 74 years old were 10–19 percent overweight, and 23.8 percent were 20 percent or more overweight. For men the values were 18.1% and 14.0% respectively. By skinfold measurements more women than men are also classified as obese. Rural populations may be more overweight than urban populations. By race, white men tend to be fatter than black men; white females are fatter than black females through adolescence but significantly thinner from age 18 through 70.

The postadolescent reversal in incidence of obesity in black and white females has been attributed to socioeconomic factors. Before puberty, girls of lower socioeconomic status are thinner (as are lower-class boys), no matter what their skin color. After mid-adolescence, women from lower income levels get heavier whereas more affluent women get slimmer. Current research has corroborated these socio-economic differences, suggesting that they are not caused by hidden biological factors or by childhood feeding practices. For example, researchers find that women of low educational status who marry into high-income families are significantly thinner than their low-income-group peers. Obviously, social factors are implied.

Concerns About Obesity

The medical, psychological, and economic costs of obesity are extremely high.

MEDICAL CONCERNS. Mortality rates for people who are above or below average weight are higher than those for people of average weight. According to 1980 data, a body weight 20% above average is associated with a corresponding increase in mortality of 20% for men and 10% for women. When obesity exceeded these levels, the risk of premature death was even greater. Estimates indicate that for every 10 percent above normal weight, life span is decreased by one year—and it has been shown that return to normal weight is accompanied by a return of normal life expectancy.

Not only are obese people more likely to die at earlier ages, but they are also more likely to become seriously ill. Conditions in which obesity may be implicated include coronary heart disease, hypertension (high blood pressure), diabetes mellitus, osteoarthritis, renal (kidney) disease, cirrhosis of the liver, pulmonary (lung)

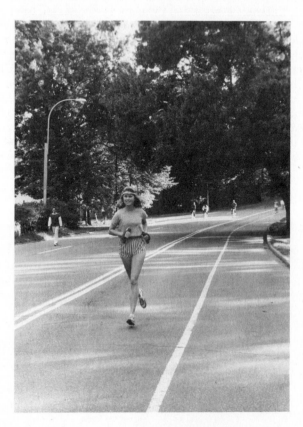

In the past large girth was often a symbol of high status, but today slim is "in."

Laimute E. Druskis

disease, and even surgical complications. Why is this so? Research suggests that being overweight places a physical burden on some systems of the body. Obesity increases the work of the heart as it enlarges with an increase in body weight. Glucose tolerance may be impaired in obese individuals and plasma concentrations of insulin may increase. There may also be abnormalities of the reproductive system; menstrual irregularity is more common in obese women. The changes seen in obese individuals may either be the result of the increased food intake or the increased body fat. Reduction of weight to desired levels may often arrest or even reverse these disease processes. For example, weight reduction alone, without medication, can reduce blood pressure in hypertensive patients who are overweight.

PSYCHOLOGICAL CONCERNS. As great as the physical costs of obesity may be, the psychological costs can be even greater for many individuals. In fact, since health warnings are notoriously poor motivators (as the continuing prevalence of cigarette smoking shows), psychological factors are more likely than physical ones to motivate people to lose weight.

Women suffer the effects of the social definition of obesity since they more than men are expected to conform to certain weight expectations. Socially defined obesity affects attitude toward weight, and attitude is a complex mixture of facts and sociocultural values.

To a greater or lesser degree most people consider themselves too fat. As part of a questionnaire on weight attitude, female health professions (both students and practitioners) were asked their present weight and what they would like to weigh. Based on the data from this nonrandom sample, the desired weight for all the women was 117 pounds. Using the same questionnaire, women aged 65 to 84 years also wanted to lose weight. Only one of fifty in the latter group thought she was too thin. Why is there such an ingrained desire to lose weight? Is it due in part to the incorrect characterization of individuals as obese by the misuse of tables, or is it due to a more general process of stigmatization, or a general Madison Avenue pitch? Ten years ago large sizes started at 20, now they start at size 12 or 14! Or is the desire to lose weight due to the fear of nonconformity? Or a concern for health? Probably a combination of all of these, since different people have different reasons.

As personal body size deviates from the social stereotype, self satisfaction decreases. Body image (our mental picture of our physical appearance plus our attitudes and feelings about our body) is different for some people. Patients with anorexia nervosa or obesity tend to overestimate their body size compared to controls. Females of all weights prefer to be thinner than the size they perceive themselves to be.

Obesity may be particularly difficult to handle in adolescence when peer pressure for conformity is the strongest and being different is equated to being inferior. Teenagers have been shown to evaluate fat figures negatively and slim figures positively. They frequently view themselves in the middle, but aspire toward the slim figure. Adolescent girls also rated an obese peer more negatively unless that obese person could offer either a physical reason for her weight or reported a recent successful weight loss.

ECONOMIC CONCERNS. Many companies still have acceptable weight standards for prospective employees. Salary level may be influenced by body weight either directly or indirectly. In one study, 40 percent of the men who earned under $20,000 were more than 10 percent overweight in contrast to only 9 percent of those who earned more than $20,000. Other data do not confirm this. There are also studies which show that tall men earn more than short men and "attractive" women earn more than plain women. Equal pay for equal work is still a long way from reality.

Etiology of Obesity: Biochemical Factors

Recognition that obesity is related to excessive food intake relative to need is ages old and so is advice to the overweight or obese person. However, in the past twenty years great strides have been made in our understanding of regulation of food intake and the etiology of obesity. In spite of this however, we are still a long way from a complete understanding. All obesity, like hypertension and cancer, does not result from the same cause. Obesity is now classified based on genetic and environmental factors.

Heredity is one such factor. There are two ways in which inheritance of corpulence can manifest itself. First there are the rare diseases which provide evidence of genetic transmission of obesity. Prader-Willi syndrome, which appears to be associated with chromosomal abnormalities, is manifested by mental retardation, obesity, hypogonadism, and hypotonia. Individuals with this disease eat uncontrollably. One of the manifestations of the Laurence-Moon-Bardet-Biedle syndrome is obesity. Hypercellular obesity may also be predominantly genetic.

Second, studies of twins and adopted children provided additional support for a more general role for genetics.

Identical twins raised in different homes have been shown to reach more similar weights than do fraternal twins raised in the same home. Another possible genetic factor is body build or somatotype, an inherited characteristic. Ectomorphs, thin individuals with long fingers, arms, and legs, rarely get fat. In contrast, endomorphs, who are rounder individuals with larger abdomens than chests, have a greater likelihood of becoming obese.

Hypothalmic obesity is very, very rare in humans, but has been shown to result from traumatic injury to the head. In rare cases, obesity may be correlated with disturbances of the **endocrine system**. An underactive thyroid gland is the usual culprit, a situation easily treated by hormone replacement therapy. However, the thyroid gland has been blamed out of all proportion to the actual incidence of this problem. Only a very small percent of obesity is due to hormonal abnormalities. Some hormonal abnormalities, moreover, are the *consequences* of weight gain, not the *causes*, and disappear following weight loss.

In animal studies, consumption of a high fat diet is very effective in making animals obese. Animals who fatten easily do not gain as much weight (fat) consuming a low fat diet illustrating the very important interaction of diet, that is environment, with the genetic tendency toward increased body weight and/or fatness.

Metabolic disturbances have also been cited as factors in obesity. These disturbances are difficult to identify because there are a number of metabolic changes which occur in *response* to obesity and they may be quite different than those which *cause* obesity. We do not have metabolic information on people before they become obese, which makes studying metabolic changes more difficult. People who are obese could regulate their food intake different than thin people, absorb or metabolize the food differently, or be less able to burn off the extra calories in the various forms of thermogenesis.

Food intake is regulated on a short-term or long-term basis. The size of a single meal is regulated by the response of receptors in the gastrointestinal tract, concentrations of certain hormones such as insulin, and the concentration of one or more

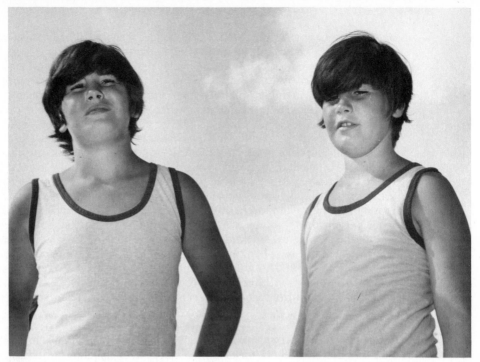

Studies have shown that identical twins raised in different homes reach more similar weights than do fraternal twins raised in the same home.

Runk/Schoenberger from Grant Heilman

compounds in the blood stream. These compounds bind with receptors in the hypothalamus and signal satiety or fullness.

Long-term regulation of food intake is an even more complex process. Don't you regulate rather well considering the quantity of food you consume in a year? Add up the amount of food you consume in one day. Four ounces of this and five ounces of that does not sound like much until you start multiplying. Eating less than three pounds of food a day would mean that you eat 1000 pounds in one year. Many people consume a ton of food a year. How does your body regulate intake? If you "pig-out" over the holidays or at a party, can you eat much the next week or the next day? Most average weight individuals who force themselves to overeat will automatically eat less and drop back to their usual weight when not forcing themselves to eat. The other side of the coin is that individuals who force themselves to undereat also gain automatically when they are not forceably trying to limit intake. This observation and others led to the development of the "Set Point Theory" which states that individuals have a programmed level or set point for body weight. This set point is usually stable, but can be changed. Overeating a high fat diet for a long period of time may lead to an elevated set point; exercise may help lower the set point.

For several years another biological explanation, the *adipose cell theory*, was proposed as a cause of some types of obesity. Certain parts of the theory still hold, namely that some individuals have a hypercellular type of obesity and once we have an increased number of fat cells, they do not seem to go away. However, why and when fat cells are recruited to start storing fat is not understood. That this occurs only in infancy and early childhood is no longer accepted. There is also less and less evidence that all fat infants will become fat adults. In one study in which the children were followed for two decades, 74 percent of obese preschool children were less than obese when they reached adulthood. The immediate environment, that is fatness of family members, plays an important role in the development of obesity.

No theory so far proposed has won widespread acceptance as a complete explanation of eating behavior. Many people are able to adjust energy intake to needs automatically, but some individuals, for reasons that are still unclear, seem to have altered control mechanisms. In some respects, we should not be surprised that eating behavior is such a complex process. If there was but a single mechanism, there would be the possibility that some people would be born with a genetic defect and starve themselves to death. We need to eat to survive, and that survival is protected by a number of backup mechanisms, making eating behavior an extremely complex process. Individuals who have been obese for many years may have to consciously control their intake by adjusting serving size and meal frequency because their metabolism does not revert completely back to "normal." People who are spontaneously obese may need to hold their intake below what an average-weight person consumes in order to maintain a lower body weight. Finally we should all remember that all our control mechanisms can be overriden by cognitive and external influences.

OTHER PHYSIOLOGICAL FACTORS. Of course, not only fat cells but also all body cells are affected by food intake. Some biological explanations of obesity propose a complex interaction of body cells and systems that results in metabolic balance for the organism. These theories emphasize the transmission within the body of "hunger" and "full" signals. **Hunger** is a strictly physiological feeling and appears to be controlled by internal mechanisms. **Appetite**, on the other hand, is cued by external stimuli—taste, smell, and social and numerous other cues—that make us feel we want—or don't want—to eat. All of us often eat when appetite is aroused, even if we are not particularly hungry at that moment. Many obese individuals may respond more readily to appetite cues and may not even feel hunger, possibly because the biochemical mechanisms producing hunger or satiety are malfunctioning.

It has been speculated that special receptors in the part of the brain known as the *hypothalamus* are sensitive to changes in the blood glucose levels. After food is eaten, blood reaching the hypothalamus contains high levels of glucose, which according to this theory, stimulate these receptors to send a "stop eating" message to the rest of the brain. A few hours later, the blood glucose level falls to a critical triggering point, the hypothalamus receptors receive less glucose in the blood, and a message of hunger is again transmitted.

Other research has suggested that the key control mechanism is located in the liver, where biochemical signals activate the release into the bloodstream of metabolites and enzymes, which are then carried to the brain. Additional candidates for hunger regulators have been proposed, including serum amino acids, lipids released from adipose stores, and a variety of hormonal and other control mechanisms.

According to theories of biochemical regulation of appetite, an imbalance in the control mechanism or process results in scrambled messages that set off eating binges. But no theory so far proposed has won widespread acceptance as a complete explanation of eating behavior. Many people are able to adjust energy intake to needs automatically, but some individuals, for reasons that are still unclear, seem to lack such a built-in control mechanism. These individuals, especially if they have been obese for many years, may have to learn to adjust their intake by using portion size and meal frequency, rather than appetite, as regulators. It does seem curious, at this late date in human development, that we still do not know for certain either how appetite is regulated or how appetite regulation relates to obesity.

Over the past few years the role of brown adipose tissue (BAT) has been investigated. BAT has been suggested as a regulator of thermogenesis or the amount of white adipose tissue.

Etiology of Obesity: Social and Psychological Factors

While biochemical factors are responsible for massive obesity, some obesity and overweight is brought about by social and psychological factors. There are times when we continue to eat despite the lack of hunger or appetite: Remember last Thanksgiving. We also may eat because the clock says it is "lunchtime" or because we are bored with studying—and for dozens of other reasons completely unrelated to our physiological state.

Some of these reasons are environmental and social. Our technologically advanced society has provided a plentiful supply of tasty food and has increased our opportunities to consume it. Our ancestors had to forage for or raise their own food supply, but we just hop into the car or walk down the street and buy whatever we choose at an amply stocked supermarket or fast-food emporium.

Then, too, our workday activities have changed. From a nation of active food producers, we have become a nation of sedentary paper pushers. The shift in activity patterns is a key contributor to the growth of our national girth. Labor-saving devices and "automobility" save time and energy and allow the kilocalories to accumulate in fat storage. Habits of inactivity develop early: Today's children play outdoors less than did children of previous generations.

Although much of our life style has changed, one tradition has continued: the American way of hospitality. Food traditionally accompanies social occasions, and this pattern has now been extended to sports events (at which we are usually observers, not participants) and even to the working day. Coffee breaks, business lunches, and office parties are common occupational hazards. After work we go home, where we may entertain at cocktails and dinner, or "get the munchies" while watching television.

Social customs influence habits and patterns of eating. The increased tendency toward snacking, "grabbing a quick bite," or grazing has deemphasized the traditional pattern of "three square meals a day." Men who ate more frequent and small meals were less likely to be obese than men who ate fewer and larger meals. However, grabbing a quick bite or having small meals may result in choices that are high in fat and limited in certain nutrients. "Fast" foods are not bad in themselves if not consumed all of the time and if some wise choices are made, such as a low-calorie beverage rather than a high-calorie shake. Frequent meals are valuable because they spread energy intake over time. But if additional meals only increase the amount of food eaten, there is no benefit.

Frequent snacking may be a product of our speeded-up life style, but it may also have psychological and emotional roots. Some individuals are likely to start nibbling when they are bored or tense. Psychologists believe that the pleasantly full sensations we get from eating take us back to the security of infancy, when our needs were fulfilled by an all-providing mother. However, the sense of satisfaction and fulfillment derived from eating is reinforced daily throughout life. Constant pairing of the act of eating with the satisfaction of biological and psychological needs is similar to the close association of other stimuli and responses in our lives. Just as we learn that turning a knob will open the door, or that carrying an umbrella will protect us from rain, so we learn that eating leaves us feeling satisfied.

All the factors discussed so far—heredity, endocrine changes, metabolic alterations, activity level, environmental and social influences, psychological needs—interact to produce a continuous pattern of increased energy intake and decreased energy expenditure (see Figure 5–2). Of course, not every obese person is affected by every factor. For some people, cultural influences are overriding; for others, physiological factors take precedence; and for many, the psychological influences predominate. The crucial factor for *all* cases of obesity, however, is the critical ratio of energy intake to energy expenditure. Whenever intake exceeds expenditure, weight gain follows inexorably.

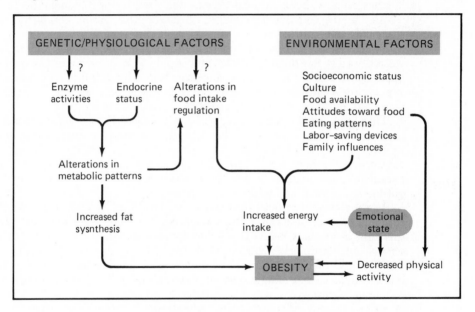

FIGURE 5-2   *Possible Causes of Obesity.*
Factors in both the internal and external environments can contribute to a state of positive energy balance resulting in obesity. The relative importance of each of these influences is not known and probably varies for each individual.

From a mathematical point of view, an intake of 100 "extra" kilocalories (420 kJ) per day will produce a 10-pound weight gain in just a year's time. One hundred kilocalories may seem like a lot, but translated into two small chocolate chip cookies, one fried egg, or a glass of low-fat milk, it becomes a mere "snack." Any food, even a recognized "low-calorie" food, has the potential to contribute to obesity if it is eaten in addition to foods that meet normal daily energy requirements. As can be seen in Table 5–4, eating just one extra apple (87 kcal) each day will add one pound of body fat in 34 days. That one-pound gain will take only 7 days if the extra is a 12-ounce milkshake (420 kcal).

TABLE 5-4. *Weight Gain Equivalents of Selected Foods When Eaten in Addition to Daily Needs*

Food Portion	Weight g	Energy kcal	BODY WEIGHT GAIN 1 lb days	25 lb weeks	1 kg days	25 kg weeks
Apple, medium, 2½" diam.	150	87	34	121	75	267
Beef roast, 1 slice 4" × 2½" × ½"	53	150	20	70	43	155
Brandy, cognac, 1 pony	30	75	39	140	87	310
Bread, 1 slice with 1 pat butter	28	96	31	110	68	242
Bread, peanut butter and jam: 1 slice, 1 tbsp, 1 tsp	38	195	15	54	33	119
Brownie with nuts 2" × 2" × ¾"	30	146	20	72	44	159
Cookies, chocolate chip, 2	22	100	30	105	65	232
Ice cream cone, ½ c dip	72	160	18	66	41	145
Martini, 3½ fluid oz	100	140	21	75	46	166
Milk, whole, 8 fluid oz	240	160	18	66	41	145
Milk, skim, 8 fluid oz	240	88	34	120	74	264
Milkshake, 12 fluid oz	345	420	7	25	15	55
Orange juice, 4 fluid oz	120	54	55	195	120	430
Peanuts, 1 oz	30	170	17	61	38	136
Pizza, ⅛ of 14" diam. pie	75	190	16	55	34	122
Potato chips, 10	20	115	26	92	56	202

Source: Adapted from F. Konishi and S. L. Harrison, Body weight-gain equivalents of selected foods, *Journal of the American Dietetic Association* 70:365, 1977 (Table 1).

Treatment of Obesity

The Last Chance Diet, the Calories-Don't-Count Diet, the Dupont Diet, the Air Force Diet, the Drinking Man's Diet, the Doctor's Quick Weight-Loss Diet, the Diet Revolution, Doctor's Quick Inches-Off Diet, the Scarsdale Diet, the Three-Day Diet, "rainbow" diet pills, Metrecal, Relaxacisor, body wrap, hormones, laxatives, diuretics, fasting, intestinal bypass, liquid protein—this plethora of weight-loss illustrates our extreme preoccupation with dieting. When caloric intake is suddenly reduced there is an initial water loss which results in a temporary weight loss in about three days. This gives many people the impression that they are losing fat and they attribute this "success" to a particular diet. Unfortunately, the weight returns when the person resumes normal intake and all the water is replaced.

Various treatments of obesity have different levels of risk. Low-risk obesity, that is BMI of 30 or below, should be treated with low-risk treatment such as diet and behavior-modifying techniques. Intermediate-risk obesity should be treated with intermediate-risk therapies such as drugs and very-low-calorie diets (under careful medical and dietetic supervision, of course). For massively obese individuals, high-risk therapies such as fasting and surgery may be considered, but they should not be the first choice for therapy.

Despite all the hard-sell promises, there is no magic way to lose pounds and inches. Diets and weight-reducing treatments that sound unbelievable are just that: unbelievable. There are several satisfactory approaches to weight loss, but all require energy intake to be lower than energy expenditure. Any sustained decrease in energy intake, with energy expenditure held constant or, better, increased, will produce weight reduction.

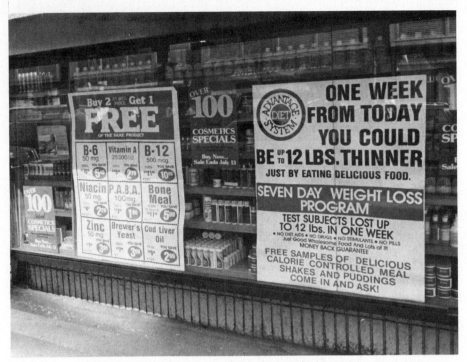

There are several satisfactory approaches to weight loss, but all require that energy intake be lower than energy expenditure.
Cecil Yarbrough

Remember, the word **diet** doesn't necessarily imply a weight-loss regimen. There are diets that promote weight gain, diets that restrict salt or fats, diets free of roughage, and diets designed to detect allergies. A diet is, simply, a prescribed regimen of eating and drinking. Most people, however, do mean "weight reduction" when they say diet. The accepted, nutritionally sound principles that apply to all weight-control regimens will be considered first, and then some efficient diet programs will be examined.

Principles of Weight Reduction

The expectation that pounds that went on slowly should be able to come off rapidly is probably the greatest diet fallacy and leads to rapid dissatisfaction and discouragement. Another fallacy is the expectation that once desired weight is achieved, prediet eating habits can be resumed. After all, those habits put the weight on in the first place. For weight reduction to be lasting, balanced intake patterns and regular eating habits must be established. Unfortunately, the vast majority of dieters are unable to maintain their weight loss. They return to their former eating patterns and, soon, to their former weights.

The regaining of weight may be partially explained by studies demonstrating that starved rats convert food to body fat more efficiently than nonstarved rats eating the same amount of food. A similar principle may be at work in some humans who have dieted. After a period of restricted intake their bodies adapt, like those of the rats, to retain energy more efficiently. Then, even when desirable weight is achieved and normal intake patterns resumed, the rate of lipid synthesis continues at the higher adaptive level, and weight gain follows. Maintaining regular eating patterns while reducing overall food intake may unwind this dietary "yo-yo."

In addition to the hazard of developing increased lipogenesis, diet methods that call for omission of breakfast and lunch are likely to fail for another reason: Often people who skip meals more than make up for it at the next meal. Whether it's because they "owe it to themselves" or because they are ravenous (and no wonder!), meal skippers are rarely as successful at dieting as meal trimmers.

More important than learning *when* to eat, however, is determining *how much* to eat. It is difficult to determine precisely the level of kilocalorie reduction necessary to produce a specified weight loss for a given individual. But there are several workable approximations. They are derived primarily from the fact that in order to lose 1 pound of fat, a 3,500-kilocalorie deficit must be achieved. Thus, to lose 1 pound per week, a dieter must have a deficit of 500 kcal per day; to lose 2 pounds (4.4 kg) per week, the deficit must be 1,000 kcal per day.

To determine the desired level of reduced caloric intake, it is first necessary to estimate the number of kilocalories needed to maintain present weight, then to subtract 500 (to lose 1 pound per week) or 1,000 (to lose 2 pounds per week). For a quick approximation, multiply present weight in pounds by 15 (assuming a moderate activity level, 15 kilocalories per day will maintain 1 pound of body weight). A young woman who weighs 150 pounds and wishes to reach her ideal weight of 130 pounds can maintain her present weight on 2,250 kcal per day (150 × 15); to lose 1 pound per week she must reduce intake to 1,750 kcal per day, and to lose 2 pounds per week intake should be reduced to 1,250 kcal per day.

Obviously, to continue losing weight at the same rate, intake levels should be readjusted downward as weight loss occurs. For example, after the 150-pound woman loses 10 pounds, she should refigure her caloric intake; her weight is now 140 pounds, and a daily intake level of 2,100 kcal (140 × 15) will maintain that weight. To continue losing weight at the rate of 1 pound per week, therefore, she should consume 1,600 kcal per day; to continue losing at the rate of 2 pounds per week, intake should be reduced to 1,100 kcal per day.

Alternately, the would-be dieter could resort to another nutritionists' rule of thumb: Multiply the ideal weight by 10 and consume that level of kilocalories per day. This, too, will surely take pounds off. Using this method, the young woman in the example would plan a diet consisting of 1,300 kcal per day. Her weight loss at the start would be about the same as she would achieve on a 1,000-kcal daily deficit, but the *rate* of weight loss would slow as she approached her ideal weight. However, she would get there—and would then be able to adjust intake upward to the level needed to maintain her ideal weight, approximately 1,950 (130 × 15) kilocalories per day.

In all weight-reduction programs, there comes a time when weight loss slows and then appears to stop altogether. This plateau is notoriously difficult for dieters. Until that time, weight loss has been a true measure of fat loss. During the plateau period, however, loss of fat apparently continues, but it does not show up (on the scales) because, for reasons that are not clearly understood, water is accumulated by the body. After a period of one to three weeks, *if reduced kilocalorie intake is maintained*, the water will be eliminated and weight will suddenly drop. But even on a lowered caloric intake, the last few pounds often do not come off. An additional reduction of intake and/or a slight increase in physical activity should help dieters to reach their goal.

"It takes the weight off *fast!*" "I actually feel less hungry when I starve myself than when I allow myself a thousand calories a day." "My morale really gets a boost when I see results by the second day of a diet." These are typical comments from enthusiasts of very low calorie diets, or VLCDs. Also called *modified fasts* (by medical personnel) and *crash diets* (by the general public), VLCDs have been hailed as safe and effective and even reasonably pleasant by some, yet have been blamed by others for serious complications such as gout flareup, uric acid stones, and cardiac arrythmias.

There is nothing new about VLCDs. In the past, many people learned from experience—perhaps quite by accident—that a few days of near starvation could cause them to lose weight, albeit water weight, almost as rapidly as complete starvation could. If this very rapid result was their immediate goal, perhaps it was of little consequence that the results were generally not long lasting. Getting into a particular dress or suit, or looking trimmer than usual for the big weekend coming up, can sometimes provide the motivation for staying with a VLCD for the short time required. If the dieter is in good health, not seriously overweight, and young, few or no health hazards may result.

Why, then, are health professionals concerned enough about the safety of such diets to issue repeated warnings about them? The answer is not necessarily related to VLCDs or weight loss per se but to the *kind* of diet, as well as the particular dieter, in the given situation under discussion. Some VLCDs, although of course deficient in food energy, provide adequate or even generous amounts of protein, essential fatty acids, vitamins, and minerals; in other words, they have extremely high nutrient density. Further, they may be administered under close medical supervision, perhaps only to carefully selected individuals who have been screened before treatment for obesity. Commonly, these individuals are the severely obese whose lives appear to be at greater risk from the obesity than from any anticipated effects of fasting. Under these conditions, a VLCD may well be justified, particularly for those who have repeatedly failed to lose weight with more traditional, moderate calorie-restriction programs.

In the 1970s a type of VLCD called the *liquid protein diet* became commercially available to the public. Virtually an invitation for people to play at being their own doctors, the liquid protein diet was hailed as a new, effective, and safe way to lose weight. New it was, but only in the sense

Nutritionists rarely recommend a weight loss greater than two, or at most, three pounds per week. Beyond this level, the body begins to metabolize body protein, producing weakness and metabolic imbalances. Ideally, weight loss occurs because of the loss of fat, not of lean body mass (muscle) or water. On an energy-restricted diet, part of the energy required to support basal metabolism and physical activity must come from the body's fat stores, which are released and burned as metabolic fuel.

But although the total food intake is drastically reduced in energy-restricted diets, all necessary nutrients should be provided—adequate amounts of vitamins and minerals, enough protein and carbohydrate, and a limited amount of fat. Thus, these are nutritionally *balanced* deficit diets. Diets of fewer than 1,000 kcal (4,200 kJ) per day are seldom advised, no matter how great the weight loss desired, because it is difficult to ingest the necessary nutrients in adequate amounts. Whenever a diet of 1,000 or fewer kilocalories per day is followed, a vitamin and mineral supplement providing RDA levels should be taken daily. Remember that nutritional adequacy is always related to the diversity of the diet; as intake of certain cat-of being nutritionally deficient in almost every respect, in contrast to the carefully balanced formulations used in hospital settings. Certainly it was effective in promoting weight loss, as would be expected of a diet providing only 200 to 300 kilocalories per day. But safe it definitely was not; by the late 1970s, over 40 deaths and more than 100 cases of serious illness had been reported in people following this diet.

Why did some of the people using liquid protein die? Some showed abnormal heart function, perhaps because of low potassium or other mineral imbalance; low blood and tissue levels of calcium and magnesium were found in some. Nevertheless, the cause of death has not been definitely established. Ketosis, diuresis (abnormal water excretion), elevated serum uric acid levels, and negative nitrogen balance all can occur with a VLCD providing only the low-quality protein, such as hydrolyzed gelatin, typical of the once-popular liquid protein preparations; any of these metabolic abnormalities could have contributed to the deaths. All these undesirable changes can be prevented by a VLCD consisting of high-quality protein supplemented with at least some carbohydrate as well as with generous amounts of vitamins and minerals.

In view of the experience with the commercial liquid protein diet of the 1970s, many nutritionists are reluctant to give even tentative approval to any VLCD. Some data suggest no significant adverse effects if the diets are used for periods of 6 to 8 weeks. Perhaps it would be best to recommend that such diets be considered as experimental treatment only and that the usual procedures applied to human experimentation, such as obtaining informed consent of the subjects, be required. Research for the future could then be directed to questions other than safety. Specifically, information on the appetite-suppressing ability of VLCDs, which implies a clear advantage over moderate calorie-restricted diets, would be of great value; if this effect is mostly psychological, the one definite advantage claimed by proponents of VLCDs would disappear. Finally, we should determine whether weight removed by VLCD regimens remains off or returns, apparently as magically as it was lost. For the one sure fact about starvation and near-starvation diets of all kinds is this: You can't adopt them as a lifetime eating pattern. Whether people can achieve permanent weight loss without permanent changes in eating habits is a crucial question that has yet to be answered.

egories of food is drastically reduced or eliminated altogether, achievement of nutrient balance becomes more and more difficult. In addition, most people cannot adhere to a severe energy-restricted diet; they feel deprived, and instead of developing sound eating habits, they tend to starve one day and "binge" the next.

Dieters should make a particular effort to choose foods that have a high nutrient content in proportion to energy content, that is, foods that have a high "nutrient density." If you do have an occasional small piece of chocolate cake, something else must go. Dieters must learn to adjust serving sizes of high-energy foods—and even so, empty calorie foods should not be eaten regularly on a weight-loss diet. When energy intake is limited to 1,000 or 1,500 kilocalories daily, it is particularly important to make those calories count in terms of their nutritional value. You may have heard that "calories don't count"—but they do!

Because fat-rich roods are "high calorie" foods, they should be eaten in moderation by dieters. But they should not be omitted altogether. Butter, margarine, salad dressings, and other fatty foods provide essential fatty acids and fat-soluble vitamins. They also add appetite appeal and reduce boredom. Fortunately for dieters, fat also has a satiety-producing effect. Thus, the inclusion of some fat in each meal will satisfy nutritional needs and leave the dieter feeling fuller longer.

Potatoes and grain products have similar hidden benefits, despite the widespread notion that bread, pasta, and other starchy foods are "fattening." A check of the energy content of a piece of bread (70 kcal, 294 kJ), even with a pat of butter (35 kcal = 147 kJ) added, shows it to be a better dinnertime addition than a second 3-ounce serving of lean roast beef (165 kcal = 693 kJ). This is not to say that protein is "fattening." Foods themselves are not fattening when taken in moderation; it is the energy we consume in excess of our daily needs that is fattening. It doesn't matter in what form the kilocalories are provided; too much from any nutrient source—whether carbohydrate, protein, and/or fat—will lead to weight gain.

What about grain products such as pizza or beer and hard liquor? Pizza is a good source of nutrients, but depending on the "extras," it can be a significant energy source. Alcoholic beverages are sources of kilocalories but not of nutrients. (Beer and wine do have slight amounts of some vitamins and minerals, but in proportion to energy content these are negligible.) Obviously, a 1,000 kilocalorie diet doesn't leave much room for beer. Does that mean that dieters can *never* drink? No, but it does mean that careful planning will be necessary. When it's going to be a long evening, they can sip club soda or mineral water with a lemon or lime wedge. Highball drinkers can make it a tall one rather than a short one (the added ice and water don't add calories) and compensate with a decrease in bread and fat intake for that day. Since having more than one may make it difficult to obtain sufficient nutrients without going over one's energy allowance, unlimited drinking of alcoholic beverages is not a way to lose weight.

Meals for weight-reduction diets can be planned in several ways. Food composition tables (see Appendix, Table H) list energy content as well as nutrient values. These can be used by themselves to plan a day's eating, or they can be used in conjunction with the two most useful food-grouping systems. The food-group system can be used to plan meals that include two servings each from the milk and the meat/alternate groups, four servings of grains/breads, and four servings of fruits/vegetables (including one citrus fruit or juice for vitamin C and one dark green or yellow vegetable for vitamin A). These choices, if prepared without additional sugar or fat, will provide about 1,200 kilocalories. Exchange lists (see Chapter 10) are also helpful for many who find it tedious actually to count calories. Table 5–5 indicates suggested distribution of exchange groups for diets at various energy-intake levels. Consult Appendix G for foods and amounts included in each of these categories.

Noting the approximate amount of kilocalories in an average serving from each of the exchange lists or basic food groups is an easy way for weight-conscious individuals to make substitutions in accordance with their personal likes and dislikes. It is important that no complete group of foods be eliminated from the diet. By including foods from all groups, an adequate supply of essential vitamins, minerals, and fatty acids, as well as necessary carbohydrate and protein, will be likely.

Serving sizes described in these lists may be distributed throughout the day. For example, two cups of milk may include ½ cup with breakfast cereal, another ½ cup taken in three cups of coffee, and a glass drunk as a snack. Options such as this, and the choices provided by the food groups or lists, allow variety in meal planning. If diets are boring, people don't stick with them. And when an individual develops a diet plan most compatible with his or her own likes and eating habits, the chances for successful weight loss are tremendously increased. Also, making choices during

TABLE 5-5. *Distribution of Exchange Groups for Diets at Various Energy Intake Levels*

Exchange List	Serving Size	Kcal per Serving	NUMBER OF EXCHANGES AT DIFFERENT ENERGY LEVELS (kcal)						
			1,000	1,200	1,400	1,600	1,800	2,000	2,200
Milk, skim	1 c	80	2	2	2	2	2	3[a]	3[a]
Vegetables	½ c	25	2	2	2	2	3	3	3
Fruit	1 small apple or equivalent	40	2	3	3	3	5	4	5
Bread/grains (cereals and starchy vegetables)	1 slice bread or equivalent	70	4	5	6	8	9	9	9
Meat/alternate (medium fat)[b]	1 oz	75	4	5	6	7	7	8	9
Fat	1 tsp margarine or equivalent	45	3	3	4	4	5	7	8

[a] To substitute whole milk for skim milk, decrease the number of fat exchanges by two for each milk exchange to keep equivalent kilocalorie content.

[b] To simplify the table, medium-fat meat exchanges have been used. Lean meats (55 kcal/oz) should be stressed in low-energy diets. High-fat meats provide 100 kcal per ounce.
Source: Exchange lists for meal planning (American Diabetes Association, and the American Dietetic Association, Chicago, 1976). (See Appendix, Table G.)

a diet is good preparation for the choices that must be made when dieting is completed.

Snacking can help reduce boredom and prevent the empty feeling between meals. Low-calorie snacks such as plain tea, bouillon, an apple, raw crunchy vegetables, tomato juice, or skim milk are good choices. Snacks should provide nutrients as well as calories. Peanut butter or cheese and crackers are nutritious snacks that can be eaten in moderation during a weight-loss program and are often more satisfying than a stalk of celery.

Another way to make choices easier while limiting energy intake is to control serving size. A dieter who can't "live" without ice cream may survive quite well on smaller portions of this favorite. Portion size assumes particular importance with high-calorie foods. Although we can't eliminate them from our diets, we can limit our intake. Three ounces of lean meat, for example, contain 165 kcal; a double-sized serving will therefore contain 330 kcal, twice as many. This may sound obvious but it's something dieters often forget. "Calorie counting" is only accurate when portion size is considered. And for many people, a reduction in serving size *alone* will produce weight loss.

The advantages of a balanced deficit diet are as follows: Weight loss is steady, foods eaten are nutritionally adequate, bizarre eating patterns are avoided, ordinary and readily available foods are utilized, and there is no medical risk. Too, there is maximal opportunity to learn new eating patterns, which are the key to continued weight maintenance. The major disadvantage of balanced deficit diets is that although weight loss is steady, it is relatively slow. Most dieters want to lose their excess weight fast. Even two pounds a week seems too slow to most overweight individuals. So they go on highly publicized diets in which the initial weight loss is rapid but, alas, impermanent. Before we discuss some of these "popular" diets, we will examine the important role of physical exercise in losing weight.

Physical Exercise

For most people, basal metabolic needs account for the greatest portion of total energy expenditure. However, individuals engaged in hard physical labor or strenuous recreational activity will have very different energy-utilization patterns. A lumberjack, or an athlete in training, may expend 4,500 or even more kilocalories in one day. Since energy intake must match energy expenditure, that individual must consume at least 4,500 kilocalories in order to maintain his or her weight. On the other hand, energy expended in sedentary activity may be insufficient to counterbalance an intake of even 1,400 kcal per day. Particularly in middle age, as metabolism slows, many individuals find that the levels of energy intake that once kept them trim now produce an uncomfortable layer of fat around the midsection. The choice is clear: Increase activity or decrease intake.

So, which would you prefer: walking, jogging, or not eating? Table 5–6 may help you to decide. This table translates the energy content of various foods into activity equivalents. Note that these equivalents are calculated by time. Thus, it would take you six minutes of running or 21 minutes of walking to "pay" for eating one serving of potato chips (ten chips). If you prefer swimming, you can work off two strips of bacon in nine minutes. And if you start bicycling for a half-hour each day *and* eliminate just one slice of bread and butter from your daily diet, you will be achieving the same effect as if you had eliminated three slices of bread and butter.

But why exercise, dieters ask, when I'm already "starving" myself? Contrary to popular notions, moderate exercise actually *decreases* appetite. Also on the positive side, exercise provides many health benefits, such as improved muscle tone (which

TABLE 5-6. *Energy Equivalents of Selected Foods and Beverages*

| Food | Kilo-calories | ACTIVITY (MINUTES) | | | | |
		Walking[a]	Riding Bicycle[b]	Swimming[c]	Running[d]	Reclining[e]
Apple, large	101	19	12	9	5	78
Bacon, 2 strips	96	18	12	9	5	74
Banana, small	88	17	11	8	4	68
Beans, green, 1 c	27	5	3	2	1	21
Bread and butter	105	20	13	9	5	81
Cake, 1/12, 2-layer	356	68	43	32	18	274
Carbonated beverage, reg., 1 glass, 8 oz	106	20	13	9	5	82
Carrot, raw	42	8	5	4	2	32
Cereal, dry, ½ c, with milk and sugar	200	38	24	18	10	154
Cheese, cottage, 1 tbsp	27	5	3	2	1	21
Cheese, cheddar, 1 oz	111	21	14	10	6	85
Chicken, fried, ½ breast	232	45	28	21	12	178
Cookie, chocolate chip	51	10	6	5	3	39
Doughnut	151	29	18	13	8	116
Egg, fried	110	21	13	10	6	85

156

TABLE 5-6. (*Continued*)

Food	Kilo-calories	Walking[a]	Riding Bicycle[b]	Swimming[c]	Running[d]	Reclining[e]
		ACTIVITY (MINUTES)				
Egg, boiled	77	15	9	7	4	59
French dressing, 1 tbsp	59	11	7	5	3	45
Halibut steak, ¼ lb	205	39	25	18	11	158
Ham, 2 slices	167	32	20	15	9	128
Ice cream, ⅙ qt	193	37	24	17	10	148
Ice-cream soda	255	49	31	23	13	196
Ice milk, ⅙ qt	144	28	18	13	7	111
Gelatin dessert, with cream	117	23	14	10	6	90
Mayonnaise, 1 tbsp	92	18	11	8	5	71
Milk, whole, 8 oz	166	32	20	15	9	128
Milk, skim, 8 oz	81	16	10	7	4	62
Orange, medium	68	13	8	6	4	52
Orange juice, 6 oz	92	18	11	8	5	71
Pancake with syrup, 1 tbsp	124	24	15	11	6	93
Peach, medium	46	9	6	4	2	35
Pie, apple, ⅙	377	73	46	34	19	290
Pizza, cheeze, ⅛	180	35	22	16	9	138
Pork chop, loin, 2.7 oz, lean & fat	314	60	38	28	16	242
Potato chips, 1 serving (10 chips)	108	21	13	10	6	83
Sandwiches						
Club	590	113	72	53	30	454
Hamburger	350	67	43	31	18	269
Tuna fish salad	278	53	34	25	14	214
Sherbet, ⅙ qt	177	34	22	16	9	136
Steak, T-bone, 3 oz	235	45	29	21	12	181
Strawberry shortcake	400	77	49	36	21	308
Beer (regular), 8 oz	100	19	12	9	5	77
Beer (light), 8 oz	70	13	8	6	4	54
White wine, 3½ oz	84	16	10	8	4	65
Dessert wine, 3 oz	124	24	15	11	6	95
Gin (80 proof), 1 oz	65	12	8	6	3	50
Rye (80 proof), 1 oz	65	12	8	6	3	50
Scotch (80 proof), 1 oz	65	12	8	6	3	50
Vodka (80 proof), 1 oz	65	12	8	6	3	50
Vermouth, dry, 1 oz	33	6	4	3	2	25
Vermouth, sweet, 1 oz	45	9	5	4	2	35
Bloody Mary, 1½ oz liquor + 6 oz juice	130	25	16	12	7	100
Screwdriver, 1½ oz liquor + 6 oz juice	175	34	21	16	9	135

Note: These values are based on the energy used by an adult male weighing approximately 154 pounds (70 kg) and should be adjusted for other individuals according to their weight and sex.
[a] Energy cost of walking for 70-kg individual = 5.2 kilocalories per minute at 3.5 mph.
[b] Energy cost of riding bicycle = 8.2 kilocalories per minute.
[c] Energy cost of swimming = 11.2 kilocalories per minute.
[d] Energy cost of running, 180 steps/min. = 19.4 kilocalories per minute.
[e] Energy cost of reclining = 1.3 kilocalories per minute.
Source: Adapted from F. Konishi, Food energy equivalents of various activities, *Journal of the American Dietetic Association* 46:186, 1965.

all by itself can make the dieter *look* slimmer) and increased circulatory efficiency. It makes people feel better psychologically. Finally, exercise can be enjoyable. Calisthenics and "diet exercises" are widely considered boring, but tennis, swimming, walking, jogging, and even rope jumping are frequently more fun.

Energy expenditure can be increased in other simple ways as well, with some advance planning. Dieters should be encouraged to park the car or get off the bus several blocks from their destination, and walk there quickly. Instead of waiting for the elevator, they should walk up a flight or two of stairs. In fact, walking at any time is an excellent exercise. It can be done virtually everywhere, requires no special equipment, and is especially suitable for people who, at least initially, find the more strenuous or competitive sports too taxing. A quick examination of daily activities can suggest many other creative ways to increase the amount of energy expended without spending a lot of time or money. This assumes, of course, that the dieter is young and healthy. Individuals who are extremely overweight, who have a history of illness, or who are middle-aged or older should consult their physician to establish an exercise program suited to their special needs.

Exercise often provides the "edge" for a dieter. Usually, dieting begins in a burst of determination, supported by quickly noticeable loss of weight and inches. But then many dieters get stuck on a plateau. Their bodies have adjusted to decreased energy intake. Physiologically, fat mobilization is still taking place, but some metabolic water is retained. This is when dieters typically get discouraged. But it is important not to give up; the weight will come off. At this point, increasing energy expenditure through exercise may speed weight loss without more rigid calorie-counting on the part of the discouraged dieter. Then, too, exercise is something positive you can do to lose weight, as opposed to the negative aspect of giving up some favorite foods.

Behavior Modification Techniques

We often eat in response not to biological cues of hunger and thirst but to various social and psychological cues. Because eating habits are learned, they can be unlearned, and more appropriate eating behaviors can be substituted for those that produce and maintain obesity. In recent years, behavior modification techniques have been used with notable success in the treatment of obesity.

Before eating behaviors can be modified, however, those habits that are destructive and should be changed must be identified. Participants in behavior modification programs work closely, often in a group situation, with a group leader or therapist and keep extensive records, which are regularly reviewed and analyzed. Clients keep a daily diary of the time and places of eating, their physical position while eating, the social aspects of the situation, other activities associated with each eating experience, the degree of hunger felt, their mood at the time, their choice of food, and the amount of each food consumed, noting its energy value. Often, the client is also asked to note what events took place immediately before eating in order to identify conditions that lead to inappropriate food intake.

After this period of data collection, the client and therapist examine the data and identify problems, such as eating while watching television, eating too quickly at meal times, or snacking when bored or tense. The next step is to plan the strategy for changing, or modifying, a particular behavior that is associated with excessive food intake. Substituting a new pattern has been found to be more successful than attempting to eliminate the negative habit altogether. A person

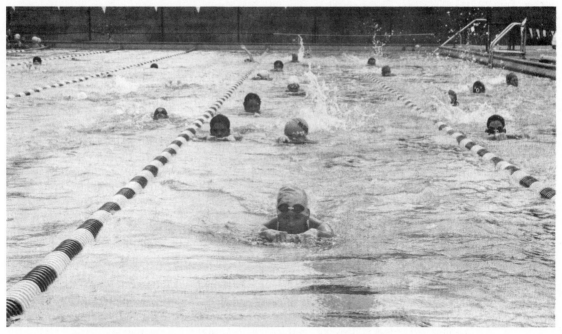

Exercise can be enjoyable: tennis, swimming, jogging, and even aerobics are frequently more fun than calisthenics or exercises.

Laimute E. Druskis

who cannot stop eating snacks completely may still be able to change her or his snacking in some way—perhaps by substituting a low-calorie, high-nutrient food such as fruit for the usual potato chips and beer. Removing tension and boredom from anyone's life may not be possible, but a client may be guided to pick up needlepoint or a crossword puzzle at such times instead of reaching for a sugar sweetened soft drink or a cookie. A similar approach may be used to increase physical activity at the same time. If weight is lost, the modifications are continued. If weight is not lost, new modifications are tried.

The changes planned in behavior modification therapy are intended to decrease both the frequency and the quantity of food intake. Such changes are effective because obese individuals frequently have eating habits that differ from those of normal-weight individuals: eating more rapidly, taking larger bites, and chewing food less thoroughly than their nonobese tablemates.

Changes will become permanent only if they are reinforced in some way. A sequence of rewards is usually built into the modification program and formalized by a "contract" between client and therapist. For instance, when a certain weight loss is achieved, or when a certain negative behavior has not been resumed for a period of time, the client is entitled to buy a new outfit in a size that fits. The goal is permanent change and permanent normal weight; the adult individual must assume full responsibility for his or her own eating behavior.

Behavior modification for children is seldom successful unless the entire family becomes involved. Each family member is shown how to aid and encourage new eating habits in the overweight child and is thus given a share of responsibility for the outcome. Otherwise, the family is likely to subvert the child's efforts to change.

So far behavior modification, in conjunction with a balanced deficit diet to ensure nutritional adequacy, seems to be an effective addition to conventional methods of weight control. However, only long-term studies will indicate its effectiveness in achieving permanent weight loss.

Alternative Methods of Weight Reduction

Having decided to lose weight, most people want immediate results. So they succumb to a succession of diets and other treatments publicized in the popular press.

The media promises are indeed appealing. "Eat all you want and still lose weight" promises one advertisement. "Lose 30 pounds in 90 minutes!!!" touts another. (This extravagant claim, explained in small print at the bottom of the advertisement, actually referred to the 18 five-minute visits to a weight-loss clinic over a period of months!) There are diet guides directed at women, at drinking men and thinking men, at chubby children and at busy executives. Devices and treatments offer to banish pounds and inches, shape the legs, trim the tummy, and otherwise alter the user's shape. Numerous over-the-counter pharmaceutical preparations promise to decrease the appetite, fill the stomach, break down fat, and speed waste products out of the body.

The Food and Drug Administration does not have authority to interfere with the promotion of such programs and products *before* they reach the marketplace. The only recourse is legal action by consumers after purchase, based on injury or ineffectiveness. Obviously, the risk of complaints is insufficient to discourage the promoters of these diet "aids." As quickly as one plan disappears from the market, another rushes in to take its place.

Many dieters, recognizing obesity as a health problem, turn to their physicians. Because few physicians have studied diet-management, all too often the result is a cursory examination and a printed diet sheet. Few of the millions of overweight Americans have ever been asked by their physicians for a diet history or instructed in any method of evaluating food-intake patterns and determining energy requirements. Or the obese turn to physicians who have developed reputations as "diet doctors," and who are just as ready as more commercial ventures to promise fast, effortless diet programs.

Weight-reduction "clinics," "medical centers," and "health spas" compete aggressively for the money to be made by promising painless loss of poundage. Their fees are generally quite high, and too often, susceptible customers sign contracts before inquiring about the actual content of their programs.

KETOGENIC DIETS. Low-carbohydrate diets have been popular for a number of years. Some of these have such impressive-sounding names as the "Mayo Clinic Diet" (a title given to several different food regimens, all of which have been disavowed by that prestigious institution) or the "Air Force Diet" (similarly disclaimed by the U.S. Air Force). In this category too are Dr. Atkin's Diet Revolution, the Stillman Diet, and many other variants. These programs have in common a severe restriction of carbohydrate intake, while they allow large or even unlimited amounts of certain high-protein foods. They differ, however, in the amount of energy intake permitted and range from being calorie-restricted to "eat all the meat you want."

Promoters of these diets assert that fat people tend to convert carbohydrates into adipose tissue more rapidly than normal people. The fat and protein in the diets they recommend, however, are said to be burned in the metabolic process and therefore cannot be stored as fat. But this is simply untrue: There is no consistent scientific evidence to indicate that energy provided from any one nutrient is utilized differently from energy from any other source.

In a low-carbohydrate diet, glycogen stores are rapidly depleted, an effect that is accelerated when calorie intake is also restricted. Fatty acids are metabolized at a rapid rate to provide energy in the form of ketone bodies for physiological functioning. Most body tissues can readily utilize the ketone bodies for energy needs, but the brain must first undergo a period of adaptation during which glucose is still required. Gluconeogenesis provides the glucose at the expense of body protein. Meanwhile, acetyl CoA is being produced more rapidly than the Krebs cycle can metabolize it, and the number of ketone bodies in the blood increases to abnormal levels.

This physiological imbalance, known as *ketosis*, is decidedly unhealthy. Ketone bodies are acids. Their overproduction upsets the body's acid-base balance, a condition that cannot be tolerated by people with kidney disease—and that may precipitate kidney problems in previously normal individuals. Electrolyte loss, which may cause cardiovascular problems, also occurs in ketosis. In addition, ketone bodies compete with uric acid for kidney excretion, increasing the risk of gout in susceptible individuals. There is one small plus for ketosis: It acts as a mild appetite suppressant, which may be somewhat helpful to the dieter.

Proponents of ketogenic diets point to the rapid and often substantial initial weight losses as evidence that these diets work. "Lose 7 to 15 pounds in the first week," they promise—and indeed the scales often bear them out. But this initial loss is a depletion of water, not of fat. The mechanism of water loss on a low-carbohydrate diet may be related to the sodium loss induced by ketosis. In any event, the water will be regained when carbohydrate intake is resumed.

Contrary to claims, actual rate of fat loss is quite slow in ketogenic diets, because fats are not metabolized efficiently in the absence of carbohydrates. Without carbohydrates to regenerate oxaloacetate, the Krebs cycle is disrupted (see Figure 5–3) and ketone bodies accumulate. For this reason, a minimum of 50 grams (200 kcal) of carbohydrate per day should be included in any weight-loss diet. Furthermore, ketogenic diets often promote excessive cholesterol and saturated fat intakes.

Because of the strange food combinations advocated in low-carbohydrate diets, few people are able to adhere to them for very long, and lost weight is often regained when regular eating is resumed. Thus, ketogenic diets often lead to the "yo-yo effect" of initial weight loss, followed by weight gain, followed by yet another unbalanced diet. This sequence may be even more dangerous than being slightly overweight.

STARVATION. Ketosis results also from the most rigorous weight-loss program, starvation or prolonged fasting. Starvation regimens are not recommended for those who should lose 35 pounds or less and they are generally used only for the massively obese. Patients should be hospitalized for the duration, at least one and perhaps two or three months; only in that way can intake be controlled and medical supervision provided. Vitamin and mineral supplements and a minimum of two quarts of water a day must be taken. The metabolic processes are essentially the same as those in the low-carbohydrate diets, with ketone bodies providing the chief energy source for all tissues. Weight loss may be as high as one pound per day. There are, however, possible severe side effects, including nausea and loss of hair. The most serious consequence is the loss of muscle protein during the fasting period; 65 percent of the weight loss produced by fasting is traceable to a loss of lean

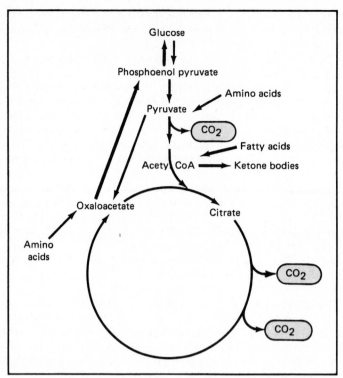

FIGURE 5-3   *Disruption of the Krebs Cycle on a Low-Carbohy-drate Diet.*

As carbohydrate intake is reduced, oxaloacetate, produced by the deamination of amino acids, is used for glucose synthesis via the intermediate PEP (phosphoenol pyruvate). Oxaloacetate is thus diverted from the reactions of the Krebs cycle. As fatty acids are metabolized to acetyl CoA, formation of citrate cannot occur. Instead, units of acetyl CoA are condensed to form ketone bodies.

body tissue and only 35 percent to loss of fat. This lean tissue loss can be avoided by administration of small amounts of protein to maintain tissue protein; on a *protein-sparing modified fast,* 3 to 6 ounces of dry milk, egg white, cottage cheese, or fish are added twice a day to the otherwise zero-calorie intake.

Although part of the rationale for prolonged fasting is that it may break the chain of dietary habits that produce obesity and thus give obese patients a clean start, this does not seem to happen. In a study of 208 grossly obese patients (192 men and 16 women) who lost weight during prolonged fasting, near normal body weight was attained in approximately 50 percent of the cases. However, within two to three years, there was a steady return to prefasting weight level in all patients, regardless of length of fasting, extent of weight loss, or age of onset of obesity. Patients who had been obese since infancy tended to regain weight to levels even *above* their prefasting point.

The presumed benefits of protein-sparing fasts have been questioned by some, and long-range studies of their effectiveness have yet to appear. However, approaches that gradually readjust the patient to the real world of eating following such a regimen have been tried and show promise. For example, the patient is weaned from the protein-sparing fast to an energy-restricted program in which regular foods are slowly introduced. Behavior modification therapy accompanies the next transition, to a normal weight-maintenance diet, with the aim of restructuring eating habits.

SURGERY, MEDICATION, AND OTHER APPROACHES. Surgical treatment of obesity should be reserved for the massively obese and patients should have tried other methods of weight reduction. Several years ago intestinal bypass surgery was a popular technique for a period. While the surgery was successful in terms of weight loss, the list of complications grew steadily. The early complications resulted from the surgery; the long term complications were metabolic and involved the liver and kidney. Gastric stapling, which reduces the size of the stomach, is now the surgical treatment of choice. While the number and severity of complications is less than with intestinal bypass, the failure rate, as measured by regaining weight or failing to lose weight, is higher with gastric stapling. Suctioning fat is not truly a technique for treatment of obesity. It can be used cosmetically to remove relatively small amounts of fat, but not a large amount because suction vacuums up blood vessels, nerves, and tissues as well as fat.

Reliance on drugs is another risky means of weight control. Americans have become so used to taking pills and potions for all sorts of major and minor problems that we expect pills to confer speedy slimness, too. Unfortunately, pills cannot do anything except suppress appetite and disrupt fluid balance and metabolism. Drugs can also be abused and become habit-forming.

Amphetamines have most often been prescribed for their appetite-depressing effects. However, these drugs are central nervous system stimulants and can lead to excitability, insomnia, constipation, and addiction. In addition, their appetite-depressing ability is short-lived, and ever-increasing amounts become necessary to maintain the same level. Newer medications attempt to suppress appetite without the side effects of the amphetamines.

Diuretics and laxatives have also been prescribed for the overweight person. Again, these substances do not attack the central problem and can lead to a temporary, and false, sense of security. Worse, they can lead to serious loss of water and electrolytes and interfere with nutrient absorption.

A placental hormone, HCG (human chorionic gonadotrophin), has been touted as an adjunct to severely energy-restricted diets. Studies have not confirmed the effect of the hormone independently of the loss of weight due to the low-calorie (500 kcal, 2100 kJ) regimen.

Finally, there is a constantly increasing assortment of devices promising to rid the body of its fat by application to the body's external surface. You might try rubber stockings that supposedly trim heavy thighs by inducing perspiration. A similar claim has been made for "Instant Trim" as well as various gloves and girdles that promise to exercise parts of your body while you are doing something else. Perspiration, it must be emphasized, has no effect on fat cells; and any garment that is wrapped or worn tightly can dangerously impede circulation. None of these devices facilitates permanent weight loss in any way although they may produce temporary dehydration. One of the gadget approaches to weight reduction is that something called "cellulite" accumulates under our skin and must be removed by controlled exercise and massage with special lotions. This, too, is nonsense. But the public spends a fortune in a vain attempt to lose those extra pounds in an easy, painless way.

Many have found that the only regimen that works for them is a combination of controlled food intake and participation in a supportive group. The growing rosters of Weight Watchers, TOPS (Take Off Pounds Sensibly), Overeaters Anonymous, and similar groups attest to the success of such supportive approaches. Regular weigh-ins, shared experiences, and the genuine interest of others in the dieter's success seem to be effective. Such programs combine balanced deficit diets, behavior modification, and social and psychological support. They encourage exercise and provide the motivation of a periodic social event and group involvement along with hope for a positive outcome.

RECOMMENDATIONS. A number of approaches to weight loss have been examined in this section. Table 5–7 shows the goals, advantages, and disadvantages of several methods. In choosing a program, it is important to determine whether its prescriptions make sense. Clearly, any progam that does not call for restricting energy intake does not make sense. Any program that stresses a single food—grapefruit, perhaps—or eliminates an entire nutrient category—"no carbohydrate"—doesn't make sense. The only sure and safe way to lose weight is to reduce the total amount of energy intake by eliminating or drastically decreasing intake of high-fat and highly sugared foods, unnecessary snacks, and alcoholic beverages; by eating smaller portions at scheduled meals; and by increasing physical exercise. Only a diverse diet provides all the nutrients necessary for continued healthy living during weight loss. Nutritionists recommend a distribution of energy intake for weight-reduction diets in the proportions of 20 to 25 percent from protein, 30 percent from fat, and 45 to 50 percent from carbohydrate. Only readjustment of eating patterns will make lifelong weight maintenance possible.

Prevention remains the best tactic of all for weight control. Balancing intake with expenditure and making adjustments throughout life as metabolic needs change during different stages of the life cycle are the keys to preventing overweight.

UNDERWEIGHT CONDITION IS NEGATIVE ENERGY BALANCE

Definition, Risks, and Treatment

Although obesity is classified as a major national nutrition problem, some individuals exhibit varying degrees of underweight. By definition, an individual who is underweight weighs less than 90 percent of the appropriate weight for his or her height, age, and body build.

Compared to the risks associated with obesity, there are fewer medical risks attached to being underweight provided the degree of underweight is not severe. A body mass index between 18 and 20 would indicate underweight without risk of severe problems. A BMI below 17 is suggestive of **anorexia nervosa** or other eating disorder or an organic problem. There is, however, a somewhat increased susceptibility to infection, including tuberculosis, particularly during adolescence. Because underweight individuals have low reserves of energy stored as adipose tissue, energy needs during periods of illness or stress, when appetite is diminished, may have to be met by drawing from lean body mass.

Probably the greatest risk associated with the underweight condition affects

TABLE 5-7. *Comparison of Various Weight-Reduction Methods*

Method	Description	Promised Goals	Advantages	Disadvantages
1. Balanced Deficit	Reduction of energy intake / Avoidance of concentrated sweets and foods of high fat content	Steady rate of weight loss	Nutritionally adequate diet / No known medical risks / Development of appropriate eating behaviors (if not below 1,000 kcal/day)	Relatively slow weight loss discouraging to some individuals
2. Weight Watchers, TOPS, and similar groups	Weekly group meetings / Reduction of energy intake by standardized meal plan	Steady rate of weight loss	Encouragement in group situation / Nutritionally adequate diet / Structured plan, beneficial for some	Relatively slow weight loss discouraging to some individuals
3. Behavior Modification	In conjunction with energy-restricted diet	Weight loss / Changes in eating behaviors	Opportunity to learn new eating behaviors / Personal preferences in foods and life styles allowed	Does not work for all individuals
4. Formula Diets	Liquid containing nutrients, usually in skim-milk base / Consumed to provide 900 kcal/day	"Easy" weight loss	Structured plan / Nutritionally adequate diet (except lacking in fiber)	Monotony / Maintenance of weight loss usually not sustained / No development of appropriate eating behaviors
5. High-protein diets (Low carbohydrate)	Meat, fish, eggs, vitamin supplement, fluid	Rapid weight loss	Short-term rapid weight loss	High fat/high cholesterol / Medical risk for some individuals / Weight loss not sustained / Low in calcium
6. Starvation	Intake restricted to water and vitamin/mineral supplements for extended period of time	Rapid weight loss	Rapid weight loss for massively obese	Hospitalization required / Medical risk / Loss of lean body mass / Maintenance of weight loss usually not sustained
7. Drugs	(a) Amphetamines	Reduction in appetite leading to weight loss	"Easy and painless" method	Weight loss not sustained / Potentially serious side effects / No development of appropriate eating behaviors
	(b) Laxatives/diuretics: excretion of nutrients, water	Weight loss	"Easy" method	Weight loss not sustained / Risk of dehydration and electrolyte imbalance / No development of appropriate eating behaviors
	(c) Thyroid hormones: induce hypermetabolic state	Weight loss	"Easy" method	Medical risk / Weight loss not sustained
8. Surgery	Reduction of volume of stomach	Weight loss	Suitability for massively obese / Steady weight loss for 1–2 years / Positive psychological benefit	Surgical risk / Serious medical side effects in many people / May not be effective long term

young women who are pregnant; they have a higher risk of not completing pregnancy and of delivering low-birth-weight infants than do women of normal weight. In addition, women may have difficulty becoming pregnant because of low body weight and may experience disturbances of their menstrual cycles. Recovery from severe illness, surgery, or other traumas may be more complicated and take longer for the underweight individual and require extensive medical treatment and nutritional therapy.

The degree of underweight common in Western society is generally not life threatening or even a significant medical risk. It is usually due to inadequate energy intake, excessive physical activity, or genetic predisposition. Of course, physical illnesses such as cancer, gastrointestinal disorders, chronic disease, or hyperthyroidism may produce serious weight loss. Illness may cause loss of appetite, leading to sharply reduced food intake, perhaps accompanied by malabsorption of energy-yielding nutrients and an increase in the rate of catabolism. In these cases, correction of the underlying condition should correct the weight problem as well. For most people who are chronically underweight, however, increased energy consumption is the key.

Increasing energy intake is not as easy as it may seem. Many underweight individuals simply do not like cakes, cookies, milkshakes, and other high-energy foods. Even for the underweight, empty calories are an unwise choice, except as supplements to a nutritionally adequate intake pattern. Nutritionists recommend instead a balanced diet of easily digested foods that are low in bulk. The goal is to increase energy without increasing the overall volume of food eaten. Raw fruit and salad, for example, will add bulk but not substantial energy and may satisfy the appetite before an adequate amount of energy-yielding food has been eaten. Fat-rich foods that increase energy without adding bulk are a good choice. Thus, it is possible to add cheese to egg dishes and sauces; cream or whole milk to soups; and butter, mayonnaise, or jams or jellies to sandwiches without significantly increasing the quantity of food to be eaten. Serving excessively fatty or sweet foods at meals can be counterproductive, however, since such foods are likely to depress appetite even further. Underweight individuals may respond more readily to the addition of snacks between their regular meals than to an addition of food at mealtimes. Thus, an afternoon snack of pie and milk or a bedtime sandwich, or muffin with butter and honey or jelly, would be a good way to add energy.

In some individuals, being underweight is associated with a rush-and-hurry life style or with a frantic, perhaps "nervous," approach to normal events and stresses. If there is a social or psychological component to an individual's lack of appetite, psychotherapy and/or behavior modification therapy may be desirable. In most cases, nutritionists find active and enthusiastic cooperation in their underweight patients, many of whom suffer serious psychological damage from their condition. Being teased about their "skinny" appearance is just as painful to underweight individuals as being teased about obesity is to many overweight individuals.

Anorexia Nervosa

Anorexia nervosa is clinically defined as self-induced starvation characterized by voluntary refusal to eat due to an intense fear of fatness. Misnamed by Sir William Gull over 100 years ago, anorexia nervosa is not truly a loss of appetite (anorexia). The prevalence of anorexia nervosa has increased rapidly in the past 15 to 20 years. According to a report published by the National Institute of Child Health and Human Development, about one of every 200 Americans between 12 and 18 years

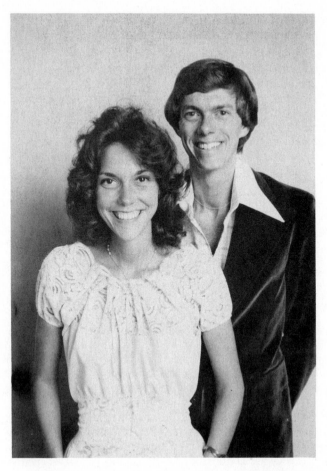

Karen Carpenter suffered from anorexia nervosa, a self-induced state of starvation that can result in death.

Steve Schapiro/SYGMA

of age will develop some degree of anorexia nervosa. The overwhelming majority of patients with anorexia nervosa are adolescents or young adult females, but it has also been diagnosed in older women and a few men. Cases have been reported in women up to age 94 years and in children under 12 years of age. Male anorectics are frequently involved in sports which necessitate lower weights, such as wrestling.

Anorexia nervosa, like obesity, is not a homogeneous disorder. Compulsive exercising may also be a manifestation of anorexia. Causation theories range from the psychoanalytic—individuals with anorexia nervosa are attempting to delay puberty—to sociocultural—an overemphasis on the ultrathin female form. The sociocultural emphasis on skinny has resulted in a syndrome roughly called "fear of obesity" which may be a new syndrome or a precursor of true anorexia nervosa. This syndrome in children has resulted in a deprivation so severe that growth was stunted and puberty delayed.

Metabolic changes which accompany anorexia nervosa include menstrual irregularities, decreased metabolic rate, slow heart rate, hypotension, hypothermia, electrolyte imbalance and decreased blood glucose concentrations. Patients with anorexia nervosa may also have abdominal pain, decreased intestinal motility, constipation, dry inelastic skin, brittle hair and nails, and lanugo, a soft fine hair covering the skin.

Bulimia

In 1980, bulimia was officially defined as a separate eating disorder, but there is still some controversy as to whether anorexia nervosa and bulimia are in fact separate disorders. Operationally, bulimia is a disorder characterized by binge eating (large amounts of food in a short period of time) usually followed by purging either by forced vomiting and/or abuse of laxatives or diuretics. For some individuals vomiting is almost a reflex action after eating. Like patients with anorexia nervosa, patients with bulimia also have an exaggerated fear of fatness. Bulimia can occur in individuals of any weight.

Bulimia may be more prevalent than anorexia nervosa, but no well-controlled studies are available. The reported prevalence ranges between 2.1 percent and 19 percent.

In a study of over 1200 females, aged 14 to 19 years, bulimic students scored higher on the body dissatisfaction and pursuit-of-thinness scales and were more likely to be chronic dieters. In an effort to control their appetite and lose weight, 5.3 percent of the students took diet pills once a week or more. Approximately 3 percent used self-induced vomiting at least once a week and almost 2 percent used diuretics once a week. Sixty-eight percent of the bulimics were currently dieting compared to 35 percent of the non-bulimic group. Thirty-three percent of the bulimic group reported they were always dieting compared to 6 percent of the non-bulimic group.

A typical bulimic is white, single, college-educated, female, normal weight for height, and in her early to mid-20s. About 10 to 13 percent of bulimics are males. About 30 to 50 percent of patients with anorexia nervosa develop symptoms of bulimia. Individuals who are bulimics can develop a number of complications from constant purging. Recurrent vomiting can result in enamel erosion by exposure of teeth to the acidic gastric contents as well as fluid and electrolyte imbalances. Laxative abuse can result in metabolic acidosis and damage to the colon. Diuretics can result in metabolic alkalosis, dehydration, and hypokalemia. Unfortunately the age group which has the highest incidence of anorexia and bulimia is the same age group who believes that they are almost indestructable and will never have health problems.

Treatment of Anorexia Nervosa and Bulimia

For the patient with anorexia nervosa, the goals of treatment are to achieve and maintain appropriate weight, resolve underlying psychological problems and improve family interactions. Initial treatment may involve hospitalization when weight loss is severe, when severe metabolic problems have developed, when outpatient treatment has failed after six months to a year, and when the patient and/or the family is in crisis. Good nutritional status must be achieved before the patient can benefit from psychotherapy. To accept weight gain, patients with anorexia nervosa need support initially from the hospital team if the patient has been hospitalized, and later from the clinic staff and family.

Success for patients with anorexia nervosa is as difficult as for the obese patient, if not more so. Combining the data from 12 major studies revealed that only 49 percent of the patients alive at follow-up were at an appropriate weight; 18 percent showed no significant change in weight. About 8 percent of the patients were dead. Mortality ranged from 3 to 25 percent and it was caused by inanition, congestive heart failure, electrolyte disturbances, and suicide. More than half the surviving patients continued to have eating disorders and about the same number showed signs of psychiatric impairment.

The goals of treatment for normal-weight bulimics are to change the patient's attitude toward food, eating, and body image and to interrupt the binge/purge cycle. Most normal-weight bulimics can be treated effectively as outpatients. Psychotherapy and behavioral treatments are used to help the bulimic cope with the anxiety, anger, and depression which triggered the binge/purge cycle. Group therapy, as with many other problems, seems to be particularly beneficial. Outcome for normal-weight bulimics apparently is better than for anorectics who binge and purge, or for those with severe bulimia. Although difficult to validate, suicide is the most common cause of death of patients with bulimia.

ON BALANCE

The principle of energy balance as applied to weight maintenance—energy taken in must be equal to energy expended—is simple enough in theory, but more difficult in practice. Foods eaten in excess, whether they have a high or low nutrient density, contribute to weight gain. Foods that are of low nutrient density may cause additional nutritional problems as well. Physical activity also plays an important role in maintaining energy balance. Eating disorders are exacerbated by our overemphasis on thinness, our lack of acceptance of variations in body weight, the almost constant hawking of food, and our decreased energy expenditure. As students you may walk a lot to and from classes, but can you go anywhere else without getting into a car? Look at the neighborhood where you and the family live. Are there sidewalks? Can you walk to a suburban shopping mall? How many times have you seen someone driving around the parking lot of a mall to find the nearest parking space and step out of the car in a jogging suit or its equivalent, or drive to the tennis courts down the block? Do we teach our children activities they can continue all of their lives? Balancing both our diets and patterns of physical activity as well as accepting a more realistic view of appropriate weight can go a long way to preventing the extremes of obesity and anorexia.

SUMMARY

The human body requires energy for each of its functions. Normal growth and development, rehabilitation following illness or stress of any kind, normal cellular metabolic processes, and our daily activities all require energy. But all these anabolic processes together consume only 30 to 40 percent of the energy our bodies derive from metabolizing food nutrients. The greatest portion of available energy is used to maintain body temperature and all our involuntary functions such as breathing.

Energy is defined as the capacity to do work, and food energy has traditionally been measured in kilocalories (also called Calories), a unit of heat energy. However, the joule, a metric nonheat measure of energy is being increasingly used. One kilocalorie (kcal) is equivalent to 4.18 kilojoules (kJ). The energy content of foods is determined by use of a bomb calorimeter which literally burns (oxidizes) a measured sample of a particular food and determines the amount of heat generated.

Energy requirements of individuals are the total of a number of components, including the basal metabolic rate or energy needs at rest, the extent and kinds of physical activity, and the quantity of energy related to the ingestion of a meal. The last is known as dietary inducted thermogenesis (DIT). All energy needs are proportionate to the size (weight and height) of the individual. Standard tables have been derived from measurements of these factors in numerous individuals, and the Food and Nutrition Board has recommended that adult American males consume 2,700 kilocalories (11,340 kJ) per day, and adult females 2,000 kilocalories (8,400 kJ).

The energy-producing nutrients are carbohydrates, fats, and protein, as well as alcohol. Of these, fats provide the most concentrated source of energy. Energy supplied in excess of that required for body functions is stored as adipose tissue. A certain amount of subcutaneous fat and energy reserve is necessary, but a marked excess is unhealthy. Obesity is excess fat and should be diagnosed on this basis. More than 30 percent of the American adult population is estimated to be obese.

The causes of obesity are varied and complex, ranging from the strictly genetic to that resulting from an interaction between genetics and environment. Our society places a premium on thinness and the millions of individuals trying to lose weight constitute a vast market for fad diets and other reducing aids. Most such methods are ineffective at best because they do not correct the underlying food habits that caused the problem, and they may be dangerous at worst. The best approach to weight control combines a balanced deficit diet (that is, balanced nutrient intake and a reduction in energy consumption) with behavior modification therapy to correct eating patterns; increasing physical activity also helps.

There is less medical risk attached to mild underweight; however, anorexia nervosa, a self-induced state of virtual starvation affecting primarily adolescent girls and caused by an underlying emotional disorder, can have severe consequences. Medical and psychological treatment is indicated to correct this disturbance.

Bulimia, another eating disorder can occur in patients of normal weight. Bulimia is manifested by binge eating and purging either by vomiting or by abusing laxatives and/or diuretics. The medical consequences of the recurrent purging can be severe. Psychological treatment is also indicated for this eating disorder.

BIBLIOGRAPHY

AMATRUDA, J.M., T.L. BIDDLE, M.L. PATTON, and D.H. LOCKWOOD. Vigorous supplementation of a hypocaloric diet prevents cardiac arrhythmias and mineral depletion. *American Journal of Medicine* 74:1016–1022, 1983.

AMES, S.R. The joule-unit of energy. *Journal of the American Dietetic Association* 357:415, 1970.

ANDERSON, A.E. Practical Comprehensive Treatment of Anorexia Nervosa and Bulimia. Baltimore, MD: Johns Hopkins Press, 1985.

ATKINSON, R.L. Very low calorie diets: Getting sick or remaining healthy on a handful of calories. *Journal of Nutrition* 116:918, 1986.

BEATON, G.H. Energy in human nutrition: Perspectives and problems. *Nutrition Reviews* 41:325–340, 1983.

BRAY, G.A. In N. Kretchmer, ed. *Adolescent Obesity in Frontiers of Clinical Nutrition.* Rockville, MD: Aspen Publications, 1986.

BRUCH, H. *Eating Disorders: Obesity, Anorexia Nervosa and the Person Within.* New York: Basic Books, 1973.

BRUCH, H. *The Golden Cage: The Enigma of Anorexia Nervosa.* Cambridge, MA: Harvard University Press, 1978.

CARNEY, R.M., and A.P. GOLDBERG. Weight gain after cessation of cigarette smoking: A possible role for adipsoe-tissue lipoprotein lipase. *New England Journal of Medicine* 31:614–616, 1984.

CASTONGUAY, T.W., E.A. APPLEGATE, D.E. UPTON, and J.S. STERN. Hunger and appetite: Old concepts/new distinctions. *Nutrition Reviews* 41:101–110, 1983.

CHARNEY, E., H.C. GOODMAN, H. MCBRIDE, B.

LYON, and R. PRATT. Childhood antecedents of adult obesity. Do chubby infants become obese adults? *New England Journal of Medicine* 295:6, 1976.

CLEARY, M.P., and J.R. VASSELLI. Reduced organ growth when hyperphagia is prevented in genetically obese (fa/fa) Zucker rats. *Proc. Soc. Exp. Biol. Med.* 167:616–623, 1981.

CORONAS, R., S. DURAN, P. GOMEX, H. ROMERO, and A. SASTRE. Modified total fasting and obesity: results of a multicentric study. *International Journal of Obesity* 6:463–471, 1982.

CUNNINGHAM, J.J. A reanalysis of the factors influencing basal metabolic rate in normal adults. *American Journal of Clinical Nutrition* 33:2372–2374, 1980.

DICKERSON, R.E. Cytochrome c and the evolution of energy metabolism. *Science American* 242:137–153, 1980.

DRABMAN, R.S., D. HAMMER, and G.J. Jarvie. Eating rates of elementary school children. *Journal of Nutrition Education* 9(2):80, 1977.

DUGDALE, A.E., G.M.S. MAY, and V.M. O'HARA. Ethnic differences in the distribution of subcutaneous fat. *Ecology of Food Nutrition* 10:19–24, 1980.

EISENBERG, E., and T.L. HILL. Muscle contraction and free energy transduction in biological systems. *Science* 227:999–1006, 1985.

FAO/WHO. Energy and protein requirements. FAO Nutrition Report Series No. 52: WHO Technical Report Series No. 522. Rome: Food and Agriculture Organization, 1973.

FELIG, P. Four questions about protein diets. *New England Journal of Medicine* 298:1025, 1978.

FERGUSON, J.M. *Habits, Not Diets: The Real Way to Weight Control.* Palo Alto, CA: Bull Publishing, 1976.

FINEBURG, S.K. The realities of obesity and fad diets. *Nutrition Today* 7(4): 23, 1972.

Food and Nutrition Board, National Research Council. *Recommended Dietary Allowances,* 9th ed. Washington, DC: National Academy of Sciences, 1980.

FRIEDMAN, M.I., and E.M. STRICKER. The physiological psychology of hunger: A physiological perspective. *Psychological Review* 83(6):409, 1976.

GARN, S.M., S.M. BAILEY, P.E. COLE, and T.T. HIGGINS. Level of education, level of income, and level of fatness in adults. *American Journal of Clinical Nutrition* 30:721, 1977.

GARN, S.M., and M. LAVELLE. Two-decade follow-up of fatness in early childhood. *American Journal of Diseases of Children.* 139:181–185, 1985.

GARRISON, R.J., M.FEINLEIB, W.P. CASTELLI, and P.M. McNAMARA. Cigarette Smoking as a confounder of the relationship between relative weight and long-term mortality in the Framingham study. *Journal of the American Medical Association.* 249:2199–2203, 1983.

GORSKY, R.D., and D.H. CALLOWAY. Activity pattern changes with decrease in food energy intake. *Human Biology* 55:577–586, 1983.

HERTZLER, A. Obesity—impact of the family. *Journal of the American Dietetic Association* 79:525–530, 1981.

HIMMS-HAGEN, J. Brown adipose tissue thermogenesis in obese animals. *Nutrition Reviews* 41:261–267, 1983.

HIRSCH, J., and J.L. KNITTLE. Cellularity of obese and nonobese human adipose tissue. Federation Proceedings 29:1516, 1970.

HOWARD, A.N. The historical development, efficacy and safety of very-low-calorie diets. *International Journal of Obesity* 5:195–208, 1981.

HUBERT, H.B., M. FEINLEIB, P.A. McNAMARA, and W.P. CASTELLI. Obesity as an independent risk factor for cardiovascular disease: A 26-year follow-up of participants in the Framingham heart study. *Circulation* 67:968–977, 1983.

JAMES, W.P.T. *Research on Obesity: A Report of the DHSS/MRC Group.* London: Her Majesty's Stationery Office, 1976.

JOHNSON, C., C. LEWIS, S. LOVE, M. STUCKEY, and L. LEWIS. Incidence and correlations of bulimic behavior in a female high school population. *Journal of Youth and Adolescence,* 13:15–26, 1984.

JOHNSON, D., and E.J. DRENICK. Therapeutic fasting in morbid obesity. Long term follow-up. *Archives of Internal Medicine* 137:1381, 1977.

JORDAN, H.A. In defense of body weight. *Journal of the American Dietetic Association* 62:17, 1973.

KELLY, J.J. Bulimia: Growing "epidemic" among women. *Postgraduate Medicine* 78:187–194, 1985.

KOLATA, G. Obesity declared a disease. *Science* 227:1019–1020, 1985.

KONISHI, F. Food energy equivalents of various activities. *Journal of the American Dietetic Association* 46:186, 1965.

KONISHI, F., and S.L. HARRISON. Body weight-gain equivalents of selected foods. *Journal of the American Dietetic Association* 70:365, 1977.

KREBS, H.A. The metabolic fate of amino acids. In HN Munro and J.B. Allison, eds, *Mammalian*

Protein Metabolism Vol. 1. New York: Academic Press, 1964.

LEVEILLE, G.A., and D.R. ROMSOS. Meal eating and obesity. *Nutrition Today* 9(6):4, 1974.

LOCKWOOD, D.H., and J.M. AMATRUDA. Very low calorie diets in the management of obesity. *Annual Review of Medicine* 35:373–382, 1984.

LOHMAN, T.G. Skinfolds and body density and their relation to body fatness: A review. *Human Biology* 53:181–225, 1981.

LOVE, S., and C.J. JOHNSON. Etiological factors in the development of bulimia. *Nutrition News* 48, 2: pp 5–7, 1985.

MAYER, J. Liquid protein: The last word on the last chance diet. *Family Health/Today's Health* 10(1):40, 1978.

MAYER, J. *Overweight: Causes, Costs, and Control.* Englewood Cliffs, NJ: Prentice-Hall, 1968.

NICHOLL, C.S., J.M. POLAK, and S.R. BLOOM. The hormonal regulation of food intake, digestion and absorption. *Annual Review of Nutrition* 5:213–239, 1985.

RACKER, E. From Pasteur to Mitchell: A hundred years of bioenergetics. *Federation Proceedings* 39:210–215, 1980.

RAVELLI, G.P., Z.A. STEIN, and M.V. SUSSER. Obesity in young men after famine exposure in utero and early infancy. *New England Journal of Medicine* 295:349, 1976.

REISINE, E., R. ABEL, M. MODAN, D.S. SILVERBERG, H.E. ELIAHOU, and B. MODAN. Effect of weight loss without salt restriction on the reduction of blood pressure in overweight hypertensive patients. *New England Journal of Medicine* 298:1, 1978.

RITT, R.S., H.A. JORDAN, and L.S. LEVITZ. Changes in nutrient intake during a behavioral weight control program. *Journal of the American Dietetic Association* 74:325, 1979.

ROSS LABORATORIES. Assessment of energy metabolism in health and disease (Report of the First Conference on Medical Research). Columbus, OH: Ross Laboratories, 1980.

ROTHWELL, N.J., and M.J. STOCK. A role for brown adipose tissue in diet-induced thermogenesis. *Nature* 281:31–35, 1979.

SCHUTZ, Y., E. RAVUSSIN, R. DIETHELM, and E. JEGUIER. Spontaneous physical activity measured by radar in obese and control subjects studied in a respiration chamber. *International Journal of Obesity* 6:23–28, 1982.

SEGAL, K.R., E. PRESTA, and B. GUTIN. Thermic effect of food during graded exercise in normal weight and obese men. *American Journal of Clinical Nutrition* 40:995–1000, 1984.

SOLOW, C., P.M. SILBERFARB, and K. SWIFT. Psychosocial effects of intestinal bypass surgery for severe obesity. *New England Journal of Medicine* 290:300, 1974.

STOFFERI, J. A study of social stereotype of body image of children. *Journal of Perspectives in Social Psychology* 7:101, 1967.

STRICKER, E.M. Biological bases of hunger and satiety: Therapeutic implications. *Nutrition Reviews* 42:333–340, 1984.

STUNKARD, A.J., ed. *Obesity.* Philadelphia, PA: W.B. Saunders, 1980.

STUNKARD, A.J., and H.C. BERTHOLD. What is behavior therapy? A very short description of behavioral weight control. *American Journal of Clinical Nutrition* 41:821–823, 1985.

VAN ITALLIE, T.B., and M.U. YANG. Current concepts in nutrition: Diet and weight loss. *New England Journal of Medicine* 297:1158, 1977.

VASSELLI, J.R., M.P. CLEARY, T.B. VAN ITALLIE. Modern concepts of obesity. *Nutrition Reviews,* 41:361–373, 1983.

WELLE, S. Metabolic responses to a meal during rest and exercise. *American Journal of Clinical Nutrition* 40:990–994, 1984.

WEINSIER, R.L., T.A. WADDEN, C. RITENBAUGH, G.G. HARRISON, F.S. JOHNSON, and J.H. WILMORE. Recommended therapeutic guidelines for professional weight control programs. *American Journal of Clinical Nutrition* 40:865–872, 1984.

WOO, R., R. DANIELS-KUCH, and E.S. HORTON. Regulation of energy balance. *Annual Review of Nutrition* 5:411–4433, 1985.

YUDKIN, J. Obesity and society. *Bibliotheca Nutritio et Dieta* 26:146, 1978.

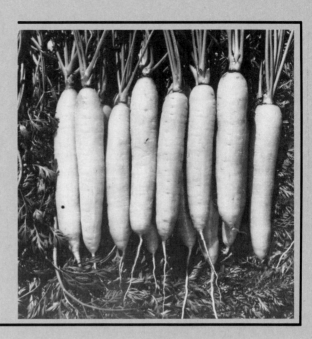

Chapter 6

FAT-SOLUBLE VITAMINS

173

That carbohydrates, fats, proteins, and certain minerals were required in the diet had been shown a hundred years ago, and researchers therefore believed that all the nutrients had been discovered. Despite the observations that unidentified "protective substances" in citrus fruits could prevent scurvy and that something in rice bran could cure beriberi, nobody made the obvious connection: As yet undiscovered substances in foods were vital to health.

However, laboratory rats stopped growing, sickened, and died when they were fed artificial mixtures containing only carbohydrates, fats, proteins, and minerals. What was the reason? Was an infectious agent present? No, because exposure of healthy animals to the sick ones did not cause the disease to be transmitted. Did the disease-producing diets contain some toxic material? Again, no, because the individual ingredients did not cause illness when given to generally well-fed rats consuming a variety of ordinary foods. There was only one logical conclusion: In contrast to diets consisting of a variety of foods, the artificial diets caused disease, not because of the *presence* of something, such as an infectious agent or a toxin, but because of the *absence* of some previously undiscovered nutrient. The concept of "deficiency disease" was thus born.

Not until 1912, however, did Casimir Funk, a Polish chemist, actually identify one of the mysterious, vital "food factors." It was neither a mineral-containing salt nor a protein but appeared to be a nitrogen-containing organic compound of rather small molecular weight. Funk called it a *vitamine*, from the Latin word *vita* (life) and the biochemical term *amine* (an organic compound containing nitrogen). As researchers began to discover other essential "food factors," however, it became apparent that not all were amines. In 1920, to avoid confusion, the British biochemist J. C. Drummond introduced the term we use today—*vitamin.*

Vitamins are, by definition, organic compounds that (1) are required in trace amounts by the body, (2) perform specific metabolic functions, and (3) are not synthesized at all in the body, or are not synthesized in adequate quantities, and so must be provided by dietary sources. Unlike the nutrients discussed thus far, vitamins do not produce energy. Also, they differ widely from one another in chemical structure and thus in biochemical function. Because no one food contains all the vitamins required by the body, a diversified diet is necessary to ensure adequate intake of each of these substances.

Vitamins are involved in a wide range of metabolic processes and may serve structural functions as well. Over and over again, the absence rather than the presence of vitamins has demonstrated their importance and specific functions. From the time of Lind's attempts to alleviate scurvy in sailors, much of what we know about vitamins has come from studies of deficiency diseases such as xerophthalmia (vitamin A), beriberi (thiamin), pellagra (niacin), and rickets (vitamin D).

Vitamin deficiencies are reflected in decreased tissue and then serum concentrations of the vitamin, followed by a decrease in the related biochemical function, leading to the clinical symptoms of the corresponding deficiency state. A *primary deficiency* results simply from inadequate consumption of the nutrient in question relative to normal physiological need. In *secondary* or *indirect deficiency,* intake is theoretically adequate but absorption may be inhibited, excretion may be accelerated, or function may be impaired in the diseased individual.

Excess consumption of certain vitamins can also have adverse effects on the normal functioning of the body. Excessive amounts of water-soluble vitamins (vitamin C and the B-complex vitamins) are readily excreted in the urine and therefore generally do not accumulate to toxic levels unless enormous overdoses are taken. Vitamins A, D, E, and K, on the other hand, are fat-soluble. Because of this property, they share a number of characteristics, including relative stability during processing, preservation, and preparation of foods; similar mechanisms of absorption and excretion; and storage in the liver and fatty deposits of the body. Because they can be stored, they do not have to be consumed on a daily basis. But for the same reason, excess consumption of vitamins A and D produces toxicity; under certain circumstances, vitamin E and some forms of vitamin K also may be toxic. These and other aspects of the fat-soluble vitamins are the subject of the present chapter.

VITAMIN A

Soon after Funk had proposed his vitamin theory, researchers at Yale University and the University of Wisconsin, working independently of each other, discovered a candidate for this new class of nutrients. They found that the source of fat in a diet fed to rats influenced growth and eye function. Removal of milkfat from a purified diet, or a diet whose only fats were lard or olive oil, produced stunted growth and eye lesions. However, with the addition of butterfat or egg yolk to the rats' diet, these symptoms were abated or even reversed.

The Wisconsin research team, Elmer V. McCollum and Marguerite Davis, named the chemically unidentified substance *fat soluble A*, based on the only property they knew it to possess. Subsequently, the yellow plant pigment carotene was shown to have the same growth-promoting properties as vitamin A, and also to be a precursor of the newly identified substance found in animal products. In 1937 the vitamin was isolated from cod-liver oil, and in 1946 it was synthesized in the laboratory.

Chemistry and Properties

Vitamin A occurs both in a preformed, active state and in a precursor form that is not active until it is converted. Preformed vitamin A exists as three biologically active variants: retinol (an alcohol), retinal (an aldehyde), and retinoic acid. As Figure 6–1 shows, the three forms are chemically identical except for the single functional group that determines its chemical behavior and how the compound is classified.

Figure 6–1 also demonstrates the chemical relationship of the three forms. Most of the preformed vitamin A in our food is the alcohol form, retinol. Retinol can be reversibly oxidized to the aldehyde form, retinal. This second form is the one involved in the visual response to dim light. Oxidation of retinal produces the acid form of the vitamin, retinoic acid. Although retinoic acid does not participate in the visual cycle and cannot be converted back to the aldehyde form, it supports growth and normal differentiation of epithelial tissue, but does not support reproductive function as do other forms of the vitamin.

Biologically active vitamin A is found almost exclusively in foods of animal origin. But all three forms of vitamin A can be produced from a group of plant pigments known as *carotenes*. These yellow-orange pigments thus serve as precursors of the biologically active forms; that is, they are provitamins. Carotenes, which give certain foods such as carrots their characteristic color, are most commonly found in the leaves of green plants, where their color is masked by the darker, green pigment chlorophyll. The most common provitamin form is β-carotene, a dark yellow-orange pigment whose chemical structure is shown in Figure 6–2.

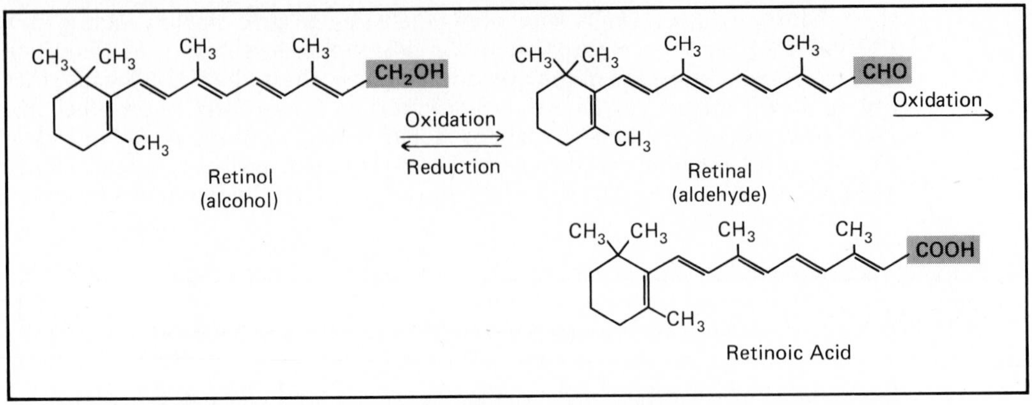

FIGURE 6-1   *Chemical Structure of Preformed Vitamin A.*

A comparison of the structure of β-carotene (Figure 6-2) with the structure of vitamin A (Figure 6-1) makes clear that two molecules of retinal can be produced by cleaving the provitamin at the position marked by the dashed line in Figure 6-2. This reaction involves molecular oxygen.

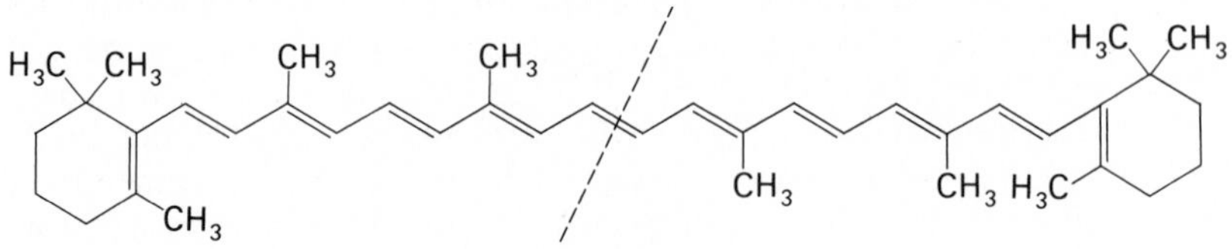

FIGURE 6-2   *Chemical Structure of β-Carotene.*

Unlike its precursors, vitamin A is colorless. Both forms are soluble in fat and fat solvents and are vulnerable to partial destruction by oxygen and ultraviolet light. They are relatively heat stable, although prolonged heat will reduce their activity.

Absorption and Metabolism

ABSORPTION.   Preformed vitamin A in foods occurs primarily as a retinyl ester—that is, as a compound of retinol and a fatty acid. In the lumen of the small intestine, pancreatic and intestinal enzymes hydrolyze it to its components. Retinol is absorbed into the mucosal cells lining the intestine, where it is rapidly reesterified (principally with palmitic acid) back to retinyl esters and "packaged" with extremely small lipid particles in the chylomicrons. In this form the retinyl esters enter the lymphatic system and then the general circulation, which ultimately delivers them to the liver, the main storage site for vitamin A.

When the diet provides the carotene precursors, which are the major source of vitamin A for most animals, the path from ingestion to storage is almost the same. In the mucosal cells of the small intestine, the provitamins are converted to retinal, assisted by a cleavage enzyme. Further conversion to retinol (by reduction) is catalyzed by another intestinal enzyme. From this point on, the processes of esterification and transport are the same as those already described.

Theoretically, every molecule of β-carotene should yield two molecules of retinal, but the conversion mechanism is not completely efficient; the implications of this fact for dietary requirements will be discussed later. Molecules of the precursor forms that remain unhydrolyzed are also packaged in the chylomicrons, along with the retinyl esters, and are transported to the liver as well. Some of the remaining β-carotene is apparently converted in the liver to retinal and then to retinyl esters, in which form it can be stored.

The absorption of vitamin A is affected by the same factors that influence fat absorption. Thus, absence of bile or any generalized malfunction of the lipid absorption system will interfere with absorption of the vitamin. Absorption can also be adversely affected by the consumption of mineral oil or of drugs that bind bile salts (such as cholestyramine, a drug used to lower blood cholesterol).

METABOLISM.   Although vitamin A is stored in the kidneys, the adipose tissue, and the adrenal glands, the primary site of storage is the liver. As noted previously, the vitamin is stored mainly in the form of retinyl esters. When vitamin A is needed by the body, esters are first hydrolyzed to retinol, which is then bound to a specific transport protein called *retinol-binding protein* (RBP) which complexes with serum transthyretin (previously called prealbumin). Bound to RBP, as retinol, vitamin A is quite stable and readily available to body tissues. But in other forms, such as retinal and particularly retinoic acid, it is quickly metabolized to products that are excreted in bile and urine. In the cytosol of many tissues there are specific proteins to bind retinol and retonoic acid.

Protein deficiency has a negative effect on vitamin A status because the synthesis of RBP is slowed or halted, and thus the serum levels of vitamin A are diminished. Zinc deficiency has a similar effect, though the actual mechanism is not understood. Liver disease such as hepatitis will decrease serum levels of both vitamin A

Development of a Bitot's spot, identified as a white patchy area on the epithelial tissue of the eyeball, is an early sign of vitamin A deficiency.
Lester V. Bergman & Associates, Inc.

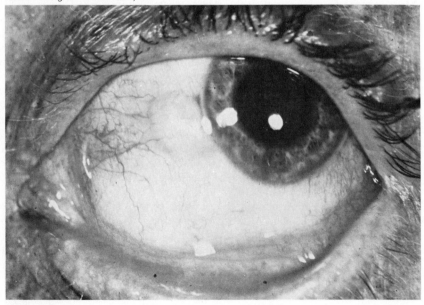

and RBP, but renal (kidney) disease actually increases the serum levels because efficiency of excretion is hampered. Among the drugs shown to affect vitamin A status are the oral contraceptives, which increase serum levels apparently by increasing RBP synthesis.

Physiological Functions

Although vitamin A is known to affect almost every tissue in the body and to have a key role in a great variety of body functions and processes, our knowledge of its biochemical activity is incomplete. There are gaps in our present understanding of vitamin A involvement in growth and tissue maintenance; its role in other metabolic processes is even less clear. In fact, the only thoroughly understood function of vitamin A is its role in the so-called visual cycle.

VISION. The mechanisms of the visual cycle were first described in detail by George Wald of Harvard University, who won a Nobel Prize in 1967 for his work. Light intensity is perceived in the retina of the eye through two types of photoreceptors or light-sensitive cells. The *rods* are sensitive to low-intensity or dim light, whereas the *cones* respond to color and high-intensity or bright light. Both types of photoreceptor contain special pigments consisting of retinal and a protein molecule called *opsin*. The pigment in the rods is *rhodopsin*, or visual purple; that in the cones is *iodopsin*, or visual violet. Slight differences in the opsin component account for the different sensitivities of the two pigments. Although the visual cycle is virtually the same for both pigments, the effects of bright light on the eye are more dramatic at night than during the day (see Figure 6–3).

The ability to see in dim light after rhodopsin has been bleached by bright light is directly related to vitamin A status. The condition called "night blindness" often results from a diminished capacity for rhodopsin regeneration. A person with night blindness will require a longer time to recover from the blinding effects of, for example, the headlights of an oncoming car. Remember that only retinol and retinal can maintain the visual cycle. Retinoic acid cannot be reduced to retinol and, therefore, cannot cure night blindness. (Vitamin A, incidentally, cannot cure color blindness, which results from the absence of some color receptors in the cones.)

Vitamin A plays an additional important role in vision by maintaining the structure of the tissues of the eye. Prolonged vitamin A deficiency can result in permanent blindness.

MAINTENANCE OF EPITHELIAL TISSUES. Epithelial tissue constitutes the external surfaces of the body—the cells that form the outer layers of the skin and the mucous membranes that line the digestive, respiratory, and reproductive tracts. These tissues produce mucus and other secretions that help to lubricate and preserve the integrity of the tissue and to protect against invasion by bacteria and other microorganisms. Vitamin A is apparently necessary for the synthesis of certain substances in mucus and other secretions.

In the absence of vitamin A, epithelial tissue does not produce mucus but becomes covered with keratin, a dry, water-insoluble protein that is the main constituent of hair and nails. Epithelial cells are gradually transformed from soft, moist tissue to hard and dry, or keratinized, areas. As more and more epithelial tissue is keratinized, there is less secretion of mucus and other protective substances. Con-

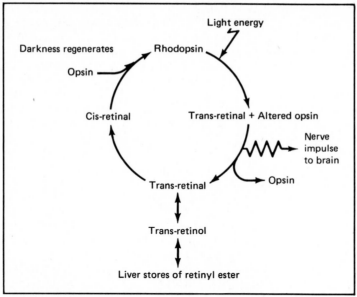

FIGURE 6-3   *Role of Vitamin A in the Visual Cycle.*

The visual cycle begins when light enters the eye and strikes the rhodopsin molecule. As the pigment absorbs the light energy, changes take place in its retinal and opsin components, causing them to dissociate. In the process, a nerve impulse is generated and sent to the brain via the optic nerve. In effect, light energy has been transformed into a signal, a nerve impulse, which carries the "visual image" to the brain.

The effect of light causing the dissociation of rhodopsin into its component parts is known as bleaching. When rhodopsin is bleached, some of the released retinal is degraded. As it is degraded, more rhodopsin must be regenerated so that the visual process can continue. Retinol released from the liver is transported by RBPs to the photoreceptor cells of the retina. Here it is oxidized to retinal and combines with opsin to form rhodopsin. Thus, new rhodopsin is always being formed to replace the rhodopsin that is broken down when visual images are transmitted. If there is not enough stored vitamin A available to participate in the regeneration process, however, rhodopsin formation is slowed or interrupted, and dim-light perception is impaired.

Source: Adapted from R. Montgomery, R. L. Dryer, T. W. Conway, and A. A. Spector, *Biochemistry: A Case-Oriented Approach* (St. Louis: C. V. Mosby Co., 1974), p. 31.

sequently the incidence of infection is noticeably greater during vitamin A deficiency. (Intestinal lining does not actually become keratinized, but its secretion of mucus decreases.) Also in vitamin A deficiency, humoral antibody production after immunization is suppressed and cell-mediated immunity is impaired. The loss of appetite noted in animals lacking vitamin A has been attributed in part to the keratinization and consequent loss of sensitivity of the taste buds. Derivatives of vitamin A have been used to treat certain forms of severe acne. These synthetic forms of vitamin A are not effective for milder forms of acne. Because of the risk of toxicity, people with acne should not attempt to treat themselves with commonly available vitamin A. Moreover, the loss of appetite noted in animals lacking vitamin A has been attributed in part to the keratinization and consequent loss of sensitivity of the taste buds.

CANCER.   The suggestion that vitamin A or its precursor may delay or prevent the development of certain types of epithelial cancer has generated a great deal of interest. Cancer, like many other diseases, can have several causes. When the term cancer is used in the following discussion, it is intended to indicate only those types which have been linked to vitamin A intake such as lung cancer.

Several large studies have associated a greater risk of cancer with lower dietary intake of beta-carotene. In the largest of these 250,000 people completed questionnaires regarding diet. After ten years, 7377 had developed cancer. Decreased risk in this group was associated with high intake of beta-carotene. Not all epidemiologic data are supportive of this correlation, however. Subjects from an area at high risk for esophageal cancer who had lesions of the esophagus had serum carotene concentrations which were not different from those subjects without lesions.

Experimental data from animal studies support a role for beta-carotene. Supplementation with beta-carotene decreased the number of tumors and increased the survival of mice inoculated with tumor cells. Oral beta-carotene also decreased the number of chemically induced skin tumors in mice. In other studies in which mice were injected with beta-carotene, growth of tumor cells was not suppressed. This suggests a role for other compounds present in green and yellow vegetables that might play a role in reducing cancer, and again points out the value of consuming foods rather than supplements as sources of vitamins and minerals.

GROWTH.   Vitamin A is required for the normal growth and development of bones and teeth. The precise mechanisms are not known, but vitamin A is believed to be an essential factor in the metabolic activity of certain specialized cells involved in the formation of these tissues.

A growing long bone contains two growth areas, or "plates," one near each end of the bone. These plates consist of layers of rapidly growing cartilaginous tissue. New bone is formed by the mineralization of the tissue at the plate edge nearest the center of the bone. This process of bone formation and growth is the function of specialized cells known as *osteoblasts*. Although the mechanism is complex and little understood, it appears that vitamin A is necessary for development of healthy osteoblasts capable of mineralizing the cartilage growth plates of bones.

Bone formation does not stop with the end of normal bone growth, however. Bone tissue is broken down and re-formed throughout the life of the individual. This continuous remodeling serves to keep the composition of bone constant. Again, osteoblasts perform the function of building new bone. The dissolution of bone is caused by enzymes released from specialized cells called *osteoclasts*. Research so far has indicated that vitamin A is apparently involved in transforming immature cells to osteoblasts and osteoclasts. Release of the enzymes that make possible the resorption of old bone also appears to require vitamin A.

Similarly, vitamin A is necessary for normal development and function of ameloblasts, specialized cells responsible for the formation of tooth enamel. In vitamin A deficiency, teeth develop imperfectly; tooth enamel is thin and tends to break or chip.

OTHER METABOLIC FUNCTIONS.   Vitamin A also has important functions in the maintenance of membrane stability, in reproduction, and in the synthesis of a number of adrenal and thyroid hormones. What little is known about the effect of vitamin A on reproductive functions indicates this influence is related to its role in the synthesis of steroid hormones.

Dietary Requirements and Recommended Allowances

UNITS OF MEASUREMENT.   Until recently, vitamin A activity in foods, as well as recommended allowances, has been expressed in **International Units (IU)**, originally defined as the amount needed to promote a specified growth rate in laboratory rats. One IU of vitamin A is equivalent to 0.3 micrograms (μg) retinol, 0.344 μg retinyl acetate, 0.6 μg β-carotene, or 1.2 micrograms of other provitamin A carotenoids. But this system, which reflects biological activity, does not take into consideration the body's absorption of the different dietary forms of vitamin A. In the form of retinol, vitamin A is completely absorbed into the body. By contrast, only one-third of dietary β-carotene (the most significant vitamin A form) is utilized, and only half of that is converted to retinol. Thus the true effectiveness of β-carotene, weight for weight, is one-sixth that of retinol; and the effectiveness of other carotenoids is one-twelfth that of retinol. Accurate specification of the total dietary activity of the vitamin, then, requires specifying the percentage from each source.

To reflect utilization more accurately, the term **retinol equivalent**, or **RE**, was introduced in 1967 by an FAO/WHO Expert Committee. By definition, one retinol equivalent is equal to one microgram of retinol or equivalent of other compounds, corrected for efficiency of utilization. The Food and Nutrition Board of the National Research Council/National Academy of Sciences has recommended adoption of the new unit. Until the transition is complete, it has also recommended that both units be used and that food analyses provide separately the different sources of vitamin A.

RECOMMENDED DIETARY ALLOWANCES.   The RDA for vitamin A is based on several factors, including the minimum amount required to eliminate clinical symptoms of deficiency, to maintain physiological function and adequate blood levels, and to promote storage. The RDA for adult American men is 1,000 RE (5,000 IU). The RDA for women has been set at 80 percent of that for men, on the basis of body weight (80 RE, or 4,000 IU). During pregnancy it is 1,000 RE (5,000 IU), and 1,200 RE (6,000 IU) is recommended for lactating mothers. For the first six months of life, the RDA is 420 RE (1,400 IU); for infants six months to one year of age, it is 400 RE (2,000 IU). The RDA for infants is based on the average content of retinol in human milk and assumes this to be the sole source for the first half year.

Dietary Sources

Considering the importance of vitamin A to health, it is fortunate that adequate amounts of this nutrient are easily obtained from a wide variety of plant and animal products (as carotenes in the former; as retinyl esters in the latter). In the United States, about half of dietary vitamin A comes from retinol and half from provitamin A carotenoids. The most concentrated sources are liver and dark green and orange-yellow vegetables, but significant amounts are provided by whole milk, butter, cream cheese, and eggs. Skim milk and its products may be fortified with the vitamin, as may margarine and other dairy product substitutes. Though plant oils contain none, fish-liver oils are highly concentrated sources of vitamin A.

Because vitamin A can be stored by the body, daily intake is not necessary. For example, as Table 6–1 shows, a single (small) serving of liver provides enough vitamin A for nine days. However, many people do not like liver and will not eat it even

TABLE 6-1. *Vitamin A Content of Selected Foods per Serving (RDA for Adults: Men 1,000 RE; Women: 800 RE)*

Food	Serving Size	IU	RE
Liver, beef, fried	3 oz	45,390	—[a]
Dandelion greens, cooked	½ c	6,084	608
Cantaloupe	½ melon	8,608	861
Sweet potato, baked	1 large	24,877	2488
Carrots, cooked, drained	½ c	15,471	1547
Collards, cooked, drained	½ c	2,109	211
Spinach, cooked, drained	½ c	7,371	737
Spinach, raw, chopped	1 c	3,760	376
Winter squash, baked	½ c	3,628	363
Beet greens, cooked, drained	½ c	3,672	367
Broccoli, cooked, drained	½ c	1,099	110
Apricots, canned in syrup	½ c	1,587	158
Tomatoes, canned	1 c	1,450	145
Apricots, dried	5 halves	1,267	126
Tomato, raw	1 medium	1,394	139
Lettuce, romaine	1 c	1,456	146
Oysters	1 c	740	—
Green peas, canned	½ c	653	65
Milk, skim or low-fat, fortified	1 c	500	140
Margarine, fortified	1 tbsp	465	141
Butter	1 tbsp	460	114
Orange juice, from concentrate	6 oz	144	12
Cream cheese	1 oz	405	124
Lettuce, Boston type	¼ head	395	40
Cheese, pasteurized, processed American	1 oz	343	82
Egg, yolk	1 large	313	94
Milk, whole	1 c	307	76
Cheddar cheese	1 oz	300	86
Yogurt, whole-milk	8 oz	280	68
Ice cream	½ c	272	66
Egg, whole	1 large	260	78
Lima beans, cooked	½ c	315	31
Banana	1 medium	92	9
Catsup	1 tbsp	210	—
Sardines, canned in oil	3 oz	190	—
Cottage cheese, creamed	½ c	170	50
Yogurt, low-fat, plain	8 oz	150	36
Apple	1 medium	74	7
Yogurt, low-fat, fruit	8 oz	104	25
Chicken, meat only	3 oz	29	9
Tuna fish	3 oz	70	—
Salmon, pink, canned	3 oz	60	—
Chickpeas	½ c	50	—
Hamburger, cooked	3 oz	30	—
Yogurt, nonfat	8 oz	16	5
Beets, canned, drained	½ c	15	—
White bread	1 slice	trace	trace

[a] Information not available.

Sources: USDA, Agricultural Research Service, *Nutritive value of foods,* Home and Garden Bulletin No. 72, rev. ed. (Washington, D.C.: U.S. Government Printing Office, 1977); and C. F. Church and H. N. Church, *Food values of portions commonly used,* 12th ed. (Philadelphia: Lippincott, 1975). Agriculture Handbooks No. 8-1, 8-4, 8-9, 8-10, (Washington, D.C.: U.S. Government Printing Office, 1976).

though it is nutritious. Thus it is important to note the many types of common foods that contain vitamin A. Since food composition tables are still expressed in IUs, it is also important to remember that the usable carotene content of foods is variable. Dark green, leafy vegetables contain carotenes, though their color is masked by the chlorophyll pigment. On the other hand, the pigments of many red or yellow-orange vegetables (kidney beans, turnips) have no significant carotene content.

In general, normal processing and cooking procedures cause little loss of vitamin A. In fact, mashing, cutting, or puréeing may increase the availability of provitamin A by rupturing plant cell walls. Also, because the vitamin is not soluble in water, there is little loss in most cooking methods. However, vitamin A oxidizes readily under the influence of high heat, and drying accelerates this reaction. To retain vitamin A, vegetables should be steamed or simmered in a small amount of water. The diet should regularly include raw or slightly cooked foods, rich in vitamin A, particularly carrots and green, leafy vegetables.

Clinical Deficiency Symptoms

Clinically significant symptoms of vitamin A deficiency are generally caused by a primary deficiency, that is, by insufficient dietary intake. Secondary deficiencies may be precipitated by absorptive disorders, including those caused by long-term use of mineral oil or prescribed drugs, or those caused by pancreatic or gall bladder disease, generally interfering with lipid metabolism. In laboratory animals, growth retardation, reproductive failure, and eye lesions are common symptoms. In humans, eye lesions and increased susceptibility to infection are the classic signs of deficiency.

Night blindness, or nyctalopia, usually the first sign of vitamin A deficiency in humans, was described as early as 1500 B.C. in ancient Egypt, and primitive "cures" for the condition have been known and used for at least 3,500 years. Ancient Egyptian documents refer to the application of liver juice to the eye as a treatment for night blindness. The question that arises, of course, is how any vitamin A could enter the body, as it must, to be effective. It has been suggested that the tear ducts of the eye may have provided the necessary entryway. This suggestion is supported by the fact that xerophthalmia in rats can be cured by the direct application of retinol to the cornea of the eye. In Java an almost identical treatment is still in use today. The one significant difference is that following local application to the eyes, the liver itself is fed to the patient. But this consumption of liver is not considered by the Javanese to be part of the treatment. It may well be that the Egyptian patients did in fact eat the liver from which the juice was derived but for some reason failed to record the fact. It is certainly known that Hippocrates, the Greek "father of medicine," prescribed eating liver as a cure for night blindness.

Of greater concern than night blindness is the progressive hardening, or keratinization, of eye tissue, which if not corrected, can result in permanent blindness. We have already discussed the role of vitamin A in the maintenance of epithelial tissue, and nowhere is its absence so obviously destructive as in the eye. *Xerosis*, or drying out of the eye tissue, is the first in the sequence of lesions associated with xerophthalmia. Epithelial cells become dry and keratinized, particularly in the cornea. Gray-white patches called Bitot's spots may appear on the surface of the eye. Keratinization of the cornea continues with prolonged deficiency and may lead to permanent blindness. These symptoms of severe deficiency are found in India and in many of the developing countries of Southeast Asia, Africa, and Latin America.

Other signs of clinical deficiency include changes in bones and nerves. In children bone growth is stunted, thereby compressing the still-growing nerves of the central nervous system (brain and spinal cord). Changes in the epithelial tissue of the gastrointestinal tract lead to diarrhea, aggravating the victim's undernutrition. Infections of eyes, ears, respiratory system, and reproductive tract are also common. Keratinization of the epithelial cells surrounding hair follicles (*follicular hyperkeratosis*) causes a bumpy, dry appearance sometimes referred to as "toad skin."

PREVENTION AND TREATMENT.   In many geographical areas foods containing vitamin A, particularly carotene-containing plants, are available; but for cultural and other reasons, they are not consumed. The need for more effective use of these dietary sources is obvious. Fortification of skim milk has helped alleviate deficiency problems. Administration of large amounts of vitamin A in single doses reverses the clinical signs and symptoms, with the exception of blindness. Preventive administration of vitamin A has been effective in reducing the prevalence of xerophthalmia.

Deficiency is more prevalent in children, as might be expected, because their tissues have not had time to build up reserves of the vitamin. Most adults eating a diverse diet have reserves that are adequate for several months to a year.

Toxicity

Paradoxically, the mechanism that protects the body against vitamin A deficiency is also the cause of its potential toxicity. The fat-soluble nature of the nutrient permits its storage in liver and other tissues. Consequently, the potential for storage of excess amounts is always present. Excess carotene intake, however, does not result in vitamin A toxicity, although the skin may turn yellow because of the high level of carotene stored in the lipid layer under the skin. This could result from consumption of a 1-pound bag of carrots every day for several weeks. Normal skin color gradually returns as carotene intake is reduced.

Serious toxic effects result from excessive intake of preformed vitamin A. Studies of pregnant animals have established that large doses of vitamin A produce severe malformations in newborn offspring: abnormalities of the central nervous system, hydrocephalus ("water on the brain"), and encephalocoele (cranial hernia). Infants may also develop hydrocephalus if fed even ten times the appropriate RDA for several weeks. **Hypervitaminosis** A in older children and adults may produce a syndrome that resembles a brain tumor: headache, nausea, vomiting, ringing in the ears, and double vision. General symptoms observed at all ages include dryness of skin and mucous membranes; thinning hair; brittle nails; enlarged spleen; anemia; and pain in the muscles, bones, joints, and abdomen. Symptoms disappear when vitamin A is discontinued.

Not more than 2,000 RE (10,000 IU) of vitamin A per day should be taken without medical recommendation and supervision. Yet, in spite of the awareness of the dangers of excessive consumption of vitamin A, hypervitaminosis A has been on the increase in recent years, with numerous reports of intakes in the range of 25,000 to 100,000 IU per day. Such quantities present a real risk to health, especially to pregnant women and the fetus. Serious toxic effects are also caused by large doses of vitamin A sometimes used in the treatment of acne. Yet clinical trials have shown that even doses in the range of 50,000 to 150,000 IU per day have no consistent or long-lasting beneficial effect on this condition. Published results from clinical trials at the dermatology branch of the National Cancer Institute, however, suggest that a vitamin A derivative, a retinoid, might be temporarily useful in the treatment of *severe* acne. The mechanism appears to be that the retinoid interferes with the production of oil by sebacious glands. The drug is still classified as experimental; moreover, caution about its teratogenic effects is advised. The new drug could not, for example, safely be given to women who are pregnant or likely to become pregnant because it is one of a class of substances known to injure embryos.

Contributory causes of hypervitaminosis A include the ease with which high-potency vitamin preparations can be obtained without a prescription; parents who act on the mistaken notion that if vitamins are good, a lot of vitamins must be even better; and the use of highly fortified "health" foods.

The biochemical mechanism of vitamin A toxicity is not known. It has been suggested that sufficiently large amounts saturate the RBP system. The unbound vitamin A then circulates as retinal in association with plasma lipoproteins. In this form it may have direct toxic effects on cells.

In summary, vitamin A is widely available in ordinary food sources, and for most people there is no need for supplementation, which may in fact be dangerous.

VITAMIN D

The identification of vitamin D and its role in human health is one of the most interesting discoveries in the history of medicine and nutritional science. The story of vitamin D, like that of vitamin A, begins in ancient times. Walking across a battlefield in 526 B.C., the Greek historian Herodotus observed a distinct difference in bone density between the Egyptian and Persian soldiers who had been opponents. The skulls of the slain Persians were fragile while those of the Egyptians were strong. The Egyptians' explanation of this difference was amazingly prophetic. They pointed out that while the Persians wore turbans to protect themselves from the sun, Egyptians went bareheaded from childhood.

Undoubtedly the Persians suffered from what we now know to be the vitamin D deficiency condition called **rickets**, which is characterized by impaired bone formation and is especially damaging during the growth years. While it must have been a common condition from the time that people began to wear clothes and live in houses, rickets was not named or described in medical literature until about 1600. By 1900, according to some estimates, 90 percent of the young children in Europe were afflicted with this disease, which killed many of them. The condition was especially common among the poor. Children who lived in cities or were born in the fall or winter were those most often affected.

As late as 1917, the cause of rickets remained unknown. The first clue came in 1918 when Sir Edward Mellanby of the University of London found that cod-liver oil and butterfat prevented the disease. Because both contained Fat Soluble A, the vitamin recently discovered by McCollum and Davis, Mellanby erroneously concluded that rickets was due to a deficiency of Fat Soluble A.

The next clue was provided by McCollum and his colleagues at Johns Hopkins University. They demonstrated that cod-liver oil retained its anti-rickets effectiveness despite being heated and oxygenated until its vitamin A content had been de-

Vitamin D Deficiency: A Disease of Civilization

Vitamin D may be the one essential nutrient that nature never intended to be a nutrient at all. A nutrient is defined in large part by its being ordinarily obtained by ingestion of foods and beverages rather than by being breathed in (as oxygen is) or by being produced in the body (like such important biochemicals as genes and hormones are). But getting adequate vitamin D by ingestion is almost impossible without the use of fortified foods, to which the vitamin has been added in unnaturally high levels; ordinary, unfortified foods are all naturally poor vitamin D sources. (Fish livers and their oils, such as cod liver oil, are rich sources, but those are hardly ordinary foods.)

Vitamin D may therefore have originally served as a biochemical other than a nutrient—perhaps a hormone or hormonelike substance. From this viewpoint, the kidneys would be considered endocrine glands because they secrete the active substance, 1, 25-dihydroxyvitamin D, or cholecalciferol. The skin produces the inactive form, or prohormone, which is fully activated only after traveling to, and being acted on by, the kidneys. After release into the bloodstream, cholecalciferol travels to the various sites at which it exerts its effects. These include the well-known effects on calcium utilization as well as other activities, including apparently an effect on insulin secretion by the pancreas.

Why then is the vitamin D deficiency disease rickets considered a dietary deficiency disease rather than a hormonal abnormality? The answer may be related to the extreme changes in living conditions that came about as people strayed progressively farther from the natural state in which humans originally developed. The original conditions—tropical or subtropical climates; little or no covering for the body; large, open, sunlit areas—could have insured adequate exposure to ultraviolet light. This in turn would have insured adequate production of vitamin D in the skin and thus of cholecalciferol in the kidneys, making provision of additional dietary supplies unnecessary. Although conditions in modern societies are obviously far different from those of our ancestors, even the much simpler earlier civilizations could have produced conditions significantly different from those of the earliest nomadic peoples. Social customs that decree that the body be covered, for purposes of modesty or to protect a child from influences such as an "evil eye," can effectively eliminate the potentially beneficial effects of the sun even in areas where sunlight is plentiful. Shelters that become sources of privacy and family gathering places, not just occasionally used places that protect people during harsh weather, may similarly decrease exposure to the sun's rays. As villages grew into cities and populations expanded, crowding undoubtedly decreased the availability of open, sunlit areas where people could walk, rest, and play. Finally, when industrialization comes to an area, the resulting air pollution may filter out the sun's rays so that going outdoors is of little benefit, even if it were not for the effects of clothing and lack of open space.

One final fact that strongly favors the argument that vitamin D might better be considered a hormonelike substance than a nutrient is the inadequacy of human milk as a vitamin D source. Even supplementation of the mother's diet fails to increase the Vitamin D content of her milk to a level sufficient to prevent rickets in the infant. Nutrients infants need are generally present in the infant's natural food, human milk; they have to be, or we would never have survived as a species in the first place. A notable exception, however, is seen in the case of vitamin D: human milk contains approximately 20 to 40 international units of vitamin D per liter, and the RDA for vitamin D is 400. Thus, human milk cannot in itself produce adequate vitamin D status in infants; the breast-fed baby must obtain additional vitamin D from supplements, from fortified milk or by internal synthesis possible through regular exposure to sunlight or to the rays of an ultraviolet lamp.

Well-meaning parents may believe that exclusively breast-fed infants get everything they need by this "natural" feeding method; they need to be informed that it took human milk and sunlight working together, not just the milk alone, to produce nature's way to health in the days before the advent of civilization.

stroyed. Moreover, they found that coconut oil, which contains no vitamin A, also prevented rickets. Apparently the "Fat Soluble A" discovered by McCollum and Davis consisted of more than one vitamin. By 1922, McCollum had demonstrated the existence of a new vitamin essential to the metabolism of bones. Because this vitamin was, by then, the fourth one discovered, it was called vitamin D.

One other puzzle remained. It was already known that sunlight, which provides ultraviolet light, could reduce and even cure rickets in rats and humans. That meant that there had to be some relationship between sunlight and the new vitamin. Indeed, shortly after McCollum's discovery, other researchers found that ultraviolet irradiation produced vitamin D in milk, yeasts, and certain other foods.

The connection between rickets as a nutritional deficiency disease, and lack of sunlight, city life, and autumn or winter birth as contributory factors, then became clear. Because their diets contained little meat or milk, the urban poor were more likely to be afflicted. Because they spent little time out of doors, and because city streets are more often shaded, city dwellers generally received less sunlight. And because of shorter days, weaker sunlight, and colder weather, infants born in the fall or winter were kept indoors and wore more clothing when out of doors during the most crucial early bone-developing period of life. We know now, too, that the rapid spread of rickets in northern European cities in the nineteenth century was one of the results of the industrial revolution, which removed people from the sunny open space of the countryside and put young children to work inside homes and factories. Even for those city dwellers who spent time outdoors, ultraviolet light was largely filtered out by the smoke from coal and wood fires.

Chemistry and Properties

Like vitamin A, vitamin D is an organic molecule composed of carbon, hydrogen, and oxygen arranged in a multi-ring structure. Certain plants, including yeast, contain a provitamin called *ergosterol*. Exposure to sunlight (ultraviolet light) converts this compound to *ergocalciferol*, or vitamin D_2. The skin of animals, including humans, contains another sterol, 7-dehydrocholesterol, which is converted by ultraviolet light to previtamin D_3 which then slowly becomes vitamin D_3, *cholecalciferol*. Both forms are equally effective in humans. As a fat-soluble substance, vitamin D is, of course, insoluble in water. When crystallized it is colorless. It is also remarkably stable; exposure to heat, light, and oxygen does not readily affect its activity.

Figure 6–4 shows one form of vitamin D and its precursor. The origin of these compounds becomes even more evident if one compares their structure with that of cholesterol.

Absorption and Metabolism

Because of its fat-soluble nature, the absorption of vitamin D into the body is similar to that of vitamin A. Vitamin D is absorbed from the jejunum in the presence of bile and enters the general circulation by means of chylomicrons transported via the lymph. The nutrient is removed from circulation and stored in the liver. The amounts stored, however, are very small, and storage does not play as important a role in vitamin D metabolism as it does in maintaining vitamin A status. As with vitamin A, factors that influence fat absorption also affect absorption of vitamin D.

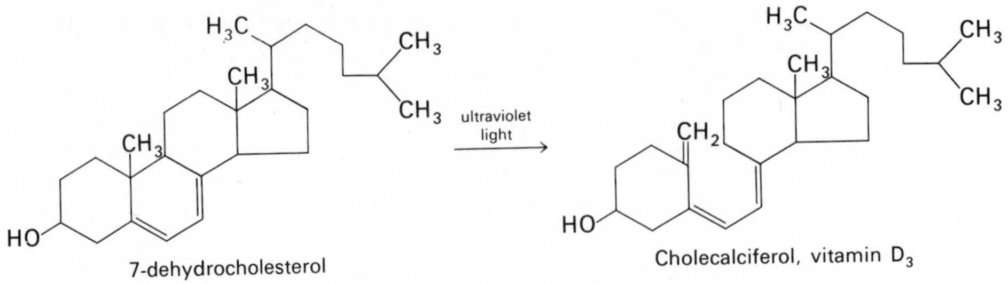

FIGURE 6-4   *Structure of Vitamin D and Precursor.*
The opening of the second ring causes a shift in location of the double bonds.

Thus impaired fat absorption, mineral oil, and drugs that bind bile acids (for instance, cholestyramine) will interfere with the absorption of vitamin D, just as with other fat-soluble vitamins.

Small reserves of vitamin D are found not only in the liver but also in the bone, brain, and skin. Some vitamin D metabolites are eliminated by excretion in the bile; others, in the urine.

Recent research on the metabolism of vitamin D suggests that it should perhaps be classified as a prohormone because it can be totally synthesized in the body and because it exerts its metabolic effect only after being hydroxylated to two more active forms, 25-OH vitamin D and 1, 25-$(OH)_2$ vitamin D.

These substances fulfill the definition of hormones: synthesis in one tissue of the body, from which they are transported through the blood to another tissue, where they exercise their specific effect. Synthesis of the prohormone form of vitamin D occurs in the skin, and then the first hydroxylation takes place in the liver, where D_3 (and ergocalciferol) is converted by a specific enzyme to 25-OH vitamin D. It is then carried in the blood by a specific transport protein to the kidneys, where 1, 25-OH vitamin D is produced by another enzymatic hydroxylation. In this form, vitamin D exerts its critical influence on the metabolism of calcium and phosphorus, and consequently on bone development. Parathyroid hormone (PTH), produced in the parathyroid glands, has a role in regulation of this process.

These and other recent discoveries concerning the biochemical activity of vitamin D continue its exciting history. They have been made possible only by the remarkable technological advances within the last two decades, including chemical synthesis of radioactive forms of the vitamin, chromatographic methods of bioassay, and high resolution mass spectroscopy.

Physiological Functions

A major function of vitamin D (that is, of 1, 25-OH vitamin D) is to increase the absorption of dietary calcium and phosphorus, both of which are needed for bone mineralization. Vitamin D also acts directly on bone, aiding bone formation and also stimulating the release of reserve calcium into the blood. An intricate network of biochemical reactions, with vitamin D as a key factor at several points, carries out these functions.

Vitamin D binds to a receptor on the intestinal cell. The receptor-bound vitamin D is transferred to the nucleus and initiates the synthesis of a specific calcium-binding protein (CaBP) that increases the absorption of calcium as well as phosphorus in the intestine. These absorption processes take place by means of *active* transport systems; that is, the mineral is carried across cell membranes by specialized carrier molecules, and metabolic energy (ATP) fuels the process.

In bone itself, vitamin D enhances mineralization through a mechanism that is not yet completely understood. However, the mechanism by which this vitamin affects *release* of bone calcium to maintain serum calcium and phosphorus at the appropriate levels is more clear. Bone tissue functions as a calcium and phosphorus reserve in a regulatory system that tightly controls the levels of these minerals in the blood. When serum calcium or phosphorus levels fall, the parathyroid glands (four small glands embedded in the thyroid gland) respond by secreting PTH. This polypeptide hormone stimulates the kidney hydroxylase enzyme that converts 25-OH vitamin D to 1, 25-OH vitamin D. By this means, the most active form of vitamin D is produced in the required quantities to perform its metabolic functions. In this way, vitamin D stimulates the release of calcium and phosphorus from the bone into the blood.

This seems paradoxical. Vitamin D is known to be necessary for the mineralization of bone. Why, then, does it also promote the process of bone resorption? The answer, apparently, is that there are optimal serum levels of calcium and phosphorus that are required for bone mineralization. By maintaining these optimal levels, vitamin D in the form of 1, 25-OH vitamin D and in the presence of PTH controls bone formation. These complex interactions are diagrammed in Figure 6–5.

Vitamin D also appears to increase reabsorption of phosphorus and calcium by the kidney and prevents excretion of phosphorus in the urine. Thus, the overall effect of vitamin D is to provide the optimal amounts of calcium and phosphorus needed for bone mineralization by increasing their availability through increased absorption and preventing the loss of phosphorus in the urine.

Dietary Requirements and Recommended Allowances

UNITS OF MEASUREMENT.   Vitamin D activity is expressed in International Units or as micrograms of cholecalciferol. One IU equals 0.025 micrograms (μg) of pure crystalline vitamin D_3. Vitamin D activity in food has historically been measured by means of the so-called line test. In this technique, rats with rickets are fed measured doses of a test material. Subsequent bone calcification can be determined through chemical staining of a longitudinal section of bone; the area of calcification is clearly visible as a line. The extent of calcification is proportional to the amount of vitamin D in the tested substance and can be compared to standardized measurements of vitamin D_3 activity.

The line test was both time-consuming and expensive and only an indirect measure of vitamin D activity. Chromatographic techniques, radioimmunoassay and competitive binding techniques can be used to measure the various forms of vitamins D in plasma. Each technique has advantages and disadvantages.

RECOMMENDED DIETARY ALLOWANCES.   A minimum dietary requirement for vitamin D is yet to be established. Sunlight, which may produce a substantial part of the amount required, is itself a variable. The amount of vitamin D formed by sunlight is dependent on various factors, including length and intensity of exposure and color of skin (the greater the pigmentation of the skin, the greater its screening effect against ultraviolet light).

The RDA for vitamin D is 10 μg (400 IU) per day from birth through 18 years

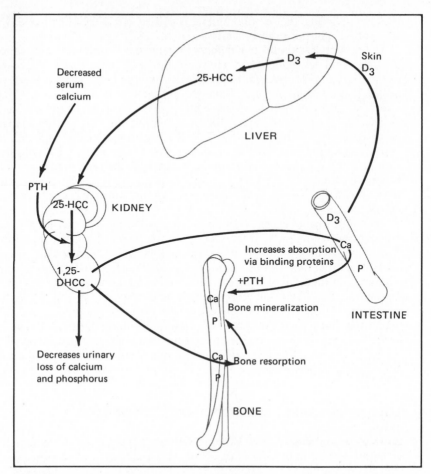

FIGURE 6-5 *Metabolic Functions of Vitamin D.*

Activated vitamin D_3 increases absorption of calcium and phosphorus from the intestine, in conjunction with parathyroid hormone (PTH) promotes both bone resorption and mineralization, and prevents loss of urinary calcium and phosphorus. When serum calcium and phosphorus levels fall, there is an increase in production of PTH by the parathyroid glands, resulting in increased 1, 25-OH vitamin D synthesis. When *both* calcium and phosphorus blood levels increase, the conversion of 25-OH vitamin D to 1, 25-OH vitamin D is diminished.

of age. A daily intake of 2.5 μg (100 IU) is sufficient to prevent rickets, but the larger amount is associated with optimal calcium absorption and growth and includes a safety margin. During late adolescence and the adult years, the RDA is 7.5 μg (300 IU) and 5 μg (200 IU), respectively. An additional 5 μg is recommended during pregnancy and lactation.

Dietary Sources

Except for certain fish and fish-liver oils, the only *significant* natural source of vitamin D is that produced by sunlight. Fortified foods and commercial preparations are the only reliable common dietary sources. Table 6–2 lists the vitamin D values

TABLE 6-2. *Vitamin D Content of Selected Foods (RDA for Adults: 5μg cholecalciferol = 200 IU)*

Food	Serving Size	Vitamin D Content IU/Serving
Sardines	3½ oz	1,150–1,570[a]
Cod-liver oil	1 tbsp	1,275
Mackerel, raw	3½ oz	1,100
Salmon, fresh	3½ oz	154–550[a]
Oysters	3–4 medium	510
Salmon, canned	3½ oz	220–440[a]
Herring, canned	3½ oz	330
Herring, fresh	3½ oz	315
Tuna, canned in water	3½ oz	250
Shrimp	3½ oz	150
Milk, whole or skim, fortified	1 c	100
Liver, chicken, raw	3½ oz	50–67[a]
Liver, pork, raw	3½ oz	45
Halibut	3½ oz	44
Liver, beef, raw	3½ oz	9–42[a]
Egg, whole	1 large	25
Egg yolk	1 large	25
Milk, human	1 c	0–24[a]
Liver, lamb, raw	3½ oz	20
Liver, calf, raw	3½ oz	0–15[a]
Cheese, cottage	½ c	10
Milk, cow, unfortified	1 c	0.7–10[a]
Cheese, cheddar	1 oz	3–8[a]
Cream, heavy	1 tbsp	8
Butter	1 tbsp	5
Ice cream	½ c	5
Clams	½ c	3
Bread, white enriched	1 slice	3
Butter	1 pat	2

[a] Ranges are given for food items in which a significant variability in vitamin D value is apparent. Values are influenced by season (amount of sunlight) in the case of dairy products. For liver, the older the animal, the longer the time available to build up vitamin stores.
Sources: C. F. Church and H. N. Church, *Food values of portions commonly used*, 12th ed. (Philadelphia: Lippincott, 1975); J. A. Pennington, *Dietary nutrient guide* (Westport, Conn.: Avi Publishing Co., 1976); and E. Yendt, in *International encyclopedia of pharmacology and therapeutics*, vol. 1 (Elmsford, N.Y.: Pergamon Press, 1970), p. 139.

of various food products. In general, egg whites, vegetable oils, unfortified dairy products, cereals, beans, fruits, vegetables, and muscle meats are poor sources of vitamin D. Relatively good sources are egg yolk, butterfat, fortified dairy products, fish oils, and organ meats.

Human milk is an unreliable source of vitamin D, as is unfortified cow's milk. Because it contains both calcium and phosphorus and is an important food for children, milk is an appropriate vehicle for fortification with vitamin D. Today almost all milk is fortified by the direct addition of vitamin D_2 or D_3 concentrates. According to estimates made in 1973, approximately 98 percent of all homogenized milk sold commercially in the United States contained vitamin D in concentrations of 400 IU per quart. Thus, growing children who drink two cups of fortified milk every day are assured of half the recommended amount from this source alone.

Because vitamin D is highly resistant to heat, light, and oxidation, it is essentially unaffected by food-processing and preparation procedures. Being fat-soluble, vitamin D is stored in the body, though to a lesser extent than vitamin A. Daily intake, therefore, is not necessary, especially for adults. But those who have limited exposure to the sun—winter-born infants, city dwellers, the elderly—should have a dietary source of vitamin D.

Clinical Deficiency Symptoms

The best known and most common deficiency condition resulting from lack of vitamin D is, of course, rickets. Metabolically, the visible symptoms of rickets are caused by inadequate absorption of calcium and phosphorus and, consequently, faulty mineralization of bones and teeth. In children lacking sufficient vitamin D, the bones remain too soft to withstand mechanical stress. The skeletal malformations characteristic of this condition include bow legs; enlargement of junctions between the ribs and their cartilaginous connection to the sternum or breast bone, forming a series of knobby protuberances sometimes called rachitic rosary; projection of the sternum ("pigeon breast"); narrow pelvis; and spinal curvature. Knock knees (enlarged knee joints), skull deformations, various muscle weaknesses, nervous irritability, and malformation of the teeth are additional symptoms of fully developed rickets.

Vitamin D deficiency in adults causes osteomalacia ("bone softening"), or adult rickets. The most common symptoms are weakening of the bone because of increased porosity and decreased density. This may result in various deformities, pain in the bones of the leg and lower back, general physical weakness including difficulty in walking, and spontaneous bone fractures. Among adults, osteomalacia generally occurs in women, especially following repeated pregnancies, and among the elderly. Again, inadequate diet and/or insufficient sunlight are the major contributory factors. Postmenopausal women sometimes have low concentrations of plasma 1, 25-OH vitamin D. An age-dependent loss of calcium absorption and of bone mass correlates with low concentrations of 1, 25-OH vitamin D. Administration of 1, 25-OH vitamin D to women with osteoporosis may help prevent the bone loss of old age, but definitive studies are needed.

The main cause of primary vitamin D deficiency is lack of sunlight. Absence of sunlight is more likely to be a significant contributory factor in premature infants and elderly people who spend very little time outdoors. Insufficient exposure to sunlight becomes increasingly important when the amount of dietary vitamin D decreases and may be a significant factor in the health of some infants. Human milk, although it is an excellent food for infants, is not a complete food, and cases of rickets in breast-fed infants continue to appear in the medical literature. Since plant foods are a particularly poor source of vitamin D, the breast-fed child of a vegetarian mother is even more at risk; cases of rickets in vegetarian children have been reported. Vitamin D supplementation is especially important for such children, unless regular exposure to sunlight is assured.

Despite adequate sunlight and dietary intake, secondary vitamin D deficiency may develop under certain conditions. Some endocrine disorders and diseases of the liver or kidney apparently interfere with the synthesis of 25-OH vitamin D and 1, 25-$(OH)_2$ vitamin D; as a result, there may develop what is known as vitamin

D-resistant rickets. The same condition can arise from a particular genetic defect as well. Various drugs also interfere with the metabolism of vitamin D. Cortisone therapy may produce osteoporosis or loss of bone tissue (as will Cushing's disease, in which there is excessive synthesis of hydrocortisone). Barbiturates and anticonvulsant drugs cause increased degradation of Vitamin D and its metabolites. As mentioned earlier, the bile necessary for absorption of vitamin D is decreased by cholestyramine, a drug used to reduce serum cholesterol in cardiovascular disease. Mineral oil also reduces absorption, as it does for all fat-soluble vitamins.

Toxicity

Because individuals vary in their sensitivity to vitamin D, a minimal toxic dose has not been determined. But excessive amounts of dietary vitamin D are definitely hazardous. Having too much of a good thing is certainly possible. The most common cause of hypervitaminosis D is dietary supplementation with cod-liver oil.

The symptoms of hypervitaminosis D are largely due to the resulting high levels of calcium in the blood (hypercalcemia). They include nausea, loss of appetite, weight loss, and calcification of soft tissues. Particularly serious injury to the kidneys can result from calcification. In children, growth may be reduced.

Sensitive infants may develop hypercalcemia on an intake of 1,800 to 2,000 IU per day, since the toxicity threshold is only four to five times the RDA. However, symptoms in adults with intakes exceeding 100,000 IU per day have also been doc-

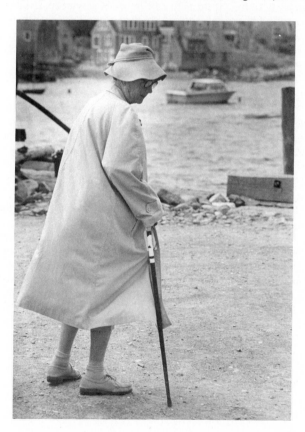

Inadequate diet and/or insufficient sunlight are the major contributory factors of osteomalacia, or adult rickets.

Ellis Herwig/Stock, Boston

umented. Moreover, because the excess vitamin is contained in stored fat tissue, hypercalcemia may last for months after intake of the vitamin has ceased. Thus it is important to remember the hazards as well as the benefits of vitamin D and to control dietary intake. Except in the case of diseases that affect vitamin D absorption or metabolism, dietary intake should be limited to 400 IU. A child (or adult) drinking a quart of milk a day should not receive vitamin D supplementation.

VITAMIN E

Vitamin E is one of the most controversial nutrients. Discovered in 1922 by H. M. Evans and K. S. Bishop at the University of California, Berkeley, it was first identified as a dietary factor essential for reproduction in rats. This function is reflected in the chemical name of the vitamin, *tocopherol*, which is derived from Greek words meaning "to bear offspring." It has since been promoted as a sex vitamin; as a cure for a number of nondeficiency diseases of the reproductive, circulatory, and nervous systems; and as a protective agent against aging and air pollution. These claims—and many similar ones—are based on inadequate evidence and are much disputed. But despite extensive research, mostly on experimental animals, the role of vitamin E in human nutrition is still not clear. Deficiency symptoms noted in animal studies have not been demonstrated in humans, although it has been established that small amounts are required by infants, especially those who are premature. Because vitamin E is found in a wide variety of foods common in the human diet, deficiencies are so unlikely in adults that none have yet been found. Nevertheless, research on the role of this vitamin continues.

Chemistry and Properties

Vitamin E is a general term for eight similar compounds. When pure, all are oily yellow liquids which are completely soluble in fats and fat solvents. By far the one with greatest biological activity and most common is α-tocopherol, whose structure is shown in Figure 6–6.

For the most part, vitamin E is highly stable. Neither boiling nor long periods of storage alone affect its activity. However, exposure to air or light, or contact with iron or copper, will cause the vitamin to decompose. The tocopherols oxidize readily—so readily, in fact, that they are oxidized before other substances in a mixture exposed to an oxidizing agent. For this reason, vitamin E is used as an antioxidant in foods to protect other substances, particularly vitamin A and polyunsaturated fatty acids (PUFA), from oxidation and in the case of fatty foods, from becoming **rancid.**

FIGURE 6-6   *Chemical Structure of α-tocopherol.*

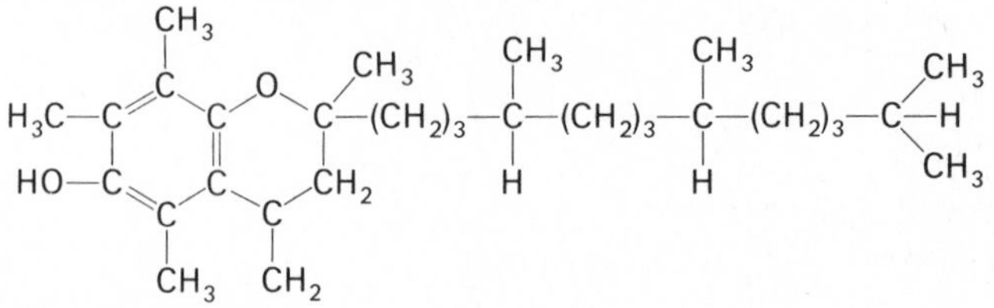

Absorption and Metabolism

The process of absorption of vitamin E is much the same as that of other fats and fat-soluble substances. It requires bile, occurs in the mucosa of the small intestine, and results in transport into the general circulation via chylomicrons and lymph.

Vitamin E is carried in the blood by lipoproteins and is stored primarily in adipose tissue, with smaller amounts found in liver and muscle tissue. The adrenal and pituitary glands contain significant concentrations of the vitamin. Vitamin E is released into the circulation whenever fat is mobilized. Its metabolites are excreted both in urine and in feces.

Absorption of vitamin E is less efficient than that of vitamin A; only 50 to 85 percent of the dietary intake of this vitamin actually enters the bloodstream. These figures are reduced by the presence of mineral oil or any of the other conditions that affect the absorption of fats generally. Efficiency of absorption is further impaired as intake increases. Tissue levels of vitamin E only double when intake is increased to ten times the RDA for the vitamin. For this reason, those who take megadoses of vitamin E are surely getting less than anticipated for their money.

Physiological Functions

Few nutrients have generated as much public interest or clinical debate as has vitamin E. If all the claims made for its curative and health-promoting effects were true, it would indeed be a wonder nutrient. To put these claims in proper perspective, note that they arose, at least in part, from a misinterpretation of research with laboratory animals, and in part from the nature of the earliest findings involving tocopherols.

Early research showed these substances to be essential for fertility in rats, and subsequent studies identified other deficiency conditions as well—for a number of laboratory animal species. But experimental animals can be fed a controlled diet and deliberately deprived of all vitamin E until a deficiency condition is produced. To produce a similar deficiency in humans would be extremely difficult. Vitamin E is widely available in a normal diet, it is stored throughout the body, and its release from storage ("turnover") is so gradual that depletion of body stores would take many months. Symptoms of vitamin E deficiency have not been identified in humans unless they had other medical disorders. Without deficiency symptoms, it is difficult to identify the function of a nutrient. Moreover, although vitamin E deficiency can produce certain conditions in animals, similar disorders in humans are unrelated to vitamin E status. For example, severe vitamin E deficiency causes a type of muscular dystrophy in animals; however, humans with this condition exhibit normal muscle tissue levels of the vitamin. Consequently, claims that vitamin E will prevent or cure muscular dystrophy in humans are simply not true. A deficiency disease induced in an animal cannot be compared with a genetic disease in humans.

Nonetheless, there is evidence to suggest that vitamin E plays an important role in a number of metabolic processes. Vitamin E may be required, although in minute amounts, for the synthesis of **heme** (a part of the hemoglobin molecule and of other metabolically important body chemicals).

The best-understood activities of vitamin E, however, result from its antioxidant activity. Tocopherol reacts with compounds that have an unpaired electron and are therefore highly reactive as oxidizing agents. These compounds are known as *free radicals*. By reacting with them, vitamin E prevents the radicals from oxidizing polyunsaturated fats, vitamin A, various enzymes, and cell membrane constituents. In forestalling oxidative damage, vitamin E increases the stability of cellular and intracellular structures, particularly membranes.

In addition to their destructive potential as oxidizing agents, free radicals are believed to participate in the formation of "aging pigments," which may contribute to the aging process in various tissues. It has therefore been theorized that by deactivating free radicals, vitamin E may be able to slow cell aging. So far, however, experimental tests on laboratory animals have not confirmed this hypothesis.

Additionally, vitamin E apparently works with certain other nutrients in complementary relationships that protect the integrity of numerous biochemical substances and cellular structures. For example, glutathione perioxidase is an enzyme that prevents oxidative destruction of PUFAs during a particular stage of cell development. Production of this enzyme requires specific proteins in association with the trace element selenium, and its function is enhanced by vitamin E as well. Since the role of this enzyme—its antioxidant activity—is similar to one of the best-understood functions of vitamin E, this involvement is not surprising.

Although the antioxidant properties of vitamin E are those most extensively studied, they do not explain all its observed efforts. Research, for example, has shown that administration of vitamin E in pharmacological doses interferes with the blood-clotting process. The postulated mechanism involves a metabolite of the vitamin tocopherylquinone, which is similar in structure to vitamin K. Vitamin K, as we shall see, promotes blood coagulation. According to the present hypothesis, tocopherylquinone acts as an antagonist to vitamin K.

Dietary Requirements and Recommended Allowances

UNITS OF MEASUREMENTS.   One milligram of d-α-tocopherol has been designated as 1 α-tocopherol equivalent (αT.E.). Values for several forms of tocopherols are

$$
\begin{aligned}
1\alpha\text{T.E.} &= 1 \text{ mg } \alpha\text{-tocopherol} \\
or & \quad\ 2 \text{ mg } \beta\text{-tocopherol} \\
or & \quad 10 \text{ mg } \gamma\text{-tocopherol}
\end{aligned}
$$

Precise activity levels of the other tocopherols are not known at present.

BASIS OF REQUIREMENTS.   The RDAs for vitamin E are based on studies of dietary intake, which are assumed to be adequate since no deficiencies have been identified. Studies have also indicated, however, that the vitamin E requirements increase directly as PUFA intake increases. In American diets, vitamin E intake varies directly with PUFA intake, since they are naturally found together in foods, for example, in vegetable oils. Because the actual requirement for vitamin E is a function of PUFA intake, which is highly variable, precise requirements cannot be established. The Food and Nutrition Board has suggested an α-tocopherol:PUFA ratio of 0.6 milligrams of α-tocopherol per 1 gram of PUFA. Actual intakes in the United States seem to approximate a vitamin E:PUFA ratio of 0.4 milligrams per gram, but no adverse effects have been identified; the Food and Nutrition Board recommendation can, however, serve as a guide. The RDAs for adult men and women are 10 and 8 mg αT.E., respectively. RDAs for other age groups will be discussed later.

Dietary Sources

Since vitamin E is generally found with PUFAs, its main sources in the American diet are oils of vegetable origin. Animal fats are not useful sources nor are animal products in general, although liver and eggs contain fair amounts. Among other vegetable foods, cereals and legumes have moderate vitamin E content. In the processing of white rice and refined flour, however, much of their vitamin E content is removed. Fruits and leafy and root vegetables contain very little vitamin E, and most of that is in a less-active form. Table 6–3 lists the tocopherol content of selected foods.

Because of its availability in the cooking oils (cottonseed, soybean, and corn) generally used in this country, not to consume the recommended dietary allowances of vitamin E would be difficult. Moreover, since vegetable oils are the major dietary source, an increase of vitamin E intake in proportion to an increase in PUFA consumption is virtually automatic, unless the oil has become rancid. Further, there is little loss of vitamin activity in most cooking procedures. High heat, however, will oxidize tocopherols. In one study, oil used repeatedly for deep-frying doughnuts was tested at intervals for tocopherol content and went from 19.4 mg per 100 g to 10.7 mg in the course of a day's cooking. But much more dramatic was the combined effect of the used cooking oil and high temperature frying on the shortening used in the doughnut batter: As mixed into the batter, this shortening contained 92.8 mg of tocopherols per 100 g; in the last batch of cooked doughnuts, tocopherol content had been reduced to 6.8 mg per 100 g. Prolonged storage, especially of foods cooked in vegetable oils, will also result in loss of tocopherols by oxidation.

Clinical Deficiency Symptoms

Because symptoms in humans have not been clearly identified, clinical deficiency can be determined only by measurement of serum levels of vitamin E or by red blood cell destruction by oxidation. Low serum levels are found in newborns generally but rise within the first month of life, especially in breast-fed full-term infants. There are reports of deficiency symptoms in premature infants fed a commercial formula with inadequate vitamin E content; these symptoms were reversed when vitamin E was administered. In adults, however, storage levels are apparently sufficient to ward off deficiencies for prolonged periods; adult male volunteers who received low-tocopherol diets for three years did not develop symptoms, although serum levels became quite low.

A few situations in which vitamin E supplementation is beneficial have been established. Several diseases, including cystic fibrosis and liver cirrhosis as well as gastric surgery, result in malabsorption of lipids. The resulting deficiencies can be effectively treated with vitamin E and the other fat-soluble vitamins. Only the treatment of hemolytic anemia in premature infants can be considered to involve a *nutritional* effect of vitamin E in human deficiency disease.

Despite various claims, tests have failed to show that vitamin E has any positive effect on athletic performance or that it provides any protection against cancer or aging. There is some evidence that it may prevent lung damage from air pollution, though it does not reverse the symptoms. And there is no reliable evidence to give vitamin E a role in either human fertility or sexual performance, unless the person is subject to a placebo effect.

TABLE 6-3. *Total Tocopherol Content of Selected Foods (RDA for Adults: Men 10 mgαT.E.; Women 8 mgαT.E.)*

Food	Serving Size	Tocopherol Content mg/serving
Wheat germ oil	1 tbsp	39.0
Baked blueberry pie, fresh	1/6 of 9" pie	28.3
Corn oil, hydrogenated[a]	1 tbsp	15.8
Soybean oil, unhydrogenated[a]	1 tbsp	15.2
Corn oil, unhydrogenated[a]	1 tbsp	15.0
Soybean oil, hydrogenated[a]	1 tbsp	11.0
Safflower oil, stabilized	1 tbsp	8.8
Safflower oil, unstabilized	1 tbsp	5.4
Wheat germ	1 oz	3.8
Yellow corn meal	½ c	3.4
Margarine, corn oil	1 pat	2.3
Oatmeal, uncooked	¼ c	1.9
Mayonnaise	1 tbsp	1.8
Salmon, broiled	3 oz	1.5
Navy beans, dry	½ c	1.5
Peas, fresh	½ c	1.5
Italian salad dressing	1 tbsp	1.4
Beef liver, broiled	3 oz	1.4
Tomato juice, canned	6 oz	1.3
Coconut oil	1 tbsp	1.2
Haddock, broiled	3 oz	1.0
Apple	1 medium	0.7
Bread, whole-wheat	1 slice	0.6
Peas, frozen, cooked	½ c	0.6
Egg	1 medium	0.5
Ground beef, fried	3 oz	0.5
Chicken, breast with bones, broiled	3 oz	0.5
Banana	1 medium	0.5
Cream cheese	1 oz	0.3
Milk, whole	1 c	0.2
Celery	1 stalk	0.2
Ice cream	½ c	0.1
Potato, raw	1 large	0.1
Lettuce	⅛ head	0.1
Corn flakes	1 c	0.1
Potato, baked	1 large	0.08
Bread, white	1 slice	0.06
Butter	1 pat	0.05
Peas, canned	½ c	0.03

[a] Hydrogenation does not systematically alter the tocopherol content of vegetable oils. Note that the tocopherol content decreases when soybean oil is hydrogenated, whereas a slight increase occurs with the hydrogenation of corn oil.

Sources: R. H. Bunnel, J. Keating, A. Quaresimo, and G. K. Parman, Alpha-tocopherol content of foods, *American Journal of Clinical Nutrition* 17:1, 1965; P. L. Harris, M. L. Quaife, and W. J. Swanson, Vitamin E content of foods, *Journal of Nutrition* 40:367, 1950; and J. A. Pennington, *Dietary nutrient guide* (Westport, Conn.: Avi Publishing Co., 1976).

Toxicity

As we saw earlier, recent studies have shown an antagonistic relationship between very high vitamin E intake and blood coagulation, with large doses slowing the clotting rate. The anti-vitamin K activity of vitamin E increases the risk of hemorrhage in patients suffering from vitamin K deficiency and is a potentially toxic effect.

Daily intakes as high as 800 mg αT.E. have not been found to be toxic. Only in recent years, however, have large numbers of people been "prescribing" vitamin E for themselves; the long-term effect is not known at present. Certainly vitamin E does not produce toxic symptoms as severe and visible as those of vitamins A and D. However, one report has noted adverse symptoms associated with excess intake for as short a time as three months, and another has reported the occurrence of hemorrhage when excess vitamin E coincided with a vitamin K deficiency. The potential for hypervitaminosis E definitely exists and should not be ignored.

VITAMIN K

K stands for *Koagulation*, the Danish spelling of the word for blood clotting, for it was discovered by a Danish scientist, Henrik Dam, in 1929. He had earlier observed a hemorrhagic disease in newborn chicks. Blood analyses showed decreased levels of prothrombin, a factor involved in blood clotting. Although the chicks' diet had appeared to be entirely adequate, Dam found that hog-liver fat or alfalfa prevented the condition. He named the antihemorrhagic factor vitamin K. In 1943 Dam received the Nobel Prize in physiology and medicine for his discovery.

Chemistry and Properties

Vitamin K is actually a group of yellowish **crystalline** (chemically pure) compounds belonging to a family of substances called *quinones*. All forms are resistant to heat, air, and moisture but are vulnerable to destruction by strong acids, alkalis, and light. Only two major forms are found in nature, and vitamin K_1 (phylloquinone) is the only form synthesized by plants (see Figure 6–7). Vitamin K_2 (menaquinone), itself a group of vitamins, is found in bacteria and in animals, in which it is a product of bacterial metabolism. The activity of K_2 is about 75 percent that of K_1. The most potent form of the vitamin, with more than twice the activity of K_2, is menadione, which is not present in nature but which can be synthesized in the laboratory. Animals convert menadione to menaquinone by adding the long side chain, which is needed for vitamin activity. Thus, it is the *ring* structure of vitamin

FIGURE 6-7   *Chemical Structures of Three Forms of Vitamin K.*

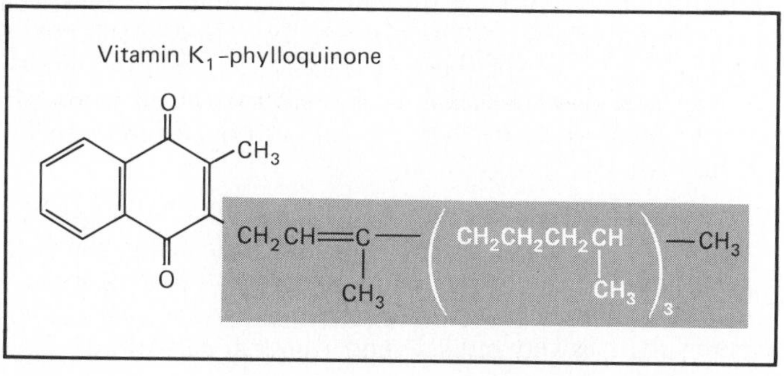

K that cannot be synthesized by animals, who therefore need an outside source for optimal health. Both diet and synthesis by intestinal bacteria contribute to the supply needed.

Absorption and Metabolism

The absorption and initial metabolism of vitamin K are much the same as those of other fat-soluble vitamins, requiring bile and other factors that promote the absorption of fat-soluble materials. Any disorder of fat absorption will interfere with absorption of vitamin K. Chylomicrons transport the vitamin to the liver, where it is combined with β-lipoproteins before entering the general circulation. Although vitamin K is concentrated in the liver for a short time, storage in the body is minimal. Small amounts appear in skin, muscle, kidneys, and heart. Metabolites are excreted in bile and urine.

One notable difference between vitamin K and the other fat-soluble vitamins is that bacterial synthesis of vitamin K_2 in the intestine is an important source of vitamin K in humans.

Metabolic Function

Our understanding of the metabolic role of vitamin K has expanded in the past 10 to 15 years. Vitamin K acts as an essential cofactor for carboxylase, an enzyme that converts specific glutamic acid residues of precursor proteins to carboxyglutamate residues in the completed protein. Among the proteins are several plasma clotting factors, prothrombin and factors VII, IX, and X as well as osteocalcin, found in bone and kidney. The role of osteocalcin is unclear; it may play a role in calcium deposition in bone matrix.

A deficiency of the vitamin or the administration of an antagonist will cause problems in blood coagulation. Blood-clotting time may be prolonged, which is normally undesirable but which may, in some circumstances, be preferred. (The mechanism of blood clotting is further discussed in a later chapter in conjunction with calcium metabolism.) Despite its great importance in blood clotting, administration of vitamin K has no therapeutic effect on hemophilia because this disease is caused by a genetic defect in another stage of the clotting mechanism, rather than by a lack of vitamin K.

Dietary Requirements and Recommended Allowances

UNITS OF MEASUREMENT.   Vitamin K activity is often expressed as micrograms of menadione, a synthetic form of the vitamin. The most common bioassay technique for measuring the vitamin activity in foods makes use of chickens in which vitamin K deficiency has been produced. Measured amounts of the test food are fed to the chicks, and the resulting increased levels of blood prothrombin are determined. These levels are then compared to those produced by known quantities of vitamin K_1.

RECOMMENDED ALLOWANCES.   Although the Food and Nutrition Board has set no RDA for vitamin K, estimated safe and adequate daily dietary intakes have been established. For adults, this estimate is 70 to 140 μg per day. Because vitamin K is found in a variety of foods and there is extensive synthesis by bacteria, inadequate vitamin status is very unlikely under normal conditions.

Dietary Sources

Since bacterial synthesis usually provides at least half the required amount of vitamin K, there is little difficulty in completing the requirement from dietary sources. A selected list of foods and their vitamin K content appears in Table 6–4. In general, green, leafy vegetables and members of the cabbage-cauliflower group are the best sources. These are followed by meats (especially liver) and dairy products, fruits, and cereals. Human milk, however, contains very little vitamin K.

Clinical Deficiency Symptoms

Although intestinal synthesis and widespread distribution of vitamin K make primary deficiency of this nutrient highly unlikely, newborn infants are an exception. Little vitamin K from the mother is received by the fetus (due to poor placental transfer), and the normal intestinal bacteria do not become established until about a week after birth. Therefore, to raise low prothrombin levels and prevent hemorrhagic disease, injection of 1 milligram of vitamin K_1 immediately after birth has become standard procedure at many hospitals.

TABLE 6-4. *Average Vitamin K Content of Selected Foods (Estimated Safe and Adequate Daily Dietary Intake for Adults: 70–140 µg)*

Food	Serving Size	Vitamin K Content µg/serving
Turnip greens	½ c	195
Broccoli	½ c	160
Lettuce	⅛ head	90
Beef liver	3 oz	78
Cabbage	½ c	56
Asparagus	4 spears	34
Spinach	½ c	27
Pork liver	3 oz	21
Tea, green	1 tsp	19
Watercress	½ c	17
Peas, green	½ c	16
Bacon	4 strips	14
Ham	3 oz	13
Cheese	1 oz	10
Pork tenderloin	3 oz	9
Beans, green	½ c	8
Cow's milk	1 c	7
Tomato	1 med.	7
Ground beef	3 oz	6
Chicken liver	3 oz	6
Egg, whole	1 large	5.5
Potato	1 large	4.7
Applesauce	½ c	2.6
Banana	1 large	2.4
Corn oil	1 tbsp	1.5
Butter	1 pat	1.5
Orange	1 med.	1.3
Bread	1 slice	1.1

Source: Adapted from R. E. Olson, Vitamin K, in *Modern nutrition in health and disease,* 5th ed., ed. R. S. Goodhart and M. E. Shils (Philadelphia: Lea and Febiger, 1973).

However, secondary deficiencies can result from a number of causes: sulfa drugs and antibiotics, which reduce bacterial synthesis; anticoagulants such as Dicumarol, which are antagonists of the vitamin; some anticonvulsant drugs, which increase the rate at which vitamin K is metabolized and eliminated; surgery involving the area of the intestine in which bacterial synthesis and absorption occur; and any condition that affects fat absorption. In situations of poor absorption, such as jaundice, patients are given vitamin K before surgery. Secondary deficiency conditions should be compensated by supplying vitamin K, *except* where an anticoagulant effect is needed to prevent blood clots in certain heart and blood vessel conditions.

The only identifiable symptom of vitamin K deficiency is decreased efficiency of blood coagulation. In extreme form, as in chronic liver disease or therapy with some drugs, decreased coagulation efficiency may result in hemorrhage.

Toxicity

In pharmacological doses for prolonged periods, vitamin K can produce hemolytic anemia and jaundice in infants. Because of its toxic effect on red blood cell membranes, the synthetic form menadione (vitamin K_3) is no longer permitted in over-the-counter preparations. The water-soluble forms of vitamin K have a greater safety margin and should be used when vitamin K supplements are indicated.

SUMMARY

Vitamins are organic compounds that (1) are required in trace amounts by the body, (2) perform one or more essential metabolic functions, and (3) must be provided at least in part from dietary sources. Much of our present understanding of these substances results from studies of the so-called deficiency diseases. Unlike other classes of nutrients, vitamins differ widely in chemical structure and, consequently, in metabolism and function.

Classifying vitamins according to their solubility in water or in fats and fat solvents is useful. Solubility affects a number of characteristics: distribution in foods, stability, absorption, metabolism, excretion, and potential toxicity. For example, the fat-soluble vitamins (A, D, E, and K) are all absorbed into the body in similar fashion from the intestine; efficient absorption requires bile and is affected by any factor or condition that affects bile or the absorption of fats. Compared to water-soluble vitamins, fat-soluble vitamins are more readily retained in the body, and their potential toxicity is therefore greater.

Vitamin A is relatively stable and occurs in three biologically active forms—retinol, retinal, and retinoic acid. Biologically active vitamin A is found almost exclusively in animal products (as retinyl esters). All three forms, however, can be derived from carotene precursors (provitamins), which are widely distributed plant pigments.

Vitamin A affects almost all tissues and functions in a great number of processes, including vision, growth of bones and teeth, maintenance of epithelial tissue, and hormone synthesis. It is readily available from many dietary sources, and significant amounts are stored in the body, especially the liver. Deficiency produces night blindness, xerophthalmia, and skin keratinization; administration of the vitamin can reverse many symptoms, especially in early stages. Conditions caused by vitamin A toxicity include birth defects, especially of the central nervous system; a syndrome that mimics brain tumor; anemia; and muscle and joint pain.

Vitamin D is chemically very stable and has two primary biologically active forms. Ergocalciferol, D_2, is derived from irradiation of a plant precursor (ergosterol), and cholecalciferol, D_3, from irradiation of 7-dehydrocholesterol, found in the skin of animals. Vitamin D serves chiefly to maintain optimum blood levels of calcium and phosphorus. This function is mediated by two metabolites of the vitamin—25-OH vitamin D and 1, 25-OH vitamin D—produced in the liver and kidneys. Commercial preparations (supplements) and fortified foods are the only reliable *dietary* sources of vitamin D. It is stored in the body, but to a lesser extent than vitamin A. Clinical conditions resulting from deficiency are rickets in children and osteomalacia in adults. Symptoms of hypervitaminosis D include hypercalcemia, nausea, loss of weight and appetite, and calcification of bone and soft tissues.

Vitamin E is highly stable (though readily oxidized) and occurs in four natural forms, the most common and biologically active being α-tocopherol. Despite numerous claims for the curative and health-promoting powers of vitamin E, its role in human nutrition is mainly as a protective antioxidant. Vitamin E is very readily available from dietary sources. The only known deficiency condition is hemolytic anemia in premature infants. In pharmacological doses the vitamin can have certain beneficial effects but may carry some risks as well. Large doses also have an anticoagulant effect; thus excessive intake could lead to hemorrhaging in certain instances.

Vitamin K is a group of relatively stable compounds belonging to the chemical family of substances called quinones. Vitamin K_1 (phylloquinone) is the only form synthesized by plants. About half the amount of vitamin K in the body is a form of K_2 (menaquinone), synthesized by intestinal bacteria. Dietary sources supply the rest. A primary function of vitamin K is as a cofactor for an enzyme involved in the production of proteins essential to blood clotting. The body stores minimal amounts of the vitamin, but it is found in many animal and plant products, and the metabolic need is for very small amounts. The only known deficiency symptom is prolonged blood-coagulation time leading to hemorrhage. In pharmalogical doses over extended periods, vitamin K can cause hemolytic anemia and jaundice in infants.

BIBLIOGRAPHY

ADAMS, J.S., T.L. CLEMENS, J.A., PARRISH, and M.F. HOLIICK. Vitamin D synthesis and metabolism after ultraviolet irradiation of normal and vitamin D deficient subjects. *New England Journal of Medicine* 306:722–725, 1982.

AUDRAN, M. The physiology and pathophysiology of vitamin D. Mayo Clinic Proceedings 60:851–866, 1985.

BIERI, J.G. AND R.P. EVARTS. Vitamin E adequacy in vegetable oils. *Journal of the American Dietetic Association* 66:134, 1975.

BRIGGS, M.H. ed. *Recent Vitamin Research.* Boca Raton, FL: CRC Press, 1984.

CAMPBELL, T.C., R.G. ALLISON, AND K.D. FISHER. Nutrient toxicity. *Nutrition Reviews* 39:249–256, 1981.

COLDITZ, G.A., L.G. BRANCH, R.J. LIPNICK, W.C. WILLET, B. ROSNER, B.M. POSNER, AND C.H. HENNEKENS. Increased green and yellow vegetable intake and lowered cancer deaths in an elderly population. *American Journal of Clinical Nutrition* 41: 32–36, 1985.

DELUCA, H.F., R.T. FRANCESCHI, B.P. HALLORAN AND E.R. MASSARO. Molecular events involved in 1, 25-dihydroxyvitamin D, stimulation of intestinal calcium transport. *Federation Proceedings* 41:66–71, 1982.

DELUCA, H.F. AND H.K. SCHNOES. Vitamin D: Recent advances. *Annual Review of Biochemistry* 52:411–439, 1983.

DRUMMUND, J.C. The nomenclature of the so-called accessory food factors (vitamins). *Biochemical Journal* 14:660, 1920.

DUBRICK, M.A. AND R.B. RUCKER. Dietary supplements and health aids—A critical evaluation. Part 1—Vitamins and Minerals. *Journal of Nutrition Education* 15:47–53, 1983.

DWIGHT, J.T., W.H. DIETZ, JR., G. HAAS, AND R. SUSSKIND. Risk of nutritional rickets among vegetarian children. *American Journal of Diseases of Children* 133:134, 1979.

ERIKSSON, U., K. DAS, C. BUSCH, H. NORDLINDER, L. RASK, SUNDELIN, J. SALLSTROM AND P.A. PETERSON. Cellular retinol-binding protein: Quantitation and distribution. *Journal of Biological Chemistry* 259:13464–13470, 1984.

FOMON, S.J. AND F.G. STRAUSS. Nutrient deficiencies in breast-fed infants. *New England Journal of Medicine* 299:355, 1978.

Food and Nutrition Board, National Academy of Sciences, National Research Council. Committee on Nutritional Misinformation. Hazards of overuse of vitamin D. *Nutrition Reviews* 33:61, 1975.

Food and Nutrition Board, National Research Council. *Recommended Dietary Allowances.* 9th ed. Washington, D.C.: National Academy of Sciences, 1980.

FURIE, B., H.A. LIEBMAN, R.A. BLANCHARD, M.J. COLMAN, S.F. KRUGER, AND B.C. FURIE. Comparison of the native prothrombin antigen and the prothrombin time for monitoring oral anticoagulant therapy. *Blood* 64:445–461, 1984.

HALL, J.G. Vitamin A: A newly recognized human teratorgen. *Journal of Pediatrics* 105:583–584, 1984.

HANDELMAN, G.J., L.J. MACHLIN, K. FITCH, J.J. WEITER AND E.A. DRATZ. Oral α-tocopherol supplements decrease plasma α-tocopherol levels in humans. *Journal of Nutrition* 115:807–813, 1985.

HARPER, A.E. and G.K. Davis, eds. *Nutrition in Health and Disease and International Development.* Symposia from the XII International Congress of Nutrition. New York: Alan R. Liss, Inc., 1981, pp 97–150.

HENRY, H.L. AND A.W. NORMAN. Vitamin D: Metabolism and biological action. *Annual Review of Nutrition* 4:493–520, 1984.

HESS, A.F., M. WEINSTOCK AND F.D. HELMAN. The antirachitic value of irradiated phystosterol and cholesterol. *Journal of Bilogical Chemistry* 63:305, 1925.

KRASINSKI, S.D., R.M. RUSSELL, B.C. FURIE, S.F. DRUGER, P.F. JACQUES AND B. FURIE. The Prevalence of vitamin K deficiency in chronic gastrointestinal disorders. *American Journal of Clinical Nutrition* 41:639–643, 1985.

LAMBERG-ALLARDT, C. Vitamin D intake, sunlight exposure, and 25-hydroxy-vitamin D levels in the elderly during one year. *Ann. Nutr. Metab.* 28: 144–150, 1984.

LANE, P.A. AND W.E. HATHAWAY. Vitamin K in infancy. *Journal of Pediatrics* 106:351–359, 1985.

LEO, M.A., M. ARAI, M. SATO, AND C.S. KIEBER. Hepatotoxicity of vitamin A and ethanol in the rat. *Gastroenterology* 82:194–205, 1982.

LIPPE, B., L. HENSEN, G. MENDOZA, M. FINERMAN AND M. WELCH. Chronic vitamin A intoxication. *American Journal of Diseases in Children* 135:634–636, 1981.

LOVINGER, R.D. Rickets. *Pediatrics* 66:359–365, 1980.

LUBIN, B. AND L.J. MACHLIN. Vitamin E: Biochemical, hematological, and clinical aspects. *Annual N.Y. Academy of Science* 393:1–5, 1982.

McCAY, P.B. Vitamin E interactions with free radicals and ascorbate. *Annual Review of Nutrition* 5:323–340, 1985.

MACHLIN, L.J., E. GABRIEL AND M. BRIN. Biopotency of α-tocopherols as determined by curative myopathy bioassay in the rat. *Journal of Nutrition* 112:1437–1440, 1982.

McCOLLUM, E.V. AND M. DAVIS. The necessity of certain lipids in the diet during growth. *Journal of Biological Chemistry* 15:167, 1913.

MASON, K.E. The first two decades of vitamin E. *Federation Proceedings* 36:1906, 1977.

MICHAELSSON G. Diet and acne. *Nutrition Reviews* 39:99–106, 1981.

MILNER, J.A. Dietary antioxidants and cancer. *Contemporary Nutrition* Vol. 10, #10, Oct. 1985.

NORDIN, B.E.C., M.R. BAKER, A. HORSMAN AND M. PEACOCK. A prospective trial of the effect of vitamin D supplementation on metacarpal bone loss in elderly women. *American Journal of Clinical Nutrition* 42:470–474, 1985.

NORMAN, A.W., B.J. FRANKE, A.M. HELDT AND G.M. GRODSKY. Vitamin D deficiency inhibits pancreatic secretaion of insulin. *Science* 209:823–825, 1980.

O'BRIEN, D.F. The chemistry of vision. *Science* 218:961–966, 1982.

OLSON, R.E. The function and metabolism of vitamin K. *Annual Review of Nutrition* 4:281–337, 1984.

ONG, D.E. Vitamin A-binding proteins. *Nutrition Reviews* 43:225–232, 1985.

PECK, G.L., R.G. OLSEN, F.W. YODER, J.S. STRAUSS, D.T. DOWNING, M. PANDYA, D. BUTKUS AND J. ARNAUD-BATTANDIER. Prolonged remission of cystic and conglobate acne with 13-cis-retinoic acid. *New England Journal of Medicine* 300:329, 1979.

PIKE, J.W. Intracellular receptors mediate the biologic action of 1, 25-dihydroxyvitamin D 3. *Nutrition Reviews* 43:161–168, 1985.

ROBERTS, H.J. Perspective on vitamin E as therapy. *Journal of the American Medical Association* 246:129–131, 1981.

SIMPSON, K.L. and C.O. CHICHESTER. Metabolism and nutritional significance of carotenoids. *Annual Review of Nutrition* 1:351–374, 1980.

SUTTIE, J.W. The metabolic role of Vitamin K. *Federation Proceedings* 39:2730–2735, 1980.

———. ed. *Vitamin K Metabolism and Vitamin K-Dependent Proteins.* Baltimore, MD: University Park Press, 1980.

WALD, G. Molecular basis of visual excitation. *Scientific American* 162:230, 1968.

WASSERMAN, R.H. AND C.S. FULLMER. Calcium transport proteins, calcium absorption, and vitamin D. *Annual Review Physiology* 45:375–390, 1983.

WATSON, R.R. AND S. MORIGUCHI. Cancer prevention by retinoids: Role of immunological modification. *Nutrition Research* 5:663–675, 1985.

WEICK, M.T. SR. A history of rickets in the United States. *American Journal of Clinical Nutrition* 20:1234, 1967.

WILLETT, W.C., B.F. POLK, B.A. UNDERWOOD, M.J. STAMPFER, S. PRESSELL, B. ROSNER, J.O. TAYLOR, K. SCHNEIDER AND C.G. HAMES. Relation of serum vitamins A and E and carotenoids to the risk of cancer. *New England Journal of Medicine* 310:430–434, 1984.

WOLF, G. A historical note on the mode of administration of vitamin A for the cure of night blindness. *American Journal of Clinical Nutrition* 31:290, 1978.

YOUNG, V.R. AND P.M. NEWBERNE. Vitamins and cancer prevention: Issues and dilemmas. *Cancer* 47:1226–1240, 1981.

ZIEL, M.H. AND M.E. CULLUM. The function of vitamin A: Current concepts. *Proc. Soc. Exp. Biol. Med.* 172:139–152, 1983.

Chapter 7

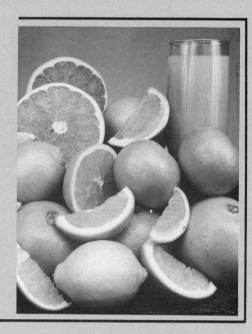

WATER-SOLUBLE VITAMINS

207

In some respects, water-soluble vitamins are similar to fat-soluble vitamins; they are organic compounds, required in very small amounts for specific metabolic functions, and are essential nutrients because the body cannot produce them in sufficient amounts and therefore must obtain them from other sources, usually dietary.

As we saw in the preceding chapter, the fat solubility of vitamins A, D, E, and K is the most important characteristic they share. Not surprisingly, the water solubility of the vitamins to be discussed in this chapter is the characteristic that most clearly distinguishes them as a group. This factor influences their absorption into and storage in the body, their rate of excretion, the frequency of intake required for health, the degree to which they are affected by food processing and preparation, and their potential for toxicity.

In addition, the two groups of vitamins differ in chemical composition. Unlike fat-soluble vitamins, which consist solely of carbon, hydrogen, and oxygen, most water-soluble vitamins contain nitrogen as well, and some also contain other elements, such as sulfur or cobalt. The water-soluble vitamins differ as much from each other in chemical structure as they do from the fat-soluble group. Water-soluble and fat-soluble vitamins differ with respect to food sources. With few exceptions, water-soluble vitamins tend to be distributed among many different kinds of foods—breads and cereals, milk and milk products, meats and meat alternates, vegetables and fruits—with modest amounts provided by *many* different foods. Exceptions are vitamin B$_{12}$, present in animal but not in plant foods, and vitamin C, found largely in certain fruits and vegetables but virtually absent from most other foods. Contrast this distribution with that of the fat-soluble vitamins, which tend to occur in high concentrations when present but to be obtainable from only a rather narrow range of foods.

In terms of metabolic activity, the distinguishing characteristic of most of the water-soluble vitamins is their function as components of specific coenzymes. (Coenzymes themselves function as components of enzyme complexes which catalyze many biochemical reactions.) Five of them—the so-called energy-producing

TABLE 7-1. *Classification of the Water-Soluble Vitamins*

B-complex	Non-B-complex
Energy-releasing	Ascorbic acid
Thiamin	
Riboflavin	
Niacin	
Biotin	
Pantothenic acid	
Hematopoietic	
Folacin	
Vitamin B_{12} (cobalamin)	
Other	
Vitamin B_6 (pyridoxine)	

vitamins—are involved in producing energy from carbohydrates, fats, and proteins. Two others—the hematopoietic vitamins—are necessary for red blood cell formation. As the classification scheme of Table 7–1 shows, these seven account for all but two of the water-soluble vitamins.

Vitamin B_6 has biological functions that are distinct from those just specified. In addition, all but one of the established water-soluble vitamins (vitamin C-absorbic acid) belong to the B-complex vitamin group. This curious-looking but useful nomenclature resulted historically from the original system of naming vitamins alphabetically as they were discovered. A newly discovered vitamin was first assigned its own letter, unless it appeared to be similar in chemical structure and dietary source to one already discovered. In the latter case, the new vitamin was assigned the same letter along with a distinguishing number (for example, B_6). When its chemical structure was determined, the vitamin was then given the appropriate chemical name. The chemical designation is the acceptable identifying name.

In the course of vitamin research, the status of some substances—the *vitamin-like factors*—has remained unclear. Moreover, certain substances, although sometimes popularly referred to as vitamins (for example, "B_{15}"), are not vitamins at all.

THIAMIN

Like vitamins A and D, thiamin has an ancient medical history. Beriberi, the disease resulting from thiamin deficiency, was known to the Chinese as early as 2600 B.C. The name itself is a doubling of the word for "weakness" in Sinhalese, the language of Ceylon, and aptly describes the major symptom of the disease. In 1855, a Japanese naval officer named Takaki effected one of the earliest known cures of beriberi by feeding his men milk and meat in addition to the sailors' usual diet, mostly refined (polished) rice. Then, shortly before 1900, Eijkman, a Dutch physician working in Java, recognized that chickens fed on polished rice developed the same symptoms as human victims of beriberi. (Polished rice has had the outer husk and bran removed in the process of milling.) Eijkman showed that the symptoms of both chickens and humans could be reversed by the addition of rice husks and bran to the diet. Eventually beriberi was observed to occur widely among peoples whose diet consisted mainly of polished rice.

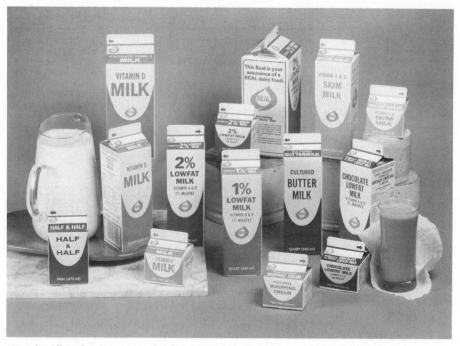

Waxed cardboard cartons are used today to contain milk so that exposure to light will not cause riboflavin to decompose.

National Dairy Council

Casimir Funk was among the first to isolate the antiberiberi factor (from rice bran and yeast), and he was also the first to realize that this substance is an essential nutrient. The new factor received the designation *vitamin B*, which it kept until subsequent research revealed that the substance actually consisted of several accessory food factors. Researchers therefore renamed the antiberiberi factor *vitamin B₁*. After the identification of its structure in 1926, vitamin B₁ received its modern chemical name, *thiamin*. (Although an *e* sometimes appears at the end of this name, the former spelling is preferred.) The vitamin was synthesized successfully ten years later.

Chemistry and Properties

Because of the amine group in thiamin, Funk coined the term *vitamine* as a general name for accessory food factors. Thiamin also contains sulfur, hence the prefix *thi*, from the Greek word for sulfur. Figure 7–1 shows the structure of thiamin. The addition of two phosphate groups produces the primary physiologically active form, thiamin pyrophosphate (TPP), as shown in Figure 7–2. This is the form in which thiamin acts as a coenzyme in energy-producing reactions. Another form, thiamin triphosphate, is possibly involved in nerve function, and its absence may be related to certain symptoms of beriberi.

In its commercially available form, thiamin hydrochloride, the vitamin is a pale yellow, crystalline substance, resistant to oxidation and highly soluble in water. In dry form, thiamin is heat-stable up to temperatures of $100\,^{\circ}C$, but in solution it be-

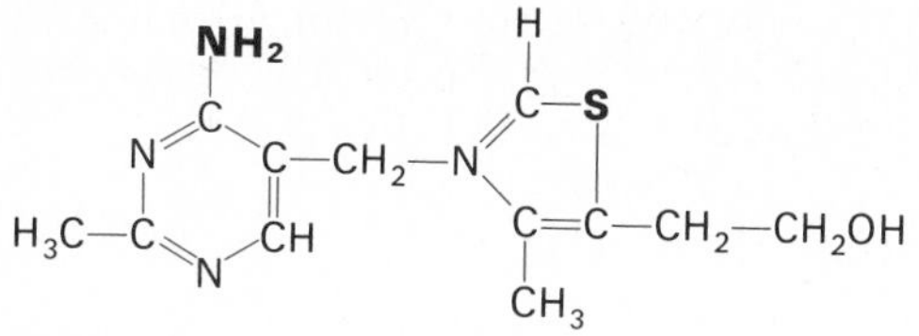

FIGURE 7-1   *Structure of Thiamin.*

Thiamin Pyrophosphate (TPP) = Cocarboxylase

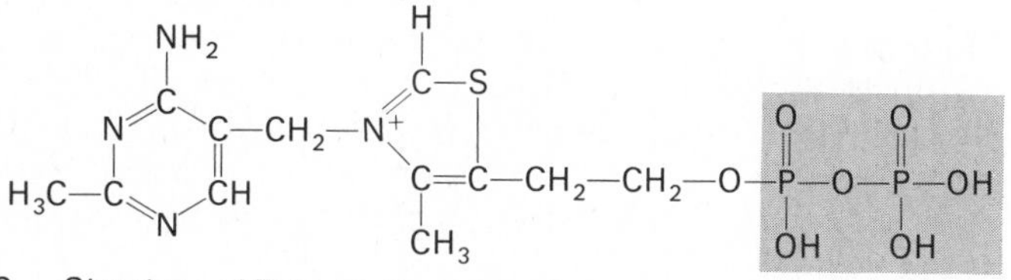

FIGURE 7-2   *Structure of Thiamin Pyrophosphate.*

comes less stable. These properties are especially relevant to the preparation of foods containing thiamin; frying and broiling such foods or cooking them under pressure for too long will destroy the vitamin. Since water will dissolve and leach the vitamin from thiamin-containing foods, washing of such foods should be brief, and only small amounts of water should be used in cooking. Thiamin becomes somewhat more heat-stable in an acidic solution but is quite vulnerable to the presence of alkali. For this reason, baking soda (sodium bicarbonate), often added to cooking water to preserve vegetable color, will decrease thiamin activity and should not be used. Because of their alkaline content, antacids consumed in large quantities may also inactivate the vitamin. Finally, the sulfur dioxide used in processing dried fruits virtually destroys their thiamin content.

Absorption and Metabolism

Absorption of dietary thiamin takes place in the upper part of the small intestine. If present in very large amounts in the intestine, the vitamin is passively absorbed. Absorption of the usual small amounts, however, is by active transport and requires energy and sodium. Thiamin apparently is converted to its active form by the addition of phosphates in the mucosal cells of the intestine. From there, the vitamin enters the general circulation via the portal vein and the liver. Barbiturates and alcohol both decrease the absorption of thiamin from the intestine.

The body stores only small amounts of thiamin, mainly as thiamin pyrophosphate; the total reserve averages about 30 milligrams. Half of it is in muscle tissue, and the remainder is stored in the heart, liver, brain, and kidneys. Excess amounts are excreted in the urine. The use of diuretics containing mercury compounds increases urinary excretion of thiamin (as well as of other water-soluble nutrients).

Physiological Function

In its most important role, thiamin is crucial to the energy-generating reactions involving carbohydrates, fatty acids, and amino acids. It participates in these reactions in its coenzyme form, thiamin pyrophosphate (TPP), also known as *cocarboxylase* (see Figure 7–2). Specifically, it catalyzes the two decarboxylation reactions shown in general form here:

1. Pyruvate $\xrightarrow{\text{TPP}}$ Acetyl CoA + CO_2

2. α-Ketoglutarate $\xrightarrow{\text{TPP}}$ Succinyl CoA + CO_2

The first reaction in effect "connects" the glycolytic to the Krebs cycle. The second reaction is part of the energy-releasing series of reactions in the Krebs cycle. Thiamin is also involved indirectly in metabolism of nucleic acids.

Altogether, thiamin participates in more than 20 different enzymatic reactions and is required for the metabolism of carbohydrates, proteins, and fats. Moreover, thiamin contributes to the body's supply of another B vitamin by assisting in the conversion of the amino acid tryptophan to niacin, as we shall see in our discussion of that vitamin.

Thiamin may play a role in nerve functioning as well, as a component of the nerve-cell membrane and in transmission of nerve impulses. If true, this hypothesis could well account for the devastating effects that thiamin deficiency has on the nervous system. But thus far, experimental research has failed conclusively to support the hypothesis. How thiamin deficiency produces its neurological symptoms remains to be demonstrated.

Recommended Allowances and Dietary Sources

As noted, the metabolism of carbohydrates, proteins, and fats requires thiamin. Therefore, the actual requirements depend on the energy content of the diet and also the distribution of calories among carbohydrate, protein, and fat. A high dietary intake of carbohydrates increases the need for thiamin; protein and fat apparently require less, thus "sparing" the vitamin to some extent. The RDA for thiamin is based on several considerations, including the excretion of the vitamin and its metabolites and the effects of measured doses on clinical symptoms of deficiency.

The allowance is usually stated in proportion to energy allowance (0.5 mg/1,000 kcal). Thus, the RDAs for adult men and women are 1.4 and 1.0 milligrams per day, respectively. Additional thiamin is recommended during pregnancy and lactation. Because some evidence suggests that older people utilize thiamin less efficiently, an intake of not less than 1 milligram per day is recommended. Daily consumption is recommended for all ages, since excess thiamin is excreted, and the body will rapidly mobilize its small reserves.

Thiamin occurs in a wide variety of plant and animal foods, but only a small number of these contain the vitamin in appreciable amounts (Table 7–2). Pork, legumes, wheat germ, and dried yeast are all excellent sources, but the last two do not represent a significant part of most American diets. Because consumption of cereal grains and enriched grain products is generally substantial, these are probably the most practical daily sources. However, much of the thiamin content of cereal grains is concentrated in the outer coat of the seed (the bran) and is removed in the milling and refining process (compare, for example, the values for brown and for unenriched white rice). In enriched bread and similar products, the thiamin, ribo-

TABLE 7-2. Thiamin Content of Selected Foods (RDA for Adults; Men 1.4 mg; Women 1.0 mg)

Food	Serving Size	Thiamin Content mg/serving
Yeast, dried brewer's	1 tbsp	1.25
Pork chop, lean, broiled	3 oz	0.87
Ham, baked, lean	3 oz	0.63
Bran flakes, 40%	1 c	0.41
Peanuts, roasted, salted	½ c	0.23
Peas, frozen, cooked	½ c	0.23
Liver, calf, cooked	3 oz	0.20
Soybeans, cooked	½ c	0.19
Oatmeal, cooked	1 c	0.19
Orange juice, frozen concentrate, diluted	6 oz	0.15
Rice, white, enriched, cooked	½ c	0.12
Orange	1 medium	0.11
Wheat germ, toasted	1 tbsp	0.11
Yogurt, nonfat milk	8 oz	0.11
Yogurt, low-fat, plain	8 oz	0.10
Milk, low-fat	8 oz	0.10
Rice, brown, cooked	½ c	0.09
Asparagus, cooked	½ c	0.09
Milk, whole	8 oz	0.09
Bread, whole-wheat	1 slice	0.06–0.09
Yogurt, low-fat, flavored	8 oz	0.08
Hamburger, 21% fat, cooked	3 oz	0.07
Yogurt, whole-milk	8 oz	0.07
Banana	1 medium	0.06
Bread, white, enriched	1 slice	0.06
Ice cream, 10% fat	1 c	0.05
Egg, whole	1 large	0.04
Egg yolk	1 large	0.04
Fish (haddock, halibut)	3 oz	0.03
Chicken, light meat	3 oz	0.03
Apple	1 medium	0.02
Cottage cheese, uncreamed	½ c	0.02
Peanut butter	1 tbsp	0.02
Rice, white, unenriched, cooked	½ c	0.02
Cheddar cheese	1 oz	0.01
Beer	8 oz	0.01
Cream cheese	1 tbsp	trace
Oils; butter; margarine	1 tbsp	0

Source: C. F. Adams, *Nutritive value of American foods in common units*, USDA Agriculture Handbook No. 456 (Washington, D.C.: U.S. Government Printing Office, 1975) and USDA Handbooks 8–1, 8–9, 8–10, 8–11, 8–12.

flavin, niacin, and iron removed by processing are restored at a later stage of manufacture; these are good sources, because most individuals consume several slices of bread a day. Not all bread, however, is enriched. Enrichment is required only for bread intended for interstate transport. Milk and milk products contribute to daily thiamin intake too, but they are not particularly rich sources. With the exception of the citrus group, most fruits and vegetables are even less useful as major sources of this vitamin.

Clinical Deficiency Symptoms

Beriberi, the disease caused by primary thiamin deficiency, is dangerous and, if untreated, lethal. The three known forms of beriberi—infantile, "wet," and "dry"—all involve impairment of the nervous, cardiovascular, and gastrointestinal systems. The chief biochemical feature of the disease is the accumulation of pyruvic and lactic acids, mainly in the blood and brain. There is a difference of opinion about whether thiamin deficiency alone causes neurologic damage, and some researchers believe that deficiencies of other B vitamins are involved as well. For this reason, supplementation with *all* B vitamins is advised as the best treatment of beriberi symptoms.

Infantile beriberi usually strikes nursing infants in the first six months of life. The cause is insufficient thiamin in the mother's milk, though she herself may show no clinical symptoms of beriberi. The disease has a rapid onset and a short course. Unless treatment begins promptly, the classic symptoms of labored breathing, bluish skin color (cyanosis), and rapid heartbeat are quickly followed by heart failure and death.

The major clinical symptoms of *wet beriberi* resemble those of congestive heart failure—edema, or swelling, of the legs and perhaps of the trunk and face as well, labored breathing, rapid heartbeat, and enlarged heart. Onset is gradual but the victim of wet beriberi runs the real danger of rapid deterioration and a fatal circulatory collapse.

In *dry beriberi* the edema of wet beriberi is absent, hence the name. Dry beriberi is a progressive, wasting disease in which the victim tires easily, the limbs feel heavy and weak, and the legs may develop areas of numbness and tingling sensations. There is difficulty in walking or in rising from a squatting position. If untreated, the disease will progress until the victim becomes bedridden and frequently dies of a chronic infection.

In areas of the world where people subsist on polished rice, and where enrichment is not a standard food-processing procedure, beriberi remains a problem. In the United States and Europe, however, it has been almost completely eliminated, although secondary deficiencies caused by drugs or malabsorptive disease sometimes occur. The most frequently seen form of secondary beriberi in Western countries is due to chronic alcoholism. The contributing factors include reduced intake of thiamin resulting from an inadequate diet, impaired intestinal absorption, and defective phosphorylation of thiamin after absorption. The extreme deficiency condition caused by alcoholism is known as the Wernicke-Korsakoff syndrome; unless diagnosed early and treated promptly, irreversible brain damage, usually requiring institutionalization, can occur. To what extent the excess alcohol intake causes the symptoms and to what extent the resulting thiamin deficiency is responsible is not clear.

Toxicity

Because of thiamin's high solubility in water, large doses of the vitamin are readily excreted. Thus, there is a large margin of safety between even supplemented consumption and the amounts needed to produce toxicity. But intravenous injections of large amounts have caused sensitization reactions in some individuals.

RIBOFLAVIN

During the 1920s researchers discovered that laboratory animals continued to grow, although not optimally, on foods in which the antiberiberi factor had been destroyed by heat. Biochemists hypothesized the existence of a heat-stable vitamin B_2 and began to look for it. In 1933 Richard Kuhn and his colleagues succeeded in extracting 1 gram of a yellow crystalline substance from 5,400 liters of milk. Even earlier, in the nineteenth century, yellowish fluorescent pigments had been discovered in milk, eggs, yeast, and liver. The name *flavin,* from the Latin word for "yellow," was given to these substances. In 1932 Otto Warburg and W. Christian found a "yellow enzyme" in yeast. It soon became apparent that the distinctively colored crystals found by Kuhn were the same as Warburg's yellow enzyme. The vitamin, which consists of a pigment, the flavin, attached to a chemical group similar to the pentose ribose, was synthesized in 1935 and named *riboflavin.*

Chemistry and Properties

Riboflavin (Figure 7–3) is a yellow-orange crystalline compound, slightly soluble in water. In solution it exhibits a yellow-green fluorescence. It is heat-stable, acid-resistant, and slow to oxidize. Because of its lower solubility in water and greater heat stability, riboflavin is less affected than thiamin by most normal cooking procedures. However, some losses do occur when vegetables are cooked for long periods of time in a large volume of water.

Riboflavin becomes unstable in alkaline solutions (caused, for example, by the addition of baking soda). Riboflavin in solution is destroyed by light. For this reason, foods cooked in uncovered vessels and exposed to light will lose some of their riboflavin content. Milk has a relatively high content of riboflavin, and opaque containers, such as waxed cardboard cartons, are generally used today to protect the vitamin from decomposition.

FIGURE 7-3　*Structure of Riboflavin.*

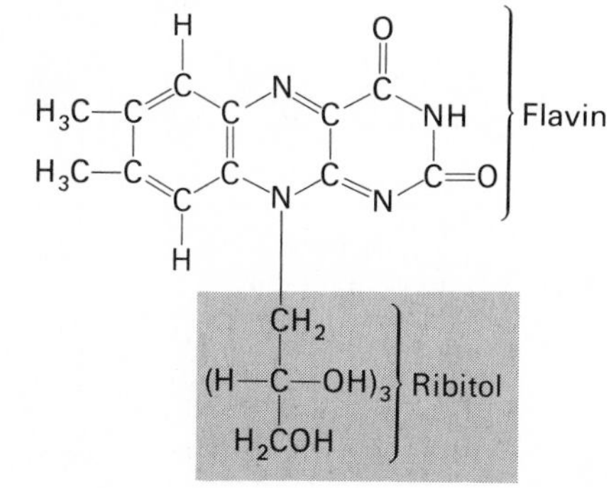

Absorption and Metabolism

Like thiamin, riboflavin is absorbed from the small intestine, phosphorylated, and then transported to the liver via the portal vein. Absorption appears to involve a specific transport system, with albumin serving as the carrier by which riboflavin reaches the liver. Further phosphorylation of the vitamin takes place in the liver and other tissues of the body. One quite curious feature of riboflavin absorption is that for reasons unknown, it increases with age.

The liver, kidneys, and heart retain small reserves of riboflavin, but the total is quite small indeed, necessitating regular intake. When intake is low, however, the body's capacity for storing riboflavin appears to be greater than that for storing thiamin.

Excess riboflavin is excreted in the urine, but an even greater amount is found in the feces. Fecal riboflavin originates not from metabolized food but from bacterial synthesis of the vitamin in the intestine. Whether riboflavin of intestinal origin is absorbed and metabolized for use by the body (as is the case with vitamin K), and if so, to what extent, is not known at present.

Riboflavin metabolism can be affected by certain drugs. For example, the antibiotic tetracycline increases urinary excretion of the vitamin. Certain types of diuretics have the same effect, as does probenecid, used in the treatment of gout. The latter drug decreases riboflavin absorption as well. Some oral contraceptives appear to lower serum levels of the vitamin but without causing any observable symptoms of deficiency. The antimicrobial sulfonamides (sulfa drugs) decrease bacterial synthesis of riboflavin, but the nutritional significance of this effect is not clear.

Physiological Function

Riboflavin, in its coenzyme form, plays a vital role in the release of energy from carbohydrates, fats, and proteins. In association with components of ATP, it enters these reactions as a component of two closely related coenzymes, *flavin mononucleotide* (FMN) (also known as *riboflavin monophosphate*) and *flavin adenine dinucleotide* (FAD). The structure of FAD is shown in Figure 7–4.

These coenzymes combine with various proteins to form active enzymes commonly known as *flavoproteins*. It is in the form of flavoproteins that riboflavin participates in the energy-producing reactions of the cell. We saw in previous chapters that the hydrogen generated (as 2H) in glycolysis and the Krebs cycle is transmitted through the electron transport system located in mitochondria, releasing H_2O and

FIGURE 7-4   *Structure of Flavin Adenine Dinucleotide (FAD).*

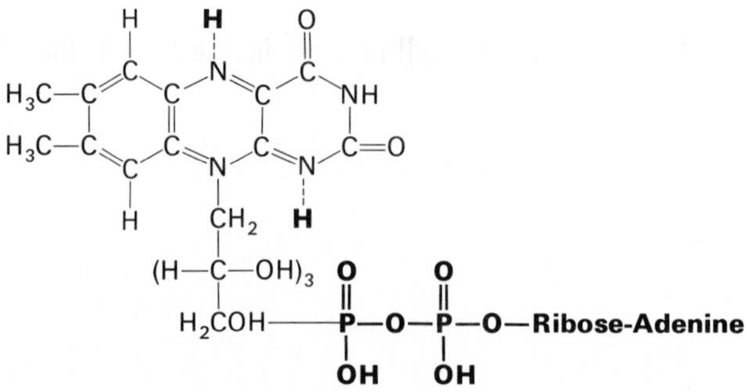

energy in the concentrated form of ATP. The flavoproteins are one of the carrier molecules to which hydrogen becomes attached as it moves through the electron transport system.

FAD has the ability to act as a carrier because it readily accepts hydrogen electrons and as readily gives them up. Thus, it exists in both reduced form ($FADH_2$) and in oxidized form (FAD). In this reaction,

$$\text{Succinic acid} \xrightarrow[\text{(Succinate dehydrogenase)}]{\quad \overset{\displaystyle FAD \quad FADH_2}{\curvearrowright} \quad} \text{Fumaric acid}$$

FAD is transformed into $FADH_2$ when it accepts hydrogen atoms from succinic acid, leaving fumaric acid to serve as substrate for the next reaction.

FAD also plays a role in the complex series of reactions in which pyruvate and α-ketoglutarate are decarboxylated. In addition, this coenzyme is important for the oxidation of fatty acids and amino acids.

In the form of FMN, riboflavin is necessary for the activity of other enzymes associated with the electron transport system, cytochrome reductase and some of the amino acid oxidases. (The cytochromes, a group of iron-containing enzymes, are another important component of the electron transport system.) Thus, the flavoproteins catalyze hydrogen-transfer reactions. Riboflavin, moreover, may play a part in the synthesis of corticosteroids and in production of red blood cells.

Recommended Allowances and Dietary Sources

Recommended allowances for riboflavin are set at 0.6 milligrams of the vitamin per 1,000 kilocalories (4,200 kJ). Assuming an average daily intake of 2,700 kcal (11,340 kJ) for adult men and 2,000 kcal (8,400 kJ) for adult women, the recommended daily allowances are 1.6 mg and 1.2 mg, respectively. Women should increase their intake to 1.5 mg/day during pregnancy and 1.7 mg/day during lactation. According to data from several recent studies, exercise increases the riboflavin requirement. An intake of 1.16 mg/1000 kcal/day was needed by young women during periods of exercise in contrast to 0.96 mg riboflavin/1000 kcal/day to achieve biochemical normality during sedantary periods.

Riboflavin, like thiamin, is found in many foods, but usually in relatively small amounts. A substantial part of daily intake is most likely to come from milk; milk products; organ meats; and green, leafy vegetables. Consequently, vegetarians, especially those who exclude milk and milk products from their diet, can ensure adequate intake through regular use of baked products containing yeast and of green, leafy vegetables and winter squash eaten in quantity. Whole grains and enriched flours and bread will increase intake also. Table 7–3 shows the riboflavin content of selected foods.

Clinical Deficiency Symptoms and Toxicity

Because B vitamins tend to occur as a group in foods, B vitamin deficiencies also tend to appear in association with one another. The clinical symptoms of riboflavin deficiency are much less dramatic than those of beriberi or niacin deficiency, and most of what we know about human ariboflavinosis comes from studies in which a riboflavin antagonist was administered to people. Observed symptoms include

TABLE 7-3. *Riboflavin Content of Selected Foods (RDA for Adults: Men 1.6 mg; Women 1.2 mg)*

Food	Serving Size	Riboflavin Content mg/serving
Liver, calf, cooked	3 oz	3.54
Yogurt, nonfat milk	8 oz	0.53
Milk, low-fat, 2% solids	8 oz	0.52
Yogurt, low-fat, plain	8 oz	0.49
Bran flakes, 40%	1 c	0.49
Milk, whole	1 c (8 oz)	0.41
Yogurt, low-fat, flavored	8 oz	0.40
Yeast, dried brewer's	1 tbsp	0.34
Yogurt, whole-milk	8 oz	0.32
Spinach, cooked	1 c	0.32
Ice cream, 10% fat	1 c	0.28
Pork chop, lean, broiled	3 oz	0.27
Ham, lean, baked	3 oz	0.22
Cottage cheese, uncreamed	½ c	0.20
Hamburger, 21% fat, cooked	3 oz	0.17
Broccoli, cooked	½ c	0.16
Egg, whole	1 large	0.15
Cheddar cheese	1 oz	0.13
Asparagus, fresh, cooked	½ c	0.11
Banana	1 medium	0.11
Peanuts, roasted, salted	½ c	0.10
Soybeans, cooked	½ c	0.08
Chicken, light meat	3 oz	0.08
Peas, frozen, cooked	½ c	0.08
Egg yolk	1 large	0.07
Fish (haddock, halibut)	3 oz	0.06
Oatmeal, cooked	1 c	0.05
Wheat germ, toasted	1 tbsp	0.05
Orange	1 medium	0.05
Bread, white, enriched	1 slice	0.05
Bread, whole-wheat	1 slice	0.03
Cream cheese	1 tbsp	0.03
Apple, raw	1 medium	0.02
Rice, brown, cooked	½ c	0.02
Winter squash, baked	½ c	0.02
Peanut butter	1 tbsp	0.02
Rice, white, cooked	½ c	0.01
Oils; butter; margarine	1 tbsp	0

Sources: C. F. Adams, *Nutritive value of American foods in common units*, USDA Agriculture Handbook No. 456 (Washington, D.C.: U.S. Government Printing Office, 1975); USDA Agriculture Handbook No. 8–1, 8–9, 8–11, 8–12 (Washington, D.C.: U.S. Government Printing Office).

growth retardation and certain abnormalities of the eyes and mouth, particularly cracks at the corners of the mouth (cheilosis); a smooth and purplish tongue (glossitis); inflamed mouth; and dry, scaly facial skin.

Some of these symptoms may result from other deficiencies of the B-complex group or even from other causes. For example, an allergy or a cold can cause cracks at the corner of the mouth. Therefore the particular symptom or condition will respond to riboflavin therapy *only if it is due to a deficiency of this vitamin.*

Riboflavin has no known toxic effects at any likely consumption levels.

NIACIN (NICOTINIC ACID, NICOTINAMIDE)

In 1867 a compound was obtained by chemical oxidation of nicotine and named *nicotinic acid*. In 1912 the same substance was identified in the antiberiberi materials extracted from rice polishings. Although Funk and others ascribed to it vitaminlike effects, the evidence to prove this ascription was not found until 1937, when Conrad Elvehjem and his colleagues found that nicotinic acid cured a condition called "blacktongue" in dogs.

The symptoms of blacktongue are similar to those of pellagra, a human disease widespread in Europe and the United States. It was first described in 1735 by Gaspar Casal, physician to Philip V of Spain, and one of the visible symptoms of deficiency bears Casal's name. Its appearance in Europe coincided with the introduction of corn (maize) from the New World to the countries bordering the Mediterranean where, in the form of cornmeal, it supplanted wheat as a staple foodstuff. The name *pellagra* comes from the Italian words meaning "rough skin"; dermatitis is one of the "four D's" that are characteristic of the disease. Diarrhea, dementia, and death are the others.

Until the early part of this century, pellagra was little known in the United States. But from 1910 to 1935, more than 150,000 cases were reported *annually*, mostly among the poor of the South. It was the worst nutritional disease outbreak in U.S. history. In 1914 Joseph Goldberger began a series of epidemiologic studies to determine its cause; these were to become a classic example of excellent epidemiological and clinical investigations of a nutritional disorder. By the end of 1917 he had succeeded in establishing the connection between pellagra and the poor diet. About the same time, blacktongue in dogs came to be recognized as the canine form of the disease. This second discovery led to the eventual identification of nicotinic acid, or niacin, as the antipellagra (pellagra-preventive) factor.

Chemistry and Properties

Niacin is a water-soluble, white, crystalline powder with a sour taste. The vitamin is very stable under a wide variety of conditions, being resistant to the degradative effects of light, heat, oxygen, acid, and alkali. Consequently, losses that occur in cooking are due largely to its solubility in water. Niacin is readily converted to nicotinamide, the physiologically active form of the vitamin which becomes part of the coenzyme synthesized from it.

Absorption and Metabolism

Absorption of niacin into the body takes place, probably by passive diffusion, in the upper part of the small intestine. The process is both rapid and efficient. The body stores only limited amounts and excretes any excess in the urine.

Niacin is distinguished from all the other water-soluble vitamins by having a dietary precursor—the amino acid tryptophan. The oxidative conversion of tryptophan to niacin requires three other B-complex vitamins—thiamin, riboflavin, and pyridoxine (B_6). On the basis of some experimental evidence, it has been estimated that 1 milligram of niacin can be synthesized from approximately 60 milligrams of dietary tryptophan. As low as this conversion rate is (compared, for example, to that of carotene to vitamin A), the tryptophan content of foods should be consid-

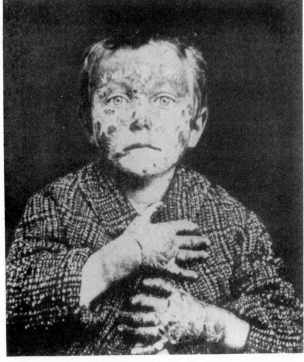

Though it still occurs in corn-eating countries of Europe, pellagra has all but disappeared in the United States.

National Medical Library, Casimir Funk. *Die Vitamine.* Wiesbaden, Bergman, 1914.

ered in estimating the dietary requirement for niacin. But the estimated rate of conversion may not always be the same. For example, conversion is probably less efficient in people who consume diets low in niacin or low in tryptophan. More than a dozen metabolites of niacin have been identified.

Physiological Function

In its role in various metabolic reactions, niacin very much resembles riboflavin. First, it functions mainly as a component of two closely related coenzymes, *nicotinamide adenine dinucleotide* (NAD) and *nicotinamide adenine dinucleotide phosphate* (NADP). The structure of NADP differs from that of NAD (shown in Figure 7–5) by addition of a single phosphate group (represented in the diagram by an asterisk). As the illustration shows, NAD contains nicotinamide, adenine, ribose, and two phosphate groups. The adenine and phosphates come from ATP.

Second, NAD and NADP combine with various proteins to form a third important group of carrier enzymes involved in the energy-producing reactions of the cell. Third, like the riboflavin coenzymes, NAD and NADP exist in both oxidized and reduced forms, enabling them to act as hydrogen carriers:

$$NAD(P) \rightleftharpoons NAD(P)H$$

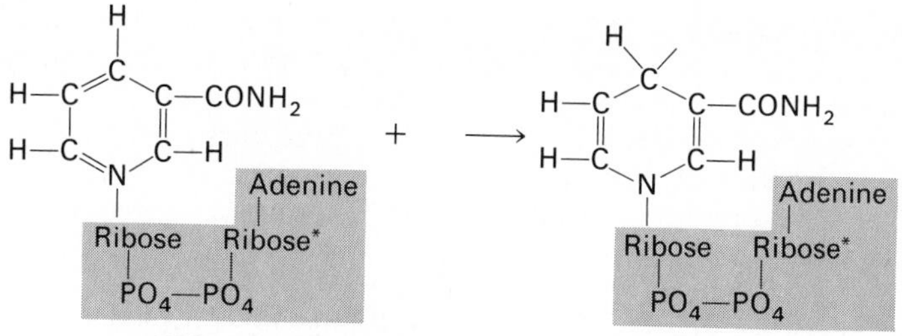

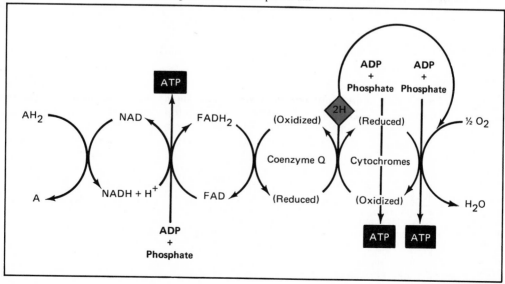

FIGURE 7-5 *Structure of NAD and NADH.*
Additional phosphate group attached to ribose in NADP (see text).

As such, the two coenzymes take part in many of the hydrogen-transfer reactions necessary for the oxidation of glucose, amino acids, and fats. NAD appears in both glycolysis and the Krebs cycle and is important in the functioning of the electron transport system (see Figure 7–6). NADP, which is produced in the pentose pathway of carbohydrate metabolism, plays an essential role in the synthesis of fatty acids and of cholesterol.

Recommended Allowances and Dietary Sources

The Food and Nutrition Board has set RDAs for niacin in relation to energy intake and recommends an allowance of 6.6 milligrams of niacin per 1,000 kilocalories (4,200 kJ); the niacin RDA for adult men is, therefore, 18 mg, and for adult women 13 mg. The Food and Nutrition Board also recommends the consumption of at

FIGURE 7-6 *The Electron Transport System.*
Water and ATP are produced through a series of reactions located in the mitochondrial membrane. Reduced substances (AH_2) such as malate and lactate are oxidized (A), and the hydrogen atoms are transferred to NAD and/or FAD and then to Coenzyme Q (ubiquinone). Electrons are transported through a series of iron-containing proteins, the cytochromes. Finally, hydrogen ions, electrons, and oxygen combine to form water. The high-energy compound ATP is generated at three places along the electron transport chain.

least 13 mg total niacin per day as a minimum, even for energy intakes below 2,000 kcal (8,400 kJ) per day. These allowances are intended to allow a substantial margin of safety. Because physiological requirements for niacin are increased during pregnancy and lactation, the RDAs have also been increased by 2 mg and 5 mg, respectively, for those situations.

The RDA is expressed as niacin equivalents because the effective niacin value of food is dependent on its tryptophan content as well. For this reason, niacin equivalents have been defined. One niacin equivalent is equal to 1 mg of preformed niacin or 60 mg of tryptophan. Both sources should be considered when estimating niacin intake.

Meat, poultry, and fish contain more niacin than do fruits, vegetables, and grains, which in turn contain more than dairy products and eggs. Although niacin was first identified as a product of the oxidation of nicotine, this component of tobacco has no vitamin activity. Cooking methods have little effect on the content of niacin, which is quite stable, unless cooking water is drained off. Table 7–4 lists the amounts of preformed niacin available in various food products and some niacin equivalents as well. Approximately 1.4 percent of animal protein is tryptophan; vegetable protein is approximately 1.0 percent tryptophan. Thus, one cup of milk, which contains 120 mg of tryptophan, can provide 2 mg of the vitamin to the body in addition to 0.25 mg of preformed niacin. Milk is therefore a better source than its low niacin content alone would indicate. So, for the same reason, are eggs.

Many foods, particularly grains, contain niacin in chemically bound forms that the body cannot metabolize. This fact explains why even some cereal-based diets may lead to niacin deficiency and pellagra. But it does not answer the fascinating question of why pellagra has never been a serious problem in Central and South America, where corn is the staple. The answer is that the treatment of corn with lime salts (a common procedure in those areas) releases the bound forms of niacin, thereby making it available for absorption. In addition, the beans that usually constitute a large part of every meal in Latin America have significant tryptophan content.

TABLE 7-4. *Niacin Content of Selected Foods (RDA for Adults: Men 18 mg; Women 13 mg)*

Food	Serving Size	Tryptophan[a] Content mg	Niacin Equivalents mg	Niacin[b] Content mg	Total Niacin Content mg
Round steak	3 oz	194	3.2	5.1	8.3
Chicken	2 pieces	125	2.1	5.8	7.9
Beans, pinto	½ c	181	3.0	2.1	5.1
Milk, whole	1 c	113	1.9	0.2	2.1
Cornmeal	½ c	34	0.6	1.2	1.8
Egg, whole	1 large	97	1.6	0.03	1.63
Banana	1 medium	31	0.5	0.8	1.3
Bread, white, enriched	1 slice	23	0.4	0.6	1.0
Ice cream	½ c	34	0.6	0.07	0.67
Orange	1 medium	5	0.1	0.5	0.6
Carrot, raw	1 medium	8	0.1	0.4	0.5
Green beans, canned	½ c	17	0.3	0.2	0.5

[a] From M. L. Orr and B. K. Watt, *Amino acid content of foods*, USDA Home Economics Research Report No. 4 (Washington, D.C.: U.S. Government Printing Office, 1968).
[b] From C. F. Adams, *Nutritive value of American foods in common units*, USDA Agriculture Handbook No. 456 (Washington, D.C.: U.S. Government Printing Office, 1975).

Pellagra, the primary clinical manifestation of niacin deficiency, results from a prolonged diet low in both niacin and protein. Since the body can synthesize niacin from tryptophan, a pellagra-producing diet must generally be deficient or marginal in the latter as well. Goldberger noted that the diet characteristic of pellagra victims in the United States in his day consisted largely of cornmeal, fatback, and molasses. The disease appeared most frequently in the spring, following a lengthy period in which the diet was likely to be particularly deficient.

Because of the key role of nicotinamide in energy metabolism, niacin deficiency affects many body systems, most dramatically the skin, gastrointestinal tract, and nervous system. The symptoms are numerous, but pellagra is best known by three of the "four D's"—dermatitis, diarrhea, and dementia. Although the onset is gradual, unless the disease is treated the fourth "D"—death—will follow. The dermatitis takes the form of a symmetrical rash on exposed areas of the body. (The phrase *Casal's necklace* is often used to refer to such a collar of dermatitis around the neck.) The mouth, tongue, and intestines become inflamed. Disturbances of the nervous system can be severe, causing mental confusion, anxiety, and psychosis. Numerous mental institutions primarily for pellagra victims were established when this disease was rampant, before it was realized that the mental symptoms were due to a nutritional deficiency disease.

Many symptoms of pellagra resemble those resulting from thiamin and riboflavin deficiencies. In fact, recent research suggests that pellagra is a "mixed deficiency" disease, and that thiamin, riboflavin, and possibly vitamin B_6 deficiencies may contribute to its development. These three vitamins are necessary for the synthesis of niacin from tryptophan, so the lack of any of them could deprive the body of a potentially significant amount of niacin.

Diets based on millet or sorghum may produce pellagra in some instances, even though these grains contain high concentrations of available niacin as well as reasonable amounts of tryptophan. But they also contain considerable amounts of leucine, an amino acid that either interferes with the synthesis of niacin from tryptophan or alters niacin metabolism in some other, as yet unidentified, way.

Secondary niacin deficiencies, due to diseases affecting ingestion, absorption, or metabolism of the vitamin, may accompany amebic dysentery, hookworm, and malaria. Cirrhosis of the liver, and therefore chronic alcoholism, can also cause secondary pellagra.

The recommended treatment for pellagra is 50 to 250 milligrams per day of nicotinamide and the other B-complex vitamins, in addition to an adequate diet. Though it still occurs in the corn-eating countries of Europe, pellagra has all but disappeared in the United States. Its disappearance was largely due to two factors: first, changes in people's economic status, and therefore diet, as the country began to recover from the agricultural and economic depression of the early 1930s; and second, a greater understanding of the vitamin and its preventive effects. For example, Figure 7–7 shows that bread enrichment, which began in 1938, further accelerated the decline in pellagra mortality.

In the period from 1920 to 1960, more than twice as many women as men succumbed to pellagra, a ratio that remained fairly constant in every year throughout this period. Is the differential due to different food habits of men and women? Do women have greater requirements for niacin? Are women more vulnerable to niacin and/or tryptophan deficiency? These questions suggest further areas for research.

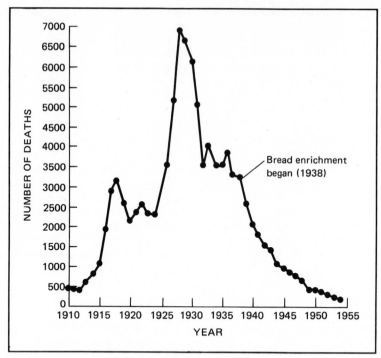

FIGURE 7-7   *Deaths from Pellagra in the United States.*

Fatalities from pellagra began climbing during World War I, briefly stabilized in the prosperity of the early 1920s, and climbed sharply as economic conditions worsened toward the end of that decade. A partial decline in fatalities followed, but not until a nationwide program of enriching bread was initiated in 1938 did mortality from pellagra begin its sharp downward plunge.

Source: National Center for Health Statistics.

Toxicity

In large amounts, niacin (not nicotinamide) produces vasodilation; tingling sensations; flushed skin, especially on the face; and liver damage. For a time, pharmacological doses of niacin (3 grams or more per day) were prescribed to lower serum cholesterol and lipoprotein levels; however, the Coronary Drug Project Research Group has stated that there is no evidence that niacin will improve the survival chances of anyone who has had a heart attack. Niacin may contribute slightly to preventing the recurrence of minor heart attack but that the side effects are serious enough to require great caution in its use. Among those side effects are increased likelihood of heartbeat irregularity and various gastrointestinal disorders.

Massive doses of niacin can cause liver toxicity and, if continued for a long period of time, may cause diabetes and activate peptic ulcers. In pharmacological amounts, then, niacin is by no means a completely harmless water-soluble vitamin.

Pharmacologic doses of niacin have also been advocated for the treatment of schizophrenia. After the publication of much conflicting data, the Canadian Mental Health Association conducted four very carefully controlled studies lasting from 6 months to 2 years. The data showed that the control groups were better adjusted in the home and the community setting than the niacin-treated group.

BIOTIN

Biotin is one of the most widely available and most scientifically elusive vitamins. Before its final identification, biotin was independently "discovered" at least three times and acquired half a dozen different names. It was originally discovered in 1901 and named *Bios* for its growth-promoting properties in microorganisms. Subsequent research showed Bios to be one component of a complex of water-soluble B vitamins, from which it could be separated. In the early 1930s, Fritz Kögl began to look for a source of this growth factor, by this time called *Bios IIb*. In 1936, a 16-stage extraction procedure and 550 pounds of dried duck-egg yolks yielded 1 milligram of a highly active growth factor, which was given the name of *biotin*.

At about the same time, other researchers found a substance they called *coenzyme R*, which stimulated growth in some bacteria, and eventually the similarity between coenzyme R and biotin was noted. In the meantime, Margaret Boas (in 1927) and others had observed that when rats were given raw egg white as their only source of dietary protein, they developed dermatitis and bleeding skin, paralysis, weight loss, and "spectacle eye," a characteristic loss of hair around the eyes. Cooking the egg whites prevented such symptoms, but so did the addition of other foods, which were presumed to contain, variously, "protective factor X" and "vitamin H."

Eventually these lines of research converged in 1940 when Paul György demonstrated that Kögl's biotin was related to his own "vitamin H." With the identification of the vitamin's chemical structure in 1942, and its synthesis the following year, biotin was officially added to the roster of water-soluble vitamins.

Chemistry and Properties

Biotin is a white crystalline substance somewhat soluble in water but quite heat-stable. The former property leads to some loss of the vitamin during cooking, whereas the latter protects it during cooking, processing, and storage. The vitamin is also alcohol-soluble and vulnerable to oxidizing substances, alkalis, and strong acids. Biotin, like thiamin, contains sulfur (see Figure 7–8).

Absorption and Metabolism

As far as is known, only one substance—the protein avidin, found in raw egg whites—will interfere specifically with biotin absorption from the intestine. Avidin combines with biotin and prevents it from being absorbed. Significant amounts of

FIGURE 7-8   *Structure of Biotin.*

* Active site, which picks up CO_2 for transfer.

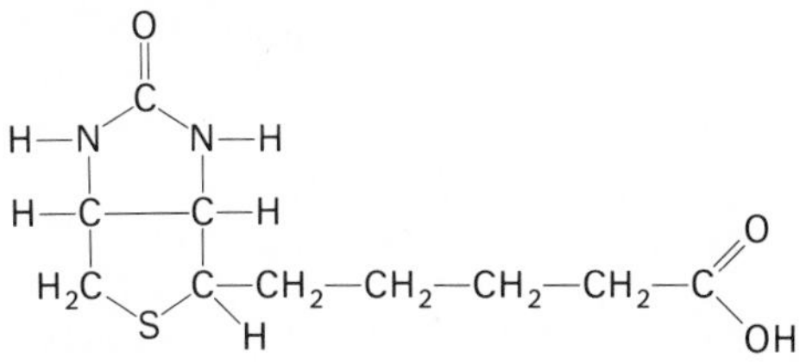

DRUG-NUTRIENT INTERACTIONS

"Take at mealtime." "Do not take with milk or milk products." Have you ever been given this advice along with your prescription medication? Why should you take some medicine with food and some without? Does food change the way the drug is absorbed, metabolized, or excreted? For some drugs, the answer is yes. Drugs can also impact on our nutritional health. They can change our desire for food as well as interfere with the normal mechanisms of nutrient absorption, function, metabolism, and excretion.

For some scientists, drug-nutrient interactions include not only the effect of diet on drug metabolism and action and the effect of drugs on nutritional processes, but also the occurrence of drugs in foods and the pharmacological uses and abuses of nutrients as drugs. Here, our discussion will deal mainly with the latter two; megavitamin therapy is discussed in its own perspective (Chapter 7) and the occurrence of drugs in foods is discussed in the perspective on additives (Chapter 14).

APPETITE. The suppression of appetite by amphetamines, sometimes prescribed in the treatment of obesity, is a well-known drug-nutrient interaction. Some other drugs (such as chloral hydrate) depress the appetite by causing nausea and gastrointestinal upset; some antibiotics decrease taste sensitivity. On the other hand, insulin, certain tranquilizers and antidepressants, oral contraceptives, and some antihistamines stimulate appetite. People given these drugs are frequently not told that carbohydrate craving or general appetite stimulation might result. Valium, librium, and elavil, commonly prescribed drugs, are among those which stimulate appetite. Whether appetite is depressed or stimulated the balance of nutrient and energy intake is upset.

NUTRIENT ABSORPTION, FUNCTION, METABOLISM AND EXCRETION. Nutrient absorption may be impaired by any of several mechanisms. Laxatives and cathartics increase intestinal motility, thereby reducing the time in which nutrients can be absorbed. Some of these pharmaceutical products interfere directly with nutrient absorption. We have already seen, for example, that mineral oil dissolves carotene, which is then eliminated in the feces. Drugs may also increase nutrient excretion by any of several mechanisms that effectively keep the nutrient from its binding sites on proteins or within tissues.

Any drug that binds bile salts or decreases their availability will greatly reduce the efficiency with which fats and fat-soluble vitamins can be absorbed. Some drugs can damage certain cells of the intestinal mucosa or directly interfere with transport mechanisms. Some cause excessive release and/or decreased synthesis of pancreatic enzymes, resulting in impaired digestion of fat, protein, and carbohydrate.

Nutrient synthesis can also be affected by drugs, as when antibiotics inhibit the manufacture of vitamin K in the intestinal tract or chloramphenicol decreases protein synthesis. Among the categories of medications that interfere with metabolism and absorption are anticholesterol drugs, such as cholestyramine; antibiotics, such as neomycin; anticonvulsants; and certain drugs that are used to treat diabetes and other conditions.

Drugs can also act as antivitamins by preventing either the synthesis of an active metabolite or conversion to a coenzyme form, by promoting retention of inactive forms, or by decreasing the natural body stores of a vitamin by increasing the activity of specific metabolic enzymes. There is considerable evidence that anticonvulsant drugs effectively counteract vitamin D by this last mechanism. Thus, epileptics on long-term anticonvulsant therapy may develop osteomalacia.

biotin are synthesized by bacteria in the body, and in this form the vitamin is very likely available for absorption and use.

Biotin occurs in all the cells of the body, although in minute amounts. The liver

Other important drug-nutrient interactions include the effect of antacids on mineral metabolism. For example, antacids containing aluminum inhibit absorption of phosphorus, ultimately increasing the excretion of both phosphorus and calcium; prolonged use may lead to significant demineralization of bone. The antacid property itself causes conversion of iron to insoluble and unabsorbable forms.

CLINICAL SIGNIFICANCE OF DRUG-NUTRIENT INTERACTIONS Individuals who already have borderline nutritional deficiencies, due to low nutrient intake and/or chronic diseases, are significantly at risk of developing clinically important effects of drug-nutrient interactions. Among the common reason for lowered nutrient intake are alcoholism, psychological stress, chronic illness, and smoking. The latter specifically lowers vitamin C and vitamin E levels. As you may imagine, these conditions involve a large number of individuals in the population. The elderly, because of lowered energy and therefore food needs, are particularly vulnerable. Moreover, they often take several drugs simultaneously. In a study of 288 long-term care, skilled nursing facilities, the average number of prescriptions per resident was 6.1. For non-institutionalized elderly, the number is less. The effects of any interaction, of course, depend on the dose and duration of drug treatment. Two or three days of medication are of no concern; neither are small doses, unless use is prolonged. Drug consumption for weeks or longer, however, is a potentially serious problem. Particularly at risk in such situations are the chronically ill who are likely to take drugs for a long time.

EFFECTS OF FOOD ON DRUGS. Conversely, some foods may interfere with drug utilization. For example, absorption of erythromycin is decreased while absorption of digoxin is delayed; effectiveness is therefore decreased if these drugs are taken simultaneously with food. Drugs are metabolized and detoxified by enzymes which need cofactors to function properly. Enzymes are proteins and the cofactors are active forms of vitamins and minerals. Therefore, adequate intake of all nutrients is essential to properly utilize and dispose of drugs. The type of foods we eat may also alter drug metabolism. Large quantities of Brussels sprouts and other vegetables of the Brassica species increase the rate of drug metabolism by the action of non-nutrient compounds.

Many people, when they think of drug-nutrient interactions, think only of prescription medication. Over-the-counter (OTC) and street drugs can also cause problems. OTCs should not be regarded lightly because they have the potential for harmful side effects. Read the label carefully and follow the directions. Abuse of certain antacids containing aluminum hydroxide results in phosphate depletion. Street drugs can cause the user to forget to eat or drain off the money needed to purchase food.

We are aware of many food-drug interactions, but many more remain to be clarified. This is an area of inquiry for scientists in a variety of fields—toxicology, pharmacology, nutrition, and medicine. The implications are important for everyone. The public and the medical profession should be aware of the possibility of these interactions, and taking drugs unnecessarily should be discouraged. When drugs are prescribed, instructions for taking them before, during, after, or between meals, and any other instructions, should be carefully followed.

and kidneys contain the highest concentrations. In plant and animal foods and in body tissues, the vitamin is protein-bound, in which form it serves its coenzymatic functions.

Excess biotin is excreted in the urine. Excretion of three to six times the amount of biotin ingested has been demonstrated, emphasizing that bacterial synthesis contributes large quantities to the body's available supply.

Physiological Function

One of the most active biological substances known, biotin functions as a coenzyme in a large number of important metabolic reactions. In particular, the vitamin acts as a carbon dioxide carrier in CO_2-fixation reactions (carboxylation), which lengthen carbon chains. Note, in Figure 7–8, the HN group in the biotin molecule to which CO_2 becomes temporarily attached in these reactions. Three important examples are

$$1.\ \text{Pyruvate} \xrightarrow{\;CO_2\;} \text{Oxaloacetate}$$

$$2.\ \text{Acetyl CoA} \xrightarrow{\;CO_2\;} \text{Malonyl CoA} \longrightarrow \text{Fatty acids}$$

$$3.\ \text{Proprionyl CoA} \xrightarrow{\;CO_2\;} \text{Methylmalonyl CoA} \longrightarrow \text{Succinate}$$

The third reaction is particularly important in the oxidation of odd-number carbon chains (such as the odd-number fatty acids).

In addition to its established role in fatty-acid synthesis, biotin has a part in several transcarboxylation reactions of amino acid metabolism and may be involved in protein and carbohydrate metabolism. Other processes that may require biotin include antibody formation and the synthesis of pancreatic amylase.

Recommended Allowances and Dietary Sources

The Food and Nutrition Board has established no dietary allowance for biotin because there is insufficient evidence on which to base an RDA. It did, however, recommend in 1979 that the daily intake be 100 to 200 micrograms for adults.

Normal dietary intake is estimated to be 100 to 300 micrograms per day. This amount, plus that from bacterial synthesis, makes the possibility of deficiency so improbable that it seems not to occur, except when large quantities of raw eggs are eaten for long periods.

Milk and various milk products are among the best sources of the vitamin since one or more appear fairly frequently in most diets. See Table 7–5 for a more extensive list. The biotin content of many foods, however, has not been determined.

Clinical Deficiency Symptoms and Toxicity

Natural biotin deficiency is not known to occur in humans except with excessive consumption of raw eggs. However, because major amounts of biotin are synthesized by intestinal bacteria, the use of antibiotics could decrease the amounts of the vitamin available for absorption from the intestine. Oxytetracycline and the sulfonamides are both known to reduce bacterial populations that synthesize biotin. Thus some of the symptoms that appear with long-term use of these drugs may in fact be symptoms of secondary deficiency of biotin or other vitamins.

Some evidence suggests that biotin deficiency may be the actual cause of two

TABLE 7-5. *Biotin Content of Selected Foods (Estimated Safe and Adequate Daily Dietary Intake: 100–200 µg)*

Food	Serving Size	Biotin Content µg/serving
Liver, beef, fried	3 oz	82
Oatmeal, cooked	1 c	58
Soybeans, cooked	½ c	22
Clams, canned, drained	½ c	20
Egg, whole, cooked[a]	1 medium	13
Salmon, broiled or baked	3 oz	10
Milk, whole	8 oz	10
Rice, brown, cooked	½ c	9
Shrimp, cooked	3 oz	9
Chicken, fried	3 oz	9
Ice cream, 10% fat	1 c	8
Sardines, canned	2 medium	7
Milk, low-fat + 2% solids	8 oz	7
Mushrooms, canned	½ c	7
Halibut, cooked	3 oz	7
Avocado	½ medium	6
Banana	1 medium	6
Beans, white, cooked	½ c	6
Peanut butter	1 tbsp	6
Cashews	6–8	5
Milk, skim	8 oz	5
Frankfurter, cooked	2	4
Rice, white, enriched, cooked	½ c	4
Hamburger, 21% fat, cooked	3 oz	3
Cantaloupe	¼ melon	3
Orange	1 medium	3
Apple, raw	1 medium	2
Carrots, cooked	½ c	2
Cottage cheese, creamed	½ c	2
Wheat germ	1 tbsp	1.3
Cheddar cheese	1 oz	1.0
Butter	1 tsp	1
Bread, whole-wheat	1 slice	0
Bread, white	1 slice	0
Oils; fats; margarine	1 tbsp	0

[a] But raw egg white consumed in quantity inhibits absorption of biotin; see text.
Source: J. A. Pennington, *Dietary nutrient guide* (Westport, Conn.: Avi Publishing Co., 1976).

types of dermatitis—seborrheic dermatitis and Leiner's disease. Biotin is highly effective in the treatment of both conditions in infants. In adults, however, neither condition responds to vitamin therapy. Experimentally induced deficiency in humans produces a grayish, dry, scaly skin; loss of appetite; lassitude; muscle pain; and nausea. Eating an occasional raw egg will not produce deficiency symptoms. According to one estimate, the avidin content of more than 20 raw eggs per day for several weeks would be required to create a biotin deficiency.

Biotin has no known toxic effects. Animals have tolerated large doses for extended periods with no signs of toxicity.

PANTOTHENIC ACID

Like biotin, pantothenic acid first appeared in the Bios complex of vitamins and was accordingly designated vitamin B_3. Roger J. Williams, who discovered the vitamin, gave it its chemical name in 1938, from *pantos*, the Greek word meaning "everywhere." The name reflects its widespread distribution in plants and animals. Pantothenic acid was synthesized in 1940.

Chemistry and Properties

Pantothenic acid (see Figure 7–9) is a yellow, oily liquid. However, calcium pantothenate, the calcium salt of pantothenic acid, is crystalline. This commercially available form is a white, alcohol- and water-soluble substance that is quite stable in neutral solution but decomposes easily in both alkaline and acid solutions. Dry heat also destroys the vitamin.

Absorption and Metabolism

Little is known about the absorption of pantothenic acid. Salts of the acid are probably absorbed from the intestines by passive diffusion. In the body tissues, the vitamin is converted to its important coenzyme form, coenzyme A (see Figure 7–10).

Modern technology makes it possible to retain the nutrients in our food sources. As a result, we are not limited to seasonal foods available locally.

Hugh Rogers/Monkmeyer Press

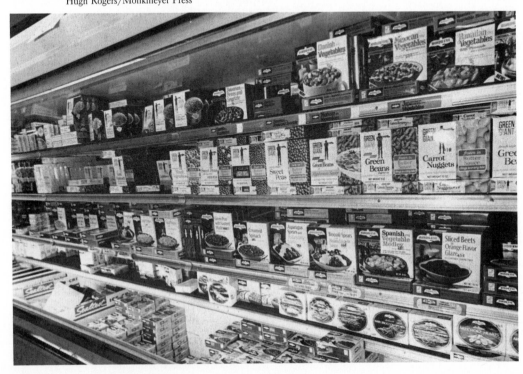

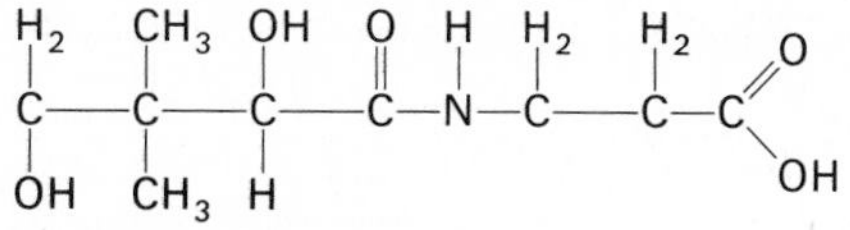

$$\underset{\text{OH}}{\overset{\text{H}_2}{\text{C}}}-\underset{\text{CH}_3}{\overset{\text{CH}_3}{\text{C}}}-\overset{\text{OH}}{\text{C}}-\overset{\text{O}}{\text{C}}-\underset{}{\text{N}}-\underset{}{\overset{\text{H}}{\text{C}}}-\overset{\text{H}_2}{\text{C}}-\overset{\text{H}_2}{\text{C}}-\overset{\text{O}}{\text{C}}\overset{}{\text{OH}}$$

FIGURE 7-9   *Structure of Pantothenic Acid.*

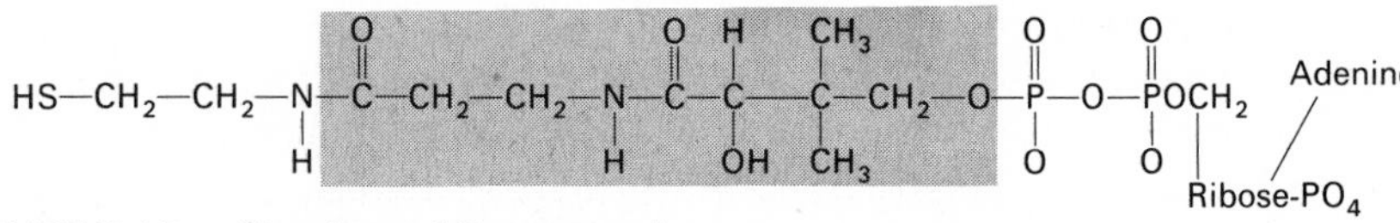

$$HS-CH_2-CH_2-\underset{H}{\overset{O}{N}}-C-CH_2-CH_2-\underset{H}{\overset{O}{N}}-C-\underset{OH}{\overset{H}{C}}-\underset{CH_3}{\overset{CH_3}{C}}-CH_2-O-\underset{O}{\overset{O}{P}}-O-\underset{O}{\overset{O}{P}}OCH_2$$ Adenine Ribose-PO$_4$

FIGURE 7-10   *Structure of Coenzyme A.*

Pantothenic acid is also a component of acyl-carrier protein (ACP), important in fatty acid metabolism.

Limited reserves of pantothenic acid are stored in the liver, adrenal glands, brain, kidneys, and heart. Little is known about excretion of this vitamin except that it is found in urine.

Physiological Function

The great importance of pantothenic acid results from its function as a component of coenzyme A and acyl-carrier protein. The extensive functions of acetyl CoA are summarized diagrammatically in Figure 7–11. ACP transports acetyl CoA from the mitochondria to the cytoplasm and participates in all the subsequent reactions of fatty acid synthesis.

FIGURE 7-11   *Sources and Functions of Acetyl CoA.*
Acetyl CoA, which derives from the oxidative breakdown of carbohydrate, protein, and fat, initiates the Krebs cycle by combining with oxaloacetate to form citric acid. Acetyl CoA also functions in the synthesis of fatty acids, sterols (including cholesterol), and porphyrin, the pigment component of hemoglobin. And in the synthesis of acetylcholine, a very important neurotransmitter, the acetyl group is provided by acetyl CoA.

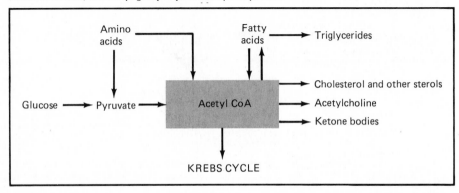

Recommended Allowances and Dietary Sources

Because of insufficient evidence concerning requirements for pantothenic acid, the Food and Nutrition Board simply suggests a dietary intake of 4 to 7 milligrams per day. Estimates place the average dietary intake of Americans at between 10 and 20 milligrams per day. Deficiency is most unlikely.

All foods contain pantothenic acid, although fruits contain only negligible amounts. Liver, eggs, yeast, salmon, and heart contain some of the highest concentrations; but other good sources include mushrooms, cauliflower, molasses, and peanuts (see Table 7-6). Although grains represent an important source of the vitamin, about 50 percent of their content is lost in milling.

TABLE 7-6. *Pantothenic Acid Content of Selected Foods (Estimated Safe and Adequate Daily Dietary Intake: 4–7 mg)*

Food	Serving Size	Pantothenic Acid Content μg/serving
Liver, beef, fried	3 oz	6,035
Mushrooms, canned	½ c	1,000
Avocado	½ medium	980
Egg, whole	1 large	864
Ice cream, 10% fat	1 c	900
Milk, skim	8 oz	806
Milk, whole	8 oz	766
Corn, cooked	½ c	720
Chicken, fried	3 oz	765
Pork, roasted	3 oz	535
Soybeans, cooked	½ c	525
Lamb leg, roasted	3 oz	510
Collard greens, cooked	½ c	400
Potato, baked	1 medium	400
Frankfurter, cooked	2 links	360
Beer, 4.5% alcohol	12 oz	360
Cantaloupe	½ melon	342
Hamburger, 21% fat, cooked	3 oz	340
Orange, raw	1 medium	328
Rice, brown, cooked	½ c	300
Banana	1 medium	296
Halibut, broiled	3 oz	255
Broccoli, cooked	½ c	225
Cottage cheese, creamed	½ c	224
Bread, whole-wheat	1 slice	184
Tuna, canned	2 oz	180
Rice, white, enriched, cooked	½ c	150
Peanut butter	1 tbsp	147
Wheat germ	1 tbsp	132
Cheddar cheese	1 oz	117
Bread, white, enriched	1 slice	92
Apple	1 medium	84
Oils; butter; margarine	1 tbsp	0
Sugar	1 tbsp	0

Note: The vitamin contents in the table are given in micrograms (μg), whereas the suggested intake is 4 to 7 mg. One mg is equivalent to 1,000 μg. But note also the many different kinds of foods which contain significant amounts of pantothenic acid.
Source: J. A. Pennington, *Dietary nutrient guide* (Westport, Conn.: Avi Publishing Co., 1976); USDA Handbooks 8-1, 8-9, 8-10, 8-11, 8-12 (Washington, D.C.: Government Printing Office).

Little pantothenic acid activity is lost in most cooking methods, but temperatures above the boiling point, as in a pressure cooker, will cause significant loss. Frozen vegetables and meats lose considerable pantothenic acid during processing and storage.

Clinical Deficiency Symptoms and Toxicity

The difficulty of establishing an RDA for pantothenic acid arises chiefly from the difficulty of identifying a clinical deficiency of the vitamin in humans. No dietary deficiency is known, and artificially induced deficiencies appear to require extended consumption of a purified diet in combination with metabolic antagonists of the vitamin. The resulting symptoms include insomnia, fatigue, irritability, numbness and tingling of the hands and feet, muscle cramps, and impaired production of antibodies. Administration of the vitamin eliminates all symptoms. Because food processing can result in vitamin losses, and because clinicians generally are not looking for pantothenic acid deficiency, concern has recently arisen that "borderline" deficiencies may occur in people who do not consume diversified diets. More study is needed. Deficiency symptoms can be produced in other species; rats, for example, develop gray hair, which may account for the false claim by some vitamin advocates that pantothenic acid will prevent graying of hair in humans. Humans, however, are very different from rats in this respect, and contrary to all claims, the vitamin has not been shown to prevent gray hair in humans.

Pantothenic acid has been used successfully in some instances to treat the neurologic symptoms of patients who have received streptomycin. More commonly, the vitamin is used to stimulate the gastrointestinal tract following surgery. However, doses of 10 to 20 grams will cause diarrhea.

No toxic effects, except for diarrhea after doses of 10 to 20 grams, are known to result from consumption of pantothenic acid in large quantities.

VITAMIN B₆ (PYRIDOXINE)

The history of vitamin B6 has been less eventful than that of most of the vitamins. Although studies of its metabolism and interaction with regulatory systems continue, the vitamin has no classic deficiency disease, such as beriberi and pellagra, associated with it. Researchers began looking for a new vitamin when they found that none of the known B vitamins was effective against acrodynia, a type of dermatitis in rats. In 1934 György reported that the "vitamin B2 complex" contained a distinct chemical substance in addition to riboflavin. This substance, isolated by several laboratories in 1938 and synthesized in 1939, was a crystalline compound which was given the name *pyridoxine*. It also proved effective against acrodynia when added to the diets of deficient rats.

Chemistry and Properties

Vitamin B6 is not a single substance but rather a complex of three closely related compounds (Figure 7–12). Structurally the vitamin molecule has a pyridine ring with an alcohol (pyridoxine, or pyridoxol), an aldehyde (pyridoxal), or an amine (pyridoxamine) group attached. All three forms are nutritionally active and can be

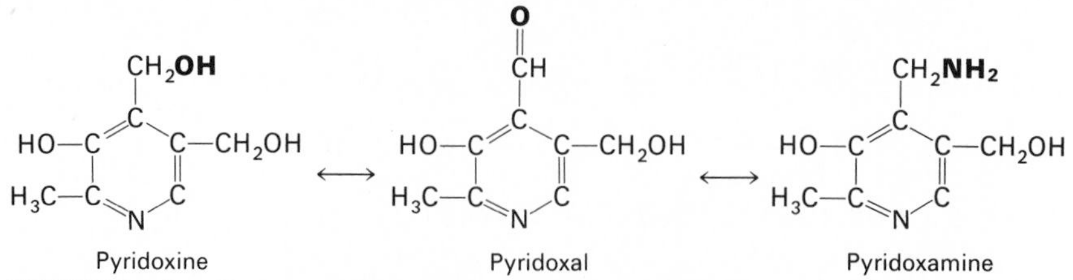

FIGURE 7-12 *Structure of the Three Forms of Vitamin B₆.*

converted to the active coenzyme form. Although *pyridoxine* is still used to refer to all three, the preferred designation is *vitamin B₆*.

Vitamin B₆ is an odorless, white, crystalline compound, soluble in both water and alcohol. Although heat-stable in acid solution, the vitamin becomes heat-labile in alkaline solution. It is also relatively vulnerable to destruction by light.

Absorption and Metabolism

Like other water-soluble vitamins, vitamin B₆ enters the body from the upper part of the small intestine. Absorption is rapid except in cases of acute infantile celiac disease (a malabsorption syndrome), chronic alcoholism (in which synthetic preparations of the vitamin appear to be more easily absorbed), and intestinal bypass operations (sometimes used as a treatment for extreme obesity).

After absorption, all three forms are converted to pyridoxal phosphate, the active coenzyme form (see Figure 7–13). Although pyridoxal phosphate is found in all the tissues of the body, there is no real storage. The vitamin is excreted in the urine, mainly as pyridoxic acid, along with small amounts of pyridoxal and pyridoxamine.

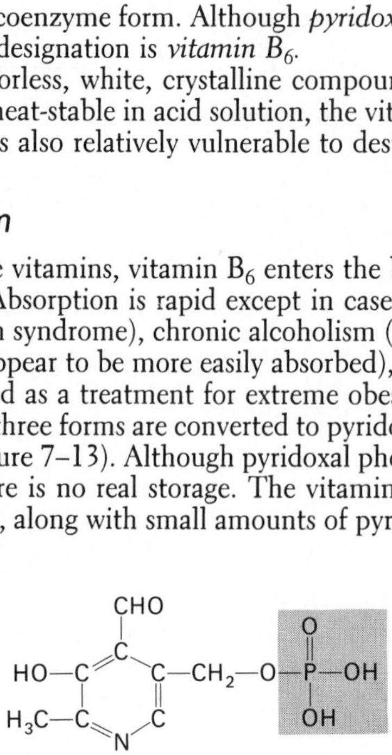

FIGURE 7-13 *Structure of Pyridoxal Phosphate (PLP).*

Physiological Functions

Unlike the water-soluble vitamins discussed so far, vitamin B₆ has no direct role in energy metabolism. Rather it functions chiefly as a coenzyme in the synthesis and breakdown of amino acids, a role that makes it of great importance in protein metabolism. In these reactions, the coenzyme is usually pyridoxal phosphate (PLP), although pyridoxamine phosphate catalyzes certain reactions. PLP is required as a coenzyme in four amino-acid-metabolizing reactions:

1. Transamination in amino acid metabolism, such as the conversion of alanine to pyruvate, the end product of glycolysis.
2. Decarboxylation in the synthesis of neurotransmitters (such as serotonin and norepinephrine) and of histamine, which acts as a vasodilator. The latter results from the decarboxylation of the amino acid histidine.

3. Transsulfuration, of which the conversion of one amino acid, serine, to another, cysteine, is an example.
4. Side-chain transfers as in conversion of methionine to cysteine.

PLP also plays an important part in other reactions. In the release of glucose-1-phosphate from glycogen in liver and muscle tissue, PLP apparently does not act as a coenzyme; instead, PLP maintains the enzyme phosphorylase in its active form so the reaction can proceed. Here a deficiency of vitamin B_6 could result in lowered blood glucose levels. As a coenzyme, PLP also affects a reaction in which a heme precursor, necessary to the formation of hemoglobin, is produced. PLP regulates the synthesis of gamma-aminobutyric acid (GABA). GABA has a role in inhibiting neurotransmitters in the brain.

Another important function of PLP is to aid in the conversion of tryptophan to niacin, discussed previously, which may explain why some of the symptoms of B_6 deficiency are similar to those of pellagra.

Recommended Allowances and Dietary Sources

Because of the association between protein metabolism and vitamin B_6, requirements for the vitamin are proportionate to protein intake. Since vitamin B_6 deficiency is not a critical health problem anywhere in the world, estimates of dietary requirements are based on data from studies of experimentally induced deficiency symptoms and from measurements of several clinical parameters. Moreover, although the vitamin occurs in a great variety of foodstuffs, albeit in small quantities, tissue levels are easily depleted by a number of physiological and pathological factors.

At present the RDA for vitamin B_6 is 2.2 milligrams per day for men and 2 milligrams per day for women. Pregnancy and lactation increase the allowances by 0.6 milligrams and 0.5 milligrams, respectively. Women using oral contraceptive agents (OCA) show abnormalities in tryptophan metabolism, a condition eliminated by large doses of the vitamin. Tryptophan metabolites were measured to indirectly determine pyridoxine status in these women. Using newer, more direct measures of pyrodixube in studies of women taking OCAs does not provide strong support for a higher requirement for pyridoxine. Therapeutic doses have also alleviated depression in some women, probably as a result of the vitamin's role in the synthesis of the neurotransmitter serotonin. But there is no reason for women generally to supplement vitamin B_6 intake.

The RDA for infants is 0.3 to 0.6 milligrams per day. These figures are derived from studies initiated more than two decades ago, when the vitamin B_6 content of a commercial infant formula was accidentally destroyed by overprocessing. The deficiency in infants fed this formula resulted in irritability and convulsions. When vitamin B_6 was administered to the affected babies, recovery was prompt.

There is evidence to suggest that the need for vitamin B_6 increases with age, but the data are insufficient to establish a firm RDA for the older age groups.

Various medical conditions and drug therapies affect vitamin B_6 metabolism and thus the requirements for the vitamin. Certain antitubercular drugs (INH) and the antibiotic chloramphenicol will bind vitamin B_6, resulting in neurological symptoms unless the vitamin is pharmacologically supplemented. Since several diuretics and hydralazine, an antihypertensive drug, increase excretion of the vitamin, supplementation may be needed in these cases as well.

Table 7–7 lists the vitamin B_6 content of selected foods. Note that the content is

TABLE 7-7. *Vitamin B$_6$ Content of Selected Food Items (RDA for Adults: Men 2.2 mg; Women 2.0 mg)*

Food	Serving Size	B$_6$ Content µg/serving
Liver, beef, fried	3 oz	569
Banana	1 medium	480
Avocado	½ medium	420
Hamburger, 21% fat, cooked	3 oz	391
Chicken, fried	3 oz	340
Halibut, broiled	3 oz	289
Lamb leg, roasted	3 oz	272
Corn, cooked	½ c	246
Beer, 4.5% alcohol	12 oz	216
Potato, white, baked in skin	1 medium	200
Collard greens, cooked	½ c	170
Spinach, cooked	½ c	161
Haddock, fried	3½ oz	140
Rice, brown, cooked	½ c	127
Peas, green, cooked	½ c	110
Walnuts	8–10 halves	109
Broccoli, cooked	½ c	107
Milk, whole	8 oz	98
Milk, skim + 2% solids	8 oz	98
Frankfurter	2	98
Orange, raw	1 medium	90
Cantaloupe, raw	¼ melon	90
Tomato, raw	½ medium	74
Wheat germ	1 tbsp	55
Ice cream, 10% fat	1 c	54
Egg, whole	1 medium	49
Peanut butter	1 tbsp	46
Cottage cheese, creamed	½ c	46
Apple	1 medium	45
Bread, whole-wheat	1 slice	41
Grapefruit	½ medium	30
Rice, white, enriched, cooked	½ c	30
Soybeans, cooked	½ c	30
Cheddar cheese	1 oz	22
Bread, white, enriched	1 slice	9
Oils; fats; margarine; butter	1 tbsp	0

Note: Vitamin content is expressed in micrograms; recommended intakes are in milligrams.
Source: J. A. Pennington, *Dietary nutrient guide* (Westport, Conn.: Avi Publishing Co., 1976).

expressed in micrograms, although the RDA is stated in milligrams. The best dietary sources include yeast, organ and muscle meats, whole grain cereals, legumes, and bananas.

Clinical Deficiency Symptoms

The only known disease condition attributable to vitamin B$_6$ deficiency is microcytic anemia, characterized by smaller than average red blood cells. Associated symptoms include muscle weakness, irritability, and difficulty in walking. Because vitamin B_6 is so widely available in food sources, deficiency cannot be produced experimentally unless an antagonist such as deoxypyridoxine is administered. Induced symptoms include nausea, neuritis, dermatitis, and mouth and tongue lesions different from those caused by riboflavin or niacin deficiency. The most extreme symptoms were observed after use of the overprocessed infant formula referred to previously. These involved severe convulsions, clearly demonstrating the importance of this vitamin in the functioning of the central nervous system.

There is increasing concern based on recent evidence that present-day normal American diets may be somewhat low in vitamin B_6. Although no clinical signs have been documented, biochemical evidence of borderline "deficiency" has been obtained in some studies. This points up the need for further study, appropriate food choices, and perhaps supplementation in some cases. Pyridoxine deficiency has been suggested as the cause of one type of premenstrual syndrome (PMS) and massive doses of pyrodoxine have been prescribed for treatment. However, large doses of pyrodoxine can result in neurologic problems as discussed under toxicity. Further, there is no definitive evidence that pyrodoxine deficiency is involved in PMS.

Because the conversion of tryptophan to niacin cannot proceed in the absence of PLP, a relative lack of vitamin B_6 may make a small contribution to a niacin deficiency and, consequently, to the development of pellagra.

Toxicity

The possibility of toxic effects from normal dietary amounts of vitamin B_6 is considered to be extremely remote. Therapeutic doses of up to 150 milligrams per day may produce slight side effects, including sleepiness. At intakes of 200 mg per day, human subjects have become metabolically dependent on large intakes of the vitamin, which can result in deficiency when the large intakes are discontinued. Intake of between 2 and 6 grams (1000–3000 times the RDA) has resulted in symptoms of unsteady gait, numb feet, and numbness and clumsiness of the hands. Patients improved dramatically after withdrawal of the vitamin although some dysfunction remained in some patients even after six months.

FOLACIN

In 1931, Dr. Lucy Wills reported finding a characteristic type of anemia in pregnant women in India. She induced the same disease in monkeys fed a diet based on polished rice and white bread and found that no known vitamin cured it. Neither did the purified liver extract used to treat pernicious anemia (see page 241). Yeast, however, which was ineffective against pernicious anemia, caused an improvement in the condition. The yeast apparently contained an antianemia factor ("Wills' Factor") that differed from the effective component of liver extract.

In 1941 a substance that promoted bacterial growth was isolated from spinach leaves and named *folic acid* from the Latin *folium*, "leaf." Folic acid was found to be an effective treatment for dietary anemias in laboratory animals and, in 1945, a cure for the megaloblastic anemia of pregnancy. It was synthesized in 1948.

Chemistry and Properties

Like vitamin B$_6$, *folacin* (a term that includes folic acid and related compounds) is actually a complex of several biologically active forms. The technical name—*pteroylglutamic acid* (PGA)—indicates its chemical composition: pteroic acid plus one, three, or up to seven glutamate molecules. Figure 7–14 shows the monoglutamate form, which is used in food supplements and therapy. The para-aminobenzoic acid (PABA) portion of pteroic acid was formerly thought to be a vitamin for humans, but we now recognize that PABA cannot be utilized by humans.

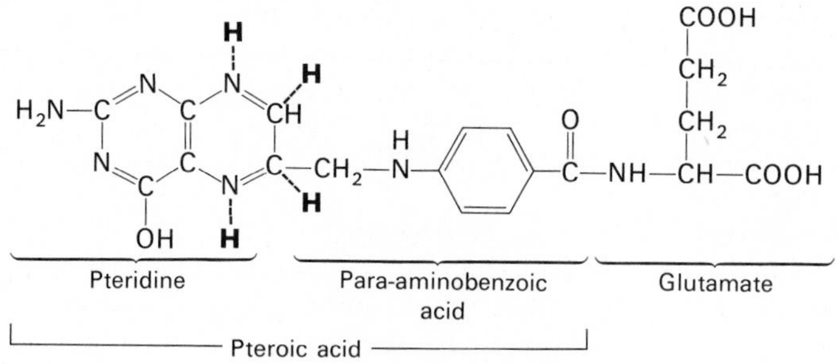

FIGURE 7-14   *Structure of Folic Acid, Monoglutamate Form.* In tetrahydrofolic acid (THFA), hydrogen ions are added as indicated.

Folacin compounds are water-soluble, yellow, and crystalline. The monoglutamate form is very heat-stable, but the vitamin becomes heat-labile in acid solution. When dry, folacin is easily destroyed by sunlight. Storage and high-temperature processing cause considerable loss of vitamin activity.

Absorption and Metabolism

Folacin is absorbed by mucosal cells in the upper part of the small intestine. But the vitamin must first be prepared for absorption by removal, with the aid of the hydrolytic enzyme folate conjugase, of most of its glutamate molecules. For this reason, the rate of absorption may vary inversely with the number of glutamates attached; studies are being conducted to determine the extent to which glutamate chain length affects the digestion and therefore the availability of the vitamin.

Once absorbed, folacin is bound to a protein for transport and storage. This form, probably methylated, occurs in all cells, but the liver contains approximately half the body's stores. Small amounts of at least one metabolite are excreted in the urine.

Several pharmaceutical compounds affect the metabolism of folacin. The antitubercular drugs aminosalicylic acid and cycloserine, certain anticonvulsants, and alcohol reduce absorption. (Chronic alcoholics, in fact, cannot absorb the common dietary forms; synthetic preparations, however, are better absorbed.) Trimethoprim and pyrimethamine, both antimalarial drugs, inactivate the vitamin, as does methotrexate, a strong folic acid antagonist used in cancer chemotherapy. Also, oral contraceptives and the hormonal changes of pregnancy produce significant decreases in serum levels of folic acid.

Physiological Function

In its principal role, folic acid is a coenzyme necessary for transferring single carbon units (such as formyl and methyl) during various reactions involved in metabolism of certain amino acids and in the synthesis of the nucleotide bases of nucleic acids. Folic acid is, first, reduced to tetrahydrofolic acid (THFA) in a reaction that requires the presence of the niacin-containing coenzyme NADPH. A 1-carbon fragment is then added to one or two of the nitrogen molecules of pteroic acid, and in this methylated form folacin participates in metabolic reactions.

Although THFA is needed for synthesis of all the nucleotides, it is particularly important in the formation of thymine, which is a distinctive component of DNA. Without THFA, thymine cannot be synthesized; and without thymine, DNA synthesis and red blood cell formation are impaired. This appears to be the ultimate cause of the megaloblastic anemia observed in folic acid deficiency.

THFA also plays a part in the conversion of histidine to glutamic acid. This reaction forms the basis of a widely used bioassay of serum levels of folic acid.

Recommended Allowances and Dietary Sources

The RDA for folacin is 400 micrograms (μg) per day for adults. During pregnancy and lactation the allowance should be increased to 800 μg and 500 μg, respectively, in view of the importance of folic acid to nucleic acid synthesis, and therefore, cell division. The allowance for infants, 30 to 45 μg per day, is easily supplied in most cases from human or cow's milk. (Goat's milk, however, is not a good source.)

Folacin occurs in most green vegetables and in a wide variety of foods, including liver, fish, poultry, most meats, and legumes. Unfortunately, there are discrepancies in the published values of the folacin content of foods because of the different assay methods used. Ideally, data for content of both the free (monoglutamate) and the total (polyglutamate) forms should be reported, because the extent to which the body utilizes polyglutamate forms remains unknown. Researchers have published both free and total folacin values for several hundred food items; some of their data appear in Table 7–8.

In its monoglutamate form, folic acid is very stable to heat. The heat stability of other forms varies considerably, however. Moreover, all forms appear to be somewhat more vulnerable to degradation by microwave cooking than by conventional methods.

Clinical Deficiency Symptoms and Toxicity

Megaloblastic anemia represents the chief disease condition caused by folacin deficiency. Other symptoms include disturbances of the gastrointestinal tract, lesions of the tongue, and retarded growth.

It is interesting to compare the types of anemia produced by deficiencies of vitamin B_6 and folic acid. A lack of folic acid, of course, interferes with DNA synthesis and therefore cell division, resulting in enlarged but undivided red blood cell precursors. Hence the term *hematopoeitic*, or "blood-forming," for this vitamin. By contrast, deficiency of vitamin B_6 (and/or iron) tends to inhibit the maturation of cells and may result in *microcytic* (small-cell) anemia.

Because folic acid metabolism occurs in close association with vitamin B_{12} (see following), some of the same symptoms appear in the absence of either of these vitamins. Folacin will cure the symptoms of anemia resulting from vitamin B_{12} deficiency, but it is ineffective against the more serious neurological symptoms. Thus a

TABLE 7-8. *Folacin Content of Selected Foods (RDA for Adults: 400 μg)*

Food	Serving Size	FOLACIN CONTENT μg/SERVING Free Folacin	Total Folacin
Yeast, brewer's	1 tbsp	14	313
Liver, beef, cooked	3 oz	—[a]	123
Spinach, raw	1 c	65	106
Orange juice, fresh or frozen, reconstituted	6 oz	63	102
Lettuce, romaine	1 c	33	98
Spinach, cooked	½ c	54	82
Beets, cooked	½ c	32	66
Orange, raw	1 medium	45	65
Avocado, raw	½ medium	36	59
Broccoli, cooked	½ c	21	44
Beans, red, cooked	½ c	—	34
Banana	1 medium	26	33
Egg, whole, raw	1 medium	20	29
Cottage cheese	1 c	—	29
Brussels sprouts	½ c	4	28
Yogurt	1 c	—	27
Tomato, raw	½ medium	14	26
Egg yolk, raw	1 medium	18	23
Wheat germ	1 tbsp	15	20
Lettuce, head or leaf	1 c	19	20
Bread, whole-wheat	1 slice	8	16
Shredded wheat	1 oz	3	14
Almonds, shelled	approx. 11	5	13
Peanut butter	1 tbsp	3	13
Apple	1 medium	5	13
Tuna fish, canned	3 oz	7	13
Milk, whole	1 c	12	12
Bread, white	1 slice	3	10
Cucumber, pared	½ small	8	10
Ham, smoked	3 oz	—	9
Mushrooms, raw	½ c	7	8
Sesame seeds	1 tbsp	4	8
Haddock, frozen	3 oz	3	8
Chicken, without skin, dark meat, cooked	3 oz	—	6
Egg white, raw	1 medium	1	5
Cheddar cheese	1 oz	<0.5	5
Pork, cooked	3 oz	—	4
Beef, ground, cooked	3 oz	—	3
Chicken, without skin, light meat, cooked	3 oz	—	3
Cornflakes	1 oz	3	3
Apricots, dried	5 halves	2	2.5
Butter or margarine	1 tbsp	<0.5	<0.5

[a] Dash indicates value not available.
Source: Adapted from B. P. Perloff and R. R. Butrum, Folacin in selected foods, *Journal of the American Dietetic Association* 70:161, 1977.

potentially lethal B_{12} deficiency could be temporarily masked by folic acid supplementation, and therefore large supplements of folacin should not be used unless the possibility of vitamin B_{12} deficiency has been ruled out.

To date, no toxic effects are known. However, folacin excess may interfere with the effectiveness of anticonvulsant drugs.

VITAMIN B$_{12}$

A form of anemia whose victims, usually older adults, invariably died within two to five years after becoming ill was identified in London in the middle of the nineteenth century and called *pernicious anemia* for its inexorable and ultimately fatal progress. In 1926 in Boston, G. R. Minot and W. P. Murphy showed that ingestion of one pound of raw liver daily cured pernicious anemia, and William B. Castle observed that anemia patients had abnormal gastric secretions. Postulating that an *intrinsic factor* (in gastric secretions) was needed for absorption of an unknown *extrinsic factor* (from food), Castle theorized that the pernicious anemia victims lacked intrinsic factor, and that a combination of extrinsic and intrinsic factors prevented the disease. When it was found that the common microorganism *Lactobacillus lactis* needed the antianemia (extrinsic) factor as much as humans did, the search for the unknown substance was greatly facilitated. A protein-free liver extract proved to be even more active in preventing the disease than liver itself, and in 1948 vitamin B$_{12}$ was isolated (independently in both England and the United States) from liver extract. Dorothy Hodgkin determined the structure in 1956. The vitamin was not synthesized until 1973.

Chemistry and Properties

Vitamin B$_{12}$ is a large, complex molecule that contains cobalt. Figure 7–15 shows the chemical structure of one of the naturally occurring forms, hydroxycobalamin. The vitamin takes several other forms in serum and tissues. One of the most potent

FIGURE 7-15   Structure of Vitamin B$_{12}$ (Hydroxycobalamin). The arrows indicate electrical force.

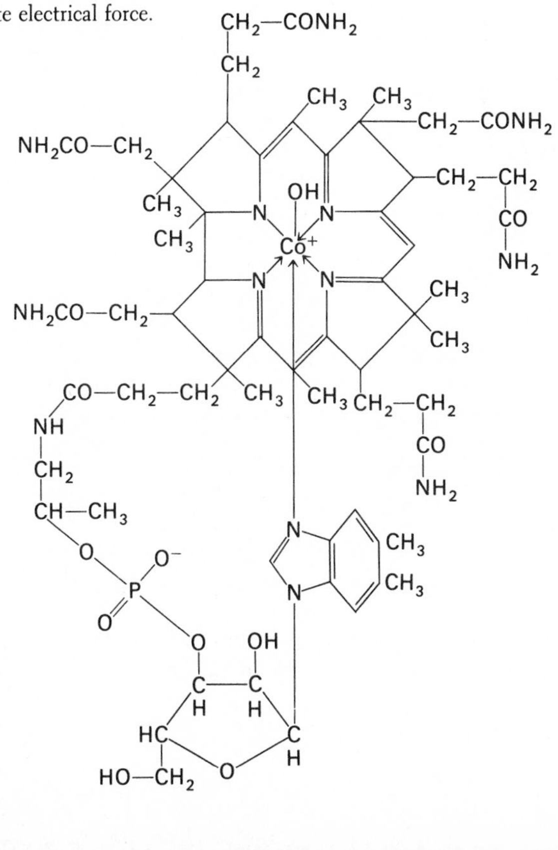

241

biological compounds to be found in the body, cobalamin is a water- and alcohol-soluble, reddish, crystalline substance. Vitamin B_{12} is stable to heat but vulnerable to strong acids, alkalis, and light.

Absorption and Metabolism

The absorption of vitamin B_{12} requires both calcium and Castle's intrinsic factor, which turned out to be a large glycoprotein secreted by the stomach wall. Intrinsic factor first combines with dietary B_{12} in the stomach and then apparently helps to attach the vitamin to receptors in the lower ileum.

Once absorbed into the mucosal lining, B_{12} is carried by a transport protein (transcobalamin) through the general circulation to the tissues. It is stored in the liver in amounts that are enormous in comparison to the quantities actually needed by the body, and in this respect differs from all other water-soluble vitamins. Cobalamin that exceeds the storage capacity is excreted in the urine.

In large concentrated doses, small but significant amounts of vitamin B_{12} are absorbed by passive diffusion (which does not require intrinsic factor). Even such small amounts—1 to 3 percent—of a large dose of such a potent compound would account for the success of Minot's and Murphy's raw liver treatment for pernicious anemia.

Iron and vitamin B_6 deficiencies, inherited deficiency of intrinsic factor, gastritis, and apparently, age, all decrease the absorption of vitamin B_{12}. Pregnancy increases absorption but also increases the need for the vitamin.

Physiological Functions

In its adenosyl or methyl forms, vitamin B_{12} is an essential coenzyme involved in reactions in all cells of the body. Along with folic acid, it is necessary for the formation of the thymine nucleotides of DNA. A lack of either of these vitamins results in megaloblastosis, or the development of red blood cells that are enlarged because normal cell division has not taken place.

Vitamin B_{12} also affects nervous system functioning, in part because it stabilizes glutathione, a component of several enzymes needed for carbohydrate metabolism. An absence of vitamin B_{12} would, therefore, interfere with the energy supply that fuels nerve cells. But this vitamin is also necessary for the formation and maintenance of myelin, the protective sheathing around the axons of nerve cells. In its adenosyl coenzyme form, vitamin B_{12} functions in the metabolism of odd-numbered fatty acids, which are important in myelin formation. This reaction also requires biotin. And the metabolism of single-carbon units (as in the conversion of homocysteine to methionine) is likewise dependent on a coenzyme of vitamin B_{12}.

Recommended Allowances and Dietary Sources

Although vitamin B_{12} is needed for such major reactions, human requirements are very small. The RDA of 3 μg (micrograms) for adults, and 4 μg for pregnant or lactating women, is more than adequately met by most diets in the United States, which contain anywhere from 7 to 30 μg. A dietary intake of 15 μg per day is recommended for those whose liver stores are depleted by illness (fever or hyperthyroidism, for example).

The best sources of vitamin B_{12} include beef and other liver, seafood, meat, eggs, and milk (see Table 7-9). Vitamin B_{12} is not synthesized by plants or animals. It is therefore available primarily in foods of animal origin because these have accumulated it from the microorganisms that make it. This raises some interesting and controversial questions pertaining to vegetarian diets.

Vegetarian diets that include milk and eggs provide an adequate source of vitamin B_{12}. But vegans, vegetarians who exclude all animal products from their diet, are ultimately at considerable risk. In several studies of vegans, serum levels of B_{12} in about half the cases measured were in the low range characteristic of pernicious anemia. Some illness and at least two deaths have been attributed to B_{12} deficiency. Yet a number of subjects tested appeared to be quite healthy despite having eaten plant foods exclusively for years. Extensive previous storage in the liver probably accounts for this; furthermore, over time the body may adapt to the minuscule amounts that might be present in plant foods because of bacterial content of soils and water.

In some foods, such as groundnuts (peanuts) and perhaps other nuts and legumes, bacterial fermentation may produce the vitamin. *Trace* amounts may be present in plants grown in very rich soil; the presence of large amounts of bacteria in the soil may enable some plants to absorb small amounts of vitamin B_{12}. Another explanation for the lack of deficiency in many vegans has been refuted; al-

TABLE 7-9. *Vitamin B_{12} Content of Selected Foods (RDA for Adults: 3 μg)*

Food	Serving Size	B_{12} Content μg/serving
Liver, beef, fried	3 oz	68
Clams, canned	½ c	19.1
Oysters, canned	3½ oz	18.0
Lamb leg, roasted	3 oz	2.63
Tuna, canned	2 oz	1.32
Frankfurter	2	1.16
Yogurt, fruit-flavored, low-fat	8 oz	1.060
Milk, skim + milk solids	8 oz	0.946
Milk, whole	8 oz	0.871
Egg, whole	1 large	0.773
Cottage cheese, creamed	½ c	0.704
Halibut, broiled	3 oz	0.85
Hamburger, 21% fat, cooked	3 oz	0.76
Liverwurst	1 oz	0.71
Shrimp, boiled	3 oz	0.59
Gruyère cheese	1 oz	0.45
Pork, roasted	3 oz	0.42
Chicken, fried	3 oz	0.36
Ice cream, 10% fat	½ c	0.31
Cheddar cheese	1 oz	0.234
Bacon	2 slices	0.11
Butter	1 tbsp	0.01
Fruits	—	0
Vegetables	—	0
Grains, cereals	—	0
Nuts; legumes; seeds	—	0
Oils; margarine	—	0

Sources: J. A. Pennington, *Dietary nutrient guide* (Westport, Conn.: Avi Publishing Co., 1976); and L. P. Posati and M. L. Orr, *Composition of foods—Dairy and egg products—Raw, processed, prepared*, USDA Agriculture Handbook No. 8-1 (Washington, D.C.: U.S. Government Printing Office, 1976).

though bacteria in the human intestine can indeed synthesize B_{12}, the vitamin is not absorbed that far down the intestine.

Interestingly, most vegetarians in India do use some animal products, particularly yogurt, and may in that way receive adequate amounts of B_{12}. Tempe, a fermented legume product, may serve the same function for vegetarians in China and Japan.

Clinical Deficiency Symptoms and Toxicity

Blood and nervous system disorders are the primary symptoms of B_{12} deficiency. The characteristic blood defect is megaloblastic anemia, or presence of large (but fewer) red blood cells. This symptom can also result from folic acid deficiency. The

Perspective On

MEGAVITAMIN THERAPY

A vitamin molecule acts in combination with a molecule of a specific body protein, such as an enzyme. Because the various specific proteins are present in small amounts, it follows that the amounts of vitamins that can combine with them completely (or "saturate" them) are also small. Therefore, in small amounts up to the saturation level, vitamins perform their normal functions as coenzymes or hormonelike compounds; above the saturation level, a vitamin becomes just another chemical. Because the metabolic machinery of a saturated cell is already working at full capacity, vitamins at above-saturation levels cannot perform their usual physiological roles.

Many people consume large amounts of vitamins in the mistaken belief that if some is good, more is better. What they actually get are small amounts (the proportion that can act in the usual metabolic roles) of vitamins and large amounts (the proportion above saturation levels) of what is generally a useless chemical at best and a dangerous toxin or drug at worst.

The use of vitamins in dosages far above the RDA is popularly known as *megavitamin therapy*, although it is not vitamin therapy at all but rather an attempt at drug therapy, with vitamins used as the drugs. Another term, *orthomolecular medicine*, coined by Linus Pauling from the Greek *ortho*, "right," describes treatments based on substances that are naturally present in the body, such as hormones and vitamins. Orthomolecular

treatment with niacin, ascorbic acid, and other nutrients has been advocated in treating schizophrenia.

The use of vitamin megadoses for schizophrenia began in the 1950s, when similarities were noted between schizophrenia and the disoriented mental state of patients with the niacin deficiency disease pellagra. Treatment of schizophrenics with massive doses of niacin appeared to be successful in at least some cases. Subsequently, orthomolecular therapy was claimed to be useful in treatment of autism, hyperactivity, alcoholism, allergies, arthritis, cancer, and a host of other conditions. Why have these claims not gained acceptance from the medical and psychiatric professions?

One reason for skepticism regarding claims of successful orthomolecular treatment of schizophrenia is that the condition is characterized by alternating periods of severe breakdown and remission, so that almost any treatment—or no treatment at all—could well coincide with a period of improvement. Also, most of the successes attributed to orthomolecular treatment of schizophrenia are based on nothing more than anecdotal testimonials or subjective impressions of improvement rather than on data derived from well-designed studies. Schizophrenia is believed to be several different conditions sharing certain symptoms of mental derangement, with multiple causes, both genetic and environmental. Bio-

nervous disorders associated with vitamin B_{12} deficiency are due both to defective synthesis of myelin and to disrupted metabolism of fatty acids.

Pernicious anemia, on the other hand, is due not to a primary vitamin B_{12} deficiency but to a lack of intrinsic factor necessary for absorption of the vitamin. It can be cured, however, by massive doses of vitamin B_{12} without intrinsic factor. This disease may be caused by an inborn error of metabolism and also is often a result of aging. Various malabsorptive conditions and surgical removal of the ileum will also prevent normal vitamin B_{12} absorption. In some areas of the world, a particular species of tapeworm found in fish has the ability to break down the B_{12}-intrinsic factor complex, thereby creating a deficiency. Daily injections of small doses (1 μg) or monthly injections of larger doses of vitamin B_{12} are often used to prevent the onset of pernicious anemia in these cases.

chemical disturbances may be involved. However, the particular substances that are abnormal, how they may act to bring about mental disorientation, and even whether the chemical abnormalities are a cause or a result of schizophrenia are all unknown. What is apparent is that mental illnesses are far too complex and baffling to be explained on the basis of nutritional deficiencies alone.

On the other hand, large doses of vitamins are sometimes helpful when used for a known medical purpose. For example, in certain inborn errors of metabolism, a vitamin megadose will stimulate an enzyme that is not fully functional or will result in adequate absorption of a nutrient when the absorptive process is defective. Large amounts of vitamin D, in the active form of DHCC, stimulate production of calcium-binding protein in the intestine. Large doses of vitamins can also compensate for effects of medications that antagonize vitamins or impair their absorption, such as anticonvulsants, oral contraceptives, and others. Here, however, the vitamin is being administered, albeit in massive amounts, for *nutritional* purposes. In such cases, it is important to maintain equilibrium between medication and vitamin megadose; otherwise, an excess of the vitamin might neutralize the effects of the drug.

Reports of the successful use of vitamins in megadosages are tantalizing, but unbiased evidence is as yet scanty. Nevertheless, many people take various high-dose vitamin preparations for their alleged benefits, ranging from increased energy and enhanced sexual performance to prevention of heart disease and cancer. All such reports should be viewed with caution; they are rarely based on scientific evidence.

Because massive doses of vitamins, especially the fat-soluble ones, have toxic effects, self-dosing is definitely not advisable. As more and more people have taken more vitamins in large quantities, more side effects have become apparent. High doses of ascorbic acid, previously thought to be totally innocuous, cause gastrointestinal discomfort and diarrhea for many people and may have other, more serious, long-term consequences. Neurological damage has also been reported to result from ingestion of high doses of pyridoxine (see Chapter 7).

Moderate supplementation of some vitamins, at levels no greater than the allowance set by the Food and Nutrition Board, may be useful for some individuals. But remember that a vitamin pill contains only one or a few vitamins; it cannot supply any of the other nutrients the body needs. For this reason, it is almost always best to obtain necessary amounts of vitamins from foods, not from pills.

In recent years nutritionists have become increasingly concerned about the effects on B_{12} status of strict vegetarian diets. The average adult has a five-to-six-year supply stored in the liver, but children eating vegetarian diets and not having accumulated such stores run a greater risk of deficiency. Even more disturbing is the potential risk to infants who are nursed by strict vegetarian mothers. The mother's milk may contain very little vitamin B_{12}, and the infant will have little stored in the liver. At least two cases of severe B_{12} deficiency in infants have been reported in the United States. Typically, the mother has been a vegan for several years before becoming pregnant. Her child, fed exclusively on breast milk, seems normal for several months but then begins to lose control of head and body movements and becomes lethargic. By six months of age, weight is lost, the infant can no longer sit up unaided, and clinical symptoms include megaloblastic anemia and even coma. Fortunately, response to vitamin B_{12} therapy is rapid.

The mothers in these cases showed only marginal deficiency of the vitamin, emphasizing the role of body storage in adults and the greater need of growing infants and young children eating vegetarian foods. Vegetarian diets for children should include milk and/or eggs; otherwise, supplementation with a vitamin preparation containing cobalamin is essential. Pregnant and lactating women who are vegetarians should also receive supplementary vitamin B_{12}.

Vitamin B_{12}, like folic acid, is not known to have any toxic effects at any reasonable intake levels.

ASCORBIC ACID

Scurvy, described as early as 1500 B.C. and much later identified as ascorbic acid deficiency, is one of the oldest known vitamin deficiency diseases. In our own day, ascorbic acid is probably the most familiar and the most controversial of the vitamins.

The story of Lind, a surgeon with the British navy, who first demonstrated a cure for scurvy and whose prescribed treatment was responsible for British sailors being familiarly known as "limeys," has been told in Chapter 1. In *A Treatise on Scurvy*, Lind tells not only of his own experiments but also the experiences of the French explorer Cartier and his party of 110 men. Stranded along the iced-in St. Lawrence River in the winter of 1535, the explorers became afflicted with the gruesome symptoms of an unfamiliar and fatal disease—swollen limbs, blotched and hemorrhaging gums and skin, loss of teeth, and severe weakness. Soon eight had died, and more than fifty others were in critical condition, until local Indians recognized the disease and told them the cure: ingestion of a solution containing pine needles and bark.

In 1907, Axel Holst and Theodor Fröhlich induced scurvy in guinea pigs, a species that, along with all primates and a few other animal species, cannot synthesize the antiscurvy factor. In 1928 Albert Szent-Györgyi isolated a highly active hydrogen carrier from the adrenal gland, cabbages, and oranges. Because Szent-Györgyi was then concerned with hydrogen reactions in cell respiration, he failed to recognize the vitamin properties of the substance and named it *hexuronic acid*. Several years later, an active crystalline substance was isolated from lemon juice and named for its antiscurvy properties (from the Latin, *scorbutus*, "scurvy"; *ascorbic* means "without scurvy"). Almost immediately, Szent-Györgyi and a colleague determined

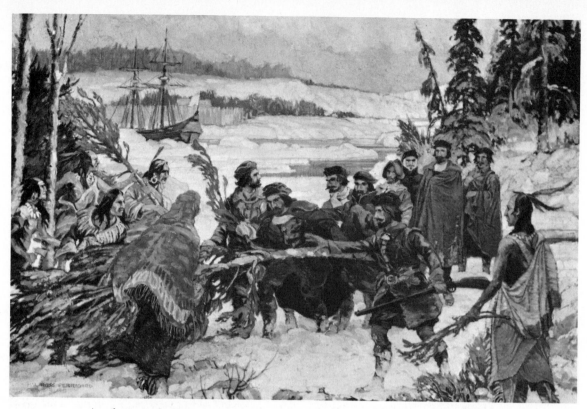

An oil painting by H. R. Perrigard depicts Indians showing explorer Jacques Cartier the source of their cure for scurvy made from the branches of the juniper tree.

Public Archives of Canada

that ascorbic acid was identical with hexuronic acid. The new vitamin was synthesized in 1933.

Chemistry and Properties

Ascorbic acid is a white, water-soluble, crystalline substance, stable when dry. However, in solution it becomes the least stable of all vitamins and oxidizes readily in light, air, and especially when heated or in alkaline solution. Oxidation is further accelerated in the presence of copper or iron. All these oxidation-enhancing factors imply potential loss of vitamin activity during many common food preparation and storage conditions.

The 6-carbon structure of vitamin C makes it chemically similar to glucose (see Figure 7–16). The biologically active forms are L-ascorbic acid and its oxidation product L-dehydroascorbic acid, which has about 80 percent of the activity of the unoxidized form. Further metabolism converts the dehydroascorbic acid to diketogluconic acid, which has no antiscorbutic activity at all (see Figure 7–16); this latter reaction is irreversible.

Absorption and Metabolism

Vitamin C is readily absorbed through the mucosa of the small intestine. From there it passes through the portal vein to the liver and is then distributed to tissues

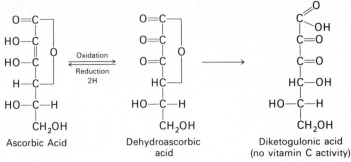

FIGURE 7-16 *Structure of Ascorbic Acid and Related Oxidation/Reduction Reactions.*

throughout the body. The transport mechanism may differ from species to species, according to whether or not a species can synthesize ascorbic acid.

In humans, body stores total about 1,500 milligrams, with moderate reserves in the liver and spleen and high concentrations but small amounts in the adrenal glands. The high concentration in the adrenal glands suggests that ascorbic acid may be involved in synthesis of adrenal steroids. Serum and tissue levels appear to be in equilibrium. Thus, white blood cells, which take up vitamin C, provide a basis for evaluating vitamin C status in humans.

The body excretes vitamin C primarily as ascorbic acid and as the metabolite oxalic acid in the urine, with very small amounts expired as carbon dioxide. The amount excreted daily represents about 3 percent of the total body reserves. Excretion increases with the administration of adrenal steroids, salicylates, sulfonamides, and tetracycline. Though the finding has been disputed, cigarette smoking appears to decrease plasma levels of vitamin C. Findings suggesting that oral contraceptives adversely affect ascorbic acid metabolism are also in dispute.

Physiological Functions

Ascorbic acid is apparently the only water-soluble vitamin that is not known to serve as a coenzyme in any metabolic pathway. Although much is known about its physiological functions, the biochemical involvements of this vitamin remain unclear.

The most important role of vitamin C is in the formation of collagen, a major component of all connective tissues in the body—skin, bones, teeth, muscle, tendon, cornea, and so on. Ascorbic acid is necessary for transformation of the amino acids proline and lysine into hydroxyproline and hydroxylysine. These hydroxy forms provide the tertiary structure which gives stability to the collagen molecule. The major symptoms of scurvy, which result from the breakdown of connective tissue, demonstrate the importance of vitamin C. Vitamin C further contributes to the formation of collagen needed for healing wounds, and therapeutic doses are sometimes used in treatment of postsurgical patients and burn victims.

Vitamin C, furthermore, apparently functions in conversion of amino acids for neurotransmitter synthesis and also enhances absorption of iron. Undoubtedly the most controversial issue concerning ascorbic acid function involves its alleged power in preventing and curing the common cold and in the treatment of cancer. The idea that vitamin C might prevent or cure the common cold was introduced in

1970 by Linus Pauling in his book *Vitamin C and the Common Cold.* Since then Pauling's hypothesis has been tested in many studies. Pauling advocated consumption of 1 to 3 grams of ascorbic acid daily, asserting that 1 gram per day would reduce the number of sick days. All in all, evidence for the effectiveness of vitamin C against the common cold is at least inconclusive. Some studies have shown that the group treated with vitamin C had fewer colds, less severe symptoms, or fewer sick days due to colds than the control group. However, the differences were often small and not statistically significant—for example, a 5 to 10 percent reduction rather than the marked decrease in number of colds. Other studies show no effectiveness whatever for vitamin C, and some even show a slight increase in the number of colds for those taking the vitamin.

Recommended Allowances and Dietary Sources

Although 10 milligrams per day of ascorbic acid are all that is needed to prevent scurvy, optimal health requires more. The RDA is 60 mg for adults, with increases to 80 mg and 100 mg for pregnant and lactating women, respectively. Because body stores are small, daily intake is advisable. Individuals with chronic illness and those recovering from surgery should receive additional amounts.

In addition to citrus fruits and their juices, which are well known as sources of vitamin C, tomatoes, green vegetables, and other fruits such as most melons and berries also contain significant quantities. Potatoes, not generally thought to provide exceptional amounts of this vitamin, may nonetheless be an important source for population groups consuming large quantities; one medium baked potato will provide about one-half of the recommended allowance for an adult. With the exception of liver, foods of animal origin generally have little or no ascorbic acid content (see Table 7–10).

Because vitamin C is so vulnerable to light, air and heat, care must be taken in food preparation to preserve its activity. Cut foods should not be left exposed for long periods; there should be as little cutting and chopping before cooking as possible; baking soda should never be added to cooking water; minimal quantities of water should be used in cooking; vegetables should be put into water that has already come to a boil and should not be overcooked. Vegetable cooking liquids should be reused in soups; and foods should be covered and stored in opaque containers.

Clinical Deficiency Symptoms

The numerous symptoms of ascorbic acid deficiency include lassitude and general weakness; swollen joints and aching bones; spongy and bleeding gums; delayed healing of wounds; muscle cramps; and dry, scaly skin. Infants with scurvy assume a characteristic "frog's leg" position, are generally irritable, have particularly sensitive lips and limbs, and have little appetite. Unless the mother is deficient, breast-fed infants rarely get scurvy. Several years ago, a case of experimental scurvy was reported. The volunteer ate a diet deficient in vitamin C for 105 days and developed the same symptoms described in spontaneous scurvy. All symptoms of scurvy disappeared over a period of 116 days during which the volunteer had a vitamin C intake of only 6.5 mg per day. Signs of scurvy did not appear until the body pool dropped below 300 mg and disappeared when the body pool was restored to that level.

In the United States, scurvy has almost completely disappeared, although alco-

TABLE 7-10. *Ascorbic Acid Content of Selected Foods (RDA for Adults: 60 mg)*

Food	Serving Size	Ascorbic Acid Content mg/serving
Orange juice, frozen concentrate, diluted as directed	6 oz	90
Strawberries, fresh	1 c	88
Broccoli, fresh, cooked	3 spears	81
Broccoli, frozen, cooked	3 spears	66
Orange	1 medium	66
Grapefruit juice, canned	6 oz	63
Cantaloupe	¼ melon	45
Grapefruit	½ medium	37
Liver, calf, cooked	3 oz	31
Asparagus, cooked	⅔ c	31
Potato, white, baked	1 medium	31
Cranberry juice cocktail	6 oz	30
Tomato juice, canned	6 oz	29
Spinach, frozen, cooked	½ c	27
Winter squash, mashed	1 c	27
Sweet potato, baked	1 medium	25
Liver, beef, cooked	3 oz	23
Avocado, raw	½ medium	16
Vegetable juice cocktail	6 oz	16
Tomato, raw	½ medium	14
Lemonade, frozen concentrate, diluted as directed	6 oz	13
Soybeans, cooked	½ c	13
Tomato soup, prepared with water	1 c	12
Banana	1 medium	12
Apricots, raw	3	11
Green beans, fresh, cooked	⅔ c	10
Clams, raw, meat only	3 oz	8
Apple	1 medium	6
Yogurt, plain	8 oz	2
Milk, whole	8 oz	2
Milk, low-fat	8 oz	2
Yogurt, fruit-flavored	8 oz	1
Bread, white, enriched	1 slice	trace
Cheddar cheese	1 oz	0
Fish	3 oz	0
Hamburger, 21% fat, cooked	3 oz	0
Poultry	3 oz	0
Oils; butter; margarine	—	0
Egg, whole	1 medium	0

Source: C. F. Adams, *Nutritive value of American foods in common units*, USDA Agriculture Handbook No. 456 (Washington, D.C.: U.S. Government Printing Office, 1975).

holics and the elderly, as well as some of those with bizarre eating habits, may show deficiency, usually because of decreased consumption of fresh fruits and juices. Interestingly, two sources of vitamin C have fallen victim to "progress," and sporadic outbreaks of scurvy have been the result. In the southern states, it was the custom, particularly among rural people, to drink the liquid in which green vegetables had been cooked; this "pot likker" was a good source of the vitamin C that long cooking and a large volume of water had leached out of greens. But a rising standard of living eliminated this dietary custom in many families, and children developed scurvy. Children also became "victims" of pasteurization, which destroys the ascorbic acid of milk along with microorganisms.

For somewhat different reasons, Eskimos, especially in the Arctic might be expected to have a relatively high incidence of scurvy, since their diet contains almost no foods of plant origin (unlike the sub-Arctic Eskimos, who do get some fruits, berries, and vegetables). Apparently the fact that the Eskimos eat much of their animal food frozen, raw, or only partially cooked preserves what little vitamin C is in their diet.

Toxicity

Because it is water-soluble and readily excreted, and because the body's capacity for storage of ascorbic acid is low, toxic effects have long been thought unlikely. Indeed, even in doses as high as several hundred milligrams per day, little toxicity has been demonstrated. But ingestion of very large doses, in the range of one to several grams per day, does have potentially serious effects for some people. There is, for example, some evidence that high intakes can cause kidney stones and gout in susceptible individuals. Other evidence has suggested that vitamin C may act as a vitamin B_{12} antagonist, although this has been challenged. The ability of ascorbic acid to enhance absorption of dietary iron may pose the threat of iron overload to sensitive individuals. A more serious problem, potentially affecting larger numbers of individuals, is that urine tests to determine desirable insulin requirements for diabetics are falsified by consumption of large doses of ascorbic acid. Very large doses may also acidify the urine and produce a burning sensation during urination.

A single case study related to megadosage of vitamin C for migraine headaches has suggested the possibility that prolonged intake of such quantities may lead to nutritional dependency. Additional evidence suggests that individuals who have been consuming large amounts of ascorbic acid should wean themselves slowly until moderate levels of intake are achieved.

Some physicians have warned that ingestion of megadoses of ascorbic acid during pregnancy may produce a vitamin C-dependent infant. In such a case, a condition known as "rebound scurvy" could develop when the infant receives only normal amounts of the vitamin after birth. Once the fetal metabolic system has adapted to the higher amounts by removing the excess vitamin C more rapidly than normal, even the normal amounts ingested by the newborn are removed at the faster-than-normal rate, depressing serum and tissue levels (Anderson, 1977).

VITAMINLIKE FACTORS

At different times in the history of vitamin research, a number of substances have been candidates for classification as vitamins. Some—like those discussed thus far in this chapter and those discussed in Chapter 6—have been "elected," so to speak. Some have been "defeated," and some elected only to be recalled later. As our knowledge of nutritional metabolism grows, one or more of these substances may yet receive recognition as vitamins. The compounds with the best qualifications are choline, inositol, ubiquinone, lipoic acid, para-aminobenzoic acid, and the bioflavinoids. At present, however, each is considered to lack one or more of the three essential criteria that characterize this nutrient class.

Choline

Choline is apparently synthesized in all plant and animal species. Its greatest importance is as a precursor of the neurotransmitter acetylcholine; dietary choline directly affects acetylcholine levels as well as the density of acetylcholine receptors in the brain. For this reason, pharmacological doses of choline have been used to treat brain disorders that are apparently related to deficiency of choline functioning, such as tardive dyskinesia and Huntington's disease. Choline is also a component of phospholipids and lecithins, which form an essential part of cell membranes and lipoproteins; deficiency produces structural and functional abnormalities in cells. And choline is needed, along with methionine, to prevent the development of fatty liver. Food sources include wheat germ, egg yolk, organ meats, and legumes; the average American diet provides about 800 milligrams, an ample supply, per day.

Inositol

This colorless, water-soluble substance, whose structure resembles that of glucose, is widely found in plants, especially in grains, nuts, fruits, and vegetables, as well as in yeast and milk. Because the body, it has been learned, apparently synthesizes enough for all metabolic requirements, inositol is no longer considered to be a vitamin. Its main function in humans is as a component of muscle phospholipids. Phytic acid, an inositol-phosphate compound found in some plants and seeds, binds zinc, iron, and calcium in the human gastrointestinal tract and therefore may significantly decrease absorption of those minerals.

Ubiquinone

Also known as Coenzyme Q, and chemically related to both vitamins E and K, this compound derives its name from its ubiquitous distribution in animals and plants. Because adequate amounts are synthesized in body cells, food sources are not necessary. Ubiquinone is a component of the phospholipids that form the mitochondrial membranes, and in this way it plays a very important part as an electron carrier in the electron transport system.

Lipoic Acid

Lipoic acid is a sulfur-containing fat-soluble molecule for which no human dietary requirement is known. Acting as a coenzyme in conjunction with thiamin, niacin, riboflavin, and pantothenic acid, lipoic acid participates in the conversion of (1) pyruvate to acetyl CoA and (2) α-ketoglutarate to succinyl CoA. Thus, it plays an important role in the metabolism of carbohydrate, protein, and fat. It is not classified as a vitamin, however, because it can be synthesized in the body in physiologically effective amounts.

Para-Aminobenzoic Acid

Para-aminobenzoic acid (PABA) functions as a growth factor for bacteria and lower animals. It is a component of folic acid and can completely satisfy the need in rats and mice for dietary folic acid. For these reasons, it was accorded vitamin status at one time. But it is not clear whether PABA has any metabolic role other than as a component of folic acid, and it is no longer considered a vitamin for humans or other animals.

Bioflavonoids

The bioflavonoids were discovered by Szent-Györgyi, in 1936, as a mixture of compounds in lemon peel and red peppers that he named *citrin* (a designation later dropped). The active component in citrin was briefly called *vitamin P* for its role in maintaining permeability of capillary membranes. Experimentally induced bioflavinoid deficiency in animals results in a syndrome marked by increased capillary permeability and fragility. This deficiency effect has some relationship to the role of vitamin C. Apparently the bioflavonoids have an antioxidant effect that protects ascorbic acid from oxidative destruction. But this is an indirect and nonessential effect. At present there is not enough evidence to include these substances among the vitamins.

NONVITAMINS

Laetrile

In 1952, the biochemist Ernst T. Krebs, Jr. (not related to Sir Hans Krebs) announced the development of a drug he called *Laetrile*, which was asserted to be a cure for cancer. Subsequently, he claimed that Laetrile was a vitamin (B_{17}).

Laetrile is found in apricot and peach pits and almond kernels; it is a glucose-related compound that contains cyanide and is known chemically as *amygdalin*. In controlled studies, Laetrile had no effect on cancer growth.

Laetrile does not meet the essential criteria for being a vitamin. It has no known metabolic function essential to nutritional health, and its absence from the diet produces no deficiency symptoms. (The only criterion that it does meet is that it is not synthesized in the human body.) More important, it is not a harmless substance. Its cyanide content is potentially lethal, and symptoms of toxicity have been reported. Some observers, however, do believe that it is harmless.

Pangamic Acid

Pangamic acid, also known as *pangamate* and as *vitamin B_{15}*, was patented in 1949 by the same people who developed Laetrile. Claims are made that it is a wonder drug that provides "extra" energy and cures a host of physical ailments besides. Pangamate's developers, however, have never furnished any proof (other than testimonials) of its vitamin properties and curative powers.

Like Laetrile, pangamate is found in apricot pits and all other seeds, hence the name given to it by Krebs, from *pan*, "all," and *gamete*, "seed." Also as with Laetrile, it does not meet the criteria for a vitamin.

SUMMARY

The water-soluble vitamins are distinguished from their fat-soluble counterparts in three major ways:

1. Solubility—their water solubility substantially determines such properties as limited body storage and excretion in urine.
2. Chemical composition—in addition to carbon, hydrogen, and oxygen, most water-soluble vitamins also contain nitrogen, and several contain sulfur, cobalt, or phosphorus.
3. Metabolic function—except for ascorbic acid, all the water-soluble vitamins are known to function as components of one or more coenzymes.

Thiamin (B_1) participates in more than 20 enzyme reactions necessary for the metabolism of carbohydrates, fats, and proteins. Its active form is a sulfur-containing molecule, thiamin pyrophosphate (TPP or cocarboxylase). Many foods contain thiamin in varied amounts. Thiamin deficiency, or beriberi, takes several forms, all involving impairment of the nervous, cardiovascular, and gastrointestinal systems.

Riboflavin (B_2) is a component of the coenzymes flavin mononucleotide (FMN) and flavin adenine dinucleotide (FAD). It combines with various proteins to form flavoprotein enzymes, which function as hydrogen carriers. A wide variety of food provides small amounts of riboflavin, usually in association with other B vitamins. Deficiency symptoms, probably associated with deficiencies of other vitamins as well, include growth retardation and various abnormalities or lesions of the eyes, mouth, tongue, and skin.

Niacin, also known as *nicotinic acid* and *nicotinamide*, resembles riboflavin in metabolic function. Niacin forms two related coenzymes, nicotine adenine dinucleotide (NAD) and nicotine adenine dinucleotide phosphate (NADP). These combine with various proteins to form enzymes that act as hydrogen carriers. Niacin is found in many foods and also is synthesized in the body from the amino acid tryptophan in a reaction that requires thiamin, riboflavin, and vitamin B_6.

The serious niacin-deficiency condition pellagra is characterized by "the four D's"—dermatitis, diarrhea, dementia, and death. Pharmacological doses may be toxic to the liver and may cause diabetes or peptic ulcer.

Biotin, a widespread and potent vitamin, was not identified chemically until 1942. It is a sulfur-containing, heat-stable growth factor which functions chiefly as a coenzyme in fatty acid synthesis (CO_2-fixation reactions) and amino acid metabolism (transcarboxylation reactions). No RDA for biotin has been established, nor have any deficiency or toxic effects been identified.

Pantothenic acid, named for its extremely wide distribution, functions mainly as a component of coenzyme A (CoA), the compound that combines with oxaloacetate to initiate the Krebs cycle, and in acyl-carrier protein. No RDA for pantothenic acid has been established, nor has any natural deficiency been identified in humans.

Vitamin B_6 (pyridoxine) has three forms, all of which are active as the coenzyme pyridoxal phosphate (PLP). Among other functions, PLP participates in reactions essential to amino acid metabolism. The only known natural clinical deficiency is microcytic anemia in infants. Therapeutic doses may cause mild toxicity, and dependency and severe toxicity may result from larger intakes.

Folacin was identified ten years after the discovery of a deficiency anemia that did not respond to any of the known B-complex factors. Its primary function is as a coenzyme involved in the synthesis of thymine, a nucleotide in DNA. Folacin deficiency produces megaloblastic anemia (immature, enlarged red blood cells).

Vitamin B_{12} (cobalamin), identified in 1948 as the antipernicious anemia factor, is a large, complex, cobalt-containing molecule. Like folic acid, vitamin B_{12} is necessary for DNA synthesis, and it is essential also for nervous system function. Since it is found only in foods of animal origin, individuals on strict vegetarian diets, especially pregnant and lactating women, breast-fed infants of vegetarian mothers, and children, should receive supplementation.

Ascorbic acid was identified as the antiscurvy factor in 1932. It functions chiefly in maintaining the structure of collagen, the major component of all connective tissue. It also enhances iron absorption. The role of ascorbic acid in prevention of the common cold and cancer is disputed. Vitamin C is found in many fruits and vegetables. Possible toxic effects may result from long-term high doses and include gout, lessened calcium retention, and vitamin dependence.

Vitaminlike factors are important biological substances that have been classified or may yet be classified as vitamins but at present lack one or more of three defining characteristics. On the other hand, Laetrile ("B$_{17}$") and pangamic acid ("B$_{15}$") are definitely nonvitamins since they satisfy none of the important criteria for vitamins.

BIBLIOGRAPHY

ALHADEFF, L., C.T. GUALTIERI, AND M. LIPTON. Toxic effects of water-soluble vitamins. *Nutrition Reviews* 42:33–40, 1984.

BAILEY, L.B., J.J. CERDA, B.S. BLOCH, M.J. BUSBY, L. VARGAS, C.J. CHANDLER, AND C.H. HALSTED. Effect of age on poly- and monoglutamyl folacin absorption in human subjects. *Journal of Nutrition* 114:1770–1776, 1984.

BELKO, A.Z., E. OBARZANEK, H.J. KALKWARF, M.A. ROTTER, S. BOGUSZ, D. MILLER, J.D. HAAS, AND D.A. ROE. Effects of exercise on riboflavin requirements of young women. *American Journal of Clinical Nutrition* 37: 509–517, 1983.

BELKO, A.Z., M.P. MEREDITH, H.J. KALKWARF, E. OBARZANEK, S. WEINBERG, R. ROACH, B. MCKEON, AND D.A. ROE. Effects of exercise on riboflavin requirements: Biological validation in weight reducing women. *American Journal of Clinical Nutrition* 41:270–277, 1985.

BORSCHEL, M.W., A. KIRKSEY, AND R.E. HANNEMANN. Effects of vitamin B-6 intake on nutrition and growth of young infants. *American Journal of Clinical Nutrition* 43:7–15, 1986.

BREEN, K.J., R. BUTTIGIEG, S. IOSSIFIDIS, C. LOURENSZ, AND B. WOOD. Jejunal uptake of thiamin hydrochloride in man: Influence of alcoholism and alcohol. *American Journal of Clinical Nutrition* 42:121–126, 1985.

BRIGGS, M.H., ed. Recent vitamin research. Boca Raton, FL: CRC Press, 1984.

CARPENTER, K.J. Effects of different methods of processing maize on its pellagragenic activity. Fed. Proc. 40:1531–1535, 1981.

CENTERWALL, B.S. AND M.H. CRIQUI. Prevention of the Wernicke-Korsakoff syndrome. A cost-benefit. *New England Journal of Medicine* 299:285, 1978.

COURSIN, D.B. Convulsive seizures in infants with pyridoxine-deficient diets. *Journal of the American Medical Association* 154:406, 1954.

DUBRICK, M.A., AND R.B. RUCKER. Dietary supplements and health aids—A critical evaluation. Part 1—Vitamins and Minerals. *Journal of Nutritional Education* 15:47–53, 1983.

GOLDBERGER, J. The prevention of pellagra. A test diet among institutional inmates. *Public Health Reports.* 30:3117, 1938.

GOLDSMITH, G.A., O.N. MILLER, AND W.G. UNGLAUB. Efficiency of tryptophan a niacin prescursor in man. *Journal of Nutrition* 73:172, 1961.

HENDERSON, L.M. Niacin. *Annual Review of Nutrition* 3:289–307, 1983.

HERBERT, V. Pangamic acid ("vitamin B$_{15}$"). *American Journal of Clinical Nutrition* 32;1534, 1979.

HILKER, D.M. AND J.C. SOMOGYI. Antithiamins of plant origin: Their chemical nature and mode of action. *Annual N.Y. Academy of Science* 378:137–145, 1982.

HODGES, R.E. Vitamin C and cancer. *Nutrition Reviews* 40:289–292, 1982.

———. J. HOOD, J.E. CANHAM, H.E. SAUBERLICH, AND E.M. BAKER. Clinical manifestations of ascorbic acid deficiency in man. *American Journal of Clinical Nutrition* 24:432–443, 1971.

HORWITZ, M.K., A.E. HARPER, and L.M. HENDERSON. Niacin-tryptophan relationships for evaluating niacin equivalents. *American Journal of Clinical Nutrition* 34:423–427, 1981.

JACOB, E., S.J. BAKER, AND V. HERBERT. Vitamin B$_{12}$ binding proteins. *Physiol. Rev.* 60:918–960, 1980.

KANTOR, M.A., J.R. TROUT, AND P.A. LACHANCE. Food dyes produce minimal effects on locomotor activity and vitamin B-6 levels in postweaning rats. *Journal of Nutrition* 114:1402–1412, 1984.

KELSAY, J.L. Effects of fiber on mineral and vitamin bioavailability. In *Dietary Fiber in Health and Disease*, G.V. Vahouny and D. Dritchevsky, eds., New York: Plenum, 1982.

LEKLEM, J.E. Vitamin B-6 requirement and oral contraceptive use—A concern. *Journal of Nutrition* 116:475–477, 1986.

MERRILL, A.H. JR., J.D. LAMBETH, D.E. EDMONDSON, AND D.B. McCORMICK. Formation and mode of action of flavoproteins. *Annual Review of Nutrition* 1:281–317, 1981.

MERRILL, A.H., J.M. HENDERSON, E. WANG, B.W. McDONALD, AND W.J. MILLIKAN. Metabolism of vitamin B-6 by human liver. *Journal of Nutrition* 114:1664–1674, 1984.

MILLER, D.F. Pellagra deaths in the United States. *American Journal of Clinical Nutrition* 31:558, 1978.

MINOT, G.R. AND W.P. MURPHY. Treatment of pernicious anemia by a special diet. *Journal of the American Medical Association* 87:470, 1926.

Nutrition Today. Report: Discovery and synthesis of vitamin B_{12} celebrated. Vol. 8(1):24, 1973.

PAULING, L. *Vitamin C and the common cold.* San Francisco: W.H. Freeman & Co., 1970.

ROSE, R.C. Transport and metabolism of water-soluble vitamins in intestine. *American Journal Physiol.* 240:G97–G101, 1981.

ROTH, K.S. Biotin in clinical medicine—A review. *American Journal of Clinical Nutrition* 34:1967–1974, 1981.

RUDOLPH, N., A.J. PAREKH, J. HITTLEMAN, J. BURDIGE, AND S.L. WONG. Postnatal decline in pyridoxal phosphate and riboflavin. Accentuation by phototherapy. *American Journal Diseases of Childhood* 139:812–815, 1985.

SAUBERLICH, H.E., Y.F. HERMAN, C.O. STEVENS, AND R.H. HERMAN. Thiamin requirement of the adult human. *American Journal of Clinical Nutrition* 32:2237–2248, 1979.

SCHAUMBERG, H., J. KAPLAN, A. WINDEBANK, N. VICK, S. RASMUS, D. PLEASURE, AND M.J. BROWN. Sensory neuropathy from pyridoxine abuse: A new megavitamin syndrome. *New England Journal of Medicine* 309:445–448, 1983.

SCHUSTER, K., L.B. BAILEY, AND C.S. MAHAN. Effect of maternal pyridoxine-HCl Supplementation on the vitamin B-6 status of mother and infant and on pregnancy outcome. *Journal of Nutrition* 114:977–988, 1984.

SEETHARAM, B. AND D.H. ALPERS. Cellular uptake of cobalamin. *Nutrition Reviews* 43:97–102, 1985.

SHANE, B. AND E.L.R. STOKSTAD. Vitamin B-12 Folate Interrelationships. *Annual Review of Nutrition* 5:323–340, 1985.

SMITH, G.F., D. SPIKER, C.P. PETERSON, D. CICHETTI, AND P. JUSTINE. Use of megadoses of vitamins with minerals in Down syndrome. *Journal of Pediatrics* 105:228–234, 1984.

SNETI, F.R. AND S.M. PILCH. Analysis of folate data from the second national health and nutrition examination survey (NHAMES II). *Journal of Nutrition*, 1986.

Special Report—Affirmative: Linus Pauling; Negative, C. Moertel. A Proposition: Megadoses of Vitamin C are valuable in the treatment of cancer. *Nutrition Reviews* 44:28–32, 1986.

SWEETMAN, L., L. SURH, H. BAKE, R.M. PETERSON, AND W.L. NYHAN. Clinical and metabolic abnormalities in a boy with dietary deficiency of biotin. *Pediatrics* 68:553–558, 1981.

SYDENSTRICKER, V.P., S.A. SINGAL, A.P. BRIGGS, N.M. DeVAUGHN, AND H. ISBELL. Preliminary observations on "egg white injury" in man and its cure with a biotin concentrate. *Science* 95:176, 1942.

WAGNER, C. Folate-binding proteins. *Nutrition Reviews* 43:293–296, 1985.

WILLIAMS, R.R. *Toward the Conquest of Beriberi.* Cambridge, MA: Harvard Univeristy Press, 1961.

YOUNG, V.R. AND P.M. NEWBERNE. Vitamins and cancer prevention. *Cancer* 47:1226–1240, 1981.

ZEISEL, S.H. Dietary choline: Biochemistry, physiology, and pharmacology. *Annual Review of Nutrition* 1:95–121, 1981.

Chapter 8

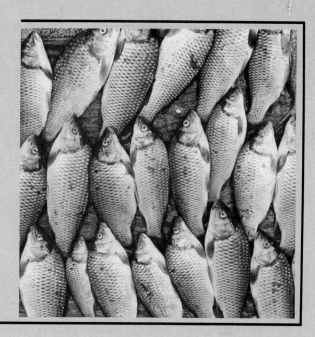

MINERALS

About 50 of the more than 100 known elements are found in body tissues and fluids, and four of these 50—carbon, hydrogen, oxygen, and nitrogen—make up 96 percent of our body weight. In varying combinations, these four elements are fundamental components of one or more of five nutrient classes: carbohydrate, protein, lipids, vitamins, and water. Twenty-one additional elements have been classified as essential nutrients; they account for most of the remaining 4 percent of body weight. Their chemical nature and similarities of function justify classifying them together as the single nutrient category, *minerals*. This class of nutrients consists of those chemical elements that (1) are known or strongly suspected to be essential for nutritional health in humans and (2) are required in milligram quantities in the daily diet. (See Appendix J, page 550 for the percentage amounts of different elements in the body.)

An additional two dozen or more elements are found in the body but have no known essential function and are therefore classified as *contaminants*. These enter the body via air, food, and water and, for the most part, pose no health problem. Under certain circumstances and in sufficient quantity, however, they can be toxic and even lethal. Three well-known examples are lead, mercury, and strontium-90.

The essential minerals can be divided into two subgroups on the basis of dietary requirement: The so-called *macro* or **major minerals** are required in amounts of 100 milligrams or more per day; **trace minerals** are required in amounts no greater than a few milligrams per day (see Table 8–1). In contrast to the much larger requirements established for carbohydrates, proteins, and lipids, the small requirements for minerals resemble those for vitamins.

Minerals have wide distribution in the tissues and fluids of the body. They occur chiefly (1) as components of various important organic molecules such as metalloenzymes (the iron-containing cytochromes), amino acids (sulfur in cysteine and methionine), and others (iron in hemoglobin, iodine in thyroid hormones); (2) as structural components of certain tissues (calcium, phosphorus, and fluorine in dental tissue); and (3) as free ions (sodium, calcium, and potassium) in blood and other body fluids. As free ions, minerals play an important part in water and acid-base balance, nerve impulse transmission, and muscle contraction, and as catalysts for enzymatic reactions. In terms of quantitative distribution most minerals function primarily as structural components of body tissues.

Most minerals are not stored by the body in significant amounts and so must be supplied in the daily diet. When dietary intake is adequate, the quantities of nearly all essential minerals found in the body and the various body compartments are closely regulated. If the body is viewed as a system with an input and an output, it becomes clear that both absorption and excretion can serve to control mineral balance. In fact, tissue levels of some minerals are controlled by the efficiency of absorption. For minerals whose absorption is almost completely efficient, the

TABLE 8-1. *The Essential Minerals*

MAJOR MINERALS	TRACE MINERALS	
Calcium	Iron	Manganese
Phosphorus	Copper	Molybdenum
Magnesium	Zinc	Selenium
Sodium	Iodine	Silicon
Potassium	Fluoride	Tin
Chloride	Chromium	Vanadium
Sulfur	Cobalt	Nickel

amounts excreted in urine are modified according to the needs of the organism. These controls protect the body against both deficiency and potentially toxic accumulations and can be described as gatekeeper mechanisms. In addition, other internal control mechanisms regulate the distribution of minerals throughout body tissues.

Chemically, minerals are the simplest nutrients found in the body. Nonetheless, nutritional scientists still have a great deal to learn about them. Until recently, research has been greatly hampered by the difficulty of measuring the minute quantities in which minerals exist in the body and in foods. However, technological advances have led to the development of new analytical techniques. With the resulting increase in knowledge has come the discovery that the functions of some minerals are interrelated. The absorption, metabolism, mode of action, and dietary requirements for many minerals may be modified by the presence or absence of other minerals.

THE MAJOR MINERALS

Of the minerals, seven are required in amounts greater than 100 milligrams per day, are present in the body in quantities representing at least 0.05 percent of body weight, or both. These major minerals are calcium, phosphorus, magnesium, sodium, potassium, chlorine, and sulfur.

Calcium

Calcium is, after carbon, hydrogen, oxygen, and nitrogen, the most abundant element in the human body. In the form of the doubly positive ion Ca^{++}, calcium is also the most abundant cation in the body. Though it is best known for its role in bone development, this mineral has other important functions.

DISTRIBUTION IN THE BODY. The calcium content of the average healthy adult is a little less than 2 percent of body weight and represents half the total mineral content of the body. Depending on their height, adult men contain 950–1300 grams of calcium; adult women, 770–920 grams. Of this amount, almost all (99 percent) is deposited in bone and dental tissue. The remaining 1 percent is located in extracellular fluid, including blood.

METABOLISM AND PHYSIOLOGICAL FUNCTIONS: ABSORPTION. Calcium is absorbed into the body from the small intestine primarily by active transport, which requires the assistance of vitamin D. Some passive diffusion also occurs. The body normally absorbs between 30 and 40 percent of ingested calcium. Active absorption appears to be controlled by a gatekeeper mechanism (see Figure 8–1). The rate of absorption increases with decreased dietary intake of calcium and with the increased physiological need for the mineral that occurs during growth, pregnancy, and lactation.

A number of other factors affect calcium absorption as well. Parathyroid hormone (PTH) increases calcium absorption by increasing the conversion of vitamin D to its active form (see Chapter 6). Amino acids appear to increase the solubility of calcium and therefore enhance its absorption. Lactose also increases the solubility of calcium. Since lactose is the primary sugar in milk and since milk is commercially fortified with vitamin D, this beverage is an excellent source of the mineral.

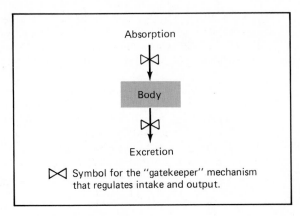

Absorption

Body

Excretion

◁ Symbol for the "gatekeeper" mechanism
that regulates intake and output.

FIGURE 8-1
The Gatekeeper Mechanism.

Factors that decrease calcium absorption include vitamin D deficiency; decreased intestinal acidity (high pH), more common in later age; diarrhea; and any condition that generally results in malabsorption. Oxalic acid, which is found in chocolate, spinach, beet tops, collard greens, and several other vegetables, combines with dietary calcium to form an insoluble compound, thereby binding calcium and making it unavailable for absorption. But normally this is not a concern because the total amount of dietary calcium greatly exceeds the amount of dietary oxalate, so that the effect of the latter is insignificant. Child and adolescent vegans should probably avoid high intakes of foods high in oxalates. Mean heights of three-to-five-year-old vegans tend to be lower than standards for the age.

Phytic acid, which is found in relatively large amounts in the outer layers of cereal grains and therefore in cereal products containing unrefined grain, also binds dietary calcium to form an insoluble complex known as **phytate**. Here again the effect is not significant unless extensive consumption of phytic acid-containing foods is accompanied by low calcium intake. This may be a concern to strict vegetarians (vegans), although a well-varied vegetarian diet should compensate for any imbalance. Free fatty acids, particularly the saturated variety, may also combine with calcium to form the type of insoluble complexes known as *soaps*.

Further, it has long been believed that the absorption of calcium is maximized when dietary calcium and phosphorus are present in approximately equal amounts. But current evidence does not support a significant effect of either wide varieties of phosphorus intake or the dietary calcium-to-phosphorus ratio on calcium retention. However, some preliminary data suggest that the form of phosphorus may influence calcium absorption. The absolute amount of calcium is probably the more important consideration.

METABOLISM AND PHYSIOLOGICAL FUNCTIONS: FUNCTIONS. Following absorption, calcium enters the bloodstream and is transported to body tissues. The major site of deposition is bone. In the process of bone mineralization, an inorganic calcium-containing complex interacts with the organic material, cartilage. The inorganic complex, *hydroxyapatite*, consists of phosphorus and hydroxide ions in addition to calcium. The organic components of cartilage are collagen and mucopolysaccharides. Bone, then, constitutes the major reservoir of body calcium, accounting for about 99 percent of the total. Readily available stores of the mineral are located particularly in the ends of long bones, known as *trabeculae*. When the trabecular stores become exhausted (which might happen as a result of prolonged dietary cal-

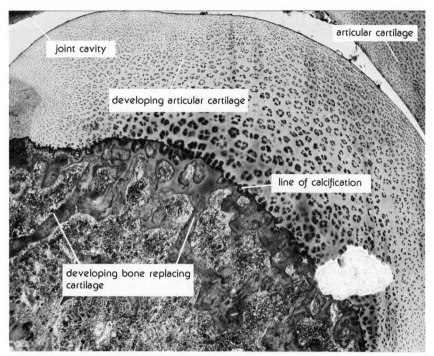

Developing bone and cartilage in the finger of a human fetus.
Lester V. Bergman & Associates, Inc.

cium deficiency) and dietary intake continues to be insufficient, calcium is withdrawn from the shafts of the bones to meet physiological needs. As calcium is removed, the bone becomes weakened.

Bone formation, or **ossification**, begins during fetal development, proceeds rapidly during the growth years, and continues throughout life as a dynamic metabolic process. Bone mineralization is mediated by bone-synthesizing osteoblasts; and bone resorption, by bone-destroying osteoclasts. Together these two types of specialized cells are responsible for the continuous remodeling of bone.

Thus calcium enters and leaves the skeleton continuously. The relative rates of mineralization and resorption are key factors in determining the structural integrity of bone. Estimates indicate that between 600 and 700 milligrams of calcium are removed from, and added to, the bones of a normal adult *every day.* At that rate, the total calcium content of the skeleton is replaced every five years.

Tooth formation, which also begins during fetal development, requires calcium. This process resembles bone formation in several respects: Calcium and phosphorus (as well as magnesium and fluorine) mineralize an organic (protein) matrix to give teeth their rigidity. (The importance of nutrients to dental health during the growth years will be discussed in Chapter 12.) Unlike bone calcium, tooth calcium cannot be replaced once it has been lost.

Calcium in very small amounts plays an important part in other processes as well. In particular, blood clotting requires calcium at several steps in a series of interconnected reactions (see Figure 8–2). Calcium is required for the absorption of

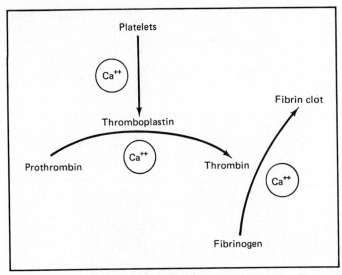

FIGURE 8-2   *The Role of Calcium in the Blood-Clotting Process.*
Calcium is a factor at three key points in the clotting process. This process begins with the exposure of collagen in the walls of the broken blood vessels, causing platelets to gather in the vicinity of the wound. In the presence of Ca^{++}, (1) platelets release thromboplastin, which in the presence of Ca^{++}, (2) activates prothrombin and causes it to change to thrombin, which again in the presence of Ca++, (3) converts soluble fibrinogen to insoluble fibrin, thus forming the hardened, protective blood clot that seals off the outside of the wound. This is a "cascade" reaction, in which each successive step is initiated by the step that immediately precedes it.

dietary vitamin B_{12} (Chapter 7); for the synthesis of the neurotransmitter acetylcholine; for activation of several important enzymes, such as pancreatic lipase; and for the regulation of muscle relaxation and contraction. For several years interest has focused on the role of sodium intake in some individuals as a cause of hypertension, high blood pressure. More recently the role of other minerals, particularly calcium, in the development of hypertension has been explored. Evidence supportive of a relationship between calcium intake and hypertension comes from both animal and human studies. Increasing calcium intake lowers blood pressure of hypertension prone animals, although not always to normal levels. In addition to hypertension, these animals also have an increase in PTH, a decrease in blood levels of free ionized calcium and an increase in urinary calcium excretion. Several population studies have shown an inverse relationship between calcium and blood pressure. Several studies have shown that giving calcium supplements has resulted in decreased blood pressure. Additional research is needed to confirm the proposed relationship between dietary calcium and blood pressure regulation.

The great importance of calcium is emphasized by the fact that serum levels of the mineral are maintained within very narrow limits. The normal range of serum calcium is 9 to 11 mg/dl. *Hypocalcemia* results in tetany, a condition characterized by stiff, contracted muscles and increased nerve activation. *Hypercalcemia,* on the other hand, produces calcium deposition in soft tissues, such as the heart and kidneys. But these conditions result from abnormalities in the regulating mechanisms rather than from dietary deficiency or excess of calcium. Hypercalcemia also results from excessive vitamin D intake.

The maintenance of serum calcium within strict limits is so important that several mechanisms exist to regulate it. (There is a similarity between this multiple regulatory system and that of blood glucose described in Chapter 2.) Serum calcium can be raised by increasing the activation rate of vitamin D and thereby increasing absorption of dietary calcium; the peptide hormone secreted by the parathyroid glands, PTH, serves this function. And vitamin D and PTH both act to release calcium from storage sites in bone and to reduce urinary excretion of the mineral. But if serum calcium exceeds optimal levels, an antagonist of PTH is produced by the thyroid gland. This antagonist, the peptide hormone calcitonin, indirectly counteracts the effects of PTH by decreasing the conversion of vitamin D to its active form, thus diminishing the absorption of dietary calcium. At the same time, calcitonin directly slows the rate of release of calcium from bone. The mechanism by which the hormone acts on the kidney to modify urinary excretion remains unclear. These controls act in combination as a gatekeeper, letting calcium in and out as needed.

METABOLISM AND PHYSIOLOGICAL FUNCTIONS: EXCRETION.   Perspiration, feces, and urine all provide routes for loss of body calcium. Under normal circumstances perspiration losses amount to 15 to 20 milligrams per day. Profuse sweating may lead to greater losses. Fecal calcium consists both of unabsorbed dietary calcium and of calcium secreted into the gut from endogenous sources such as digestive juices. Fecal loss of endogenous calcium ranges from 125 to 180 milligrams per day; variable amounts of dietary calcium are lost in the feces, depending on dietary intake.

Calcium loss through urinary excretion, usually 100 to 200 milligrams per day, appears to be fairly constant for any one individual but varies widely from individual to individual. Research has demonstrated that urinary loss is influenced by either the total amount of protein or the amount of sulfur-containing amino acids consumed in the diet—the higher the intake of protein, the greater the loss of urinary calcium. Moreover, increased consumption of calcium does not compensate for the losses resulting from high protein intake, since the additional calcium is not absorbed in proportion to urinary excretion. Because the average American diet contains a large amount of protein, additional protein intake may have an adverse effect on calcium status. High protein intake probably explains, at least in part, why Eskimos, who commonly ingest as much as 200 grams of protein per day, have a high incidence of osteoporosis, a condition characterized by bone resorption and weakening.

A summary of calcium metabolism is presented in Figure 8–3.

DIETARY ALLOWANCES.   The present RDA for adults is 800 milligrams. This value was established by adding the average daily losses and correcting for the average absorption rate:

$$\left.\begin{array}{l} 175 \text{ mg (urine)} \\ + \ 125 \text{ mg (feces)} \\ + \ \ 20 \text{ mg (perspiration)} \end{array}\right\} = 320 \text{ mg/day} \div 40\% = 800 \text{ mg/day}$$

Some nutritionists consider the RDA to be unrealistically high, since many people appear to be in good health although consuming less calcium. The Food and Agricultural Organization recommends a daily intake of only 400 to 500 milligrams for adults. Others consider the present RDA to be too low, especially for women. There is some evidence that a daily intake of 1,000 to 1,500 milligrams is necessary to maintain calcium balance in this group. Although there is a theory that adapta-

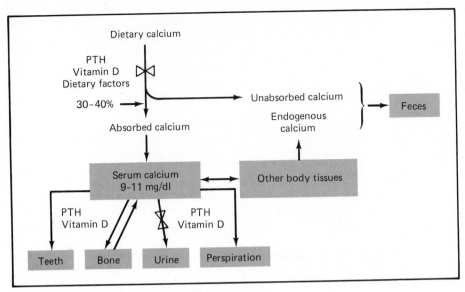

FIGURE 8-3   *Summary of Calcium Metabolism.*

tion to low intakes occurs, the effects of long-term suboptimal intake may only begin to appear in later life. Assessing the bone status and fracture rate of two communities matched for ethnic origin, physical activity, and living conditions, but very different calcium intakes, has provided one of the most important studies of long-term low intake. In the community consuming a high-calcium diet, both men and women had greater bone mass and bone density. Among the men in the high calcium district, there was a lower incidence of hip fractures; after age 59, the same was true for the women. Given these considerations, and in view of the high protein intakes in the American diet, there have been suggestions that the calcium RDA should be increased.

DIETARY SOURCES.   The primary sources of dietary calcium are dairy products (with the exception of butter), which provide 75 percent of the calcium in the American diet. Milk, cheese, ice cream, and yogurt are significant sources.

Other foods of high protein content provide variable amounts of this mineral. Clams, oysters, shrimp, and canned salmon (including the soft bones) are moderately good sources, although they are not eaten frequently or in large amounts by most people. Red meats, poultry, and most fish are not good sources. Liver, many readers will be pleased to learn, is *not* a good source. By contrast, tofu, or soybean curd, contains significant amounts of calcium. Nuts, seeds, and legumes are good sources and with vegetables constitute the primary source of calcium for vegetarians. Spinach, collard greens, beet greens, and other leafy, dark green varieties provide the largest amounts of calcium among vegetables. Fruits contain smaller quantities. Bread and grain products contribute some calcium, especially if the mold-preventive calcium propionate and dry milk solids have been added.

Table 8–2 indicates the calcium content of selected food items. In contrast to some sources of vitamins, no one food can provide the RDA for calcium in a single serving. This table does not indicate, however, a number of nondietary sources,

TABLE 8-2. *Calcium Content of Selected Foods (RDA for Adults: 800 mg)*

Food	Serving Size	Calcium Content mg/serving
Yogurt, plain, low-fat	8 oz	415
Sardines, Atlantic, in oil	1 can = 3¼ oz	402
Milk, low-fat + protein-fortified	1 c	352
Yogurt, fruit-flavored, low-fat + milk solids	8 oz	345
Milk, skim	1 c	302
Milk, whole	1 c	291
Salmon, red, canned	3½ oz	285
Yogurt, whole-milk, plain	8 oz	274
Cheddar cheese	1 oz	204
American cheese, pasteurized, processed	1 oz	174
Tofu (soybean curd) processed with calcium sulfate	1 cake (2½″ × 2¾″ × 1″)	154
Oysters, raw	½ c	113
Collard greens, cooked	½ c	110
Spinach, frozen, cooked	½ c	100
Ice cream, 10% fat	½ c	88
Beet greens, cooked	½ c	72
Soybeans, cooked	½ c	66
Molasses, medium	1 tbsp	58
Orange	1 medium	54
Beans, navy type, cooked	½ c	48
Clams, raw, meat only	4 or 5	48
Beans, green, cooked	⅔ c	42
Beans, red kidney, cooked	½ c	35
Egg	1 large	28
Egg yolk	1 large	26
Bread, whole-wheat	1 slice	25
Lentils, cooked	½ c	25
Cottage cheese, uncreamed	½ c	23
Bread, white, enriched	1 slice	21
Bran flakes, 40%	1 c	19
Yeast, dried brewers	1 tbsp	17
Halibut, broiled	3 oz	15
Apple, 3″ diameter	1	12
Apricots, dried	5 medium halves	12
Broccoli, frozen, cooked	3 spears	12
Liver, calf, cooked	3 oz	11
Hamburger, 21% fat, cooked	3 oz	9
Peanut butter	1 tbsp	9
Chicken, white meat, cooked	2 pieces	6
Egg white	1 large	4
Sugar, brown	1 tsp	3
Butter or margarine	1 pat = 1 tsp	1
Vegetable oil	1 tsp	0
Sugar, white	1 tsp	0

Sources: C. F. Adams, *Nutritive value of American foods in common units*, USDA Agriculture Handbook No. 456 (Washington, D.C.: U.S. Government Printing Office, 1975); L. P. Posati and M. L. Orr, *Composition of foods—Dairy and egg products—Raw, processed, prepared*, USDA Agriculture Handbook No. 8-1 (Washington, D.C.: U.S. Government Printing Office, 1976).

such as water supply, rocks used for grinding and cooking (for example, in Mexico, South America, and Japan), and contaminants in many of the foods available in traditional societies.

METABOLIC DISTURBANCES.   Hypocalcemia and hypercalcemia may result from disturbances in the calcium-regulating system. **Osteoporosis**, which can be defined as reduction of total bone mass and must be distinguished from osteomalacia (adult rickets, see Chapter 6), is particularly common among the elderly in all parts of the world, including the United States. Calcium deficiency is now considered to be one (but not the only) factor contributing to the development of osteoporosis. Animals fed diets deficient in calcium develop osteoporosis, and increasing the calcium intake to adequate amounts reverses the condition. The long-term study in humans which was mentioned earlier provides the best direct evidence of the role of long-term low intake in the development of osteoporosis.

Progressive alveolar bone disease leading to tooth loss has been suggested as a manifestation of osteoporosis. Loss of alveolar bone with age parallels that of finger bone, but losses started earlier in alveolar bone. Two preliminary clinical trials show that increasing calcium intake decreases alveolar bone loss; this research must be confirmed.

Phosphorus

The presence of phosphorus in the activated forms of various energy-releasing vitamins and ATP gives some indication of just how important this mineral is in the physiology and biochemistry of the body. But phosphorus has not received as much attention as other nutrients. This neglect may be due to the fact that phosphorus occurs in all plant and animal cells, and therefore in all foods. As a result, deficiency is almost unknown in humans except under certain unusual circumstances.

DISTRIBUTION IN THE BODY.   Phosphorus, the second most common mineral in the body, represents 0.8 to 1.2 percent of human body weight, or about half the amount of body calcium. Bones and teeth contain 80 to 90 percent of body phosphorus, the remainder being found in body cells and the blood.

METABOLISM AND PHYSIOLOGICAL FUNCTIONS: ABSORPTION.   Dietary phosphorus is absorbed into the body as soluble phosphate ions (PO_4^-). Combination of phosphorus with iron and magnesium will decrease its absorption. Similarly, the phosphorus-containing phytic acid found in whole-grain cereals combines with calcium to form phytate, which because it is insoluble, prevents both the calcium and phosphorus from being absorbed. Altogether, as much as 30 percent of dietary phosphorus passes through the gastrointestinal tract without being absorbed. As it does with calcium, vitamin D increases absorption of phosphorus from the intestine.

METABOLISM AND PHYSIOLOGICAL FUNCTIONS: FUNCTIONS.   The 70 percent or more of dietary phosphorus that enters the body functions in a variety of roles:

1. In the mineralization of bones and teeth (as a major component, along with calcium, of hydroxyapatite). Decreased mineralization of bone can result as much from phosphorus deficiency as from calcium deficiency.
2. As a component of various compounds essential for energy metabolism, including the phosphorylated vitamins (thiamin, niacin, riboflavin, pyri-

doxine) and ATP, the production of which also requires phosphorus-containing intermediates.

3. In absorption and transport of nutrients. Glucose must be phosphorylated in order to be absorbed from the intestine and to enter the cells of the body. Phospholipids represent the chief means of transporting lipids throughout the body fluids.
4. As components of the nucleic acids (DNA and RNA), which are vital to heredity and protein synthesis.
5. In the regulation of acid-base balance. Phosphate compounds are effective buffers.

Serum levels of phosphorus range from 35 to 45 mg/dl. Like calcium, phosphorus remains in dynamic equilibrium between cells and fluids and is continuously released from and incorporated into bone.

METABOLISM AND PHYSIOLOGICAL FUNCTIONS: EXCRETION. In contrast to calcium, for which absorption is controlled, urinary excretion provides the gatekeeper mechanism for regulating the amount of phosphorus in the body. Relatively small amounts, representing nonabsorbed and endogenous phosphorus, are excreted in the feces. As Figure 8–4 indicates, both vitamin D and PTH affect the rate at which the kidneys reabsorb phosphorus to increase serum levels of the mineral. Vitamin D increases reabsorption from the kidney, whereas PTH increases urinary excretion of phosphorus.

DIETARY ALLOWANCES. Except for infants, the recommended allowances are the same as those for calcium—that is, 800 milligrams for adults. For newborn infants, the allowances for calcium and phosphorus are 360 and 240 milligrams, respectively. Infants are at risk of developing hypocalcemia and possibly tetany not only because of the depressing effect of phosphorus on calcium absorption but also because in the first months of life PTH is not produced quickly enough or in adequate quantity in response to lowered serum calcium levels. Therefore, to prevent neonatal tetany (or neonatal hypocalcemia), the recommended allowance is lowered for phosphorus to give a calcium:phosphorus ratio of 1.5:1.0 in newborns.

FIGURE 8-4   *Summary of Phosphorus Metabolism.*

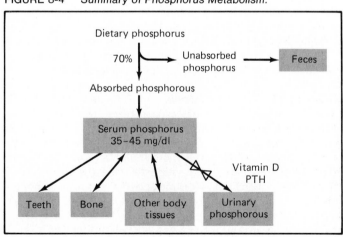

DIETARY SOURCES.   Because of the widespread distribution of phosphorus in foods, primary deficiency is highly unlikely. The milk and meat groups provide the most important sources of the mineral. High protein foods in general are good sources. Table 8–3 lists the phosphorus content of a variety of foods. The phosphorus values given in food composition tables include the amounts present in phytic acid, which may not all be biologically available. However, during the leavening and baking of whole-wheat bread, phosphorus is released from phytic acid, increasing calcium and phosphorus absorption. Habitual consumption of unleavened bread, in which the phytic acid remains intact, may contribute to the development of bone disease, particularly when vitamin D and calcium intakes are low.

METABOLIC DISTURBANCES.   Although primary deficiency of phosphorus is rare, excessive and long-term use of antacids that contain aluminum hydroxide can produce symptoms of hypophosphatemia—weakness, anorexia (loss of appetite), and bone demineralization. Other factors and conditions, including use of anticonvulsants (for example, phenobarbital), vitamin D deficiency, certain metabolic abnormalities, and inadequate reabsorption by the kidneys, can produce symptoms of phosphorus deficiency. Hyperphosphatemia can result from renal disease.

Magnesium

The characteristic purgative effects of magnesium became known, almost two centuries before the element itself was identified, with the accidental discovery of a pool of bitter-tasting water in the village of Epsom, England, in 1618. People who drank the water felt healthfully purified, and later in the century its salts were crystallized and marketed, to great acclaim. Sir Humphrey Davy isolated magnesium, the key component of Epsom salts, in 1808, and since then this element has become well known for its use in photographic flashes, flares, and incendiary bombs and as a metal greatly valued for its lightness in space-age technology.

Magnesium is to plants what iron is—as we shall see—to animals. Just as iron is the "core" atom of hemoglobin, magnesium is the "core" atom of chlorophyll, the green pigment that enables plants, in the presence of light, to transform carbon dioxide and water into carbohydrates. It thus has some claim to being, after carbon, the element most important to life.

DISTRIBUTION IN THE BODY.   The human body contains considerably less magnesium than it does either calcium or phosphorus. The total magnesium content of an adult weighing 70 kilograms (154 lb) averages between 20 and 28 grams. Of this total, a little over half occurs in bone; slightly more than one-quarter in muscle; and the remainder in other soft tissues, serum, and red blood cells.

METABOLISM AND PHYSIOLOGICAL FUNCTIONS.   The body absorbs about 35 to 40 percent of dietary magnesium by active transport from the intestine. However, the percent absorbed varies inversely with dietary intake. That is, as dietary magnesium increases in quantity, the efficiency of absorption decreases. In this respect magnesium resembles calcium and may even share the same transport system. Many of the factors that influence calcium absorption also affect the absorption of magnesium, though to a lesser degree; the intestine apparently is not a major control point in magnesium metabolism. Also, there is little fecal excretion of endogenous magnesium.

The physiological importance of magnesium is clearly reflected in the number

TABLE 8-3. *Phosphorus Content of Selected Foods (RDA for Adults: 800 mg)*

Food	Serving Size	Phosphorus Content mg/serving
Liver, beef, cooked	3 oz	405
Yogurt, low-fat + milk solids	8 oz	326
Yogurt, fruit-flavored + milk solids	8 oz	271
Chicken, cooked	3½ oz	266
Milk, skim	1 c	247
Milk, 2% fat	1 c	232
Milk, whole	1 c	228
Yogurt, plain, whole-milk	8 oz	215
American cheese, pasteurized, processed	1 oz	211
Haddock, fried	3 oz	210
Tuna, canned	3½ oz	188
Swiss cheese	1 oz	171
Soybeans, cooked	½ c	161
Hamburger, 21% fat, cooked	3 oz	159
Cheddar cheese	1 oz	145
Bran flakes, 40%	1 c	125
Potato, baked in skin	1 medium	101
Egg	1 large	90
Egg yolk	1 large	86
Peas, green, cooked	½ c	79
Frankfurter	1	76
Cottage cheese, uncreamed	½ c	75
Ice cream, 10% fat	½ c	67
Peanut butter	1 tbsp	61
Bread, whole-wheat	1 slice	57
Collard greens, cooked	½ c	50
Broccoli, cooked	½ c	48
Avocado	1 half	47
Raisins	small box = 1½ oz	43
Spinach, cooked	½ c	34
Orange	1 medium	33
Cola beverage	6 oz	30
Rice, cooked	½ c	28
Bread, white, enriched	1 slice	28
Banana	1 medium	27
Tomato	1 medium	25
Carrots, cooked	½ c	24
Green beans, cooked	½ c	23
Egg white	1 large	4
Butter	1 pat = 1 tsp	1
Margarine	1 pat = 1 tsp	0.7

Sources: C. F. Adams, *Nutritive value of American foods in common units*, USDA Agriculture Handbook No. 456 (Washington, D.C.: U.S. Government Printing Office, 1975); L. P. Posati and M. L. Orr, *Composition of foods—Dairy and egg products—Raw, processed, prepared*, USDA Agriculture Handbook No. 8-1 (Washington, D.C.: U.S. Government Printing Office, 1976).

and variety of its functions in the body. Many of these functions depend on the mineral's ability to interact with calcium, phosphate, and carbonate ions. In a complicated relationship, magnesium plays an important role in bone metabolism. Equally important, this mineral catalyzes many essential enzymatic reactions, playing a crucial role in glucose and fatty acid metabolism, amino acid activation, and synthesis of ATP. Protein synthesis also requires magnesium, directly or indirectly, at several different stages. Magnesium is important (along with calcium, sodium, potassium, and phosphorus) in nervous activity and muscle contraction. At certain stages of neuromuscular activity, the interaction between magnesium and calcium is antagonistic; at others, synergistic (enhancing). Such interactions are particularly significant because the metabolism of calcium, sodium, and potassium are all affected by any deficiency of magnesium.

Serum levels of this essential mineral are controlled by urinary excretion, which is influenced by the adrenal hormone **aldosterone** (see Chapter 9). When usual amounts of magnesium are ingested, urinary excretion normally amounts to 100 to 200 milligrams of the mineral per day. This amount, however, is rapidly diminished if intake decreases, and as quickly increases in response to more ample supplies.

DIETARY ALLOWANCES.   Because the magnesium content of foods is highly variable, dietary intakes of the mineral are also variable. According to current estimates, typical American diets provide from 180 to 480 mg of magnesium per day, or 120 mg per 1,000 kcal. Various studies have led to the establishment of RDAs of 350 mg for adult males and 300 mg for adult females. Thus, intake of 300 mg of magnesium would require a 2,500 kcal intake. Many individuals, therefore, especially women, may not consume the recommended amounts of magnesium. However, it appears that women lose less of the mineral and are able to maintain equilibrium levels on lower intakes than men. Symptoms of magnesium deficiency are not prevalent, and the body may well adjust to less than optimal intakes.

DIETARY SOURCES.   Dairy products are the best sources of magnesium, followed by breads and cereals, vegetables, meats and poultry, and fruits. Of the vegetables, green, leafy types are best because of their chlorophyll content. Legumes and whole grains also contain significant amounts. Some loss of the mineral results from food processing and preparation, including loss when cooking water is discarded. Table 8–4 gives the magnesium content of selected foods.

Milk of magnesia should not be considered a dietary source of magnesium. Commonly used as a laxative, it acts by drawing water from cells into the intestine and by increasing intestinal motility. The use of milk of magnesia as an antacid (to neutralize stomach acidity) may produce diarrhea as a side effect. Because of its effect on water balance, overuse of this substance represents a potential hazard to those with kidney problems.

METABOLIC DISTURBANCES.   Because of the mineral's wide availability in foods and because of the body's reserve in bone, depletion of body stores proceeds slowly. This may mask a borderline deficiency, and magnesium deficiency may be more common than is generally recognized.

Primary deficiency can result from dietary insufficiency; malabsorption; and prolonged, severe diarrhea and vomiting. Secondary deficiency can be caused by diuretics, overconsumption of alcohol, kidney disease, acute pancreatitis, and cirrhosis of the liver, among other disease conditions. Regardless of cause, magnesium deficiency produces clinical symptoms indistinguishable from hypocalcemic tetany—mainly muscle contraction and nervous irritability. Other common symptoms include tremor, disorientation, and confusion.

TABLE 8-4. *Magnesium Content of Selected Foods (RDA for Adults: Men 350 mg; Women 300 mg)*

Food	Serving Size	Magnesium Content mg/serving
Peanuts, roasted	¼ c	63
Banana	1 medium	58
Beet greens, raw	1 c	58
Avocado	1 half	56
Molasses, blackstrap	1 tbsp	52
Cashew nuts	9 medium	52
Milk, 2% fat, protein-fortified	1 c	40
Swiss chard, raw	1 c	37
Milk, whole	1 c	33
Yogurt, fruit-flavored + milk solids	8 oz	33
Collard greens, raw	1 c	31
Milk, skim	1 c	28
Peanut butter	1 tbsp	28
Spinach, raw	1 c	28
Oysters, raw	6 medium	27
Yogurt, plain	8 oz	26
Macaroni, cooked	1 c	26
Pork, fresh, roasted	3 oz	25
Turkey, light meat, roasted	3 oz	24
Wheat bran	1 tbsp	20
Wheat germ	1 tbsp	20
Hamburger, lean, cooked	3 oz	20
Haddock, fried	3 oz	20
Bread, whole-wheat	1 slice	19
Carrots, raw	1 medium	19
Yeast, brewer's	1 tbsp	18
Chicken, broiled w/o skin	3 oz	16
Orange, peeled	1 medium	15
Apple, 3″ diameter	1	14
Beans, green, frozen	½ c	14
Ice cream, 10% fat	½ c	9
Cheddar cheese	1 oz	8
American cheese	1 oz	6
Bacon, cooked	3 strips	6
Egg, whole	1 large	6
Bread, white	1 slice	5.5
Cornflakes	1 c	4
Egg yolk	1 large	3
Egg white	1 large	3
Mushrooms, raw	¼ c	2
Butter	1 pat = 1 tsp	trace
Vegetable oil	1 tbsp	0

Sources: C. F. Adams, *Nutritive value of American foods in common units*, USDA Agriculture Handbook No. 456 (Washington, D.C.: U.S. Government Printing Office, 1975); L. P. Posati and M. L. Orr, *Composition of foods—Dairy and egg products—Raw, processed, prepared*, USDA Agriculture Handbook No. 8-1 (Washington, D.C.: U.S. Government Printing Office, 1976); Consumer and Food Economics Institute, *Composition of foods, raw, processed, prepared*, USDA Handbook No. 8, rev. ed. (Washington, D.C.: U.S. Government Printing Office, 1963).

Sodium

Although sodium can be obtained from a variety of foods, by far the best-known source is common table salt, or sodium chloride (NaCl). This compound is unique in that its historical importance has been much greater than its undeniable value as a source of nutrients would seem to justify. Wars have been fought over salt deposits. Women and children have been traded for salt. Long before similar methods were known in Europe, the Chinese had developed sophisticated techniques for obtaining salt from underground deposits that were too deep to be mined directly. And today salt is the one mineral source for which the demand is so great that the production of dietary salt constitutes a significant industry in itself.

Herbivorous animals (cattle, deer, horses) are attracted to salt licks, but carnivores are not. Meat-eating animals apparently get adequate amounts of sodium with the flesh they consume. The early human diet, consisting largely of animals, provided an adequate sodium supply. When agriculture developed, dietary intake of grains and vegetables increased. Additional sources of salt therefore became important.

Human sodium intakes can vary tremendously. Some people consume none other than that occurring naturally in the foods they eat. Others put salt "on everything," whereas the majority steer a course somewhere between these two extremes.

DISTRIBUTION IN THE BODY.   The adult body contains about 120 grams of sodium. Approximately half of the total is found in body fluids outside the cells, with an additional third bound to the skeletal surface. Intracellular sodium represents about 10 percent of the total body content.

Herbivorous animals (cattle, deer, horses) are attracted to salt licks to satisfy their sodium requirements.
Paul W. Nesbit/Photo Researchers

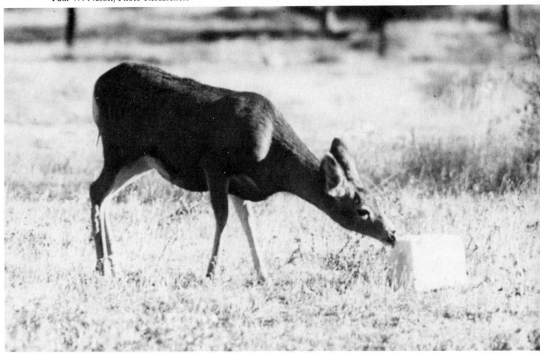

METABOLISM AND PHYSIOLOGICAL FUNCTIONS.   Dietary sodium is absorbed rapidly and with almost perfect efficiency, very little being lost in the feces. Absorption, therefore, does not regulate sodium metabolism.

The concentration of sodium (and other ions) in the different body fluids affects the direction of fluid movement between body compartments. In turn, the control of fluid volume is directly related to blood pressure.

Sodium also functions in the control of acid-base balance, plays a part in both carbohydrate and protein metabolism, and has a major role in the generation of nerve impulses. (A nerve impulse arises, in part, from the electrical change produced by the sudden flow of sodium ions across the nerve-cell membrane—from the outside to the inside of the nerve cell.)

The kidneys represent the main regulatory means for controlling the sodium content of the body. Except for losses through perspiration, the amount excreted in the urine usually balances dietary intake. Since the gatekeeper mechanism in this case is reabsorption in the tubules of the kidneys, the kidneys are able to maintain sodium balance over a wide range of dietary intakes. As Figure 8–5 indicates, however, ultimate control lies in the adrenal glands, which produce aldosterone. This hormone increases reabsorption of sodium by the kidney. Some medications also modify urinary excretion. Diuretics, for example, increase sodium loss.

Loss of sodium through perspiration depends on the volume of sweat. Normal losses range from 230 to 575 milligrams per day, but heavy sweating can result in losses as great as 8 grams per day! Cystic fibrosis, a disease that affects the exocrine glands such as the sweat glands, also leads to large losses of the mineral.

DIETARY ALLOWANCES AND SOURCES.   The Food and Nutrition Board has not established an RDA for sodium. The average daily intake of salt, which is the chief source of dietary sodium, ranges from 6 to 24 grams. Since sodium constitutes 40 percent (by weight) of salt, this intake is equivalent to 2.4 to 9.6 grams of the mineral per day. (A pinch of salt contains about 300 mg of sodium; 1 teaspoon, over

FIGURE 8-5   *Summary of Sodium Metabolism.*

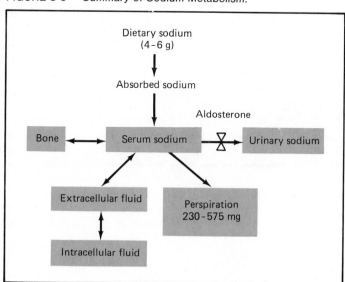

2,000 mg.) Studies have indicated that the average individual *requires* only 0.5 to 1.0 grams for nutritional health. However, this is a minimal amount, and the Food and Nutrition Board recommends a daily intake of 1,100 to 3,300 mg for adults (or 1.1 to 3.3 g).

Most dietary sodium comes from table salt, but it is found also in other inorganic salts used during some food-processing procedures. Sodium is found in a wide variety of foods as well (see Table 8–5)—so readily found, in fact, that it is quite difficult to eliminate this mineral from the diet. Meats and many dairy products are naturally rich in the mineral, and most processed foods contain sodium either as salt added to enhance flavor or in a variety of preservative compounds. Moreover, salt is commonly added to food during cooking and also at the table. Drinking water contains variable amounts of salt, possibly including "road salt" used to melt snow and ice in winter. Many drugs contain sodium as well. Considering this multiplicity of sources, sodium deficiency is a rather remote possibility.

METABOLIC DISTURBANCES.   Lowered serum levels of sodium can result from insufficient production of adrenocortical hormones and from prolonged, excessive sweating. Prolonged diarrhea and vomiting can also produce sodium depletion. Addition of salt to drinking water (1 g NaCl/1 liter H_2O) or to food quickly relieves deficiency symptoms, which include nausea, giddiness, muscle cramps, and vomiting. In extreme cases, sodium deficiency can cause circulatory failure.

Potassium

DISTRIBUTION IN THE BODY.   Functionally, potassium is closely associated with sodium. But in contrast to sodium, potassium is concentrated inside the cells. Nerve and muscle cells are especially rich in potassium. Fluid outside the cells contains less than 5 percent of the total body amount (approximately 250 g).

METABOLISM AND PHYSIOLOGICAL FUNCTIONS.   The body absorbs potassium efficiently, and very little potassium appears in the feces.

The main functions of potassium are the same as those of sodium: maintenance of fluid balance and volume. Other functions include a role in carbohydrate metabolism, enhancement of protein synthesis, and muscle contraction and nerve impulse conduction.

The mechanism for regulating body potassium is urinary excretion, which removes excess amounts of the mineral. Aldosterone increases excretion of potassium, just the opposite of its effect on sodium. The body cannot conserve potassium as efficiently as sodium, and the potential for deficiency is thus greater. Potassium is also lost through perspiration; heavy exercise in hot conditions can cause potassium losses that exceed 6 grams per day. For a summary of potassium metabolism, see Figure 8–6.

DIETARY ALLOWANCES AND SOURCES.   Although the Food and Nutrition Board has not yet established an RDA for potassium, it recommends a daily intake of 1,875 to 5,625 mg for adults. The typical American diet provides 2 to 6 grams per day.

Because the mineral is widely distributed in foods (see Table 8–6), obtaining sufficient dietary potassium presents no difficulty. Meat and dairy products (other than cheese, from which potassium is lost in the whey) are good sources. Fruits,

TABLE 8-5. *Sodium Content of Selected Foods* (*Estimated Safe and Adequate Daily Dietary Intake for Adults: 1,100–3,300 mg*)

Food	Serving Size	Sodium Content mg/serving
Soy sauce	1 tbsp	1,319
Bouillon	1 cube	960
Olives, green, large	10	926
Ham	3 oz	770
Frankfurter	1	627
Cottage cheese, creamed	½ c	425
American cheese, pasteurized, processed	1 oz	406
Rice, cooked in salted water	½ c	383
Tomato juice, canned	6 fl. oz	364
Salad dressing, Italian	1 tbsp	314
Table salt	1 pinch	267
Bran flakes, 40%	1 c	207
Peas, canned, cooked	½ c	200
Beets, canned, cooked	½ c	200
Cheddar cheese	1 oz	176
Liver, beef, cooked	3 oz	156
Bacon, cooked	3 slices	153
Haddock, cooked	3 oz	150
Milk, 2% fat, protein-fortified	1 c	145
Bread, white, enriched	1 slice	134
Bread, whole-wheat	1 slice	132
Milk, skim	1 c	126
Milk, whole	1 c	120
Peanut butter	1 tbsp	97
Egg, whole	1 large	69
Chicken, meat only	3½ oz	64
Ice cream, 10% fat	½ c	58
Celery	1 stalk	50
Egg, white	1 large	50
Hamburger, 21% fat, cooked	3 oz	49
Spinach, cooked	½ c	45
Margarine, salted	1 pat	41
Butter, salted	1 pat	41
Tuna fish	3½ oz	41
Beets, fresh, cooked	½ c	36
Carrots, cooked	½ c	26
Raisins	small box = 1½ oz	12
Egg yolk	1 large	8
Broccoli, cooked	½ c	8
Potato, baked	1 large	6
Avocado	1 half	5
Soybeans, cooked	½ c	2
Orange	1 medium	2
Peas, fresh, cooked	½ c	1
Banana	1 medium	1

Sources: C. F. Adams, *Nutritive value of American foods in common units*, USDA Agriculture Handbook No. 456 (Washington, D.C.: U.S. Government Printing Office, 1975); L. P. Posati and M. L. Orr, *Composition of foods—Dairy and egg products—Raw, processed, prepared*, USDA Agriculture Handbook No. 8-1 (Washington, D.C.: U.S. Government Printing Office, 1976).

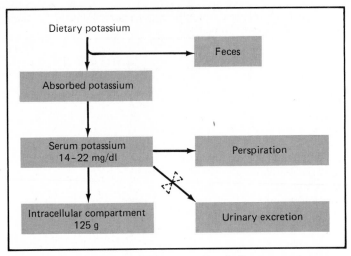

FIGURE 8-6   *Summary of Potassium Metabolism.*

vegetables, and whole-grain products are also good sources of potassium; these foods have the added advantage of being low in sodium.

Preparation and cooking cause some potassium loss. Water leaches out the mineral, and the loss increases with the amount of surface area exposed. To conserve potassium, food should not be finely cut, cooked in a large amount of water, or cooked in water for an extended period of time. On the other hand, these methods provide a way to reduce the potassium content of foods for those on restricted diets, as in the case of kidney disease; potatoes, for example, are cut into small cubes, soaked in water which is discarded, and finally cooked in additional water.

METABOLIC DISTURBANCES.   Potassium deficiency is rare but may result from starvation, drugs that increase its urinary excretion (such as diuretics used in the treatment of hypertension), diarrhea, and adrenal tumors (which increase the production of aldosterone). Aldosterone production is also increased when physiological or emotional stress stimulates the anterior pituitary gland to release **ACTH** (the "stress hormone"), with consequent potassium loss. Clinical symptoms of deficiency include nausea, vomiting (which itself can result in potassium loss), muscle weakness, tachycardia (rapid heart beat), and—in extreme cases—cardiac failure.

Hyperkalemia, or excess potassium in the blood, occurs in cases of renal failure because the kidneys lose the ability to excrete the mineral. Severe dehydration will also produce hyperkalemia. The consequences of this condition are muscle weakness and cardiac arhythmias that lead to heart failure.

Chloride

DISTRIBUTION IN THE BODY.   As the chloride ion (Cl^-), chlorine is the primary anion found in fluid outside the cells and particularly in cerebrospinal fluid. Less than 15 percent of the body's total of 74 grams (for adults) is in intracellular fluid. Chloride is mostly associated with sodium but also occurs in protein-bound forms.

TABLE 8-6. *Potassium Content of Selected Foods (Estimated Safe and Adequate Daily Dietary Intake for Adults: 1,875–5,625 mg)*

Food	Serving Size	Potassium Content mg/serving
Potato, baked in skin	1 medium	782
Avocado	1 half	680
Yogurt, plain, low-fat + milk solids	8 oz	531
Soybeans, cooked	½ c	486
Yogurt, fruit-flavored + milk solids	8 oz	442
Banana	1 medium	440
Chicken, meat only	3½ oz	412
Milk, skim	1 c	406
Milk, 2% fat + milk solids	1 c	397
Milk, 2% fat	1 c	377
Milk, whole	1 c	370
Yogurt, plain	8 oz	351
Raisins	small box = 1½ oz	328
Liver, beef, cooked	3 oz	323
Haddock, fried	3 oz	300
Spinach, cooked	½ c	291
Orange	1 medium	291
Tuna, canned	3½ oz	276
Collard greens, cooked	½ c	249
Tomato	1 medium	222
Hamburger, 21% fat, cooked	3 oz	221
Broccoli, cooked	½ c	207
Apple	1 medium	165
Carrots, cooked	½ c	162
Peas, green, fresh, cooked	½ c	157
Bran flakes, 40%	1 c	137
Celery	1 stalk	136
Ice cream, 10% fat	½ c	128
Frankfurter	1	125
Peanut butter	1 tbsp	100
Green beans, cooked	½ c	95
Bread, whole-wheat	1 slice	68
Coffee, prepared	1 c = 6 oz	65
Egg, whole	1 large	65
American cheese, pasteurized, processed	1 oz	46
Egg, white	1 large	45
Bacon, cooked	2 slices	35
Bread, white, enriched	1 slice	33
Rice, cooked	½ c	28
Cheddar cheese	1 oz	28
Cottage cheese, uncreamed	½ c	24
Cranberry juice	6 oz	19
Egg yolk	1 large	15
Butter or margarine	1 pat = 1 tsp	1

Sources: C. F. Adams, *Nutritive value of American foods in common units,* USDA Agriculture Handbook No. 456 (Washington, D.C.: U.S. Government Printing Office, 1975); L. P. Posati and M. L. Orr, *Composition of foods—Dairy and egg products—Raw, processed, prepared,* USDA Agriculture Handbook No. 8-1 (Washington, D.C.: U.S. Government Printing Office, 1976).

METABOLISM AND PHYSIOLOGICAL FUNCTIONS. The body absorbs almost all dietary chloride. The most usual source of dietary chloride is as a component of common table salt.

Chloride helps maintain the acid-base balance of the blood. It is also a component of the hydrochloric acid in gastric juice and is therefore involved in the digestion of dietary protein and absorption of vitamin B_{12}. Other functions include the mineral's role in maintaining the flow and composition of body fluids and the activation of amylase enzymes that accelerate the digestion of starch.

The control of chloride levels involves the same mechanism that regulates sodium—reabsorption in the tubules of the kidneys. Excess chloride appears in the urine. Variable amounts are lost via the feces and sweat. Because of its presence in hydrochloric acid, significant amounts of the mineral may be lost through vomiting.

DIETARY ALLOWANCES AND SOURCES. No RDAs have been established for chloride, but the Food and Nutrition Board has recommended an intake of 1,700 to 5,100 mg per day for adults. Intake is usually adequate as long as sodium intake is sufficient. The amount of salt in the average diet assures a more than adequate dietary supply.

METABOLIC DISTURBANCES. Abnormal chloride metabolism commonly occurs in association with disturbances in sodium metabolism. Vomiting and diarrhea can produce chloride loss, resulting in hypochloremic alkalosis. The latter may also accompany hypokalemia.

Because the kidneys excrete excess chloride, *dietary* chloride has no known toxicity. (Note the emphasis on "dietary"—chlorine gas is deadly!)

Sulfur

DISTRIBUTION IN THE BODY. All body cells contain sulfur, chiefly as a component of the amino acids methionine and cysteine found in many proteins. Sulfur also occurs in a number of important metabolic compounds, including acetyl CoA and the water-soluble vitamins thiamin and biotin. Because of the specific structural amino acids they contain, the proteins of hair, skin, and nails are especially high in sulfur content.

METABOLISM AND PHYSIOLOGICAL FUNCTIONS. The body absorbs sulfur mainly in the form of sulfur-containing amino acids and absorbs the remainder as inorganic sulfate.

The important functions of sulfur include its roles as a component of (1) sulfur-containing amino acids; (2) the sulfur groups of various compounds essential to certain oxidation-reduction reactions: coenzyme A, thiamin, biotin, glutathione; (3) insulin and certain other hormones and the anticoagulant heparin; (4) such compounds as the mucopolysaccharides and sulfated lipids that are components of the structural tissues of the body; and (5) taurocholic acid, a bile acid derived in part from the amino acid cystine.

Sulfur is excreted in the urine as inorganic sulfate. Urinary output averages 2 grams per day and is proportional to nitrogen excretion (because most of the sulfate is derived from amino acid metabolism). Small amounts are excreted in the feces.

DIETARY ALLOWANCES AND SOURCES. No RDA has been established for this mineral. The sulfur content of foods parallels that of methionine and cystine. Adequate intakes are not a problem in the average American diet, with large protein intake from varied sources. Approximately 1 percent of dietary protein is sulfur. However, the amino acid composition of protein must be considered by strict vegetarians, since grains are low in the sulfur-containing essential amino acids (see Chapter 4). Vegetarians who consume a variety of foods in addition to grains are not likely to be at risk in developing a sulfur deficiency.

TRACE MINERALS

Although essential trace elements differ chemically from vitamins, they resemble the latter in several important respects: They are required by the body in very small amounts; they influence biochemical reactions, functioning either as components or activators of enzymes, vitamins, or hormones; and their nutritional function is influenced by other members of the same nutrient class.

The main problem facing researchers who study these micronutrients is the accurate determination of optimal nutritional requirements. The problem is important because many trace elements can be toxic in larger amounts. (Copper and fluoride are two well-known examples.) The difficulty of determining requirements is aggravated because trace minerals are effective in such tiny amounts in the body and because absorption is affected dramatically by the composition of the diet (fiber, phytates, and other nutrients). Only in recent years have new techniques of biochemical assay begun to analyze and accurately measure these elusive substances. In addition, the widespread use of processed foods from which trace minerals have been removed is of concern to nutritionists because inadequate intakes may result if people eat nothing but highly processed food.

Each micronutrient can be classified in one of three groups, depending on what is known about its dietary requirement: (1) those for which a well-defined allowance has been established (iron, zinc, and iodine); (2) those for which "provisional" allowances have been suggested (copper, chromium, manganese, molybdenum, fluoride, and selenium); and (3) the "newer" trace elements, which occur in such minute amounts that present analytical techniques do not permit even an estimate of dietary requirement (cobalt, silicon, tin, vanadium, and nickel).

Iron

The importance of iron as part of hemoglobin in red blood cells is well known, although iron has other functions as well. Iron-deficiency anemia is a widespread health problem in the United States, particularly among children and women of childbearing age regardless of socioeconomic status. Iron-deficiency anemia is rightly a major nutritional concern.

DISTRIBUTION IN THE BODY. Despite its great importance, the total body content of iron averages no more than several grams (0.004 percent of body weight). All body cells contain some iron, but the mineral is concentrated in red blood cells. For men, the average total body concentration ranges from 40 to 50 milligrams per kilo-

Perspective On

MINERALS AND HYPERTENSION

In humans, the principle determinate of blood pressure is change in peripheral resistance. Hypertension, or high blood pressure, develops as the result of a number of factors, including genetic predisposition, cigarette smoking, environmental stresses, a "high-strung" or "Type A" personality, and obesity. Epidemiological and research data suggest a role for several minerals, such as sodium, calcium, and magnesium in the development of hypertension.

SODIUM. Epidemiologic data show a relationship between sodium intake and high blood pressure. Populations with low intakes have stable blood pressure throughout life. In contrast, in countries with higher intakes, such as the United States where an estimated 20 percent of the adult population has hypertension, blood pressure increases with age. Examining the data carefully reveals that not everyone is equally susceptible to hypertension; even while consuming a high sodium intake, apparently it develops only in predisposed individuals.

The relationship between sodium and elevated blood pressure is based on sodium's ability to "attract" water; that is, the more sodium present in the body, the more water is retained along with the sodium. The retention of the additional water serves to dilute the sodium concentration in the body and more specifically, in the bloodstream. However, it also increases the total blood volume, and this greater volume exerts greater pressure on blood vessel walls.

Dietary sodium intake is not the only factor in sodium concentration of the blood. Individuals with heart or kidney diseases have a greatly decreased ability to excrete sodium in the urine; as a result, sodium and fluid are retained.

Finally, sodium in foods is not the only source of sodium. Drinking water may provide up to 10 percent of the total intake. Many drugs, particularly nonprescription drugs, also contain sodium, either as part of an active ingredient or as an inert vehicle with which the active drug is mixed. Although the total amount of sodium ingested by this route by the average American cannot be measured accurately, drugs can be a significant source of sodium in the diet.

Just as hypertension has no single cause, so it has no one means of treatment. Dietary restriction of sodium and weight loss are generally part of the treatment; the loss of excess weight in itself can often lower moderately elevated blood pressure even without reducing sodium intake. Drugs that increase sodium excretion (diuretics) or that modify tone and flexibility of blood vessels are often prescribed for hypertension.

Salt substitutes should be used with caution. Many are not really substitutes; as much as 50 percent of the product may be ordinary salt or sodium chloride. Moreover, the replacement is often potassium chloride, which can lead to excessive blood potassium levels and place an ad-

gram of body weight. Of this amount, 60 to 70 percent is present in hemoglobin, 30 percent is stored, and the remainder functions as a component of various substances, in particular the cytochrome enzymes of the electron transport system (see Chapter 7). Hemoglobin and storage levels of iron are generally lower for women than for men, the total body iron for women ranging from 35 to 50 milligrams per kilogram of body weight.

METABOLISM AND PHYSIOLOGICAL FUNCTIONS: ABSORPTION. Absorption provides the gatekeeper mechanism for regulating iron metabolism. Since the body has no effective means of eliminating iron, and excess amounts are toxic, the body strictly regulates the quantities permitted to enter. Indeed, absorption of iron—which may

ditional burden on the kidneys, a dangerous situation for those with kidney disease. For similar reasons, ammonium-containing salt substitutes should not be used by those with liver disease. If these products are used at all, it should be only with a physician's approval. Those who are advised to decrease their salt intake can find helpful ideas in the many good low-salt diet cookbooks now available. The use of alternate seasonings—lemon juice, garlic, herbs, and spices—will add flavor and variety to meals; a low-salt diet does not have to be boring and bland.

CALCIUM. While long recongized for its role in skeletal muscle contraction and relaxation, more recent research has suggested a role for calcium in regulation of blood pressure. In 1960, the first epidemiological observation linking calcium content of water and cardiovascular disease was observed by Schroeder. Since that time some data support the hypothesis and other data does not. Some of the inconsistencies of the results may be attributed to the small amount of calcium coming from drinking water compared to the amount coming from dietary sources.

Support of a role for calcium in hypertension comes from a variety of studies. Women with osteoporosis, who are typically in negative calcium balance, are more likely to have hypertension than women without osteoporosis. Several studies have shown that greater consumption of calcium is related to lower blood pressure. Experimental evidence for the role of calcium in hypertension comes mainly from studies of a type of rat which develops hypertension spontaneously. Supplementing the diets of these rats with calcium results in a significant decrease in their blood pressure. Conversely, removing or lowering the amount of dietary calcium results in increased blood pressure. Thus for small studies of supplementation of humans with hypertension have been positive, but further studies are needed both on the direct effects of calcium supplementation and on sodium/calcium interactions. The mechanism by which calcium affects blood pressure has not been demonstrated at this time.

MAGNESIUM. There is also evidence from animal studies that hypomagnesemia (low concentrations of magnesium in the blood) results in an elevation of blood pressure. Epidemiological data suggest a decrease in dietary intake of magnesium. The two types of evidence support a possible role for magnesium in human hypertension, but more direct evidence is necessary before making any suggestions regarding intake.

The above data herald an interesting and hopefully productive period in the study of mineral metabolism. Eventually we will have a better understanding of which minerals are involved in the control of hypertension and their interactions with each other.

vary from 2 to 40 percent of intake, with an average in the 5 to 15 percent range—is a complex process which is not completely understood.

Many factors influence the amount of iron absorbed. Of major importance are (1) metabolic need, which increases when iron stores are low, following hemorrhage or blood donation, and during pregnancy, lactation, and growth; (2) the nature of the dietary iron; and (3) the presence or absence of other dietary nutrients that influence the absorption of iron. But to understand just how these factors affect absorption requires some understanding of the general regulatory mechanism involved.

There are two types of dietary iron, *heme* and *nonheme*. Heme iron is found in hemoglobin (hence its name) and muscle myoglobin and is obtained exclusively from meats. The one factor that appears to determine absorption of organically bound or heme iron is iron status. If body stores are adequate, approximately 25 percent of ingested heme iron will be absorbed. Absorption can be as high as 35 percent if stores are depleted. Thus, absorption of dietary heme iron is inversely proportional to iron status.

Absorption of nonheme iron, found in both animal and vegetable foods, is a much more complex process than that of heme iron. Inorganic iron occurs in foods primarily in oxidized form as the ferric ion (Fe^{+++}). The reduced form, ferrous iron (Fe^{++}), is more readily absorbed, however, because it is more soluble in digestive juices. Thus factors that affect the reduction of iron also affect its absorption. Particularly important in this respect is the pH or acidity of the stomach and the upper part of the small intestine. The presence of both ascorbic acid and fructose increases absorption by enhancing the conversion of ferric to ferrous ion.

Another absorption-enhancing factor for nonheme iron is present in meat, poultry, and fish as an otherwise unidentified "meat factor." Protein per se does not enhance absorption of nonheme iron, but beef, lamb, liver, pork, chicken, and fish do and are therefore considered to contain the "meat factor" (in addition to the heme iron that is absorbed). Milk, cheese, eggs, and some other foods may actually decrease absorption. Specific factors known to decrease the availability of nonheme iron include antacids, tannic acid (in tea), phytates, phosvitin (in egg yolk), and calcium and phosphate salts.

Both heme and nonheme iron enter the mucosal cells lining the upper intestine. Heme iron is first absorbed as part of the porphyrin component of hemoglobin, then released to join the "pool" of inorganic iron on which the body draws as necessary. The iron binds with a specific protein to form a compound known as *ferritin*. This molecule acts as a "holding bin" of sorts and never actually leaves the mucosal cell. Ferritin is lost when the mucosal cells are sloughed off into the intestinal lumen. Iron is transported by the protein transferrin, which circulates in the blood. When body stores are adequate, the transferrin molecules are "fully booked" with iron and will not accept any more iron "passengers" from the mucosal cells. When body stores are low, however, the transferrin molecules contain less iron and will more readily pick up more iron atoms from ferritin molecules in the mucosal cells. Thus, only a small portion of absorbed iron actually enters the circulation. That portion varies according to the amount being carried by the circulating transferrin molecules, which in turn depends on the iron stores. Clearly, iron absorption is a tightly regulated process.

Transferrin delivers iron to the bone marrow, where red blood cells (erythrocytes) are synthesized, and to such storage sites as the spleen and liver, where iron is stored as the proteins ferritin and hemosiderin. Transferrin also shuttles iron to other tissues, as well as between tissues, of the body.

Unlike other cells, erythrocytes lose their nuclei in the course of maturation. Because they are therefore lacking any DNA, cell replication and protein synthesis cannot occur. This is why they become "old" and "die" and must be replaced by new red blood cells synthesized "from scratch." This process begins in the bone marrow, where stem cells are produced (see Figure 8–7). These in turn give rise to white blood cells and erythroblasts, the nucleus-containing cells. Each erythroblast divides, in the presence of vitamin B_{12} and folic acid, to form two new cells, which in the presence of vitamin B_6, incorporate iron into hemoglobin. Every second 2.5 million erythrocytes, 20,000 white blood cells, and 5 million platelets are sent into the circulation.

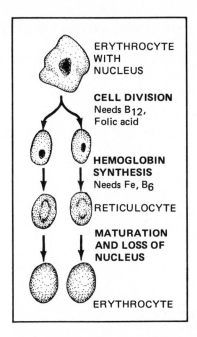

ERYTHROCYTE
WITH
NUCLEUS

CELL DIVISION
Needs B_{12},
Folic acid

**HEMOGLOBIN
SYNTHESIS**
Needs Fe, B_6

RETICULOCYTE

**MATURATION
AND LOSS OF
NUCLEUS**

ERYTHROCYTE

FIGURE 8-7
*Normal Production of Red
Blood Cells.*

METABOLISM AND PHYSIOLOGICAL FUNCTIONS: FUNCTIONS.   The major function of iron is oxygen transport. It accomplishes this as a component of two different transport molecules, hemoglobin in red blood cells and myoblobin in muscle. Four heme groups combine with the protein globin to form a single molecule of hemoglobin. Each red blood cell contains over 250 million hemoglobin molecules, which means that a single cell can transport to the body more than a billion molecules of oxygen from their entry point in the lungs. The oxygen is required by the body for energy production by aerobic metabolism. Hemoglobin also transports CO_2, a byproduct of cellular metabolism, back to the lungs for excretion.

The amount of iron in myoglobin is only one-quarter that in hemoglobin, or one atom of iron per molecule of myoglobin. This protein functions as a temporary oxygen reserve in muscle metabolism.

As a component of cytochromes in the electron transport system, iron has an important role in cell respiration. Other essential iron-containing compounds include such enzymes as catalase and xanthine oxidase. The latter is involved in the catabolism of purines, one of the components of nucleic acids, thereby giving iron a part in cell division and protein synthesis. Other functions of iron have been proposed on the basis of changes which occur in individuals with iron deficiency anemia. Two areas of particular interest are immune function and learning ability. How iron affects these functions is not completely clear at this time.

METABOLISM AND PHYSIOLOGICAL FUNCTIONS: EXCRETION.   Red blood cells have an average life span of 120 days. As they die, their iron is recycled very efficiently by the body (see Figure 8–8). The regeneration process begins with the removal of the red blood cells by the liver, bone marrow, and spleen, where breakdown of the hemoglobin molecule into heme and globin occurs. Globin is then broken down into its constituent amino acids, which are recycled into the body's available pool of

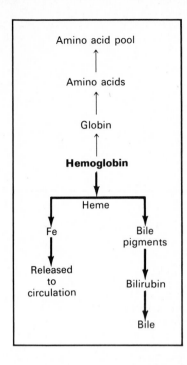

FIGURE 8-8
Recycling of Hemoglobin Components.

amino acids. The iron in heme may be stored in the spleen and liver or released into the circulation, to be picked up by transferrin and transported back to the bone marrow for incorporation into new red blood cells. The noniron portion of heme is converted to bile pigments, primarily bilirubin, which can be reutilized in the synthesis of new erythrocytes or is excreted in the bile.

So efficient is this recycling process that very little iron is excreted on a daily basis—less than 0.1 milligram in the urine, 0.5 milligram from the intestine, and even smaller amounts in perspiration and sloughed skin. Most of the iron present in feces represents *unabsorbed* dietary mineral, though a small part of fecal iron comes from sloughed mucosal cells and digestive juices. A summary of iron metabolism is presented in Figure 8–9.

DIETARY ALLOWANCES. Although the body requires relatively little iron to replace daily losses, it absorbs only a small portion of the dietary amount. For this reason, and because of the complex interactions involved in absorption, dietary allowances for iron have been based on measurements of the amounts excreted. For adult men, body losses of iron normally amount to 1 mg per day. Women, however, because of their additional losses in menstruation, have an average iron loss of 1.8 mg per day. Correcting these figures for an average absorption rate of 10 percent, allowances have been established at 10 and 18 mg per day for men and women, respectively.

Estimates indicate that the average American diet supplies 6 mg of iron for every 1,000 kcal of food. Thus, men should be able to meet the RDA for iron by consuming 1,700 kcal per day, well below the amount of food eaten by the average man. Women, on the other hand, would have to consume food totaling 3,000 kcal per day, much more than most women can, should, or want to eat. Not surpris-

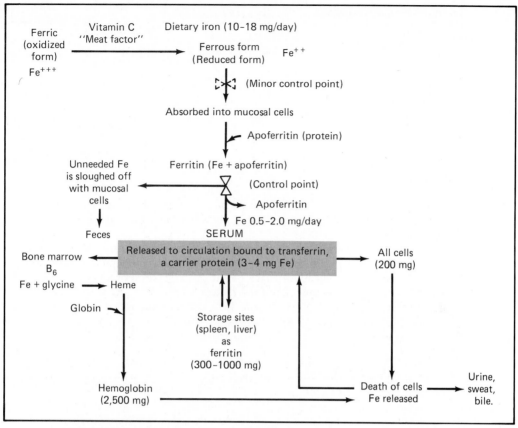

FIGURE 8-9   *Summary of Iron Metabolism.*

ingly, a rather high proportion of American women do indeed have iron deficiencies of varying degrees.

Determination of actual iron needs and provision of adequate iron for women are difficult because the amount of dietary iron that is absorbed depends on a number of factors, including the amount of stored iron in the individual and the kinds of foods served at a given meal. (Remember, absorption of nonheme iron is in direct proportion to the ascorbic acid and "meat factor" present in the same meal, whereas both nonheme and heme iron are absorbed in inverse proportion to body stores).

A working estimate of absorbable iron can be calculated from the amounts of five components in a given meal: total iron; heme iron; nonheme iron; ascorbic acid; and amount of meat, poultry, or fish. On the basis of these determinations, a meal can be classified as one of high, medium, or low availability of iron (see Table 8-7).

The average individual cannot, of course, be expected to work out these calculations. A realistic guideline for obtaining adequate absorbable iron is based on estimates that a minimum of 25 milligrams of ascorbic acid in a meal will double the amount of iron absorbed, and 1 gram of meat tissue has the approximate effect of 1 milligram of ascorbic acid. For most people, then, the simple addition of a source

TABLE 8-7. *Iron Availability in Three Types of Meals*

Low Availability	Medium Availability	High Availability
Less than 1 oz meat, poultry, or fish	1–3 oz meat, poultry, or fish	More than 3 oz meat, poultry, or fish
Or	*Or*	*Or*
Less than 25 mg ascorbic acid	25–75 mg ascorbic acid	More than 75 mg ascorbic acid
		Or
		1–3 oz meat, poultry or fish, plus
		25–75 mg ascorbic acid

Source: E. R. Monsen et al., Estimation of available dietary iron, *American Journal of Clinical Nutrition* 31:134, 1978.

of ascorbic acid—tomato juice, green pepper, a piece of melon—to every meal, and/or consumption of 3 ounces of meat, poultry, or fish will significantly enhance the availability of iron in their diet.

Vegetarians, however, cannot enhance availability with "meat factor" foods and must depend on larger quantities of ascorbic acid-containing foods to compensate. A high-available-iron vegetarian meal might include kidney beans with tomato sauce, broccoli, and pineapple. (And the factors that may hinder absorption—such as egg and tea—should be considered as well; drinking tea with a high-availability meal will transform it into a poorer source of absorbable iron.) In order to meet their needs, women should try to consume two "high-availability" meals per day.

DIETARY SOURCES.   Food-composition tables reflect *total* iron content and do not distinguish between heme and nonheme iron or otherwise indicate the amount of absorbable iron. Meat, poultry, and fish contain anywhere from 30 to 60 percent of their iron in the heme form. Fruits, vegetables, milk, eggs, and dairy products contain nonheme iron only. Dried fruits, legumes, and meats (especially liver) and seafood are generally good sources of iron; milk is a very poor source. Table 8–8 indicates the iron content of a variety of foods.

Certain dietary factors, such as phytate and fiber, decrease the absorption of iron. The method of preparing iron-containing foods can also affect iron availability. Boiling in water, for example, will leach significant amounts of the mineral, which is then lost if the water is discarded. Cast-iron cooking vessels, on the other hand, can be an important supplementary source of the mineral. Iron cooking vessels have been used for centuries throughout the world, and the Chinese wok and Mexican *comal* or tortilla griddle have certainly added to the dietary supply of this

TABLE 8-8. *Iron Content of Selected Foods (RDA for Adults: Men 10 mg; Women 18 mg)*

Food	Serving Size	Iron Content mg/serving
Bran flakes, 40%	1 c	12.4
Liver, beef, cooked	3 oz	7.5
Oysters	½ c, raw	6.6
Clams	4–5 raw	5.3
Molasses, blackstrap	1 tbsp	3.2
Hamburger, 21% fat, cooked	3 oz	2.6
Beans, navy, cooked	½ c	2.6
Soybeans, cooked	½ c	2.5

TABLE 8-8. (*Continued*)

Food	Serving Size	Iron Content mg/serving
Beans, red kidney, cooked	½ c	2.2
Split peas, cooked	½ c	2.1
Shrimp, canned	½ c	2.0
Spinach, cooked	½ c	2.0
Tuna fish, canned	3½ oz	1.6
Raisins	small box = 1½ oz	1.5
Chicken, meat only	3½ oz	1.4
Molasses, medium	1 tbsp	1.2
Potato, baked in skin	1 medium	1.1
Frankfurter	1	1.1
Egg, whole	1 large	1.04
Apricots, dried	5 medium halves	1.0
Egg yolk	1 large	0.95
Rice, cooked, enriched	½ c	0.9
Haddock, cooked	3 oz	0.9
Collard greens, cooked	½ c	0.8
Bread, whole-wheat	1 slice	0.8
Banana	1 medium	0.8
Avocado	½ fruit	0.7
Bread, white, enriched	1 slice	0.6
Cranberry juice	6 oz	0.6
Lobster, cooked	½ c	0.6
Orange	1 medium	0.6
Broccoli, cooked	½ c	0.6
Tomato	1 medium	0.5
Crabmeat, canned	½ c	0.5
Carrots, cooked	½ c	0.5
Bacon, cooked	3 slices	0.5
Green beans, cooked	½ c	0.4
Apple	1 medium	0.4
Cottage cheese, uncreamed	½ c	0.3
Salami	1 slice = 1 oz	0.3
Peanut butter	1 tbsp	0.3
Bread, white, unenriched	1 slice	0.2
Coffee, prepared	1 c = 6 oz	0.2
Cheddar cheese	1 oz	0.19
Yogurt, low-fat, fruit-flavored	8 oz	0.16
Milk, 2% fat + protein	1 c	0.15
Milk, whole	1 c	0.12
Milk, 2% fat	1 c	0.12
American cheese, pasteurized, processed	1 oz	0.11
Yogurt, plain	8 oz	0.11
Milk, skim	1 c	0.10
Celery	1 stalk	0.10
Ice cream, 10% fat	½ c	0.06
Swiss cheese	1 oz	0.05
Butter	1 pat = 1 tsp	0.01
Egg white	1 whole	0.01

Sources: C. F. Adams, *Nutritive value of American foods in common units*, USDA Agriculture Handbook No. 456 (Washington, D.C.: U.S. Government Printing Office, 1975); L. P. Posati and M. L. Orr, *Composition of foods—Dairy and egg products—Raw, processed, prepared*, USDA Agriculture Handbook No. 8-1 (Washington, D.C.: U.S. Government Printing Office, 1976).

mineral in their native lands. In North America and Europe, the mid-twentieth-century shift to aluminum, stainless steel, and enamel vessels may well have increased the risk of iron-deficiency anemia.

IRON DEFICIENCY.   In iron deficiency, body stores are depleted, and consequently the ability to synthesize hemoglobin is drastically reduced. Clinical anemia is the result of a long-term deficiency, since the elimination of all iron stores is a slow process.

Clinically, decreased serum iron, which follows tissue depletion, is reflected in decreased saturation of transferrin and less than 10 to 12 grams of hemoglobin per 100 milliliters of serum. Symptoms include chronic fatigue, headache, and pallor. The characteristic symptoms of iron-deficiency anemia are also symptomatic of numerous other conditions, including depression. Therefore, clinical iron-deficiency anemia can be determined only by a variety of blood tests to evaluate iron status.

Iron deficiency can arise from several different causes: decreased intake, decreased absorption, hemorrhage or abnormal bleeding (including bleeding because of hookworm infestation), and excessive blood donations (1 pint of blood contains 250 mg of iron). Iron deficiency, however, is not the only cause of anemia, which by definition represents a decreased number of red blood cells. Folate and vitamin B_{12} deficiencies cause anemia of a different kind (as we saw in Chapter 7), resulting

When cast iron cooking vessels were used regularly, iron deficiency was rare.
New York Public Library Picture Collection

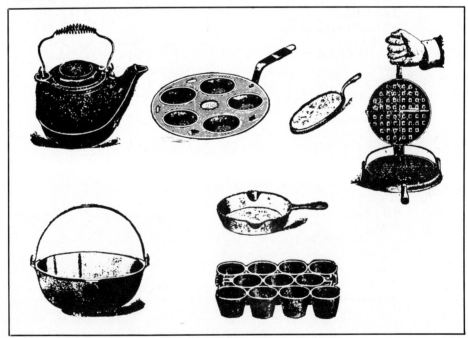

from changes in the shape and development of red blood cells. Severe pyridoxine and protein deficiencies also cause anemia.

Infants, young children, adolescents, and women of childbearing age are especially susceptible to iron-deficiency anemia. Iron supplements, usually in the form of ferrous salts with ascorbic acid added to increase absorption, can be used to build up iron stores. For many women, this is indeed advisable. However, because of individual variation, not all women need iron supplementation, even if their dietary intake falls below the recommended allowance of 18 milligrams per day. Unfortunately, by the time a clinial deficiency can be identified, iron stores have been depleted. A special effort should be made, therefore, to include iron-rich foods in the diet on a daily basis.

IRON TOXICITY. For a small percent of the population, iron accumulation and not deficiency is a problem. Because the body lacks a mechanism for excreting excess iron, the mineral accumulates in the body, particularly in soft tissues such as liver, lungs, and pancreas. Iron accumulation causes necrosis, or cell death, because it distorts the structure of the cells of these tissues.

The resulting condition, known as *hemosiderosis*, appears to involve aggregates of ferritin molecules (hemosiderin), formed when large amounts of iron are complexed to ferritin. Hemosiderosis occurs frequently among Bantu men of South Africa as a result of the high iron content of their beer, which is fermented in iron pots. Absorption is facilitated by the acid content of the beer as well as of other dietary items. This demonstrates that the regulation of iron absorption is not absolute, and in fact fails at very high levels of iron intake.

Hemosiderosis also results from types of anemia characterized by excessive breakdown of red blood cells. Because the iron and amino acids of hemoglobin are reutilized, transferrin can become completely saturated in the case of excessive erythrocyte turnover, with the result that iron unable to attach to transferrin will be deposited in soft tissues. Hemosiderosis may also occur following excessive blood transfusion.

Hemochromatosis, an abnormal increase in iron deposition in tissues, is an advanced state of hemosiderosis. It is associated with pathological changes in tissue structure and function and may lead to liver damage, diabetes, and heart failure if untreated. Hemochromatosis is caused by a disturbance in the control of iron absorption. Termed *idiopathic hemochromatosis*, this unexplained increase in absorption of iron from a normal diet is of genetic origin.

Treatment for both of these rare but dangerous conditions includes administration of an iron-binding agent to solubilize the iron so that it can be excreted in the urine, or phlebotomy (medically supervised bleeding).

Copper

This mineral is of increasing interest to nutritionists for its importance in iron metabolism, contributing to iron absorption and the formation of hemoglobin. The recognition that bottle-fed infants may under certain circumstances develop anemia that is more responsive to copper treatment than to iron therapy has spurred research on this essential nutrient.

DISTRIBUTION IN THE BODY. The human body contains 75 to 150 milligrams of copper. All body tissues contain some copper, but the greatest concentrations are found in the liver, brain, heart, and kidneys. Blood copper is apportioned in roughly equal amounts between red blood cells and plasma. In plasma, copper occurs as the copper-protein complex called *ceruloplasmin*.

METABOLISM AND PHYSIOLOGICAL FUNCTIONS. Absorption takes place in the duodenum of the intestine, but relatively little is known about regulatory control of the process. Approximately 30 percent of dietary copper is absorbed. Molybdenum, zinc, cadmium, and other trace minerals interfere with absorption. Following uptake of absorbed copper from the intestine, the liver stores the mineral or releases it as ceruloplasmin, which accounts for 95 percent of the copper found in serum. Albumin binds the remaining 5 percent.

Ceruloplasmin is involved in various stages of iron metabolism. In particular, it is necessary for the conversion of ferrous to ferric iron, important during various stages of iron metabolism. Copper enhances iron absorption and stimulates the mobilization of iron from stores in the liver and other tissues. Copper-containing enzymes play a part in various oxidation reactions in energy metabolism and in the metabolism of fatty acids. The mineral itself activates certain enzymes. The major route of copper excretion is via the bile.

DIETARY ALLOWANCES AND SOURCES. The Food and Nutrition Board has established provisional recommended ranges for dietary intake of copper but not RDAs. From copper balance studies in adults, it has been determined that the body needs from 1.5 to 2.0 mg/day. The provisional recommendations by the Food and Nutrition Board are 2 to 3 mg/day for adults. The interactions of copper with other trace minerals, and the lack of sufficient data, compound the difficulty of setting a reliable RDA for copper.

The average diet contains 2 milligrams or more copper per day. Drinking water may be a source of variable amounts as well. The richest sources of the mineral include nuts, shellfish, liver, kidney, raisins, and legumes. Just as it is a poor source of iron, milk is a poor source of copper.

A number of factors influence the copper content of foods. Environmental factors include copper content of soil, geographic location (such as nearness to industrial complexes that may release copper-containing wastes), use and kind of fertilizers, origin of water supply, and the season. Handling and processing also affect copper content. Water, equipment, and various contaminants may introduce copper, whereas milling, grinding, and cooking in water tend to remove it.

It should be noted that laboratory analyses of foods have produced a wide range of copper values, and consequently the copper contents of foods reported in the literature vary widely. The values listed in food composition tables are approximations only. Table 8–9 gives the copper content of selected foods. Consumption of a diversified diet should ensure sufficient intake of the mineral.

DEFICIENCY AND TOXICITY. The broad scope of copper's functions can be judged by the range of symptoms that result from deficiency: anemia, cardiovascular lesions, degeneration of the nervous system, skeletal defects, various hair abnormalities, and loss of taste acuity. Copper-deficient infants exhibit low serum copper levels, anemia, and bone demineralization. Copper imbalances usually result from genetic defects in control mechanisms. One such inherited defect produces a fatal condition called Menke's syndrome (or kinky-hair disease), caused by defective absorption of copper from the intestine. Symptoms include rapid degeneration of nerve tissue, skeletal abnormalities, a "steely" texture of the hair, vascular lesions,

TABLE 8-9. *Copper Content of Selected Foods (Estimated Safe and Adequate Daily Dietary Intake for Adults: 2.0–3.0 mg)*

Food	Serving Size	Copper Content mg/serving
Oysters	6 medium	14.2
Lobster	1 c	2.45
Liver, beef, cooked	3 oz	2.38
Bran flakes, 40%	1 c	0.51
Avocado	1 half	0.49
Potato, baked in skin	1 medium	0.36
Soybeans, cooked	½ c	0.30
Banana	1 medium	0.26
Haddock, cooked	3 oz	0.16
Apple	1 medium	0.14
Chicken, meat only	3½ oz	0.14
Spinach, cooked	½ c	0.13
Peas, green, cooked	½ c	0.12
Tuna, canned	3½ oz	0.12
Raisins	small box = 1½ oz	0.11
Tomato	1 medium	0.11
Green beans, cooked	½ c	0.09
Peanut butter	1 tbsp	0.09
Milk, whole	1 c	0.09
Broccoli, cooked	½ c	0.08
Bacon, cooked	3 slices	0.08
Bread, whole-wheat	1 slice	0.06
Bread, white, enriched	1 slice	0.06
Carrots, cooked	½ c	0.06
Egg, whole	1 large	0.05
Egg yolk	1 large	0.05
Milk, skim	1 c	0.05
Frankfurter	1	0.05
Beef, ground	3 oz	0.05
Coffee, prepared	6 oz	0.04
Swiss cheese	1 oz	0.03
Cheddar cheese	1 oz	0.03
Celery	1 stalk	0.03
Ice cream, 10% fat	½ c	0.03
Rice, cooked	½ c	0.02
American cheese	1 oz	0.02
Cottage cheese	½ c	0.01
Egg white	1 large	0.01
Margarine	1 pat = 1 tsp	trace
Butter	1 pat = 1 tsp	0

Source: J. T. Pennington and D. H. Calloway, Copper content of foods, *Journal of the American Dietetic Association* 63:143, 1973.

and subnormal body temperature. Copper deficiency can also arise from malnutrition, diarrhea, malabsorption, and kidney disease.

Toxicity due to an excess of dietary copper is rare. Daily intakes of more than 20 milligrams of copper, however, produce nausea and vomiting. An inherited condition, Wilson's disease, produces chronic copper toxicity because of defective excretion. Ceruloplasmin levels decrease and copper gradually accumulates in the tissues. The symptoms of this progressive disease include tissue necrosis (especially in the liver), mental deterioration, tremor, and loss of coordination. Patients with this condition are treated with a low copper diet and a drug which binds the copper and allows it to be excreted in the urine.

Zinc

Although long known to be essential for animals, the importance of zinc in human nutrition began to be appreciated only about 25 years ago. The impetus for the revised view of zinc's relevance to human nutrition came with evidence of zinc deficiency in Iran and Egypt in the early 1960s.

DISTRIBUTION IN THE BODY. The human body contains 2 to 3 grams of zinc. It occurs in all tissues, with highest concentrations in the choroid membrane of the eye and the male reproductive organs. The liver, skeletal muscle, and bone contain somewhat lower concentrations. Zinc also occurs in blood (mostly in erythrocytes) and in the pancreas as a component of insulin.

METABOLISM AND PHYSIOLOGICAL FUNCTIONS. Absorption of zinc from the upper part of the small intestine is about 30 percent efficient. Although the mechanism of absorption remains to be identified, it is thought that the process is energy-dependent and increases with body size, physiological need, and dietary zinc content. Calcium, phytate, and dietary fiber interfere with absorption.

As a component of insulin, a hormone that regulates carbohydrate metabolism, zinc is extremely important to nutritional health. It is also a component of at least 200 metalloenzymes—including carbonic anhydrase (necessary for CO_2 transport from cells to the lungs), carboxypeptidase (needed for peptide digestion), and alcohol dehydrogenase as well as other dehydrogenase enzymes. It plays an essential part in the synthesis of DNA, RNA, and proteins. Mobilization of vitamin A from the liver requires zinc, and the mineral also plays a part in healing wounds, perhaps in the synthesis of collagen.

According to one study, zinc appears to be a necessary activator of the conjugase enzyme associated with absorption of the polyglutamate forms of folic acid. Polyglutamate absorption was decreased by approximately half when zinc depletion was experimentally induced. Further research is needed to clarify the role of zinc in other physiological systems.

In addition to fecal excretion of unabsorbed zinc, the daily loss of endogenous zinc amounts to 2 to 3 milligrams. Urine and perspiration account for about 0.5 milligrams per day each, and the remainder is lost in pancreatic and intestinal secretions. The control points of zinc metabolism remain to be identified.

DIETARY ALLOWANCES AND SOURCES. Metabolic studies indicate that a dietary intake of 12.5 milligrams per day produces a positive zinc balance in adults. Correcting for absorption, the adult RDA has been set at 15 milligrams. This figure is supported by limited research.

Data on dietary sources also are limited. As Table 8–10 shows, oysters are by far the richest source of zinc. High protein foods, such as meats and egg yolks, contain valuable amounts. Fruits, vegetables, and egg whites are poor sources of zinc. Milling cereals reduces their zinc content, and the zinc found in whole-grain products may be largely unavailable because of the presence of phytic acid. The interrelationships among dietary zinc, copper, calcium, and protein are only beginning to emerge.

TABLE 8-10. *Zinc Content of Selected Foods (RDA for Adults: 15 mg)*

Food	Serving Size	Zinc Content mg/serving
Oysters, fresh	6 medium	124.9
Turkey, dark meat, cooked	3 oz	3.7
Liver, beef	3 oz	3.31
Lima beans, canned, cooked	½ c	2.72
Pork, lean, cooked	3 oz	2.6
Beef, ground, cooked	3 oz	2.12
Turkey, light meat, cooked	3 oz	1.8
Yogurt, fruit-flavored	8 oz	1.68
Yogurt, plain	8 oz	1.34
Bran flakes, 40%	1 c	1.3
Almonds	¼ c	1.24
Peanuts, roasted	¼ c	1.17
Swiss cheese	1 oz	1.11
Milk, skim	1 c	0.98
Milk, whole	1 c	0.93
Wheat germ	1 tbsp	0.9
Cheddar cheese	1 oz	0.88
Whole egg	1 large	0.72
Ice cream, 10% fat	½ c	0.71
Egg yolk	1 large	0.58
Potato, baked	1 medium	0.44
Cottage cheese, uncreamed	½ c	0.34
Lentils, cooked	½ c	0.18
Spinach, cooked	½ c	0.17
Cream cheese	1 oz	0.15
Orange juice	6 oz	0.13
Lettuce, chunks	1 c	0.12
Banana	1 medium	0.04
Egg white	1 large	0.01
Butter or margarine	1 pat = 1 tsp	trace

Sources: L. P. Posati and M. L. Orr, *Composition of foods—Dairy and egg products—Raw, processed, prepared,* USDA Agriculture Handbook No. 8-1 (Washington, D.C.: U.S. Government Printing Office, 1976); H. H. Sandstead, Zinc nutrition in the United States, *American Journal of Clinical Nutrition* 26: 1,257, 1973.

DEFICIENCY AND TOXICITY. The major symptoms of zinc deficiency are delayed growth and maturation, including sexual maturation. Other symptoms include delayed healing of wounds and impaired taste acuity (hypogeusia). These symptoms reflect the importance of zinc in nucleic acid and protein synthesis. Most studies of zinc deficiency have been of boys. Girls suffer growth retardation, but no studies have been done on the effect of zinc deficiency on sexual maturation in girls. In animals zinc deficiency during the critical period of brain development is expressed by behavioral changes in later life and altered concentrations of neurotransmitters. What role, if any, maternal zinc deficiency may play in the development of the human infant is not known. Concern has recently been expressed that suboptimal intake may be more common than previously thought.

Zinc apparently has no significant toxic effects, although vomiting, diarrhea, and abdominal cramping have been reported following consumption of beverages stored in galvanized containers. However, because long-term effects of prolonged high consumption are not known, zinc supplements should be taken only when prescribed for therapeutic reasons.

Iodine

As a nutrient, iodine is well known for its association with iodized salt and the unsightly iodine-deficiency condition called *goiter*. Although the causal connection between iodine and goiter was established only about a century ago, iodine-containing substances were used long before that by the Chinese, Egyptians, and Incas to treat the goitrous condition.

DISTRIBUTION IN THE BODY.   The total amount of body iodine averages between 20 and 30 milligrams, of which 75 percent is found in the thyroid gland. The thyroid gland is a two-lobed structure that lies across the trachea and which has as its major function the synthesis and storage of thyroid hormones. The remaining 25 percent of body iodine is found in all body tissues, and especially in skeletal muscle, blood, and the ovaries.

METABOLISM AND PHYSIOLOGICAL FUNCTIONS.   The body absorbs dietary iodine (primarily as iodides) with nearly 100 percent efficiency. After entry into the blood and distribution throughout the extracellular fluid, about 30 percent of the ab-

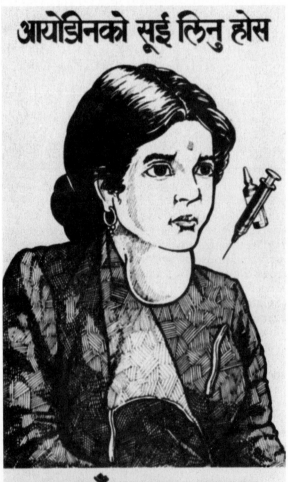

In Nepal, a poster prepared by UNICEF shows a woman with goiter.
Unicef/NYT Pictures

sorbed iodine is trapped by the thyroid. Since there is no mechanism for the conservation of additional iodide, the remainder of the absorbed iodine is excreted in the urine.

Iodide functions in the synthesis of two thyroid hormones—thyroxine (T_4) and triiodothyronine (T_3)—which are essential for normal metabolism. Synthesis of these hormones begins with the formation of a large iodine-containing protein called *thyroglobulin*, which contains many tyrosine molecules (Figure 8–10). Enzymatic hydrolysis of thyroglobulin releases the hormones into the blood, which distributes them to all tissues.

The two thyroid hormones accelerate biochemical reactions in all cells of the body, causing greater utilization of oxygen and an increased metabolic rate. Consequently these hormones have a profound and far-reaching influence on growth and development, protein synthesis, and energy metabolism. The mechanisms by which thyroid hormones produce these effects have yet to be clearly identified. The hormones also play a part in the conversion of carotene to vitamin A and in the synthesis of cholesterol.

The thyroid gland is able to compensate for low dietary iodine intake by expanding its activity (and size), thereby maximizing the use of the limited supply. The most important regulator of thyroid activity is a pituitary product called *thyroid-stimulating* or *thyrotropic hormone* (TSH). The regulation of thyroid hormone synthesis and release by TSH involves a number of feedback mechanisms.

The condition known as **hypothyroidism** (or underactive thyroid) results in subnormal levels of thyroid hormones in the blood, a consequence of insufficient synthesis. The form of hypothyroidism known as *myxedema* produces a clinical picture of coarse hair, yellowish skin, decreased tolerance to cold, and a tendency to be overweight. Although rare, this condition is the basis for the claim that obesity results from an underactive thyroid. Myxedema, however, does not stem from iodine deficiency but rather from a metabolic error in hormone synthesis.

FIGURE 8-10

Substitution of iodine for 3 or 4 hydrogen atoms on two linked tyrosine molecules produces T_3 or T_4, respectively.

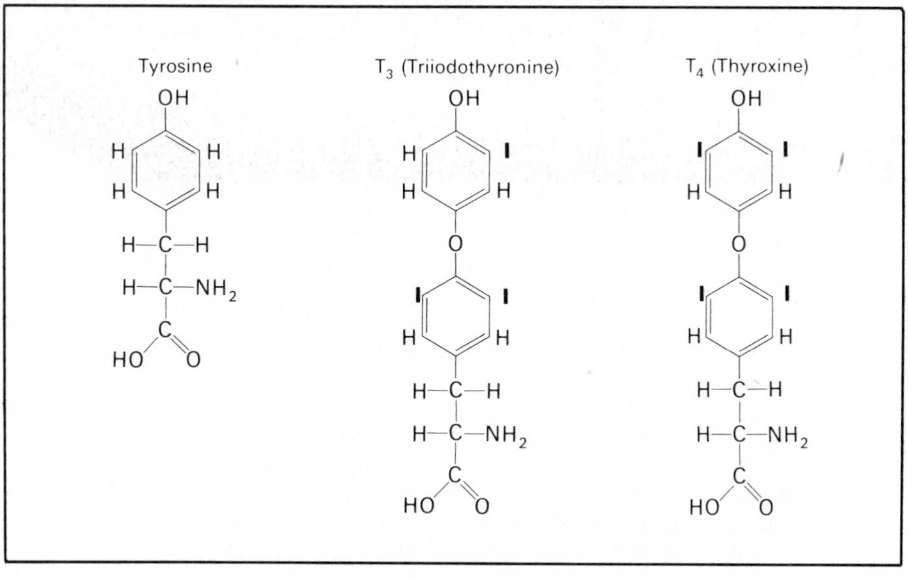

On the other hand, **hyperthyroidism**, or overactive thyroid, occurs when the regulatory mechanisms that control thyroid hormone synthesis do not function. A person with Graves' disease, as one type of hyperthyroidism is called, is nervous, has a voracious appetite but loses weight, demonstrates an increased metabolic rate, and cannot tolerate heat. A frequent symptom, known as exophthalmia ("pop-eye"), is a visible protrusion of the eyeballs.

Thyroid hormones are sometimes suggested as a part of weight-loss regimens because of their effect in increasing the metabolic rate. But this method of treating obesity is potentially dangerous and can cause cardiac failure. Moreover, the hormones are not permanently effective against weight gain.

DIETARY ALLOWANCES AND SOURCES. The RDA for iodine for both men and women has been set at 150 micrograms per day, with increases recommended during pregnancy and lactation.

In the United States important sources of the mineral are iodized salt and bread to which iodine-containing dough conditioners have been added. In recent years, the dietary intake of iodine appears to have increased, although the sources of the additional amounts remain to be determined. Present iodization of table salt adds 100 milligrams of potassium iodide for each kilogram of sodium chloride. Thus 1 teaspoon of table salt contains far more than the RDA for iodine.

Drinking water supplies variable amounts of the mineral and tends to reflect the amount present in the soil. Iodine content of foods varies considerably according to the type of soil, animal feed, fertilizers, and processing methods used. Because of the variability of iodine content in foods, and because it is present in such small amounts, accurate determinations are not available for most food items. Fish, seafoods, and seaweeds are usually good sources. Bread and dairy products may be good sources as well, as will any prepared foods containing iodized salt. A single pinch of iodized salt contains about 50 micrograms of iodine, as does an 8-ounce glass of milk—fully one-third the RDA. Most vegetables contain little iodine: Spinach, broccoli, and potatoes all contain less than 10 micrograms per serving.

DEFICIENCY. The most common consequence of iodine deficiency is simple **goiter**, or swelling of the thyroid gland. In response to decreased serum levels of thyroid hormones caused by a lack of dietary iodine, TSH is released. TSH controls thyroid metabolism in part by increasing the number and size of thyroid cells. This in turn increases the efficiency of the gland's iodine-trapping mechanism and enables it to accelerate synthesis and release of its hormones. Thus, simple goiter is a useful compensatory mechanism and generally does not pose any serious medical problem. Development of goiter was for centuries a sign of puberty in girls and considered normal and desirable. In fact, goiter was so common that many Renaissance paintings depict the beautiful women of the day showing enlarged thyroids among their other physical endowments. Today we know that estrogen alters thyroid hormone metabolism, and thus may result in goiter if iodine intake is marginal. In extreme cases a goiter may become so enlarged as to interfere with breathing.

Goiter may also develop from ingestion of "goitrogens"—compounds that compete with iodine for thyroid uptake or that interfere with thyroid hormone synthesis. Such goitrogens are to be found in cabbages and brussels sprouts. Another goitrogen, thiocyanate, occurs in cassava, a dietary staple in areas in Africa that have a high incidence both of goiter and of **cretinism**. Cretinism is a much more serious form of thyroid hormone deficiency. This condition is present at birth in infants who were deprived of iodine during fetal development because their mothers had a profound deficiency of thyroid hormone due to severe and prolonged iodine deficiency. The symptoms of cretinism include lethargy (as a result of very low basal metabolism), mental retardation, stunted growth, enlarged tongue, and dry skin.

Congenital hypothyroidism also produces the same symptoms but is the result of a genetic defect rather than of iodine deficiency. In both these conditions, mental and physical retardation can be prevented if thyroid hormones are administered soon after birth. Since early diagnosis is essential, mandatory screening of all newborn infants for hypothyroidism has been suggested.

Recently concern has developed that dietary intake of iodine may be excessive. Over a long period of time, ingestion of large amounts of iodine (25 to 50 times the recommended levels) can suppress the synthesis of thyroid hormones, resulting in a hyperactive and enlarged thyroid, a condition known as *iodide goiter*. Indeed, the sensitivity of the thyroid gland makes iodine one of the very few nutrients of which both excess and deficiency can produce the same effect.

Fluoride

The body contains less than 1 gram of fluoride, which has an interesting history in relation to dental health. The presence of fluoride in bones and teeth was discovered early in the last century. Dentists in Colorado Springs had observed that people living in the area had unusual teeth: Their teeth had dark brown stains (so-called mottled enamel) but the incidence of dental caries was exceptionally low. The stains, although esthetically unappealing, had no adverse effects on health. By 1931 investigators established that naturally occurring fluorides in the water supply were responsible for both the observed effects.

METABOLISM AND PHYSIOLOGICAL FUNCTIONS. Passive absorption of fluoride is rapid and takes place primarily in the stomach, but some may be absorbed from the intestine as well. Efficiency of absorption ranges from 75 to 90 percent of the amount ingested, with approximately half retained in the teeth and bones.

The function of fluoride appears to be the protection of bone and—especially—dental tissue, an influence that it exercises primarily during prenatal life, infancy, and childhood. Fluoridated water, however, is of some benefit to adults as well as to children. There is also some evidence that an adequate dietary intake of the mineral throughout life protects against osteoporosis in the elderly.

The body excretes fluoride mainly in the urine, although small amounts are lost in sweat and feces. Urinary loss is very rapid, the excess amount being excreted within 24 hours.

DIETARY ALLOWANCES AND SOURCES. Although RDAs for fluoride have not been established, the Food and Nutrition Board provisionally recommends that water supplies be fluoridated at a level of 1 ppm (or 1 mg/liter) to provide 1.5 to 4 milligrams per day for adults.

The amounts of fluoride from dietary sources other than fluoridated water are unreliable. Most plant and animal foods reflect the variable contents of soil, water supply, and other factors and contain only minor amounts of the mineral (Table 8–11). Fish products and seaweed (important components of Japanese diets) are exceptions, and tea provides 0.3 milligrams per cup. Grains and vegetables are sometimes good sources, as are bone meal, meats, fish, and dairy products. As an

TABLE 8-11. *Range of Fluoride in Selected Foods*

Food	Fluoride Content μg/g
Spinach	0.1 –20.3
Cheese	0.16– 1.71
Potatoes	0.4 – 5.20
Fish	1.0 – 8.0

example of the variability of fluoride content of food, nuts usually have anywhere from 0.3 to 1.45 micrograms per gram, but values as high as 7.8 micrograms per gram have been recorded. Fluoridated water used during processing and preparation increases the fluoride content of food, as does cooking with Teflon vessels. Boiling water in aluminum ware, on the other hand, greatly reduces fluoride content.

Because the mineral occurs in such small amounts in foods and is so rapidly excreted, fluoride toxicity is rare. In areas where fluoride is naturally present in the water supply at levels approximating 6 to 8 ppm, tooth enamel becomes mottled, but no adverse effects on health have been documented. In rare instances in which fluoride has been ingested, usually accidentally, in amounts greater than 2,500 times recommended levels, fatal poisoning has resulted. Chronic ingestion of more than 50 milligrams per day, which may result from environmental pollution, can produce bone and tooth malformations. However, it has been thoroughly documented that the levels provided by artificially fluoridated water pose no health hazard and in fact are beneficial.

Other Trace Elements

Until quite recently, little has been known about the functions in the body of a number of trace elements, but in the past few years evidence has accumulated that minute amounts of a number of minerals are essential to human health and must be provided in the diet. As a result, provisional allowances have been set for manganese, molybdenum, selenium, and chromium. These elements, along with cobalt, are now known to be integral constituents of essential body compounds. Silicon, tin, vanadium, and nickel are being carefully studied, because they are also potentially essential nutrients. Valid methods of analysis are critical for all of these trace elements since they are present in such low concentrations. Contamination of samples can occur very easily. Much of the early data of concentrations in tissues and body fluids is probably invalid due to either poor instrumentation or contamination.

CHROMIUM. Because chromium was implicated as a participant in glucose metabolism in 1959, it has been more actively studied than most of the other trace elements, and evidence for its essentiality has continued to accumulate. The total amount of this mineral found in the human body averages less than 6 milligrams but is highly variable. The hair, spleen, kidney, and testes contain the highest concentrations; heart, pancreas, lungs, and brain have lower concentrations. There is still disagreement regarding the normal range of plasma chromium. The amount of chromium in the body declines with age, possibly as a result of depletion of body stores, but most likely because of decreased dietary intake.

Absorption—in the organically bound form known as *glucose tolerance factor* (GTF)—is 10 to 25 percent efficient. However, the body absorbs only about 1 percent of inorganic chromium from the diet. Daily loss, mainly via urinary excretion, averages between 200 and 500 nanograms (1 nanogram equals one-billionth of a gram).

The major function of chromium is to enhance the activity of insulin in the metabolism of glucose and particularly in maintaining the rate at which glucose is removed from blood for uptake into cells. Chromium also activates several enzymes and may play a role in protein and lipid metabolism.

Small quantities, approximately 50 micrograms, of chromium are consumed each day. Based on available information about need and utilization, the Food and Nutrition Board offers provisional allowances of 0.05 to 2.0 milligrams (50 to 200 μg) per day for adults. In a recent study, a small group of elderly people had an average intake of about 25 micrograms per day and on the whole were in chromium balance. Good sources include yeast, beer, liver, cheese, bread, and beef. Black pepper contains chromium but is seldom consumed in amounts sufficient to make this a useful dietary source. Refining of sugar and flour removes most of the chromium contained in these sources. Even good sources contain varying amounts of the mineral in different samples tested because of variations in water and soil content and methods of processing and preparation.

Impaired glucose tolerance results from chromium deficiency in both animals and humans. Some studies show that supplementation of chromium for humans results in improvement of glucose intolerance. In other studies there are no changes. Supplementation for humans also results in improvement of their lipoprotein profile in some studies, but not all. The differences may be due in part to the form of chromium given as the supplement, the age of the subject, and the lipid and glucose status of the subject at the start of the study. Symptoms shown by laboratory animals have included growth retardation, hyperglycemia, glycosuria, and elevated serum cholesterol, along with a generally reduced ability to cope with psychological stress. Severely malnourished children have shown improved glucose removal following chromium therapy. Some researchers feel that many elderly Americans may have a chronic deficiency. Consuming a high intake of simple sugars was shown, in one study, to result in a higher excretion of chromium. However, evidence is far from sufficient to offer a clear-cut theory of how chromium exerts its effects or, indeed, precisely what those effects are. Although no evidence exists of toxicity from dietary sources, until more is learned about this trace mineral, supplements are not advised.

COBALT. The first evidence for a nutritional role for cobalt came about 45 years ago when an anemialike disease of cattle in Australia and New Zealand was cured by administration of iron compounds. It was subsequently demonstrated that the effective portion of the compound was a cobalt salt and, eventually, that it functioned as part of vitamin B_{12}. This is still the only known role for cobalt, although there is some evidence that it has an effect on thyroid function.

Dietary cobalt can be utilized only in its physiologically active form, cobalamin, or vitamin B_{12}; inorganic cobalt is excreted and has no known function. (Inorganic cobalt is needed in diets of cattle, however, because vitamin B_{12} is produced by gastrointestinal microorganisms during the ruminant digestive process. But because intestinal synthesis of vitamin B_{12} is limited or nonexistent in humans, cobalt must be obtained in the active form.) Thus it is the vitamin B_{12} content of foods, and not their cobalt content, that supplies human needs for this element. Although cobalt is present in a variety of foodstuffs (meats and dairy products and, to a lesser extent, in cereals, grains, and vegetables), the physiologically active form (as described in Chapter 7) must be consumed.

The body of the average human male contains only 1.1 milligrams of cobalt. Small amounts are lost in feces, sweat, and hair, but urine is the main excretory route. Cobalt shares the same transport route as iron and is absorbed in proportion to iron need. Although at times cobalt absorption may, for this reason, be relatively great in proportion to human need for cobalamin, toxicity is rare. Excessive intakes may have a thyroid-stimulating effect and cause stimulation of the bone marrow, resulting in excessive production of erythrocytes (polycythemia). For most persons, however, cobalt toxicity is not likely to occur.

MANGANESE. The total body content of this mineral is about 10 to 20 milligrams, which is distributed throughout all tissues but with the highest concentrations occurring in the pancreas, liver, kidneys, and intestines. Manganese absorption tends to be inefficient (less than 20 percent) and varies inversely with the amount of dietary calcium and iron. Little is excreted in the urine, the major excretory route being the bile.

Studies of laboratory animals have shown that manganese is required for normal growth, nervous function, and lipid and carbohydrate metabolism. Although the mineral appears to function much the same way in humans, further study is needed. For example, animal research data have clearly established that manganese has a role in glucose metabolism and is a cofactor or component of many enzymes in the body. Many metabolic pathways require manganese, although its mechanism of action remains unclear.

Dietary intake of manganese averages between 2.5 and 7 milligrams per day. Because manganese deficiency is almost unknown in humans, the Food and Nutrition Board has established a provisional requirement of only 2.5 to 5 milligrams per day for adults.

As Table 8–12 shows, a wide range of foods contains generous amounts of manganese. Whole grains and tea are especially rich in the mineral, but nuts, vegetables, and fruits are also good sources. As with other trace minerals, the manganese content of foods depends in large part on agricultural and processing conditions.

To date, manganese deficiency has been demonstrated only in animals, whose requirements are far greater than those of humans. Deficiency in animals affects bone, brain tissue, and reproductive function. Because substantial amounts of manganese are found in many common foods, intakes for most people probably far exceed need. But the possibility of manganese deficiency should be considered in certain cases. In particular, pregnant women consuming diets high in calcium and low in manganese may risk deficiency because of the requirements of the developing fetus. Growing children, who may require more of this mineral, and adults on weight-reduction diets may also develop deficiencies. (Deficiencies of other minerals occur in such cases as well.)

Toxicity from dietary intake appears to be highly unlikely. However, miners of manganese ores may develop a syndrome from inhaling ore dust. The symptoms resemble those of viral encephalitis. Tremor and loss of coordination characterize severe cases. But this is not associated with an excess of dietary manganese.

MOLYBDENUM. Total body content of this mineral is very small, as is the provisional daily allowance of 150 to 500 micrograms. As a component of xanthine oxidase, molybdenum plays an essential role in the metabolism of the purine

TABLE 8-12. *Manganese Content of Selected Foods (Estimated Safe and Adequate Daily Dietary Intake for Adults: 2.5–5 mg)*

Food	Serving Size	Manganese Content μg/serving
Tea	1 c (1 tsp tea)	400–2,700
Raisins	small box = 1 ½ oz	201
Rice, cooked	½ c	146
Spinach, cooked	½ c	128
Carrots, cooked	½ c	120
Broccoli, cooked	½ c	119
Orange	1 medium	52
Peas, green	½ c	51
Bran flakes, 40%	1 c	48
Apple	1 medium	46
Milk, whole	1 c	46
Milk, skim	1 c	46
Swiss cheese	1 oz	37
Bread, white	1 slice	36
Eggs	1 large	30
Tomato	1 medium	30
Chicken, meat only	3 ½ oz	21
Green beans, cooked	½ c	15
Liver, beef, cooked	3 oz	14
Butter	1 pat = 1 tsp	5
Beef, ground, cooked	3 oz	4

Note: The mineral contents in the table are given in micrograms (μg), whereas the provisional requirement is 2.5 to 5 milligrams (mg). One milligram is equivalent to 1,000 μg.
Source: Adapted from H. Q. Schroeder, J. J. Balassa, and I. H. Tiptin, Essential trace metals in man: Manganese, *Journal of Chronic Diseases* 19:545, 1966.

components of nucleic acids and the formation of uric acid. It is also a cofactor for various flavoprotein enzymes. High sulfate intakes decrease absorption and increase urinary excretion of the mineral.

The estimated dietary intake of 45 to 500 micrograms per day probably more than meets human requirements. Although present in small amounts, molybdenum is widely distributed in foods. Whole-grain cereals, legumes, and organ meats are good sources of the mineral.

No deficiency of molybdenum is known in humans. Since the mineral competes with copper, excess molybdenum produces symptoms of copper deficiency in animals. Increasing the sulfate content of the diet prevents copper deficiency by increasing excretion of molybdenum.

SELENIUM.   The body content of this mineral, totaling only a few micrograms, is distributed throughout the body tissues, with highest concentrations in the kidney, liver, spleen, pancreas, and testes. It is readily absorbed and is excreted in urine and feces. Absorbed selenium is transported primarily bound to plasma proteins.

Because selenium and vitamin E were known to spare each other, it was long thought that the mineral must function as an antioxidant. This has been confirmed by the finding that selenium specifically functions as a component of glutathione peroxidase, a powerful antioxidant that protects cell membranes from destruction.

Dietary deficiencies of selenium and/or vitamin E can cause a variety of disorders in animals including dysfunctions of the brain, cardiovascular system, liver, muscles, and fetus. The role of selenium in certain diseases of humans is not clear.

Evidence from epidemiological studies links low selenium status with certain types of cancer. High, but not toxic, intakes can inhibit carcinogenesis in some experimental animals. These data suggest a role for selenium in human cancer, possibly related to its function as an antioxidant.

Areas of low selenium status also have an increased incidence of cardiovascular disease suggesting the possibility of a link. The Chinese have reported a disease of selenium deficiency, Keshan disease. Keshan disease is characterized by multiple focal myocardial necrosis throughout the heart muscle. Post-weaning infants, children, and women of child-bearing age are most affected. There are significant annual and seasonal variations. Patients with Keshan disease have lower blood selenium values than people anywhere else in the world. Oral selenium supplements have been very effective in reducing the incidence. Children with genetic diseases of protein metabolism who must consume special diets have low blood selenium concentrations, close to, but not quite as low as found in China. These children may be at risk for deficiency should they suddenly have an increased need for selenium.

Little is known about the dietary requirement for selenium—estimated to be 75 micrograms—and no RDA has been set. Provisional allowances of 50 to 200 micrograms per day have been recommended. In general, the selenium content of foods varies with their protein content. Meats, seafoods, egg yolk, and milk are good sources. Cereals are not reliable sources since their selenium content depends on the amount of this mineral in the soil. Milling of grains causes little loss, but the addition of sugar in processing appears to produce significant loss of selenium. Cooking has little effect on selenium content, but boiling the few vegetables that do have high content, such as mushrooms and asparagus, will leach the mineral. Generally, though, fruits and vegetables are poor sources.

Selenium can be toxic. Cattle that graze on selenium-rich land develop a condition with the descriptive name "blind staggers." Increased dental caries have been reported among schoolchildren living in areas of selenium-rich soil. Selenium also produces chronic fatigue, irritability, and damage to such tissues as nails and hair. However, long-term ingestion of 2,400 micrograms or more daily would be required to produce these effects.

SILICON, TIN, VANADIUM, AND NICKEL. All these minerals, originally believed to be contaminants (like lead), have been reappraised since the inducement of deficiency conditions in experimental animals. If a nutrient is essential to one or more species of mammals, there is a good chance that humans require it too.

Silicon, after oxygen the most common element on earth, is found only in trace amounts in the body. The highest concentrations are found in the connective tissues generally and in the collagen of skin and bone.

Deficiency studies of animals suggest that silicon may have an essential role in bone calcification and the synthesis of mucopolysaccharides. Confirmation of the latter role would mean that silicon participates in other processes involving growth and maintenance of connective tissue, embryonic development, and healing of wounds. Silicon may play a part in aging—the silicon content of skin, aorta, and thymus decreases with age, whereas that of other tissues remains constant throughout life. The human requirement for silicon is unknown.

Tin has been found to be an essential mineral for rats. Induced tin deficiency in rats resulted in poor growth, loss of hair, and other symptoms. At present, where and how tin functions in the human body remain to be determined. It occurs in water and some foods and especially in canned foods.

Vanadium deficiency has been induced in rats and chickens. Symptoms include impaired growth and abnormal bone development. Research data indicate that vanadium functions in iron and lipid metabolism and perhaps in development of bones and teeth. Its site and mode of function in humans remain to be determined. Vanadium is found in root vegetables, nuts, seafood, some grains, and vegetable oils.

Nickel deficiency has been induced in several different species of laboratory animals, variously affecting growth, serum cholesterol levels, and red blood cell count, and having other effects as well. The organ most usually affected is the liver. Nickel, like vanadium, appears to be involved in lipid metabolism, but its function in humans has not been established. It occurs in legumes, tea, pepper, cocoa, grains, and a variety of fruits and vegetables.

Knowledge of these trace elements is still evolving. The bioassay techniques to measure the involvement of the minute quantities in which these elements occur in the human body are themselves still evolving as well. The need for these elements is already clear, however, and emphasizes the importance of consuming a diversified diet. Foods fortified with vitamins and iron do not necessarily contain trace minerals, nor do the vitamin supplements available at health food stores or drugstores. We cannot meet our requirements for them through artificial sources. Our food supply contains *all* the many nutrients we need—including those for which the need cannot yet be measured.

SUMMARY

In addition to carbohydrate, lipid, protein, and vitamins, the body requires a group of some 20 elements called *minerals*. Each of the *macrominerals* is required in amounts of 100 milligrams or more per day, contributes at least 0.05 percent of body weight, or both; each *trace* element is required in amounts of no more than a few milligrams per day.

The minerals commonly occur as components of important organic molecules such as hemoglobin, thyroid hormone, and metalloenzymes. They also form inorganic compounds (as in bone) and function as free ions in the blood and other body fluids. The minerals help to maintain acid-base and fluid balance; act as catalysts of reactions in hormonal and metabolic processes; are involved in muscle contraction and nerve-impulse transmission; and are components of essential body compounds, both structural and functional.

The seven major minerals are calcium, phosphorus, magnesium, sodium, potassium, chlorine, and sulfur.

Calcium functions chiefly as a component (with phosphorus) of hydroxyapatite, the main structural component of bone and dental tissue, and plays an important part in blood coagulation, synthesis of the neurotransmitter acetylcholine, activation of certain enzymes (for example, pancreatic lipase), regulation of muscle contraction, and nerve-impulse transmission.

Phosphorus, like calcium, functions in the mineralization of bones and teeth. Energy metabolism requires phosphate-containing compounds (for example, ATP and certain phosphorylated vitamins), as does the absorption of glucose. Phosphorus is an essential component of phospholipids in membranes and of nucleic acids; phosphates are also effective buffers.

Magnesium interacts with calcium and with phosphate and carbonate ions in many of its functions, which include bone metabolism, catalysis of many enzyme reactions (including glucose, fatty acid and amino acid metabolism, and protein synthesis), muscle contraction, and nerve activity.

Sodium maintains osmolarity and acid-base balance, and affects extracellular fluid volume (and thus blood pressure) and nerve-impulse transmission. Because of the very widespread distribution of sodium chloride in natural and processed foods, and its extensive use as table salt, sodium deficiency is rare. Excessive intake, however, is associated with high blood pressure in some individuals.

Potassium, like sodium, functions in maintaining fluid balance and osmolarity, muscle contraction, and nerve activity. It also plays a role in carbohydrate metabolism (particularly glycogen synthesis and glucose oxidation) and, indirectly, in protein synthesis.

Chloride also helps to maintain acid-base balance and osmolarity. As a component of hydrochloric acid in gastric juice, chloride has an important part in digestion. The mineral also activates amylase (which hydrolyzes starch and glycogen) and functions in nerve activity.

Sulfur has a variety of functions as a component of sulfur-containing amino acids, compounds associated with oxidation-reduction reactions (for example, CoA, thiamin, biotin), insulin and other hormones, and structural compounds (mucopolysaccharides and sulfated lipids).

The trace minerals about which most is known are iron, copper, zinc, iodine, and fluoride. Much less is known about chromium, cobalt, manganese, molybdenum, selenium, and even less about silicon, tin, vanadium, and nickel.

Iron functions chiefly as a component of oxygen-transporting hemoglobin found in red blood cells. It is also a component of myoglobin (for oxygen reserve in muscle) and such enzymes as catalase, xanthine oxidase, and the cytochrome enzymes of electron transport and as a cofactor of aconitase in the citric acid cycle.

The classic disease condition resulting from deficiency is iron-deficiency anemia (although anemia can have a number of causes). Excess iron produces hemosiderosis, characterized by necrosis of the liver and other soft tissues.

Copper, as a component of ceruloplasmin, is essential for incorporation of iron in hemo-globin. It also increases iron absorption and stimulates iron mobilization from tissue stores. Copper-containing enzymes function in energy metabolism and the metabolism of fatty acids and connective tissues.

Zinc is a component of at least 20 metalloenzymes; its more important functions include CO_2 transport and peptide digestion. Zinc also has a part in protein and nucleic acid metabolism, mobilization of vitamin A from the liver, and healing of wounds. Deficiency of the mineral retards growth and sexual maturation and delays healing.

Iodine functions in the synthesis of two thyroid hormones (thyroxine and triiodothyronine), which are "metabolic accelerators" and which are essential to normal metabolism. Iodine deficiency results in the classic symptom of goiter. Hypothyroidism (underactive thyroid), of which myxedema is a form, and hyperthyroidism (Grave's disease) are not related to dietary intake but represent metabolic errors.

Fluoride protects bone and especially dental tissue. An increased number of dental caries results from inadequate fluoride intake.

Little is known about the other trace minerals. *Chromium*—as GTF—enhances the activity of insulin and several other enzymes. *Cobalt's* only known function is as a component of vitamin B_{12}, the only form of this mineral the body can utilize. *Manganese* appears to be essential for growth, nervous function, and metabolism of lipids and carbohydrates. *Molybdenum* functions in purine metabolism. *Selenium* has antioxidant properties and functions as a component of glutathione oxidase, which destroys lipid peroxides. The mineral can be toxic, causing the "blind staggers" in animals and a variety of chronic symptoms in humans who live in areas where selenium-rich soils transfer large amounts of the mineral to plant foods.

Silicon, tin, vanadium, and *nickel* have yet to be established as essential nutrients, although there is some evidence that they have roles in maintenance of nutritional health. Silicon appears to be needed for structure and maintenance of connective tissue; and tin, vanadium, and nickel also appear to be involved in growth, the latter two elements possibly involved in lipid metabolism.

BIBLIOGRAPHY

ALLEN, L. H. Calcium bioavailability and absorption: a review. *American Journal of Clinical Nutrition* 35:783–808, 1982.

ALTURA, B. M. Role of magnesium ions in regulation of muscle contraction. *Federal Proceedings* 40:2645–2679, 1981.

The American Dietetic Association. Position paper on the vegetarian approach to eating. *Journal of the American Dietetic Association.* 77:61–69, 1980.

BELIZAN, J. M., J. VILLAR, O. PINEDA, A. E. GONZALEZ, E. SAINZ, G. GARGERRA, and R. SIBRIAN. Reduction of blood pressure with calcium supplementation in young adults. *Journal of the American Dietetic Association* 249:1161–1165, 1984.

BRONNER, F., and J. W. COBURN, eds. *Disorders of Mineral Metabolism, Vol. 2.,* New York: Academic Press, 1982.

BURK, R. F. Biological activity of selenium. *Annual Review of Nutrition* 3:53–70, 1983.

CARLISLE, EDITH M. The Nutritional essentiality of silicon. *Nutrition Reviews,* 40:193–198, 1982.

CHANDRA, R. K., ed. Trace elements in nutrition of children. *Nestle Nutrition Workshop Series, Vol. 8.* New York: Raven Press, 1985.

CHARLTON, R. W., and T. H. BOTHWELL. Iron absorption. Annual Review of Medicine 34:55–68, 1983.

COOK, J. D., ed. *Iron. Vol. 1.* New York: Churchill Livingston, 1980.

COOK, J. D., and M. E. REUSSER. Iron fortification: An update. *American Journal of Clinical Nutrition* 38:648–659, 1983.

CZAJKA-NARINS, D. M. Absorption of nonheme iron. In *Biochemistry of the Elements, Nonheme Iron Biochemistry Vol. 1,* A. Bezkorovainy, ed. New York: Plenum Publishing Co., 1980.

DALLMAN, P. R. Diagnosis of anemia and iron deficiency: Analytic and biological variations of laboratory tests. *American Journal of Clinical Nutrition* 39:937–941, 1984.

DELUCA, H. F., and C. S. ANAST, eds., *Pediatric Diseases Related to Calcium.* New York: Elsevier North-Holland, 1980.

DISILVESTRO, R. A., and R. J. COUNSINS. Physiological ligands for copper and zinc. *Annual Review of Nutrition* 3:261–288, 1983.

DUBRICK, M. A., and R. B. RUCKER. Dietary supplements and health aids—A critical evaluation. Part 1—Vitamins and Minerals. *Journal of Nutritional Education* 15:47–53, 1983.

ESKEW, D. L., R. M. WELCH, and E. E. CARY. Nickel: An essential micronutrient for legumes and possibly all higher plants. *Science* 222:621–623, 1983.

FINCH, C. A., and J. HUEBERS. Perspectives in iron metabolism. *New England Journal of Medicine* 306:1520–1528, 1982.

FISCHER, P. W., A. GIROUX, and M. R. L'ABBE. The effect of dietary zinc on intestinal copper absorption. *American Journal of Clinical Nutrition* 34:1670–1675, 1981.

Food and Nutrition Board, National Research Council. *Recommended dietary allowances,* 9th ed. Washington, D.C.: National Academy of Sciences, 1979.

FORBES, R. M., and J. W. ERDMAN, JR. Bioavailability of trace mineral elements. Annual Review of Nutrition 3:213–231, 1983.

FREGELY, M. J. Sodium and potassium. *Annual Review of Nutrition* 1:69–83, 1981.

GARN, S. M., A. S. RYAN, and S. ABRAHAM. The black-white differences in hemoglobin levels after age, sex, and income matching. Ecol. Food Nutr. 10:69–70, 1980.

GARN, S. M., and A. S. RYAN. Relationship between fatness and hemoglobin levels in the national health and nutrition examinations of the U.S.A. Ecol. Food Nutr. 12:211–215, 1983.

GOLUB, M. S., M. E. GERSHWIN, L. S. HURLEY, A. G. HENDRICKS, and W. Y. SAITO. Studies of marginal zinc deprivation in rhesus monkeys: Infant behavior. *American Journal of Clinical Nutrition* 42:1229–1239, 1985.

HALBERT, L. Bioavailability of dietary iron in man. *Annual Review of Nutrition* 1:123–147, 1981.

HEANEY, R. P., J. C. GALLAGHER, C. C. JOHNSTON, R. NEER, A. M. PARFITT, and G. D. WHEDON. Calcium nutrition and bone health in the elderly. *American Journal of Clinical Nutrition* 36 (Suppl.): 986–1013, 1982.

HEANEY, R. P., R. R. RECKER. Osteoporosis-related nutritional influences on bone calcium. In H. F. DeLuca, ed., *Osteoporosis: Recent Advances in Pathogenesis and Treatment.* Baltimore: University Park Press, 1981.

HEGSTED, M., S. A. SCHUETTE, M. B. ZEMEL, and H. M. LINKSWILER. Urinary calcium and calcium balance as affected by level of protein and phosphorous intake. *Journal of Nutrition* 111:553–562, 1981.

HOOPER, P. L., L. VISCONTI, P. J. GARRY, and G. E. JOHNSON. Zinc lowers density lipoprotein-cholesterol levels. *Journal of the American Medical Association* 244:1960–1961, 1980.

HURLEY, L. S. Trace metals in mammalian development. *John Hopkins Medical Journal* 148:1–10, 1981.

KELSAY, J. L. Effect of diet fiber level on bowel function and trace mineral balances of human subjects. Cereal Chemistry 58:2–5, 1981.

KELSAY, J. L., K. M. BEHALL, and E. S. PRATHER. Effect of fiber from fruits and vegetables on metabolic responses of human subjects, II. Calcium, magnesium, iron and silicon balances. *American Journal of Clinical Nutrition* 32:1876–1880, 1979.

KIDD, P. S., F. L. TROWBRIDGE, J. B. GOLDSBY, and M. Z. NICHAMAN. Sources of dietary iodine. *Journal of the American Dietetic Association* 65:420, 1974.

KOHRS, M. B., C. KAPICA-CYBORSKI, and D. CZAJKA-NARINS. Iron and chromium nutriture in the elderly. In D. Hemphill, ed. *Annual Conference on Trace Substances in Environmental Health,* XVIII, pp. 476–486, Columbia, MO: University of Missouri, 1984.

LANE, H. W., and J. J. CERDA. Potassium requirements and exercise. *Journal of the American Dietetic Association* 73:64, 1978.

LONNERDAL, B., A. CEDERBLAD, L. DAVIDSON, and B. SANDSTROM. The effect of individual components of soy formula and cows' milk formula on zinc bioavailability. *American Journal of Clinical Nutrition* 40:1064–1070, 1984.

LUO, X., H. WEI, C. YANG et al. Selenium intake and metabolic balance of 10 men from a low se-lenium area of China. *American Journal of Clinical Nutrition* 42:31–37, 1985.

McCARRON, D. A., C. H. CHESNUT III, C. COB, and D. J. BAYLINK. Blood pressure response to pharmacologic management of osteoporosis. *Clinical Research* 29:274A, 1981.

McGEE, C. D., M. J. OSTRO, R. KURIAN, and K. N. JEEJEEBHOY. Vitamin E and selenium status of patients receiving short-term total parenteral nutrition. *American Journal of Clinical Nutrition* 42:432–438, 1985.

MATKOVIC, V. K., I. KOSTIAL, R. SIMONOVIC, A. BUZINA, J. BRODAREC, and B. E. C. NORDIN. Bone status and fracture rates in two regions of Yugoslavia. *American Journal of Clinical Nutrition* 32:540–549, 1979.

MENEELY, F. R., and H. D. BATTARBEE. Sodium and potassium. *Nutrition Reviews* 34:225, 1976.

MERTZ, W. Mineral elements: New perspectives. *Journal of the American Dietetic Association* 77:258–263, 1980.

MILLS, C. F. Dietary interaction involving trace elements. *Annual Review of Nutrition* 5:173–193, 1985.

MORRIS, E. R. An overview of current information on bioavailability of dietary iron to humans. Federal Proceedings 42:1716–1720, 1983.

NIELSEN, F. Ultratrace elements in nutrition. *Annual Review of Nutrition.* 4:21–41, 1984.

NORDIN, B. E. C., M. R. BAKER, A. HORSMAN, and M. PEACOCK. A Prospective trial of the effect of vitamin supplementation on metacarpal bone loss in elderly women. *American Journal of Clinical Nutrition* 42:470–474, 1985.

OFFENBACHER, E. G., and F. X. PI-SUNYER. Beneficial effect of chromium-rich yeast on glucose tolerance and blood lipids in elderly subjects. *Diabetes* 29:919–925, 1980.

OSKI, F. A., and S. A. LANDAW. Inhibition of iron absorption from human milk by baby food. *Am. J. Dis. Child.* 134:459–460, 1980.

POLLITT, E., and R. L. LEIBEL. *Iron Deficiency: Brain Biochemistry and Behavior.* New York: Raven Press, 1982.

POTTER, J. O., S. P. ROBERTSON, and J. D. JOHNSON. Magnesium and the regulation of muscle contraction. Federal Proceedings 40:2653–2656, 1981.

RAO, G. S. Dietary intake and bioavailability of fluoride. *Annual Review of Nutrition* 4:115–135, 1984.

REISIN, E., R. ABEL, M. MODAN, S. S. SILVERBERG, H. E. ELIAHOU, and B. MODAN. Effect of weight loss without salt restriction on the reduction of blood pressure in overweight hypertensive patients. *New England Journal of Medicine* 298:1, 1978.

RICHMOND, V. L. Thirty years of fluoridation: A review. *American Journal of Clinical Nutrition* 41:129–138, 1985.

ROGOFF, G. C., R. B. GALBURT, and A. E. NIZEL. *Calcium in Biological Systems.* New York: Plenum, 1984.

ROMSLO, I. Intracellular transport of iron. In A. Jacobs and M. Worwood, eds., *Iron Biochemistry and Medicine, II.* London: Academic Press, 1980, pp. 325–362.

ROSENBERG, I. H., and N. W. SOLOMONS. Biological availability of minerals and trace elements: A nutritional overview. *American Journal of Clinical Nutrition* 35:781–782, 1982.

RUDE, R. K. and R. R. SINGER. Magnesium deficiency and excess. *Annual Review of Medicine* 32:245–249, 1981.

SANDSTEAD, H. H. Copper bioavailability and requirements. *American Journal of Clinical Nutrition* 35:809–814, 1982.

SANDSTEAD, H. H. Zinc: Essentiality for brain development and function. *Nurtition Reviews* 43:129–137, 1985.

SCHAMSCHULA, R. G., and D. E. BARNES. Fluoride and health. *Annual Review of Nutrition* 1:427–435, 1981.

SIMOPOULOS, A., and F. BARTTER. The metabolic consequences of chloride deficiency. *Nutritional Reviews* 38:201–205, 1980.

SLAVIN, J. L., and J. A. MARLETT. Influence of refined cellulose on human small bowel function and calcium and magnesium balance. *American Journal of Clinical Nutrition* 33:1932–1939, 1980.

SIIMES, M. A., L. SALMENPERA, and J. PERHEEN-TUPA. Exclusive breast-feeding for 9 months: Risk of iron deficiency. *Journal of Pediatrics* 104:196–199, 1984.

SPENCER, H., L. KRAMER, M. LESNIAK, M. DE-BARTOLO, C. NORRIS, and D. OSIS. Calcium requirements in man: Report of original data and a review. *Clinical Orthopedics* 184:279–280, 1984.

SPIRO, T. G., ed. *Zinc Enzymes.* New York: John Wiley, 1983.

STEKEL, A., ed. Iron nutrition in infancy and childhood. *Nestle Nutrition Workshop Series: Vol. 4.* New York: Raven Press, 1984.

VAN RJJ, A., C. THOMPSON, J. MCKENZIE, and M. ROBINSON. Selenium deficiency in total parenteral nutrition. *American Journal of Clinical Nutrition* 32:2076–2085, 1979.

VETTER, J., ed. Adding nutrients to foods: Where do we go from here? St. Paul, MN: *American Association of Cereal Chemists*, 1982.

WACKER, W. *Magnesium and Man.* Cambridge, MA: Harvard University Press, 1980.

WEINSIER, R. L., and D. NORRIS. Recent developments in the etiology and treatment of hypertension: Dietary calcium, fat and magnesium. *American Journal of Clinical Nutrition* 42:1331–1338, 1985.

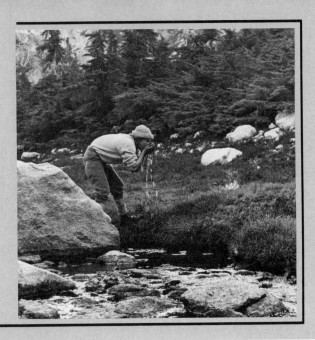

Chapter 9

WATER BALANCE

From the beginning of recorded history, water has been the source of life, the healer of illness, the secret of immortality. The water serpent of the Pueblo Indians; the river Lethe whose waters, according to Greek mythology, brought forgetfulness; the Christian ritual of baptism—these are only a few examples of the universal recognition given to water throughout human existence.

Water was generally believed to be the primordial environment in which living cells, which would give rise to all subsequent life forms, first appeared. Biologically speaking, we haven't strayed too far from those origins. The millions of cells that make up our bodies may be viewed as tiny fluid-filled aquatic organisms, moving in a sea of flowing body fluids. Body fluids—mostly *water*—normally comprise from 45 to 60 percent of the weight of healthy adults and a similar proportion of the weight of every other kind of living organism. Body fluids are never static. Water enters the body with ingested foods and beverages and is excreted in perspiration, respiration, feces, and urine. As it travels through the various body systems, it is constantly assisting or participating in biochemical reactions or otherwise facilitating essential body processes.

Water intake and output are normally in equilibrium, and about 2,400 milliliters (2.5 quarts) are ingested and excreted by the average adult every day. Interrelated regulatory systems in the brain, kidneys, and endocrine glands maintain water balance between intake and output and control the distribution of water within the body as well. Normally there are no significant fluctuations in body water levels. Although the body can tolerate a loss of most of its fat and carbohydrate content, and of about 50 percent of its protein, a loss of only 10 percent of body water is life threatening, and deficits greater than 20 percent are invariably fatal. Tales of survival after weeks of starvation are common, but more than a few days' survival without water is rare.

WATER AS A CHEMICAL

Water is a vital nutrient, and yet its role is quite different from that of the other nutrients previously studied. It is not digested before being absorbed from the intestine. It does not supply energy for growth, maintenance, or physical work. But as a substance with unique chemical and physical properties, it provides a suitable **medium** for the chemical reactions that occur in the body. In addition, water participates in biological reactions and plays an important role in regulation of body temperature.

A water molecule is triangular in shape, with one oxygen atom attracting the electrons from the two hydrogen atoms, which then become relatively positive in charge (Figure 9–1). The electronegative oxygen atom can attract other positive ions (cations), and the hydrogen atoms attract negative ions (anions). This chemical property decreases the strength of attraction between cations and anions and permits them to dissolve in a water solution. Since most biological compounds have areas of positive and negative charge, water is an excellent **solvent.**

Another fascinating property of water is that it remains liquid at room—and body—temperatures, although its component elements are gases at these same temperatures. If it were not for the strong attraction water molecules have for *one another*, water would be a volatile substance under normal living conditions. Large amounts of heat are needed to break the hydrogen bonds that allow water to

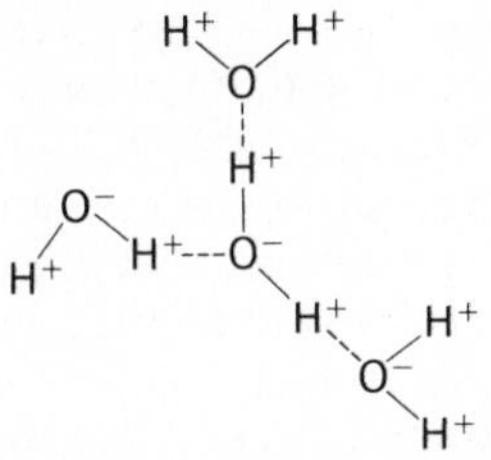

H^+ H^+
O
H^+
O^-
H^+ H^+---O^-
H^+ H^+
O^-
H^+

FIGURE 9-1   *Model of Four Water Molecules Joined by Hydrogen Bonds.*

"stick" to itself, accounting for the observation that water has a high *heat capacity;* that is, it takes a relatively large amount of heat to increase the temperature of water. As a result, water is a relatively poor conductor of heat. This property is important in the economy of the body; although water helps to distribute heat evenly throughout the body, it absorbs the heat produced without becoming "hot" itself.

Compared to other molecules of the same size, water has a high *latent heat of vaporization,* the amount of heat necessary to produce a vapor from a liquid. Only at 212°F (100°C) are all the hydrogen bonds between water molecules broken, allowing water to boil up to form water vapor. This special property of water is important, because one of the ways the body dissipates excess heat is through evaporation of water from the skin. If water were vaporized at lower levels of energy (heat), humans could not survive the external heat of tropical climates or the internal heat of high fevers: The body's fluid supply would quickly sizzle away.

HOW WATER FUNCTIONS

The chemical properties of water are responsible for its functions in the body.

Regulation of Body Temperature

Metabolic reactions produce energy, some of which is trapped as ATP and some of which is released as heat. A portion of this heat is useful for maintaining body temperature. But the body must dispose of excess heat, which would otherwise inactivate enzymes necessary for vital metabolic processes. The major routes for loss of excess heat at low environmental temperature and humidity are radiation and conduction. Smaller amounts of heat are dissipated as "insensible perspiration." Six hundred kilocalories are used in the evaporation of every liter of fluid from the surface of the body. As a result, loss of water by insensible perspiration, estimated to be 20 to 30 milliliters per hour, results in loss of heat of about 12 to 18 kilocalories per hour. The amount of heat lost by insensible evaporation is in direct proportion to body surface area and in inverse proportion to the amount of subcutaneous fat. This layer of fat acts as an insulator, preventing effective heat transfer—a bonus in winter and a detriment in summer.

When environmental temperature or humidity rise, body heat cannot be effectively lost by radiation and conduction. If the ambient temperature is greater than that of the skin, the body actually gains heat. Under this condition, the only way for the body to cool itself is by sweating (sensible perspiration). When environmental temperature and humidity become so high that perspiration cannot evaporate and exert its cooling effect, heat stroke may result, with body temperatures soaring as high as 107° to 110°F (42° to 43°C). Ambient temperatures higher than 90°F (32°C) and relative humidity greater than 80 percent may produce this condition, particularly during exertion. Heat stroke is life-threatening not only because of water loss due to continued sweat production but also because elevated body temperatures inactivate cellular enzyme systems. Irreversible cell damage may follow.

The temperature-regulating capacity of water is also apparent when a fever "breaks," which is signalled by heavy perspiration. As water evaporates from the skin, it has a cooling effect, and body temperatures start to subside. Prolonged fevers are dangerous because the body's heat cannot be released to the external environment. As in heat stroke, irreversible cell damage occurs when the body temperature exceeds 106°F (41°C).

Solvent for Biochemicals

The solvent properties of water underlie some of its other functions and are nutritionally important in several ways. Enzymes, hormones, and coenzymes are dissolved in watery body fluids and act on metabolites (amino acids, carbohydrates, vitamins, minerals) that are similarly dissolved. Water also serves as a solvent for waste products—urea, carbon dioxide, and various electrolytes—destined for excretion. As a solvent containing these substances, water assists in their transport to and from all cells of the body.

Lubrication

Water serves as a lubricant in digestion and other body processes. The water in saliva facilitates chewing and swallowing, ensuring that foods will slide easily down the esophagus. Water in other digestive fluids sustains movement throughout the gastrointestinal system. The watery fluid surrounding such body parts as joints and eyeballs helps them to move smoothly.

Hydrolysis and Other Biological Reactions

Water is an active participant in hydrolysis, a major chemical process. During this process water molecules separate into hydrogen (H^+) and hydroxyl (OH^-) groups, each of which reacts with other substances. Sucrose, for example, is hydrolyzed into fructose and glucose, forms in which it can be utilized by body cells (see Chapter 2). In addition, water serves as a reactant in intracellular reactions and plays an important role in the maintenance of electrolyte balance.

DISTRIBUTION OF BODY WATER

The proportion of water in the body varies with age, tissue composition, and sex. It is highest in earliest life; a human embryo is an average 97 percent fluid, and the body of a newborn baby is about 77 percent water. Dehydration proceeds slowly but steadily throughout life. In an adult male of normal weight, water represents about 60 percent of body weight. Loss of water in all tissues continues and is probably involved in many of the physical alterations associated with aging.

Although water is present in all tissues, its relative proportion varies. Bone is 10 percent water, teeth only 5 percent, and adipose tissue 25 to 35 percent. In comparison, muscle tissue is 72 percent water. Thus, as body fat increases, the relative percentage of body water decreases. In lean, muscular adults, water accounts for 70 percent of total body weight, but in obese adults, only 50 percent. Because women of normal weight have a higher percentage of adipose tissue than men, they have a lower percentage of body water.

Compartmentalization

Approximately 60 percent of the body's total water content is contained inside the cells and is said to make up the **intracellular compartment.** The remaining 40 percent, located in the many areas outside the cells, makes up the **extracellular compartment,** which has two major subdivisions as shown in Figure 9–2. **Intravascular fluid,** representing 20 percent of the extracellular fluid in the body, is the liquid component of blood and is present in the heart, arteries, veins, and capillaries. **Interstitial** and **transcellular fluid,** accounting for 80 percent of the extracellular fluid in the body, includes the fluids bathing all the cells, as well as such diverse substances as cerebrospinal fluid, the ocular fluid lubricating the eyes, the synovial

FIGURE 9-2   *Fluid Compartments of the Body.*

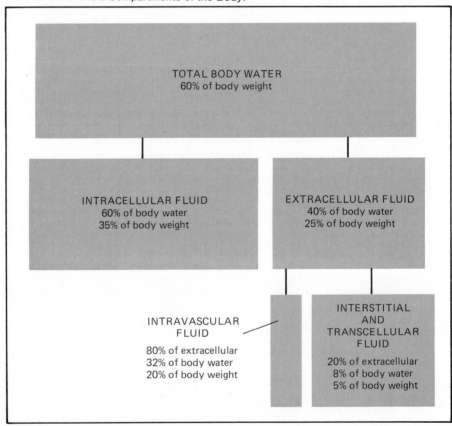

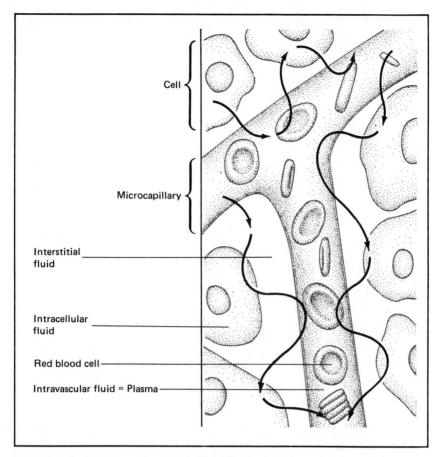

FIGURE 9-3 *Relationship of Body Fluid Compartments.*
Interstitial fluid is the vehicle for the exchange of nutrients, oxygen, and metabolic waste products between the microcapillaries and the cells.

Source: Adapted from J. R. Robinson, Water, the indispensable nutrient. *Nutrition Today* 5(1):16, 1970.

fluid that lubricates joints, various secretions (saliva, bile, gastric juice, mucus), and lymph.

The locations of body fluid are considered separate compartments, but they do not exist in isolation. Rather, compartmentalization is dynamic, with a constant exchange of fluid and other substances between compartments (see Figure 9–3). A variety of forces maintains the equilibrium of fluids and body chemicals in all compartments. Operation of these forces depends to a large extent on the content of the different body fluids.

CONTENT OF BODY FLUIDS.   In addition to fluid, every cell in the body contains the various nutrients required for all metabolic processes. Substances dissolved in the body fluids are **solutes.** Three categories of solute affect movement of body fluids: electrolytes, large molecules such as the plasma proteins, and smaller molecules such as glucose and urea.

Electrolytes are molecules that dissociate in a water solution into anions (negatively charged particles) and cations (positively charged particles). Chloride, bicarbonate, phosphate, and sulfate are the major anions; sodium, potassium, calcium, and magnesium are the most important cations contained in body fluids (see Table 9–1).

Within each compartment the total concentration of cations equals the total concentration of anions, making the solutions electrically neutral. By far the most common cation in extracellular fluid is sodium, and chloride is the most common anion. In intracellular fluid, however, potassium is the most common cation, and phosphate the most common anion. Extracellular fluid has a high sodium:potassium ratio, about 28:1, whereas intracellular fluid has a potassium:sodium ratio of approximately 15:1. Body fluids, then, differ in electrolyte content and concentration according to their location and function (see Table 9–2).

Fluid and Electrolyte Balance

Cell membranes are selectively permeable, allowing water and some solutes, but not others, to pass through. Several mechanisms control the flow of these substances within and among body tissues. Water is constantly flowing across—entering and leaving—every cell membrane; as much as 100 times the cell volume passes through the membrane every second, and yet total cell volume remains unchanged. The movement of water molecules through a membrane is known as **osmosis**. The specific electrolyte content and concentration in the fluids on either side of the membrane control the flow of water; fluid moves from the area of low to high electrolyte concentration in order to equalize the concentrations on both sides of the membrane.

The primary mechanisms underlying water transport through cell membranes are osmosis and **filtration pressure**. The greatest part of fluid exchange in the body takes place through the capillaries, whose walls are so thin that fluid and small solute particles pass through easily. Thus water, urea, and glucose move readily across capillary membranes, whereas hemoglobin and serum albumin, being large molecules, are retained within the capillaries. These large plasma protein molecules within the capillaries create *colloidal osmotic pressure* that tends to retain water in the capillaries and prevent its transfer into the interstitial spaces. Meanwhile, water and small particles are "pushed" out of the capillaries by the hydrostatic or filtration pressure exerted by the beating heart. This exchange is constantly occurring.

Under normal circumstances, despite the constant flow of body fluids, the electrolyte balance characteristic of each compartment and kind of cellular or extracellular location is maintained. Cell membranes keep specific proportions of different ions or other solutes in their respective places at a great expense of energy. Water balance, then, is maintained by the varied distribution of osmotically active solutes in the different compartments and cells. Overall volumes of blood and intracellular fluids are stabilized, even, if necessary, at the expense of interstitial fluid, which in effect serves as a "resource" for the maintenance of blood and cell fluid volumes.

Changes in permeability of membranes also affect water movements. The physiological state of an individual can alter membrane permeability, largely through the effects of hormones.

Under normal circumstances, the lymphatic circulation serves as an additional control mechanism, draining moderate amounts of excess fluid from the tissues and eventually returning them to the blood circulation. Under some pathological circumstances, however, this balance is thrown off, and excess fluid is retained in the interstitial space, resulting in **edema**. A sharp increase in blood pressure is one of

TABLE 9-1. *Electrolytes*

Major Cations	Major Anions
Sodium Na^+	Chloride Cl^-
Potassium K^+	Bicarbonate HCO_3^-
Calcium Ca^{++}	Phosphate HPO_4^{--}
Magnesium Mg^{++}	Sulfate SO_4^{--}

TABLE 9-2. *Ionic Concentration of Body Fluids*

Cation	Anion	EXTRACELLULAR FLUID		INTRACELLULAR FLUID	
		Cation, mEq/l	Anion, mEq/l	Cation, mEq/l	Anion, mEq/l
Na^+		142		11	
K^+		5		164	
Ca^{++}		5		2	
Mg^{++}		3		28	
	Cl^-		103		
	HCO_3^-		27		10
	HPO_4^{--}		2		105
	SO_4^{--}		1		20
	Protein		16		65
	Organic acids		6		5
Total		155	155	205	205

$$mEq = \frac{\text{Weight of Substance (mg)}}{\text{Molecular weight} \div \text{Valence (charge)}}$$

Source: Adapted from D. A. Black, *Essentials of fluid balance*, 4th ed. (Philadelphia: Lippincott, 1968), p. 9.

several reasons why this might occur. Other causes are infections of the lymph vessels and severe protein malnutrition. In this last instance, the concentration of the plasma proteins becomes so low that fluid is not drawn back into the capillaries and instead accumulates in interstitial fluid, leading to the characteristic bloated appearance of victims of kwashiorkor.

WATER BALANCE

Water, like the nutrients previously discussed, is at the center of a metabolic system that comprises sources of intake, body uses, and routes of output (see Figure 9–4).

Sources of Intake

Dietary fluids and foods constitute the primary sources of water. Consumption of soda, coffee, tea, juice, alcoholic beverages, milk, and just plain tap water typically tallies up to about 1,100 to 1,200 milliliters per day (1 to 1¼ quarts). Solid foods contribute another 500 to 800 milliliters of water each day. All foods, except pure fats such as vegetable oil, contain water, some foods having higher water content than others. Table 9–3 presents the water content of a variety of common foods.

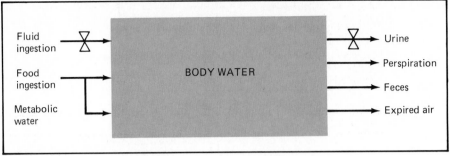

FIGURE 9-4   *Normal Routes of Water Intake and Output.*
Major regulatory controls are indicated. Thirst sensations increase fluid ingestion, and several mechanisms influence urine volume.

TABLE 9-3. *Water Content of Selected Foods*

Food	Serving Size	WATER CONTENT ml/serving	WATER CONTENT ml/100 g
Milk, skim	1 c	222.6	90.6
Cantaloupe	¼ 5″-diam. melon	217.0	91.2
Milk, low-fat, 2% solids	1 c	214.0	87.0
Milk, whole	1 c	213.3	87.4
Yogurt, plain	1 c	193.0	85
Yogurt, fruit-flavored	1 c	170.2	75
Orange	1 medium	129.0	86
Apple	1 medium	126.6	84.4
Banana	1 medium	113.5	75.7
Spinach, frozen, cooked	½ c	87.2	91.8
Beans, green, cooked, drained	½ c	59.7	91.8
Fish, haddock, cooked	3 oz	56.1	66.0
Soybeans, cooked	½ c	55.3	73.7
Rice, cooked	½ c	54.4	72.5
Chicken, light meat, cooked	3 oz	54.2	63.8
Hamburger, 21% fat, cooked	3 oz	46.1	54.2
Carrots, raw	½ large	44.1	88.2
Egg	1 large	42.0	73.7
Ice cream	½ c	41.7	63.2
Lettuce	½ c chunks	35.3	95.4
Cream cheese	1 oz	14.3	51.1
Cheddar cheese	1 oz	10.4	37.1
Bread, whole-wheat	1 slice	8.4	35.0
Bread, white, enriched	1 slice	8.2	35.6
Apricots, dried	5 halves	4.5	25.0
Corn flakes, dry	1 c	1.0	3.6
Butter	1 tsp	0.8	16.0
Margarine	1 tsp	0.8	15.5
Popcorn	1.5 c	0.8	3.8
Peanut butter	1 oz = 2 tbsp	0.5	1.8
Margarine, whipped	1 tsp	0.5	15.5
Saltine crackers	2	0.3	4.3
Oils	1 tsp	0.0	0.0

Source: C. F. Adams, *Nutritive value of American foods in common units,* USDA Handbook No. 456 (Washington, D.C.: U.S. Government Printing Office, 1975).

Note that vegetables, fruits, and fluid milk products contain more than 75 percent water, whereas meats and fish provide from 50 to 65 percent. Breads (approximately 35 percent water) and dry cereal products (less than 5 percent) contribute only small amounts of water.

Metabolism itself provides an additional 300 to 400 milliliters of water each day; when protein, carbohydrate, and fat are oxidized, they yield approximately 0.4, 0.6, and 1.1 milliliters of water per gram, respectively. Catabolism of fat stored in the body, as well as dietary fat, is a source of water, producing approximately 1 liter of water for 1 kilogram of adipose tissue. This metabolic water is formed by combining hydrogen removed from nutrients with oxygen obtained by breathing air.

Mechanisms of Loss

Urine production in the kidneys accounts for most of the body's water output. The lungs, skin, and feces also provide routes for water loss.

THE KIDNEYS. The body's total volume of blood passes through the kidneys many times each day, at a rate of about 1¼ quarts (1,200 ml) per minute. In this short time a specific part of the kidney's functional units known as *nephrons* (each kidney contains 1 million nephrons!) acts as a filter, producing a protein-free filtrate containing water, glucose, amino acids, minerals, metabolic waste products, and very small amounts of the myriad of other substances present in body fluids.

The filtrate then passes into long tubules whose cells selectively reabsorb most of the glucose, amino acids, and electrolytes in the filtrate, along with some 80 percent of the water. This complex separation and reabsorption process produces urine containing primarily sodium, urea, and other waste products of metabolism dissolved in water. Ordinarily, there is no glucose in the urine. The kidneys have a highly efficient active transport system that passes glucose back into the blood. Only when blood glucose exceeds approximately 160 mg/dl does it surpass its renal threshold and spill into the urine.

Active transport mechanisms also move additional quantities of potassium, hydrogen, and other ions from the blood capillaries across the cells of the kidney tubules, where they are secreted into the urine. This secretion process serves the important function of adjusting acid-base balance in the body. The kidneys' combined filtration, reabsorption, and secretion systems help to regulate the osmotic pressure of body fluids, to control fluid and electrolyte balance, and to maintain acid-base equilibrium.

Under normal circumstances, urine production in the kidneys ranges from 900 to 1,400 milliliters per day, depending on fluid intake. However, metabolic disturbances and altered dietary intake are quickly detected by the kidneys. If there is a decrease in extracellular fluid volume (as in hemorrhage), the kidneys respond by decreasing urine volume. If water consumption is excessive, urine volume is increased. High-protein, high-salt, and low-carbohydrate diets all tend to increase urine volume, because they present the kidneys with a large solute load of urea, sodium, and ketone bodies, respectively. Increasing water intake with these diets will dilute solute concentrations but increase urinary output. Conversely, low-protein, low-salt, and high-carbohydrate diets are useful in situations where water intake and output must be minimized.

FECAL WATER LOSSES. Of the approximately 8 liters of water secreted into the gastrointestinal tract as part of digestive juices per day, only about 200 milliliters is excreted in the feces. Much of the water of digestive fluids is normally reabsorbed in the colon. Diarrhea and high-fiber diets decrease reabsorption and thus increase fecal water loss.

THE LUNGS. Another 300 milliliters of water vapor is exhaled through the lungs each day. High altitudes and strenuous exercise increase the respiration rate to meet the body's oxygen needs. Under these conditions, respiratory water loss also increases. Dehydration and physical debilitation are often experienced by mountain climbers at high altitudes, when several liters of water may be expired in the course of a day.

THE SKIN. Each day from 400 to 500 milliliters of water is lost through the skin as "insensible" perspiration, the nonvisible sweating that occurs even when the body is at rest. Insensible perspiration increases in dry climates. In the pressurized cabins of airplanes, for example, very dry air and rapid air circulation combine to cause large insensible losses of water, contributing to the feelings of lethargy and fatigue known as "jet lag." Although beverages are usually served to passengers, fluid intake may not be sufficient to replace the quart or more of water lost through insensible perspiration even on short flights. The heavy perspiration that we experience in hot, humid weather contributes to water losses through the skin in addition to normal loss.

Taken together, normal water losses through the urine, feces, insensible perspiration, and respiration total about 1,900 to 2,400 milliliters per day for an adult living in the temperate zones, closely matching the average daily fluid input. Under normal conditions, the water intakes and outputs are balanced.

REQUIREMENTS

There is no RDA for water. Needs vary from individual to individual in response to changes in both the external and internal environments. Age, activity level, health status, air temperature, and even the time of day influence water requirements. The Food and Nutrition Board indicates that "under ordinary circumstances," a reasonable daily water allowance for adults would be 1 milliliter per kilocalorie, providing about 2.5 to 3 quarts, including that contained in foods. The daily allowance for infants is 1.5 milliliters per kilocalorie (0.5 to 1.5 quarts in the first year), an approximate reflection of the higher water content of the body at younger ages, the increased surface area in relation to body weight, and the high basal metabolic rate of infants.

REGULATION OF WATER BALANCE

Water is unique among nutrients because the body has a set of intricate warning mechanisms that detect negative balance. Of course, the body also has hunger warning systems, but they do not indicate specific nutrient deficits. When people

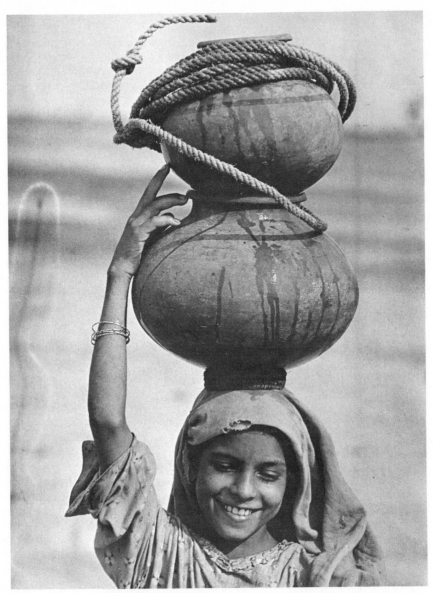

Water is a vital nutrient. In most of the developing nations, water must be drawn by hand and carried to the home, often from a distance.

Lynn McLaren, Rapho/Photo Researchers

feel hungry, they know the body is calling for food, but they usually don't know which specific carbohydrates, proteins, fats, vitamins, or minerals are lacking. Thirst, on the other hand, means just one thing: Take a drink. Whether one chooses milk, tea, coffee, or any other fluid, the basic nutrient supplied is still water, just what the body ordered.

Regulation of Intake

The thirst warning system involves a complex network of signals and responses. Dehydration and decreased blood volume increase electrolyte concentration in extracellular fluids, thus raising the osmotic pressure of the blood. A decrease of normal body fluids by as little as 1 percent causes thirst. Three interrelated sensing systems become activated, making the individual aware of the need for water intake.

The most familiar sensing system consists of the nerve endings in the mouth and pharynx. As body fluid levels decrease, secretion of saliva decreases as well, and these nerve endings perceive the increasing dryness of the mouth.

Another sensing system consists of thirst receptors in the hypothalamic portion of the brain. Decreases in fluid in the extracellular compartment result in higher electrolyte levels and greater osmotic pressure. As the osmotic pressure draws fluid from the intracellular compartment, cells become dehydrated. This signals the thirst center of the hypothalamus, which also triggers drinking behavior.

A third network is activated when sodium content of extracellular fluid is depleted. As water leaves that compartment to raise the sodium concentration, blood volume diminishes, and fluid levels in the intracellular compartment are increased. The fluid-filled cells do not, however, send nonthirst signals. Rather, the decrease in blood volume stimulates volume receptors in the heart, which in turn signal the hypothalamic thirst center. This might happen, for example, on a low-sodium diet or as a result of hemorrhage, prolonged diarrhea, or vomiting.

As ingested water enters the system, it is rapidly dispersed into the blood stream. As the extracellular compartment regains its fluid volume, osmotic balance between compartments is achieved. The various thirst receptors are no longer stimulated, and the sensations of thirst vanish until the cycle begins again.

Regulation of Output

The kidneys are the primary control mechanism for regulating water output, and they function chiefly by adjusting urine volume. (See Figure 9–5.) As decreased extracellular fluid volume results in an increase in osmotic pressure, cells of the posterior pituitary gland are stimulated to secret antidiuretic hormone (ADH). This polypeptide, also known as *vasopressin*, acts on the tubules of the kidneys to cause increased reabsorption of water, resulting in the production of more concentrated urine. As reabsorption causes fluid volume levels of extracellular fluid to rise, osmotic pressure becomes equalized, cells regain their full fluid volume levels, and ADH secretion is halted.

Another hormone, aldosterone, also acts in the kidneys to help maintain water balance. A steroid hormone produced in the adrenal gland, *aldosterone*, is released in response to sodium depletion, reduced blood volume, or increased extracellular potassium concentration. In the kidney, aldosterone increases reabsorption of sodium, leading to greater sodium concentration inside kidney cells. As a result, the cells of the tubules reabsorb additional water. These increased quantities of sodium and water move from the kidney into the plasma, increasing plasma volume and sodium content.

Recall that the sodium:potassium ratios characteristic of the intracellular and the extracellular compartments must be maintained. When the decrease of sodium or increase of potassium in the blood results in an increase in aldosterone produc-

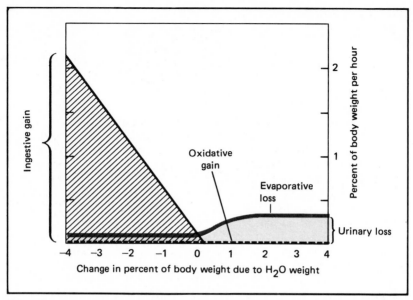

FIGURE 9-5   *How Water Balance Is Maintained.*
The maintenance of water balance is shown in this diagram devised by E. P. Adolph of the
University of Rochester. When the body is dehydrated (left of zero water load), gain by
drinking (hatched area) exceeds water loss via urine excretion and evaporation from lungs
and skin. When there is an excess of water in the body (right of zero water load), urine output increases and drinking stops so that water loss exceeds the small gain from the oxidation
of the hydrogen of food (indicated by broken line). These regulatory processes compensate
for deficits or excesses of water and tend to bring the body to a zero water load, where the
curves of total gain and loss cross.

Source: A. V. Wolf, Body water, *Scientific American* 199(5):125, 1958.

tion, potassium is drawn from the blood into the kidneys, where it enters the urine
for excretion. Release of aldosterone, then, results in retention of sodium and water
and excretion of potassium.

DISTURBANCES IN WATER BALANCE

Regulatory systems in the kidneys, hypothalamus, and several other glands ordinarily function in remarkable harmony, finely tuning water and electrolyte balances
throughout the body and within its numerous parts (see Figure 9–6). But a number
of external and internal conditions may overtax these mechanisms. Because water
balance is critical, any condition resulting in significant depletion or excess is dangerous and must be corrected promptly.

Dehydration

Dehydration may result from unusual fluid loss as well as from decreased fluid intake. Hemorrhage, diarrhea, vomiting, or ADH insufficiency directly diminish

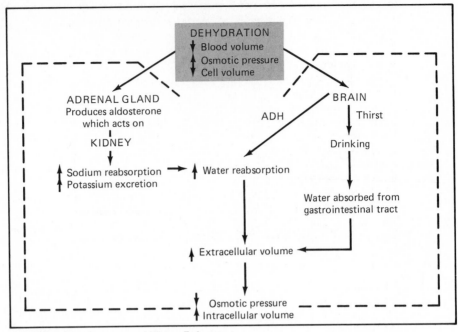

FIGURE 9-6 *Summary of Water Balance.*
Dehydration results in water conservation, mediated by behavioral (thirst) and hormonal (aldo-sterone and ADH) mechanisms. Restoration of water balance turns off the signals to the brain and adrenal gland.

blood volume. Abnormal sweating, or seepage from extensive burns or other severe wounds, represents loss of interstitial fluid.

Fluid loss consists not only of water but of electrolytes as well. Because the body's fluid compartments are contiguous and interdependent, water and electrolyte losses in any compartment have an impact throughout. Vomiting, for example, causes loss of hydrochloric acid as well as water from the stomach and results not only in dehydration but also in electrolyte imbalance. The loss of acid directly causes an excessive concentration of sodium and potassium ions in the remaining body fluids.

In diarrhea the fluid loss from the intestines includes sodium-containing bile, pancreatic secretions, and intestinal secretions. The result is dehydration. The changed osmotic pressure because of this electrolyte imbalance causes more water and sodium to move from the intravascular and interstitial areas into the gastrointestinal tract. Blood volume and cell volume decrease, and too little water is available for the kidneys. These organs respond by increasing sodium retention by the aldosterone mechanism previously discussed, so that water will also be reabsorbed. Meanwhile, to maintain the potassium:sodium ratios, potassium ions move out of cells into interstitial spaces. At the same time, the kidneys are recycling the retained sodium back into the blood to increase the *volume* of blood. Potassium must move out of the blood, to be lost in the urine. This deprives muscles of the potassium ions needed for contraction, producing weakness and diminished reflex responsiveness. Severe potassium depletion will affect the functioning of heart muscle and may result in cardiac failure.

For most adults, the mild diarrhea that accompanies occasional stomach upsets or viral infections does not cause significant risk. Even mild diarrhea, however, may have severe consequences for the very young and the elderly, as may any other dehydrating condition. Although the bodies of infants and children contain a higher percentage of water than adults' bodies do, their total water content is, of course, quite small. Because of their high metabolic rate and increased surface area, their water requirements are relatively high. This makes infants quite vulnerable to sudden water losses. Because the elderly have a low percentage of body water, and renal mechanisms for water reabsorption may be impaired, they also are at risk. Metabolic losses of nutrients may be significant as well. When any dehydrating condition exists, at any age, care should be taken to restore fluid and electrolyte balance by ingestion of fluids—water, weak tea, bouillon, orange juice, gelatin dessert, or soft drinks. With the very young or the elderly, fluids may have to be forced or administered intravenously. Even in healthy young adults, if the condition is severe or prolonged, it may be necessary to administer fluid and electrolytes intravenously.

CHOLERA. An extreme dehydrating condition is cholera, a gastrointestinal disturbance caused by toxin-producing microorganisms. The rapid and voluminous watery diarrhea of cholera creates a sudden and significant loss of both fluid and electrolytes. Therapy limited to antimicrobial agents may kill the infecting organism but does not combat the severe dehydration that is the primary cause of fatalities from cholera. Immediate and constant therapy with a solution of water and electrolytes is essential.

PROFUSE SWEATING. Profuse sweating represents water loss from the interstitial spaces; sodium and chloride, the major electrolytes of interstitial fluid, are lost as well. Although intense thirst may be perceived, it is not advisable to drink more than 2 quarts of tap water in this situation. Rapid ingestion of plain water further

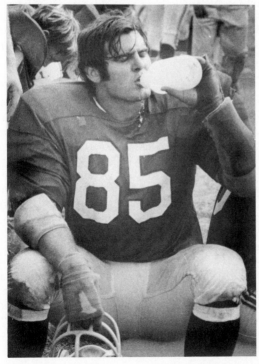

A football player should drink to maintain adequate hydration and optimum performance, not merely to satisfy thirst.

Ellis Herwig/Stock, Boston

323

dilutes the depleted salts in the extracellular compartment. In order to equalize electrolyte concentrations, water enters the cells. Cellular overhydration leads to painful muscle contractions ("heat cramps"), weakness, and a decrease in blood pressure. The Food and Nutrition Board recommends that when more than 4 quarts (approximately 4 liters) of water have been consumed to replace sweat losses, additional water intake should be accompanied by 2 grams of sodium chloride for each quart.

The need for salt is related to water replacement, not to the amount of perspiration. Individuals not adapted to heavy work or exercise in a hot environment may experience salt-depletion heat exhaustion because of inadequate replacement of *salt* following heavy perspiration. This is a hazard of which many vacationers are not sufficiently aware, as they spend hours on the tennis courts or otherwise overexert on the first day at a semitropical resort. This condition may also occur in individuals who attempt to carry on a normal activity load during a heat wave or in athletes, such as football players, who train during the summer.

Water Intoxication

Several years ago there appeared reports about a woman who died after drinking too much water in a misguided attempt to "cleanse" her body of impurities. At about the same time, a young victim of child abuse also died after her father forced her to consume excessive quantities of water. Both deaths were due to **water intoxication**, an intake of fluid that exceeds the maximal rate of urinary flow. As hard as the kidneys work, they cannot keep up with tremendous influxes of water. Fluid volume of cells increases, and cellular constituent substances become diluted. Cells in all parts of the body, including the brain, are affected.

The light-headedness, confusion, and poor coordination that result resemble inebriety and give the condition its name. More severe symptoms follow: throbbing headache, nausea and vomiting, weakness, tremors, convulsions, coma, and finally, death. These symptoms are due primarily to the relative lack of salt in the body. Administration of salt in early stages of water intoxication can halt or prevent muscular and other symptoms. Cessation of fluid intake is, of course, essential.

Other Influences on Water Balance

The body is a remarkable machine, but there are limits to its ability to sustain external or internal insults. Under normal conditions the interacting water regulatory mechanisms keep in fine balance. But any of several normal, disease, and accidental conditions can cause fluid imbalance. In each case the regulatory systems are upset, but in different ways.

WATER RETENTION AND FEMALE HORMONES.   We have seen that maintenance of water balance involves the hormones ADH and aldosterone. However, other hormones act in concert with these. The thyroid hormones, for example, increase reabsorption of sodium in the kidney tubules; other hormones modify the action of ADH. Estrogen and progesterone, the two primary female hormones, are of particular interest in relation to their effects on fluid regulation.

Many women are aware of greater fluid retention immediately prior to and at the start of their menstrual periods and during the last trimester of pregnancy. Premenstrual edema was once thought to be due to high progesterone levels at these times. However, it now appears that progesterone is an aldosterone antagonist, in-

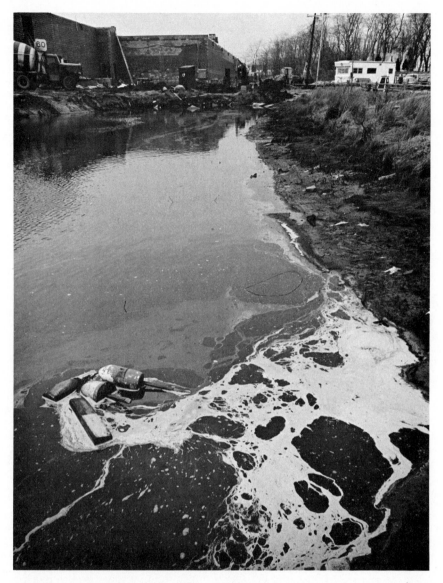

The EPA sets standards for water quality and conducts tests to detect contamination. Despite safeguards, contaminants continue to enter our water supplies.

Gordon S. Smith/Photo Researchers

creasing sodium and water excretion and causing retention of potassium. Sodium loss, and therefore water loss, caused by progesterone production in physiological amounts are transient effects.

Estrogen, on the other hand, has a slight resemblance to aldosterone and initially causes water loss followed by a period of sodium, and therefore, fluid retention. Premenstrual edema is a complex phenomenon, with variable effects in

Perspective On

NUTRITION FOR ATHLETES

Athletes, whether amateur or professional, pursue an unending search for that tantalizing "edge" in competition, the reserve and endurance that will put them out front, surging ahead of their opponents. In pursuit of that extra something, many have turned to supernutrition or even to drugs. Careful attention to nutrition can indeed help athletes achieve their bodies' full potential, while undernutrition will surely hinder athletic ability. But whether supernutrition can create super performance is debatable. And taking drugs for purposes of extending endurance or building protein in athletic competition is physiologically dangerous as well as unethical.

Nevertheless, many athletes, coaches, and trainers advocate certain nutritional supplements and dietary regimens to increase strength and endurance. Although there may be a factual basis for some recommendations, most perceived benefits are more psychological than physiological in origin. Research has shown, for example, that beyond a particular high level of athletic performance, additional physiological manipulations rarely have an influence. Subjectively, however, athletes seldom know why they perform well one day and poorly the next and may well attribute success or failure to a food eaten prior to the event. The strength of such a belief may aid performance, or deprivation of a favored food or regimen may impair performance because an athlete is insecure without it. Many sports superstitions focus on one particular nutrient category as the key to improved performance.

ENERGY. Modern athletes are a heterogeneous group with varying energy and nutrient needs based on age, sex, weight, height, metabolic rate, and the type, intensity, frequency, and duration of the activity. Energy needs of the athlete can exceed 6000 to 7000 kilocalories per day. In addition to "the event" athletes train long hours. If the athlete is still growing, additional calories are required to maintain that growth. Body weight and body composition affect performance: some sports favor greater weight and more body fat; while others favor those of lower body weight and fat. Gymnasts and dancers do better at lower body fat while those in the football line do well with extra pounds and fat. If a change in body weight is desired, gain or loss should occur slowly. In order to qualify for a particular weight class, young wrestlers sometimes abuse themselves by using drugs, vomiting, and sweating to produce dehydration which is manifested by weight loss. This practice should not be tolerated by parents or coaches. Ballet dancers, known to emphasize thinness, have been shown to consume unbalanced diets low in calories. In fact, the caloric intake was considered suboptimal for strenuous exercise.

PROTEIN. A popular training practice is consumption of great quantities of meat, intended to replace protein losses presumably incurred during strenuous muscular exertion or to confer the strength of the animal on the human depending on which myth you believe. This long-lived belief is at least as old as the original Olympic games. Because wrestlers were not classified by weight in ancient Greece, heavyweights had a distinct advantage. Trainers who introduced weight-increasing meat diets (which would be high in kilocalories) had observable success. Their method has had long-lasting repercussions: Vasily Alexeev, the 345-pound Russian Olympic gold-medal winner in weight-lifting, reportedly consumes 1,500 grams of protein each day, more than ten times the RDA, even for a man of his height, massive build, and high activity level. Nutritionists speculate that this diet has produced tremendous hypertrophy of Alexeev's liver and kidneys.

Excessive protein can deprive the body of more useful fuel and is expensive as well. Metabolism of excess protein produces excess body heat, which is detrimental to athletes. And water loss will be increased as well, as the increased urea production must be excreted in urine—at best a nuisance in athletic performance, and possibly dangerous as a potential source of severe water imbalance and increased likelihood of cramping.

Protein degradation increases during exercise and 5 to 15 percent of the oxidative metabolism of muscle comes from amino acids. Therefore, the protein needs of the athlete are slightly higher than those of a sedentary person. During the early stages of training 1.2 grams of protein per kilogram of body weight per day are recommended to allow for increased synthesis of body proteins. For the athlete who participates in intensive training, an intake of about 2 grams of protein per kilogram of body weight daily are suggested. These increased needs (197 grams of protein) are usually met by the average daily intake of most athletes; there is no need to take a protein supplement. A carefully planned vegetarian diet can also meet these requirements.

FAT. Fat-containing foods are concentrated sources of energy and are usually consumed in relatively large amounts to meet the unusual energy needs of athletes. Because they delay gastric emptying, however, there is good reason to avoid consuming fatty foods immediately before strenuous activity. The current recommendation is that an athlete in training have 30 to 35 percent of the kilocalories from fat.

Dietary fat should not be confused with *body* fat. Body fat is a reserve source of energy and may contribute as much as 70 percent of the energy required during prolonged aerobic work. But even the leanest athletes have adequate body fat to meet this sporadic metabolic demand.

CARBOHYDRATE. Carbohydrate is the most efficient fuel for energy production during maximum exertion. The body ordinarily contains limited stores of carbohydrate in the form of liver and muscle glycogen. These glycogen stores are essential for the repeated muscular contractions athletes perform. Some "single-effort" sports, such as diving, broad jumping, pole vaulting, and short-duration sports, such as sprinting and skiing, do not tax the usual stores of glycogen. However, the sustained effort required by sports, such as long-distance running, that involve endurance or extreme or prolonged stress may eventually deplete glycogen stores. Once depleted, muscles fail to contract. The result is exhaustion, a form of fatigue familiar to marathon runners, wrestlers, and rowers.

Research has shown that, over a period of time, decreased carbohydrate intake accompanied by exercise greatly reduces glycogen stores in the body. After several days on a low-carbohydrate regimen, an abrupt increase in carbohydrate intake dramatically increases glycogen stores and, consequently, physical stamina. This intake sequence is known as *carbohydrate loading.* While successfully increasing muscle glycogen, this regimen had a number of side effects. A modified technique is now recommended to achieve increased muscle glycogen and with no side effects. Following this regimen the athlete routinely consumes 50 percent of the kilocalories from carbohydrate. Three days before an event, the dietary pattern is changed so that 70 percent of the kilocalories are coming from carbohydrate and training is tapered down. Diets high in complex carbohyrdrates lead to greater muscle glycogen synthesis.

VITAMINS AND MINERALS. There is no evidence that vitamin intake in excess of body requirements confers any physiological benefit. In fact, high intake of some vitamins (fat-soluble A and D) carries a danger of toxicity. Athletes who take megadoses of various vitamin and mineral preparations are not receiving any significant benefit.

The ample diet required to provide high energy content ensures adequate intake even of those vitamins and minerals that are depleted during strenuous activity. Consumption of wholegrain or enriched bread products, for example, supplies adequate quantities of the B-complex vitamins necessary for metabolism of carbohydrate, protein, and fat. Supplements are unnecessary. Female dancers however rely on vitamin-mineral supplements to make up for the deficiencies in their low-calorie diets.

Reports of special benefits from particular vitamins are not scientifically valid. Vitamin E, for example, has been called a "supernutrient" by some trainers. But despite some early, promising reports, no consistent effect of this vitamin on physical endurance has been demonstrated.

Mineral supplementation is also commonly found in the athletic regimen. This practice, unlike vitamin supplementation, does have some physiological basis. Heavy exercise causes sweating, which can deplete the body's stores of sodium, potassium, and other minerals. Potassium deficiency is particularly damaging in athletes, since it interferes with glycogen formation in muscle tissue and results in cramping. This can be avoided by inclusion of potassium-rich foods such as oranges and bananas in the diet. Ingestion of salt tablets is not necessary and may be dangerous. Because excessive salt intake traps water in the extracellular compartments of the body and depletes intracellular fluid, water imbalance with potentially serious effects may result. Salting one's food to taste will replace losses.

Some female athletes (approximately 5 percent) experience excessive menstrual flow during strenuous exercise and may therefore lose more iron than other women. Supplements are often recommended during menstrual periods as well as careful attention to consumption of iron-rich meals at all times. This is not a universal problem, however; a significant number of female athletes fails to menstruate at all during times of heavy physical exertion. The reduction of body fat as a percentage of total body weight in well-trained female athletes most likely results in the observed amenorrhea. Exercise is usually considered to have a positive effect on calcium status. However, in a recent study, the bones of ballet dancers were shown to be less dense than expected, probably due to their low calcium intake.

FLUIDS. Exercise-induced sweating produces significant loss of water, particularly in hot, humid environments. A 2 to 3 percent loss of body water can impair performance; losses in excess of that amount greatly increase risk of dehydration and heat injury. Water cools the body as well as replaces losses. Further, it can be the vehicle of small amounts of readily usable carbohydrate when needed.

Because athletes have a larger than normal percentage of muscle tissue which contains a high percentage of water, water constitutes a larger percentage of their body weight. For this reason, they may find their after-exercise thirst is slaked by drinking fluids in amounts that do not fully replace lost fluid. Athletes should, therefore, drink according to a schedule to maintain adequate hydration and optimum performance and not merely enough to satisfy thirst. The American College of Sports Medicine recommends that fluids consumed during competition contain less than 2.5 grams of glucose per 100 ml water and less than 10 meg of sodium and 5 meg potassium per *liter* of solution. This is more dilute than most beverages given to athletes.

DRUGS. Perhaps the most controversial drugs currently taken by athletes are oral anabolic-androgenic steroids. These drugs are synthetic analogues of testosterone and other male hormones. Research has shown that androgens are involved in the anabolic processes of protein building and nitrogen retention. The higher concentration of androgens in males is responsible for their greater strength and muscle mass. Research studies do show a substantial risk of side effects ranging from inconvenient to serious. These include, in male athletes, decreased testicular size and function and decreased sperm production, and, in female athletes, delayed puberty, masculinization, voice changes, hirsutism (excess body hair), and menstrual disorders. Abnormal liver function, with various complications, has also been noted. Although many of these side effects may be benign and reversible, long-range effects are unknown, and several drug-related deaths have been reported.

Acknowledging these maximal risks and minimal benefits, the American College of Sports Medicine issued a position statement on the use and abuse of anabolic-androgenic steroids: In the absence of conclusive scientific evidence that these drugs either aid or hinder athletic performance, the reported benefits were classified as ''placebo effects'' generated by positive expectations on the part of trainers and athletes.

different women, and even in an individual woman, at different times of life. Changes in water balance during the menstrual cycle, pregnancy, and the use of oral contraceptives are clearly caused by changing relationships of estrogen and progesterone, but the mechanism causing these effects is not fully understood. Other hormones may be involved as well.

DIABETES.   The dynamics of water and electrolyte balance have particular significance for individuals with diabetes, heart disease, and of course, kidney failure. Diabetes mellitus, characterized by spillage of glucose into the urine, was discussed in Chapter 2. Another type of diabetes is known as *diabetes insipidus,* because of the bland, diluted quality of the urine, as opposed to the honeylike urine of the condition associated with lack of insulin. Diabetes insipidus is caused by abnormalities in ADH production or response, and it results in the production of enormous quantities of urine (5 to 15 liters per day) and feelings of extreme thirst. When the condition is caused by deficient production of ADH by the pituitary, it can be treated with ADH replacement. Patients with diabetes insipidus caused by kidney cells that are unresponsive to the action of ADH are less fortunate and must rely on drinking large amounts of water to compensate for the extreme urinary loss.

DIURETICS.   Edema, or fluid accumulation within the tissue spaces, accompanies various conditions, including congestive heart failure. Diuretic drugs are used to help correct this imbalance. Many diuretics inhibit the action of aldosterone, increasing sodium loss in the urine and drawing water away as well. As water is lost, accumulated interstitial fluid moves out of the tissues and into the vascular compartment on the way to the kidneys. Some diuretics also cause potassium depletion, an unwanted side effect. To counteract this, patients taking these drugs are advised to ingest potassium, either in the form of supplements or in foods, such as bananas and citrus fruits, that are rich in this mineral (see Chapter 8).

Some people use diuretics to promote weight loss. Diuretics rid the body of electrolytes and water, not of fat. Any weight loss that might follow indiscriminate use of diuretics may fool the mind of the dieter but not the body. Dehydration, potassium deficits, and other undesirable situations may follow. Meanwhile, the fat is unaffected.

Ethanol, the alcohol found in beverages, acts as a diuretic and inhibits the secretion of ADH by the pituitary gland. The increased volume of urine observed following a cocktail party is due not only to the fluid volume of the beverages consumed but also to their inhibition of ADH secretion. Instead of being reabsorbed in the kidneys, fluid goes directly into the urine. The persistent thirst felt several hours later, and the headachy "hangover" characteristic of "the morning after," signal the need to replenish the fluids lost the night before. The effect depends on the amount of alcohol in the blood, which in turn is directly related to the amount consumed and inversely related to the length of time over which the alcohol is imbibed. Symptoms can be partially prevented by drinking some water before retiring.

SUMMARY

Water is the most vital of all the nutrients, and yet it functions differently from the rest of them.

Water absorbs heat, thus helping to regulate body temperature. Evaporation of water from the skin in the form of sweat also serves this function. As a major component of the fluids involved in digestion, absorption, and metabolism, water serves as a solvent for metabolites and other substances and is an ion donor and recipient in numerous biochemical reactions. In addition, it is the transport medium in which digestive products and wastes move through the body. It is essential for the maintenance of electrolyte balance. Finally, water serves as a lubricant for body tissues.

The amount of water in the body varies with age, body composition, and sex. A newborn baby's body is 77 percent water and that of a normal adult male, about 60 percent. Adipose tissue is 25 to 35 percent water, and muscle tissue is 72 percent water. Therefore lean muscular individuals have proportionately more fluid than do the obese, whose bodies are only about 50 percent water. Women's bodies have less water than men's, and the percentage of body water is lowest in old age.

About 60 percent of the body's water is contained inside cells in the *intracellular compartment*. The *extracellular compartment* contains the remainder, of which some 20 percent is *intravascular fluid*, the liquid component of blood, and 80 percent is *interstitial* and *transcellular fluid*. Although these locations of body fluid are considered separate for conceptual purposes, in reality compartmentalization is dynamic, with fluids and their contents constantly flowing between the compartments.

Various organic molecules and the inorganic electrolytes are contained in body fluids. Electrolytes are minerals that ionize in water solution; anions are negatively charged, and cations are positively charged.

Chloride, bicarbonate, phosphate, and sulfate are the primary anions; sodium, potassium, calcium, and magnesium are the most abundant cations.

In each compartment, body fluids have a distinctive electrolyte composition. Water tends to flow from one compartment to the other until electrolyte concentration is equalized. Sodium and potassium, in particular, tend to draw water from areas of low salt concentration to areas of higher concentration; this principle is commonly expressed as "water follows salt." Cell membranes are selectively permeable, and water and various solutes enter and leave. The major influence on movement of water molecules through cell membranes is *osmotic pressure*, which increases when concentration of electrolytes and other solutes increases.

The amount of water in the body is kept at a relatively constant level. Water intake from beverages, foods, and metabolic oxidative processes is balanced by water outflow through the urine, the feces, insensible perspiration, and respiration. Although there is no RDA for water, the Food and Nutrition Board recommends an intake of 1 milliliter per kilocalorie.

When the body needs more water, saliva production decreases, and thirst warning centers sense resultant mouth dryness, increased extracellular electrolyte concentration, and decreased blood volume. These effects trigger drinking and the release of antidiuretic hormone (ADH). The kidneys respond by increasing reabsorption of water and producing more concentrated urine. Aldosterone and other hormones also participate in the control process.

Rapid water losses because of hemorrhage, diarrhea, vomiting, ADH insufficiency, extensive burns, or excessive perspiration may overwhelm regulatory mechanisms and lead to impaired cellular function due to electrolyte losses. Water intoxication because of excessive drinking is also damaging. Diuretic drugs may help to reverse fluid accumulation and its consequences in some cases.

BIBLIOGRAPHY

ALTURA, B.M., B.T. ALTURA, A. GEBREWOLD, H. ISING AND T. GUNTHER. Magnesium deficiency and hypertension correlation between magnesium-deficient diets and microcirculatory changes in situ. *Science* 223:1315–1317, 1984.

American College of Sports Medicine. Position statement on heat injuries. *Medical Science Sports* 7:vii, 1985.

ANDERSSEN, B., L. G. LEKSELL, AND M. RUNDGREN. Regulation of water intake. *Annual Review of Nutrition* 2:73–89, 1982.

AUKLAND, K. AND G. NICOLAYSEN. Interstitial fluid volume: Local regulatory mechanisms. *Physiological Review* 61:556–643, 1981.

BELIZAN, J.M. AND J. VILLAR. The relationship between calcium intake and edema- proteinuria-, and hypertension-gestosis: An hypothesis. *American Journal of Clinical Nutrition* 33:2202–2210, 1980.

BELIZAN, J.M., J. VILLAR, P. PINEDA, A.E. GONZALEZ, E. SAINZ, G. GARRERA AND R. SIBRIAN. Reduction of blood pressure with calcium supplementation in young adults. *Journal of the American Medical Association* 249:1161–1165, 1983.

BIE, P. Osmoreceptors, vasopressin, and control of renal water excretion. *Physiological Review* 60:961–1048, 1980.

BUSKIRK, E.R. Some nutritional considerations in the conditioning of athletes. *Annual Review of Nutrition* 1:319–350, 1981.

CHEN, L. C. Control of diarrheal disease morbidity and mortality. *American Journal of Clinical Nutrition* 32:2284, 1978.

CLEMENT, D.B. AND R.C. ASMUNDSON. Nutrition intake and hematological parameters in endurance runners. *The Physician and Sports Medicine* 10:37–43, 1982.

COHEN, J.I., I. POTOSNAK, O. FRANK AND H. BAKER. A nutritional and hematological assessment of elite ballet dancers. *The Physician and Sports Medicine* 13:43–50, 1985.

COSTILL, D.L., R. COTE, AND W.J. FINK. Dietary potassium and heavy exercise: Effects on muscle water and electrolytes. *American Journal of Clinical Nutrition* 36:226–275, 1982.

CZAJKA-NARINS, D.M. Water and Electrolytes in Food, *Nutrition and Diet Therapy* 7th ed. M.V. Krause and L.K. Mahan, eds. Philadelphia PA: W.B. Saunders Co. 1984.

DYCKNER, T. AND P.O. WESTER. Effect of magnesium on blood pressure. *British Medical Journal* 286:1847–1849, 1983.

FINBERG, L., R.E. KRAVATH AND A.R. FLEISCHMAN. *Water and Electrolytes in Pediatrics.* Philadelphia, PA: W.B. Saunders Co. 1982.

Food and Nutrition Board, National Research Council. *Recommended Dietary Allowances,* 10th ed. Washington, DC: National Academy of Sciences, 1979.

Food Power: A Coach's Guide to Improving Performance. National Dairy Council, 1983.

GOODMAN, M.N. AND N.B. RUDERMAN. Influence of muscle use on amino acid metabolism. In R.L. Teryung, ed, *Exercise and Sports Science Reviews.* Vol. 10. Philadelphia, PA: Franklin Institute Press, 1–26, 1982.

HANDLER, J.S. AND J. ORLOFF. Antidiuretic hormone. *Annual Review of Physiology* 43:611–624, 1981.

HAYMES, L.M. Protein, vitamins and iron. In

M.W. Williams, ed. *Ergogenic Aids in Sport.* Champaign, IL: Human Kinetics, pp. 27–55, 1983.

JOHNSON, R.E. Water and osmotic economy on survival rations. *Journal of the American Dietetic Association* 45:124, 1964.

LEHNINGER, A.L. Principles of Biochemistry. New York: Worth, 1982, pp. 67–93.

MCCARRON, D.A., C.D. MORRIS AND C. COLE. Dietary calcium in human hypertension. *Science* 217;267–269, 1982.

MOLHMAN, H.T., B.J. KATCHMAN, AND A.R. SLONIM. Human water consumption and excretion data for aerospace systems. *Aerospace Medicine* 39:396, 1968.

NARINS, D.M., S. SAPALA AND R. BELKENGREN. Nutrition for the growing athlete. *Pediatric Nursing* 9:163–169, 1983.

NIH Workshop on Nutrition and Hypertension. Proceedings from a symposium. M.J. Horan, M. Blaustein, J.B. Dunbar, W. Kachadorian, N.M. Kaplan, A.P. Simopoulos, eds. New York: Biomedical Information Corporation, 1985.

Nutrition for Sports Success. Washington, DC: The Nutrition Foundation, 1984.

O'BRIEN, D.F. The chemistry of vision. *Science* 218:961–966, 1982.

OLSON, R.E. The function and metabolism of vitamin K. *Annual Review of Nutrition Reviews* 4:281–337, 1984.

ONG, D.E. Vitamin A-binding proteins. *Nutrition Reviews* 43:225–232, 1985.

PARROTT-GARCIA, M. AND D.A. MCCARRON. Calcium and hypertension. *Nutrition Reviews* 42:205–213, 1984.

PECK, G.L., R.G. OLSEN, F.W. YODER, J.S. STRAUSS, D.T. DOWNING, M. PANDYA, D. BUTKUS AND J. ARNAUD-BATTANDIER. Prolonged remission of cystic and conglobate acne with 13-cis-retinoic acid. *New England Journal of Medicine* 300:329, 1979.

PHILLIPS, M.I., W.E. HOFFMAN, AND S.L. BEALER. Dehydration and fluid balance: Central effects of angiotensin. *Federation Proceedings* 41:2520–2527, 1982.

PIKE, J.W. Intracellular receptors mediate the biologic action of 1, 25-dihydroxyvitamin D 3. *Nutrition Reviews* 43:161–168, 1985.

RICHMOND, V.L. Thirty years of fluoridation: A review. *American Journal of Clinical Nutrition* 41:129–138, 1985.

ROBERTS, H.J. Perspective on vitamin E as therapy. *Journal of the American Medical Association* 246:129–131, 1981.

ROLLS, B.J. AND E.T. ROLLS. *Thirst.* New York: Cambridge Press, 1982.

SCHOELLER, D.A., VAN SANTEN, D.W. PETERSON, W. DIETZ, J. JASPAN AND P.D. KLEIN. Total body water measurement in humans with ^{18}O and ^{2}H labeled water. *American Journal of Clinical Nutrition* 33:2686–2693, 1980.

SCHRIER, R.W. AND T. BERL. Non-osmolar factors affecting renal water excretion. *New England Journal of Medicine* 292:81–88, 141–145, 1975.

SCHROEDER, H.A. Relation between mortality from cardio-vascular disease and treated water supplies. *Journal of the American Medical Association* 172:1902–1908. 1960.

SHERMAN, W. M. AND D. L. COSTILL. The marathon: Dietary manipulation to optimize performance. *American Journal of Sports Medicine* 12(1):44–51, 1984.

SHORT, S.H. AND W.R. SHORT. Four-year study of university athletes' dietary intake. *Journal of the American Dietary Association* 82:632–645, 1983.

SIMPSON, K.L. and C.O. CHICHESTER. Metabolism and nutritional significance of carotenoids. *Annual Review of Nutrition* 1:351–374, 1980.

SMITH, N.J. *Food for Sport.* Palo Alto, CA: Bull Publishing Co., 1976.

STUMBO, P.J., B.M. BOOTH, J.M. EICHENBERGER AND L.B. DUSDIEKER. Water intakes of lactating women. *American Journal of Clinical Nutrition* 42:870–876, 1985.

SUTTIE, J.W. The metabolic role of Vitamin K. *Federation Proceedings* 39:2730–2735, 1980.

SUTTIE, J.W. ed. *Vitamin K Metabolism and Vitamin K-Dependent Proteins.* Baltimore, MD: University Park Press, 1980.

WALD, G. Molecular basis of visual excitation. *Scientific American* 162:230, 1968.

WASSERMAN, R.H. and C.S. FULLMER. Calcium transport proteins, calcium absorption, and vitamin D. *Annual Review Physiology* 45:375–390, 1983.

WATSON, R.R. AND S. MORIGUCHI. Cancer prevention by retinoids: Role of immunological modification. *Nutrition Research* 5:663–675, 1985.

WEICK, M.T. SR. A history of rickets in the United States. *American Journal of Clinical Nutrition* 20:1234, 1967.

WILLETT, W.C., B.F. POLK, B.A. UNDERWOOD, M.J. STAMPFER, S. PRESSELL, B. ROSNER, J.O. TAYLOR, K. SCHNEIDER AND C.G. HAMES. Relation of serum vitamins A and E and carotenoids to the risk of cancer. *New England Journal of Medicine* 310:430–434, 1984.

WOLF, G. A historical note on the mode of administration of vitamin A for the cure of night blindness. *American Journal of Clinical Nutrition* 31:290, 1978.

YOUNG, V.R. AND P.M. NEWBERNE. Vitamins and cancer prevention: Issues and dilemmas. *Cancer* 47:1226–1240, 1981.

ZIEL, M.H. AND M.E. CULLUM. The function of vitamin A: Current concepts. *Proc. Soc. Exp. Biol. Med.* 172:139–152, 1983.

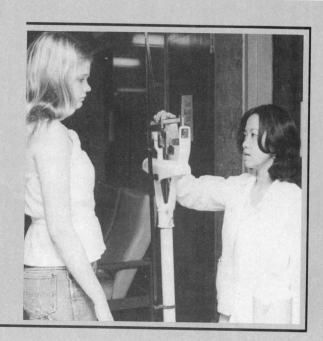

Chapter 10

We are all food *consumers*. As economic consumers, we select and purchase food. As biological consumers, we ingest, digest, absorb, and metabolize it. Both processes have become centers of attention. Books, magazines, newspaper articles, and radio and television programs provide a constant flow of information about food budgeting, "healthful eating," wise marketing, menu planning, and gourmet cookery. But despite our preoccupation with food and demand for information about it, and despite the fact that we have an abundance of food in this country, many people, either through ignorance or neglect, choose foods that do not provide adequate supplies of key nutrients.

Nutrition has also become an increasing concern to professionals involved with preventive as well as curative health care, as evidence mounts to implicate dietary factors in the incidence of heart disease, cancer, diabetes, and other illnesses. Poor nutritional status is sometimes associated with prolonged recovery periods following illness or injury, adding to the duration and cost of hospitalization.

Since good nutrition is consonant with good health, nutritional shortcomings and disorders and nutrient-related problems must be identified, not only in patient populations but in the presumably healthy general public as well. Four major methods—anthropometric, clinical, biochemical, and dietary—are used to assess nutritional status. The particular measurements used in the assessment depend on whether it is a minimal or screening assessment of an essentially healthy individual; whether it is a detailed and specific assessment of a patient who is unhealthy and may need complex support systems; or whether it is an examination of a population to determine the incidence of malnutrition. Because a particular finding may be due to any of several causes, no one of these methods is sufficient to diagnose a nutritional deficiency state. A child's failure to achieve an adequate rate of growth, for example, could be *documented* by anthropometric measurements but might be *caused* by heredity, disease, nutrition, or other factors. Only biochemical, clinical, and dietary data could confirm that the growth failure was caused by inadequate nutrient intake or some other factor.

These assessment tools are also used to identify individuals or populations who are "at risk" of developing nutritional deficiencies, as well as to evaluate the effectiveness of nutrition education or supplementary feeding programs. They can also determine relationships between nutrient intake and the onset or prevention of chronic nutrition-related disease, such as coronary heart disease, diabetes, and some forms of cancer. No association between a disease condition and nutritional factors can be determined if food intake patterns are not known. These methods can also help to identify nutrients that may be inadequately provided by the available food supply and necessary dietary changes can be instituted.

In this chapter we will examine not only the different means by which professionals assess nutritional status but also some of the aids to nutritional choice that have been designed to assist the general public in making good nutritional choices. Educated consumers are the key to improving nutritional status on a broad scale.

TOOLS FOR ASSESSING NUTRITIONAL STATUS

In a particular individual, clinical symptoms of nutrient deficiency and abnormalities of growth, development, or physiological function are the ultimate results of long-standing deprivations. Visible signs of nutritional deficiency do not appear until the body's stores of nutrients have been depleted. For most nutrients this will happen only after daily intake has fallen far short of need for a prolonged period of time. Examination of an individual's food behaviors may suggest the existence of a nutritional deficiency, and laboratory tests may confirm the tentative diagnosis. On the other hand, biochemical data can indicate tissue depletion of nutrients before clinical signs become apparent, and a study of food intake patterns may then strengthen the argument. A variety of standardized anthropometric, clinical, biochemical, and dietary assessment techniques are therefore necessary to determine nutritional status of individuals and groups. Each of these methods has advantages and disadvantages, but taken together they can confirm suspicions and provide the factual basis for corrective measures.

Anthropometric Assessment

Anthropometric (human measurement) assessments provide a gross indication of over- or undernutrition. Anthropometry cannot be used to detect short-term nutrient-specific disturbances in nutritional status. Anthropometric measurements are relatively easy to make, but they must be made very carefully in order to be useful. Measurements of many individuals representative of the total population provide standards against which data for an individual can be compared. Individual anthropometric measurements that vary significantly from standards may therefore indicate a nutrition-related problem, although they are not definitive.

HEIGHT AND WEIGHT. A person's potential for overall growth and body build is determined by heredity, but nutritional and other environmental factors can modify this potential considerably. Especially for young children, measurements of height or, for infants, length are reliable indicators of normal growth and development and imply adequate nutritional status. Similarly, height measurements also indicate subnormal growth that may be caused by dietary deficiency.

Current standards for evaluating the height and weight of children from two to 18 years of age were published in 1976 by the National Center for Health Statistics. These standards are based on measurements of large numbers of boys and girls from birth through age 18, who were selected from diverse geographical areas and cultural backgrounds and who represent the national population as it currently exists. Growth charts based on data of this type provide guidelines against which individual growth rates and patterns can be compared.

Data used for the growth curves of infants and young children from birth to 36 months are based on data from the Fels Research Institute and are older and less representative of the general population than the data for older children. Breast-fed infants are very under-represented in the Fels population and the data were collected at a time when early introduction of solid foods was common. These growth charts continue to be used as a frame of reference because of their general acceptance, but the limitations should be remembered when evaluating growth of infants, particularly those under one year of age.

Since genetics is an important factor in the final height of the individual, use of mid-parental height (the average of the heights of the parents) has been suggested to better evaluate growth of infants and children. A specific child is evaluated relative to other children of similar parental stature. Tables and equations are available to adjust the child's measured length or stature according to the parental stature. The presence of chronic disease may make growth assessment of some children more difficult, but some data are available for alternate methods of assessment of height or length.

NUTRITION SURVEYS IN THE UNITED STATES

For decades, information on agricultural production and sale of food products has been collected in the United States. These statistics, known as disappearance data, reflect the amounts of various foods absorbed into the economy. As such, they are useful in planning farm production, imports, exports, and food assistance programs. However, they do not describe the actual food intakes of the real people who make up our population. To do that would require a nationwide dietary survey.

Collecting intake data from the entire population would obviously be impossible. Therefore, sampling methods similar to those used by polling organizations are utilized to select a random sample of people whose food consumption patterns and other nutritional characteristics are then studied. From the resulting data, statistics are projected which are accurate, with a small margin of error, for a much larger group.

The 1960–70 study known as the Ten State Nutrition Survey, or TSNS, conducted by the Nutrition Program of the U.S. Department of Health, Education and Welfare (now Health and Human Services), was the largest nutrition survey ever done in this country until then. Impetus for the study came from an outpouring of public concern after congressional hearings in 1967 disclosed an unexpectedly high incidence of hunger and malnutrition in Americans, and numerous cases of starving children and emaciated elderly people were reported in the media. Because malnutrition in low-income groups was the focal point of the study, the sample was composed mostly of low-income families. The population studied was not therefore a representative sample of the entire population of the United States, or even of any individual state.

The sampling technique identified 30,000 families that were believed to be suitable for study; of these, 24,000 families, comprised of more than 86,000 individuals, were finally studied in detail. Each examination included a medical history; anthropometric measurements (height and weight, as well as selected diameters and circumferences); dental evaluation; and serum tests for anemia. Dietary intake was evaluated based on data obtained from a 24-hour dietary recall. High-risk subgroups of infants, young children, adolescents, pregnant and lactating women, and elderly people were assessed in particular detail.

The TSNS confirmed dramatically that a significant proportion of low-income groups was malnourished, and showed that specific nutritional problems varied in different subgroups. Overall, malnutrition was highest among migrant workers of Texas and low-income blacks. Generally, the incidence of malnutrition increased as income levels declined. The one specific nutrition deficiency present in all racial, age, and income groups was iron deficiency. Adolescents generally had the highest incidence of dental caries as well as the greatest number of indicators of

Growth, as measured in terms of weight for age or height for age, reflects the sum total of what has occurred up to that point in time. An alternate way to evaluate growth is to examine it per unit of time, that is, velocity or rate of growth. Velocity growth is more sensitive to changes in nutritional status. However, standards to evaluate velocity growth are not readily available, particularly for growth during the first few months of life. Published tables of normal adult weight, categorized by sex and height, also exist. Many of these are based on insurance company surveys of policyholders. Users of the tables should be aware that insurance studies do not include the total population and that although the sample is very large (4.2 million in the case of the latest revision) it is not random. The sample used was people who could and did buy life insurance. Weights for height in the 1983 Metropolitan tables are slightly higher than in the 1959 version. This has aroused considerable

malnutrition. The study concluded that poor food choices and inequitable distribution of food among family members, and not simply lack of food, were underlying causes of the nutritional problems observed.

The findings of the TSNS suggested the need for other surveys, more representative of the entire American population. Therefore, in 1971 the first Health and Nutrition Examination Survey, or HANES, was begun, using a random sample of subjects aged 1 to 74 years from all parts of the country. All subjects underwent complete clinical examinations, anthropometric assessments, and biochemical determinations on blood and urine. In addition, a subgroup of subjects completed a 24-hour food recall and a food history questionnaire. A second HANES study was then undertaken in 1976–79 and the third is in the planning stages. The mass of data collected in these studies is still being analyzed, but preliminary findings indicate the following:

1. Iron deficiency, evident from both dietary and biochemical findings, is prevalent in all segments of the U.S. population, with biochemical deficiency especially common in young children. The only subgroup with mean iron intake above the RDA was the 18- to 74-year-old male group.
2. Blacks 18 to 75 years old had lower intakes than whites for numerous nutrients: women had lower intakes than men. Those who took supplements had higher intakes than those who did not except for black males and low-income males who had lower dietary intakes.
3. White women in general and black women age 45 to 74 are more likely to be obese than are men; white men are more often obese than black men.

Interesting changes are seen when HANES data are compared with older survey results. For example, an unexpected and as yet unexplained decrease has occurred in serum cholesterol levels of middle-aged women over the past decade. Changes such as this illustrate the impossibility of ever obtaining once-and-for-all answers to questions regarding nutritional status in the United States, and point out the need for ongoing surveillance of the population.

Who to include in the survey, what nutrients to measure and how the status of specific nutrients can best be evaluated are all important questions. Perhaps future surveys should limit themselves to known significant variables and to carefully selected population subgroups. Nutrients presently considered important in public health nutrition are protein, iron, zinc, calcium, folic acid, thiamin, ascorbic acid, and vitamin A. Energy intake must also be considered as well because of the high incidence of obesity in the United States. But priorities change, because conditions change, and the principal nutrient concerns of today will surely give way to a different set of problems to be identified and studied in future nutrition surveys.

controversy. However, the relationship of obesity to mortality is not that clearcut and unless an individual has hypertension, diabetes, or a predisposition to diabetes, mortality may not be increased.

All insurance tables, including the present one, classify weight by frame size in addition to height. Unfortunately, frame size is not easy to determine. In the past, wrist circumference (either measured or estimated) was used, but reference data were not easily available. For the most recent tables a method of determining frame size by measurement of elbow breadth is given. Using this method, the individual places the thumb and index finger of one hand on the two prominent bones on either side of the elbow of the other arm, then removes the fingers from the elbow and puts them against a ruler or tape measure, reads the value and compares it to the values given in a table of elbow breadths. Keeping one's fingers the proper distance apart while moving them from the elbow to the tape measure is difficult. A better method, using a frameter, measures the elbow breadth directly. Bony chest breadth, measured on x-rays, has also been suggested as a method of determining frame size. At this point in time bony chest breadth is only of potential, not practical value.

Current data are not entirely satisfactory for anthropometric assessment of elderly persons. The large national surveys do not include individuals over 74 years of age in the sample, in spite of the fact that the most rapidly growing segment of the population is over 75 years of age. Data on the elderly are particularly difficult to interpret due to variations in the normal aging process from individual to individual. Reduction in stature, changes in the amount and distribution of body fat, and changes in tissue elasticity and compressibility make assessment more difficult. Limited reference data have been published, including a suggested method for calculating stature from knee height to correct for the reduction in height seen in many elderly persons. Weights of the elderly are not that difficult to obtain, but the answer to the question "How much should an elderly person weigh?" is not that easy. In the past the recommendation was that the weight at 25 years of age should be maintained. There are really no scientific data to back up that recommendation. Since the elderly are at greater risk for various diseases, they may be better protected if they weigh more.

Despite the limitations mentioned, height-weight tables are useful in defining extremes and are particularly useful in monitoring an individual over a period of time. Marked changes in an individual's weight (or in the case of children, changes in the *pattern* of growth and development) may indicate a nutritional problem. A child whose height and weight were at the median level (at the 50th percentile) at birth and during the preschool years, but whose growth rate decreases to the 25th percentile at age 10, should be examined for the presence of disease or other factors, including malnutrition, that retard growth.

OTHER ANTHROPOMETRIC INDICES.   Body mass index (BMI) or Quetelet index (weight in kilograms divided by the square of the height in meters) is being used more frequently in assessment of patients, particularly hospitalized patients. BMI is highly correlated with body fat. Frequently used cutoff points for obesity are 25 for men and 27 for women; with a cutoff of 20 for underweight. Only recently have values been published for the whole spectrum of weights. BMI less than 15 would indicate emaciation; 15 to 18.9 underweight, 19 to 24.9 normal weight, 25 to 29.9 overweight, 30–39.9 obese and 40 or above, severely obese. These values were determined using an Australian population and might be different for other populations. The 5th percentile for BMI for women aged 65 is about 20 and does not drop to 18.9 until age 85. Individuals with BMIs below 19 are not necessarily ill, but this value should alert the health professional of a potential problem. Measurement of skinfold thickness, midarm muscle circumference, and chest and head circumferences, as well as the use of X-rays to determine wrist bone development, are also helpful in identifying abnormal growth. In certain situations, they can provide significant additional data about an individual's condition. Their disadvantage, in comparison to more easily and inexpensively obtained height and weight measures, is that they require specialized equipment and personnel trained in their use.

The increased precision of these techniques does not guarantee better diagnosis of nutritional problems, however. The most complex and sophisticated anthropometric measurements are nonspecific. That is, although they may indicate signs of general undernutrition, they cannot pinpoint specific deficiencies or metabolic dis-

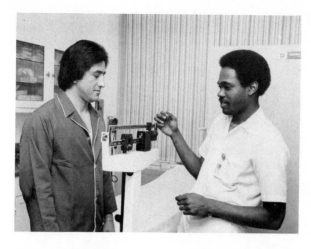

Marked changes in an individual's weight may indicate a nutritional problem.
Ken Karp

orders. With obesity, for example, overweight reflects excess energy intake but does not indicate the nature of the underlying causes. Similarly, unplanned weight loss can be due to many factors. These measurements may add little to what can be learned by simple height, weight, or weight/height ratios which have the additional advantages of being easily performed by a trained individual using equipment that is checked regularly and is readily available in clinics, physicians' offices, or other health care facilities.

Clinical Assessment

Anthropometric data collected during routine physical examinations reflect general health status. The physician uses this information as a guide and supplement in the clinical examination, a more thorough search for visible signs that reflect long-term disease processes. Severe nutritional deficiencies cause characteristic signs, directly related to the biochemical function of the nutrient involved, which can be observed during the physical examination. The most important of these have been mentioned in earlier chapters. Among the most apparent deficiency conditions are bone abnormalities due to lack of vitamin D or calcium, changes in eye appearance and function due to lack of vitamin A, and goiter resulting from lack of iodine. Such dramatic physical effects reflect long-term dietary deficits; a nutritionally inadequate diet for a few days or even a few weeks will not produce them. And in developed nations, nutritional deficiencies such as kwashiorkor, beriberi, and pellagra are rarely seen, in free-living populations. Hospitalized patients or patients with chronic diseases do exhibit clinical signs of deficiencies. Some clinical observations and their nutritional causes are listed in Table 10–1.

Although such symptoms seem easy to identify, many are puzzling when they do appear. There is a large area of subjectivity in all clinical observation. What looks like emaciation to some physicians may be "thinness" to others. This is a significant problem in clinical surveys of large populations, which depend on diagnostic reports from many physicians. Many physicians are not alert to signs of nutritional deficiency. Careful training and exact specification of clinical criteria are required if errors by examiners are to be avoided. Nevertheless, clinical observation is useful assessment method for screening large groups or institutionalized patients for signs of overt nutritional deficiency. Cinical assessment is quick, causes

TABLE 10-1. *Some Clinical Observations Used in Nutritional Assessment*

Part of Body	Observation	Deficiency/(Excess)
Hair	Dry, brittle	Protein
	Can be plucked easily	Protein
	"Flag sign"	Protein
Eyes	Dryness of conjunctiva and cornea	Vitamin A
	Increase in blood vessels in cornea	Riboflavin
Lips and mouth	Cheilosis (cracking)	Niacin, riboflavin
	Smooth, dark tongue	Niacin
	Magenta (purple) tongue	Riboflavin, folacin
	Bleeding gums	Vitamin C
	Dental caries	Fluoride/(carbohydrate)
		Protein
		Calcium
	Mottled enamel	(Fluoride)
Neck	Goiter	Iodine/(iodine)
Skin	Roughness at base of hair follicle	Vitamin A, essential fatty acid
	Dermatitis with sun sensitivity	Niacin
	Nasolabial dermatitis	Pyridoxine, riboflavin
	Pinpoint hemorrhages	Vitamin C
	Paleness	Iron
Nails	"Spoon-shape"	Iron
Extremities or torso	Edema	Protein, niacin
	Rachitic rosary	Vitamin D, calcium
	Scorbutic rosary	Vitamin C
	Frog legs	Vitamin C
	Bowed legs	Vitamin D
	Emaciation, muscle wasting	Energy, protein
	Obesity	(Energy)
	Abnormal reflexes	Thiamin, vitamin B_{12}

Note: These observations suggest, but do not prove, that malnutrition is the cause. Dry hair, bleeding gums, dental caries, dermatitis, edema, emaciation, abnormal reflexes, and many other clinical signs may result from genetic abnormalities, endocrine diseases, infections, exposure to toxins, or numerous other factors, as well as from malnutrition.

relatively little discomfort or inconvenience to the patient and, when done by a skilled practitioner, correlates well with more objective measures of undernutrition. Since there are many oral manifestations of deficiencies, dentists should be as aware of the clinical signs as other health professionals.

A number of extensive clinical studies have been designed to provide information about nutritional status and to identify populations at risk for nutritional deficiency. Documentation of clinical signs associated with malnutrition requires immediate intervention, since by the time a clinical sign of deficiency is apparent, underlying tissue depletion and metabolic disruption have already occurred.

Such studies can also be of value in conjunction with other assessment data, particularly in the identification of populations at risk of developing nutritional deficiencies. If a particular symptom or set of symptoms is noted with unusual frequency in the group being examined, this indicates the need to seek out other members of that population who are not yet affected or who may have less obvious **subclinical signs** of deficiency that would be overlooked in an ordinary physical examination.

Clinical assessment, by itself, cannot confirm a diagnosis of a specific nutritional deficiency or risk of deficiency. Most clinical signs are *nonspecific*. For example, dermatitis may be related to deficiency of B vitamins, vitamin A, protein, or essential fatty acids or to factors totally unrelated to nutrient deficiency, including colds and allergies. The list of observations in Table 10–1 may include some that are personally familiar to you, but that does not necessarily mean your diet is inadequate. Dry hair or pale complexion, for example, may reflect genetic or environmental factors. On the other hand, if these signs coincide with anthropometric indicators and with the biochemical signs presented next, diet may indeed be the causative factor.

Biochemical Assessment

Biochemical tests, which are based on knowledge of the metabolism and function of nutrients, are a useful adjunct to anthropometric and clinical assessment. They confirm suspicions of existing long-term deficiencies, are the most objective measures of nutritional status, and provide an early warning of clinical deficiency symptoms. Body measurements and clinical assessments reflect long-term and previous nutritional status, but biochemical analyses reflect the most recent situation, status of stores, or functional effects.

Most biochemical measurements are static indicators of concentrations of nutrients which are affected by a multitude of biological and technical factors. Over the past ten years there has been increased interest in functional indices of nutritional status. Areas of functional competence likely to be affected by malnutrition are cognitive ability, disease response, reproductive competence, physical activity and work performance, and social behavior performance. The true significance of nutritional deficiency is in the impairment of these types of functions.

Inadequate intake, inefficient digestion, disturbances in metabolism, or altered excretion of nutrients shows up quickly in the chemical composition of body fluids. Blood and urine, therefore, provide an accessible window on current nutritional status. Most nutrients and/or their metabolites can be detected in either or both of these fluids. A sample of blood, for instance, contains all the substances that are currently circulating to every cell in the body. A urine sample contains wastes and byproducts that indicate how those substances have been used in the cells. For example, a low urinary level of a particular substance may reflect inadequate intake, abnormal metabolism, or malabsorption from the digestive tract (in which case, the fecal content of that substance will be abnormally high, a situation that can be detected by different biochemical tests). A high urinary level, on the other hand, may suggest an excessive supply of certain nutrients or physiological abnormalities.

Generally, decreased levels of nutrients or their metabolites in blood and urine reflect depleted tissue reserves of the nutrient in question. However, this is not always the case: Under certain conditions, vitamin A stores in the liver may not be released into the blood, and blood levels of the vitamin will be abnormally low even though tissues are not depleted.

Analysis of nutrient levels in various body tissues such as liver or muscle would also provide this information, but that would involve the discomfort of having a tissue sample removed, as well as a certain amount of risk. For this reason, routine biochemical assessments utilize less invasive techniques, biopsies being requested only as a last resort or to confirm other findings implicating particular organs.

BLOOD ANALYSES. Measurements of the constituents in the blood provide clues about the level of nutrients in the body. Concentrations of some nutrients— vitamins, protein, lipids, and some minerals and other substances—can be measured directly.

Blood samples taken after an overnight fast are preferred, since concentrations of many nutrients are affected by meals and some also exhibit a diurnal variation. Concentrations in the blood can be altered by factors other than nutrition. For example, in patients with infection, serum iron is low because iron moves out of the blood and into the tissues, not because of iron deficiency per se.

In addition to directly measuring the concentrations of nutrients in blood, the concentrations of compounds which require specific nutrients for their proper function can be measured. For example, iron is an essential component of hemoglobin and if not present in sufficient amounts in the body, will result in less hemoglobin being produced. Therefore, measuring hemoglobin will provide information regarding iron status. Furthermore, if the precursor of hemoglobin, erythrocyte protoporphyrin, is not used to make hemoglobin, its concentration in blood increases. If not enough hemoglobin is being produced due to lack of iron, red blood cells are smaller and less red than normal (microcytic and hypochromic). This can be detected when the red blood cells are examined under a microscope. One of the most frequently used tests of nutritional status, hematocrit, is a ratio of the packed cell volume to the total volume of the sample. In patients with iron deficiency anemia the red blood cells get smaller and fewer in number, the packed cell volume goes down and the hematocrit is lower than that of a healthy person. All of these changes can be caused by problems other than iron deficiency: therefore, other measurements must be used to confirm the diagnosis of iron deficiency anemia.

Another method of measuring the nutritional status of some nutrients, usually vitamins, is to measure the activity of enzyme systems which require that specific nutrient as an essential cofactor for the reaction. Thiamin status is frequently measured using this technique. While direct measurement of thiamin or its phosphate ester in blood is now possible, the most useful and reliable method of assessing thiamin status is to measure the activity of the enzyme transketolase in red blood cells. A sample of blood is added to an incubation mixture which contains all components necessary for the reaction except thiamin. The amount of thiamin present will affect how much of the substrates are used or how much product is produced. Similarly, glutathione reductase activity is used to evaluate riboflavin status.

A knowledge of the regulatory mechanisms controlling each nutrient is important for accurate interpretation of biochemical results. For example, abnormal serum calcium levels do not usually result from a dietary deficiency of this mineral; rather, they are more likely to reflect a disturbance in one or more of the interconnected mechanisms that maintain calcium homeostasis, such as vitamin D, or they may be secondary to protein status.

URINE ANALYSES. Analysis of urine can detect normal or abnormal amounts of some nutrients or of their metabolites. Direct analysis can be done for a number of substances; glucose and albumin are among the most common. In addition, tissue reserves of water-soluble nutrients can be estimated by means of a "load" or "saturation" test: For example, administration of a large dose of ascorbic acid is followed by measuring the urinary excretion of vitamin C. With adequate tissue reserves of the vitamin, a large percentage of the administered dose will be excreted. Conversely, if the body's tissue reserves are low, a high percentage of the loading dose will be retained in the body, and therefore less will appear in the urine (see Figure 10–1).

Indirect, functional measures are also employed in urinalysis. For example, a "loading" dose of tryptophan, which is converted to nicotinic acid, may be administered before urine is collected for evaluation of vitamin B_6 status. Vitamin B_6 is

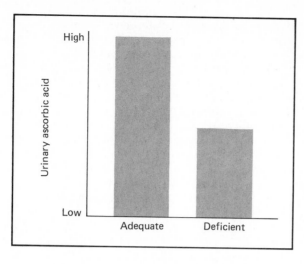

FIGURE 10-1
*Urinary Ascorbic Acid
Excretion after Load Dose
of Vitamin C.*

required in the conversion of xanthurenic acid to nicotinic acid (niacin), a step in the normal metabolism of tryptophan. Therefore, in patients with B_6 deficiency, a load dose of tryptophan will create an accumulation of xanthurenic acid, which will be excreted in the urine because there is insufficient vitamin B_6 available to convert it further to nicotinic acid.

Collection of urine samples is, surprisingly, more difficult than collection of blood samples. Although the momentary discomfort of drawing blood is avoided, the inconvenience factor is substantially increased. Ideally, biochemical tests are performed on a 24-hour sample of urine, which reflects the quantitative daily output of many substances rather than the relative output at any one time of day. Few subjects are willing to take the time and care required to collect 24-hour, or even 12- or 6-hour, urine samples. In most cases, a single specimen must suffice, from which quantitative estimates of daily excretion are calculated in reference to excretion of creatinine.

OTHER BIOCHEMICAL ANALYSES. Other samples may also be collected and studied to complement the biochemical data obtained from blood and urine analyses. Although stool examination for parasites, blood, and fats is useful, stool sampling is unpleasant and not generally used for routine nutritional assessments. It is, however, essential for detection of a number of gastrointestinal disorders.

Hair samples have been analyzed by measuring their diameter and by measuring concentrations of various components. At the present time, hair analysis is only valid to check concentrations of certain heavy metals. There are some data on concentrations of some trace minerals under a variety of conditions, hair analysis is not yet a routinely accepted measure of nutritional status. Eventually, it may prove to be a useful tool to assess status of a limited number of trace minerals such as zinc.

Immunologic responses are primarily used to provide information on the hospitalized, malnourished patient. The most frequently measured indicators of cell-mediated immunity are the total number of lymphocytes and skin.

Major disadvantages of many biochemical tests are the specialized equipment and carefully trained technicians needed to administer them. For these reasons such tests are often expensive. Many cannot be routinely used in field studies. Another drawback is that people often object to collecting urine samples or being "stuck" to give a blood sample. And finally, many biochemical analyses can show only what is *in* the body—not how it got there or why.

Biochemical studies do provide more specific information about nutrient status than the other methods described previously. Whereas anthropometric and clinical measures can only describe an individual's external appearance, biochemical tests are a "window" on the inner workings of the body.

Dietary Assessment

The three assessment techniques described thus far—anthropometric, clinical, and biochemical—can provide a great deal of data about an individual's physiological status. But they do not answer an important question: What is the food and nutrient intake? Dietary surveys do just that.

Conducting a dietary survey is more than a matter of asking a large number of people what they ate the day before. Some subjects will not remember at all, and many will omit one or more food items, either intentionally or unintentionally. The problems involved in learning about usual intake are even greater.

Dietary assessment can also suggest which biochemical tests should be performed and also enable health care professionals to compare the food patterns of an individual or group with a desirable standard, usually the RDA. This might be important, for example, in analyzing the nutritional status of a particular ethnic or socioeconomic group or of an individual. Also, dietary surveys make it possible to note trends in consumption patterns of specific population subgroups, as in the study of growth patterns and diets of children consuming vegetarian diets.

Several evaluation techniques are used. **Dietary recall** is a simple, rapid assessment method particularly useful for surveying large population groups. Typically, subjects are asked what foods, in what portions, were consumed in the previous 24-hour period. A particular advantage of the recall method is that respondents will not have had the opportunity to modify their usual food behaviors, something that frequently happens when people realize someone is interested in what they eat. Even though an individual's responses may be somewhat inaccurate or unrepresentative of typical intakes (the previous day may have been a birthday or the respondent was sick), the responses of the group as a whole provide a good qualitative estimate of general dietary behaviors in that particular population.

Because asking about yesterday's meals does not really provide very accurate information, specific kinds of dietary surveys have been developed for specific purposes. To obtain accurate dietary information about long-term patterns of consumption, *household* or *population assessment* methods are used. In **household surveys** a trained interviewer typically visits the home to record all the foods on hand at the start of the study and tells family members how to record all purchases made during the study. At the end of the study, the amounts and kinds of foods remaining in the house are also noted. Adjustments for food wasted within the home, that used for animal food, and that contributed by meals eaten outside the home must be made as well. Calculations estimate the nutrients available to the household during the study period. Adjustments are made for the number, age, and sex of people in the household, but they may not always correct for possible uneven distribution among family members. In addition, there is always the possibility that the food purchaser has altered usual buying habits during the study.

On a larger scale, the same type of survey could be used to record the quantities of foods produced in a particular region, city, or country; the amounts imported or

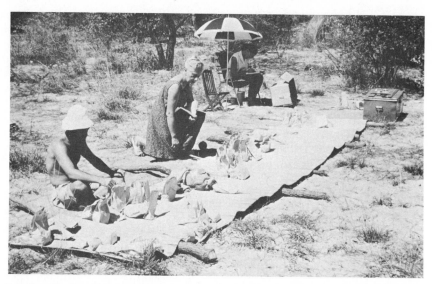

Samples of foods in the diets of peoples around the world are analyzed to determine their nutrient content. Here anthropologist Marjorie Whiting supervises the preparation of plant samples which must be dried, packaged, and labeled for analysis.
Nancy DeVore

exported; and the amounts lost in processing or allocation to animal feed. This information can serve to identify general consumption trends or ethnic or socioeconomic food habits, to predict food shortages and surpluses, and to diagnose inadequacies in a population's available diet.

To obtain accurate dietary information about a specific individual, other methods are used. **Food intake records** are written reports of foods eaten during a specified length of time, typically three to seven days. Although this reporting method minimizes the problem of atypical days, it introduces the problem of long-term diligence. Record keeping can be boring, and boredom increases with time. Not surprisingly, accuracy decreases as the duration of record keeping increases. In one study, few subjects kept accurate records for more than four days. Only well-educated, highly literate subjects maintained accuracy for a longer period. Thus, the need for diligence and literacy is a distinct disadvantage of dietary records; however, some way of motivating the subjects (visits or phone calls from a trained interviewer or a reward of some kind) often helps.

In both the recall and record methods, respondents must be advised about portions. Use of plastic food models, or description of portions in common household measures, increases the accuracy of the data obtained.

Weighed diets are carefully quantified records of the weights of all foods served to an individual or family, with the weight of uneaten food subtracted. Proponents of the weighed diet technique argue that the weighing process ensures accuracy, even with bored or poorly educated subjects. However, weighing foods and keeping records is tedious and time-consuming; unless highly motivated, the average person will not do it for a long period. Weighed diets are more feasible in an institutional setting, and studies in hospitals, prisons, and the uniformed services have used this method. Analysis of a duplicate sample of the food eaten is the most precise method of determining intake, but is seldom used, even in research studies, because of the expense involved in running the analysis.

Diet histories are interview or questionnaire surveys of subjects' usual dietary pattern. A diet history does not determine the precise foods eaten on a given day or week. Rather, it describes the kinds and amounts of foods typically eaten and the frequency of their consumption in a specified period of days, weeks, or months. Subjects frequently receive a check-off list of many different foods and drinks and a set of food models to be used in estimating portions. They simply search the list for foods they have eaten during the particular time period and then estimate the number and sizes of portions consumed. An interviewer can also elicit information about food likes and dislikes, usual number of meals consumed per day, and other pertinent information. Comparison of subjects' current diet histories with earlier patterns of consumption can provide an important measure of dietary changes that may relate to diseases or environmental variables. In addition, a dietary history can also be used to substantiate information obtained from a 24-hour recall and food intake record.

After individual, family, or group intakes have been determined, the quantity of food consumed must be translated into the quantity of nutrient intake. Then these levels can be compared with a standard, usually the RDA.

Generally, consistent intake of less than two-thirds of the RDA for one or more nutrients has been shown to be associated with risk of nutritional deficiency in an individual or population. Anthropometric, clinical, and biochemical data would, however, be needed to confirm suspicions. Figure 10–2 diagrams the interactions of the primary assessment techniques.

Of course, mere identification of current or changing consumption patterns does not benefit health. Intervention must follow. In cases of severe deficiency, immediate refeeding and medical care is, of course, urgent. Planning, redistribution of food supplies, and nutritional education programs are required for individuals and groups at risk. In addition, some attention must be paid to those not known to be at risk. Education programs and maintenance of food supplies will help to ensure that currently adequate nutritional status will continue in the future.

FIGURE 10-2   *Development of Nutrient Deficiency and Tools for Assessment.*
Source: Adapted from W. A. Krehl, *Med. Clin. N. Am.* 48:1129, 1964.

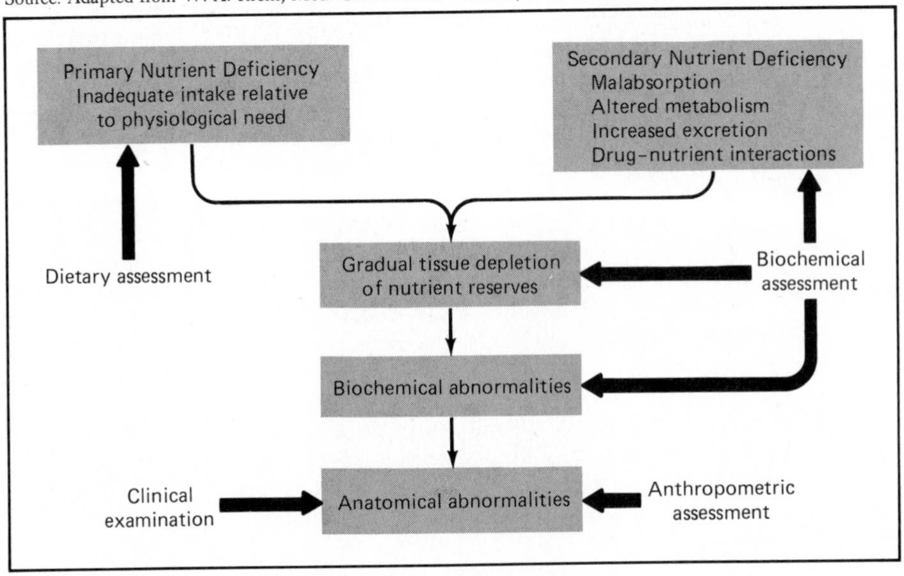

PLANNING AN ADEQUATE DIET

Our discussion of dietary assessment indicated the need for estimates of adequate and suboptimal nutrient intake based on standardized information. To obtain these measurements, nutritionists first had to determine average levels of nutrients contained in various foods, since after all, nutrients are almost never ingested in pure form. To complicate matters further, both naturally grown and manufactured foods tend to vary in their nutrient content. In metabolic nutrition research this natural variability is neutralized by laboratory analysis of samples of any food to be eaten by the subject being studied. But this procedure is impractical for large-scale research or field studies. Food composition tables provide average nutrient values, based on quantitative analysis of many samples of each food item.

Food composition tables are widely used by professional nutritionists. With the RDAs, they provide a means of planning diets and menus to meet the needs of individuals of all ages under normal conditions, and under some special conditions as well. Because these guides are too complex for everyday use by most people, meal-planning aids for the general public and for particular purposes have also been devised.

Food Composition Tables

In 1869, Wilbur Atwater chemically analyzed Indian corn, which was the first American food to be studied for its nutrient content. By 1880 tables of food composition had been issued for numerous European products. In 1892 Atwater and Woods published the results of their investigations of about 900 foods, most of them meats. In the same year the USDA issued its Bulletin No. 11 summarizing the composition of more than 3,000 food items, mostly animal feeds, which had been analyzed before 1890. *The Chemical Composition of American Food Materials*, USDA Bulletin No. 28, by Atwater and Woods in 1896, is considered the classic American food table. This first comprehensive list of more than 600 edible items included their content of protein, carbohydrate, fat, ash, and water.

Tables in use at present are compiled not only by the government but by educational and industrial research groups as well. Most include data for a minimum of five vitamins and five or more minerals now known to be essential nutrients, as well as food energy, protein, and lipid content. The new tables reflect the increasing variety of foods available in this country, and they also provide data on the different forms in which they are consumed. Although early tables gave data only for food in its raw form, tables issued by the USDA since 1940 have included values for fresh, canned, dried, and cooked forms of foods. More recently, values for frozen and commercially prepared foods have been added.

As new nutrients have been discovered and new assay methods developed to identify them in foods, tables have been issued that focus on one nutrient or a group of related nutrients; excerpts from some of these have appeared in previous chapters. In 1968, for example, when enough data had been accumulated to publish recommended dietary allowances for seven new nutrients (vitamins E, B_6, B_{12}, and folacin and the minerals phosphorus, iodine, and magnesium), there was a demand for information on their occurrence in foods.

Changing commercial and home-cooking or processing methods also affects the nutrient content of foods. Cooking by moist or dry heat, freeze drying as opposed to flash freezing, fast microwave roasting as compared with slow oven baking, all present the need for reevaluation of nutrient content. In addition, yesterday's carrot may not be the same as today's. Vitamin content of a food can vary with the season, geographical area where it was produced, growing conditions, and genetic factors; mineral content is affected by soils, weather, and water supply. Garden-to-table time, storage facilities, and cooking methods also affect nutrient content. As scientific breeding practices produce new strains, nutrient composition is altered. It has been estimated, for example, that young frying chickens sold during the 1960s contained about one-tenth more water, about half as much fat, and about 30 percent fewer calories than young chickens sold 40 years earlier. Differences in breeding, feeding, and processing account for much of this change. Another familiar product, commercial white bread, has also changed significantly. Unlike the bread of the 1920s, which was made with water, white bread today is mixed with milk and contains calcium-rich mold inhibitors. As a result, today's bread has nearly three times the calcium content of the bread Grandma used to eat.

Then, too, new foods must be analyzed. "Health" foods and foods of ethnic groups—Chinese, Italians, Mexicans, Cubans, native Americans, black Americans, and others—have become increasingly popular today in all segments of the population. Many of the foods characteristic of these groups remain to be evaluated for nutrient content. In addition, recent discoveries concerning inborn errors of metabolism and other metabolic disorders have led to a demand for information about the distribution and amount of specific amino acids in foods.

In recent years, methods of laboratory analysis have increased in accuracy and reliability. Food chemists are repeating tests to obtain specific or more useful data, as well as testing newly developed or currently popular items. But some of the nutrient contents may not actually be used by the body. Many of the factors affecting this nutrient **bioavailability** are still unknown. Certain gastrointestinal disorders and ingested drugs reduce absorption from the intestine and thus limit nutrient bioavailability. The factors affecting utilization of micronutrients can be complex, as in the case of iron. As knowledge increases about the ways in which nutrients and other chemicals present in foods (phytates, for example) interact, new research must identify these substances in foods, and food tables must make the new data available.

Health care professionals and many consumers are acquainted with a printed format that can be kept for frequent reference. Since publication of Atwater's USDA Bulletin No. 28, and its revisions in 1899 and 1906, the USDA has issued many food composition tables. The most recent major revision is Handbook No. 8, *Composition of foods—Raw, processed, prepared.* To make available the information that has become known since 1963, a revised Handbook No. 8 is now being prepared. Sections are released as they are ready: 8–1, *Dairy and Egg Products;* 8–2, *Spices and Herbs;* 8–3, *Baby Foods;* 8–4, *Fats and Oils;* 8–5, *Poultry Products;* 8–6, *Soups, Sauces, and Gravies;* 8–7, *Sausages and Luncheon Meats;* 8–8, *Breakfast Cereals;* 8–9, *Fruits and Fruit Juices;* 8–10, *Pork Products;* and 8–11, *Vegetables and Vegetables Products.* Table 10–2 presents the data for an egg as shown in Handbook 8–1.

The complete revision of Handbook No. 8 is scheduled to contain information on more than 4,000 food items. In addition to previous sections, information on the following categories is being included: nuts and seeds; legumes; fish and shellfish; beef; lamb and game; bakery products; sugars and sweets; beverages; and mixed dishes. The data tabulated are for water, energy, protein, fat, total carbohydrate, fiber and ash, mineral elements (calcium, iron, magnesium, phosphorus, po-

TABLE 10-2. Nutrient Composition of a Whole Chicken Egg, Fresh or Frozen Raw (Adapted from Handbook 8–1)

NUTRIENTS AND UNITS		AMOUNT IN EDIBLE PORTION OF COMMON MEASURES OF FOOD	
		Approximate measure and weight	
		1 egg = 50 g[a]	1 c = 243 g
PROXIMATE			
Water	g	37.28	181.20
Food energy	kcal	79	384
	kj	330	1,606
Protein (N × 6.25)	g	6.07	29.50
Total lipid (fat)	g	5.58	27.09
Carbohydrate, total	g	.60	2.92
Fiber	g	0	0
Ash	g	.47	2.28
MINERALS			
Calcium	mg	28	136
Iron	mg	1.04	5.08
Magnesium	mg	6	30
Phosphorus	mg	90	438
Potassium	mg	65	316
Sodium	mg	69	336
Zinc	mg	.72	3.50
VITAMINS			
Ascorbic acid	mg	0	0
Thiamin	mg	.044	.211
Riboflavin	mg	.150	.731
Niacin	mg	.031	.151
Pantothenic acid	mg	.864	4.197
Vitamin B_6	mg	.060	.292
Folacin	mcg	32	158
Vitamin B_{12}	mcg	.773	3.759
Vitamin A	RE	78	379
	IU	260	1,264
LIPIDS			
Fatty acids:			
Saturated, total	g	1.67	8.14
4:0	g		
6:0	g		
8:0	g		
10:0	g		
12:0	g		
14:0	g	.02	.07

NUTRIENTS AND UNITS		AMOUNT IN EDIBLE PORTION OF COMMON MEASURES OF FOOD	
		Approximate measure and weight	
		1 egg = 50 g[a]	1 c = 243 g
16:0	g	1.23	5.98
18:0	g	.43	2.08
Monounsaturated, total	g	2.23	10.83
16:1	g	.19	.90
18:1	g	2.04	9.93
20:1	g		
22:1	g		
Polyunsaturated, total	g	.72	3.52
18:2	g	.62	3.01
18:3	g	.02	.08
18:4			
20:4	g	.05	.23
20:5	g		
22:5	g		
22:6	g		
Cholesterol	mg	274	1,331
Phytosterols	mg		
AMINO ACIDS			
Tryptophan	g	.097	.472
Threonine	g	.298	1.449
Isoleucine	g	.380	1.846
Leucine	g	.533	2.591
Lysine	g	.410	1.992
Methionine	g	.196	.953
Cystine	g	.145	.703
Phenylalanine	g	.343	1.666
Tyrosine	g	.253	1.227
Valine	g	.437	2.124
Arginine	g	.388	1.888
Histidine	g	.147	.713
Alanine	g	.354	1.723
Aspartic acid	g	.602	2.926
Glutamic acid	g	.773	3.757
Glycine	g	.202	.982
Proline	g	.241	1.171
Serine	g	.461	2.242

[a] Weight applies to large egg.

Source: L. P. Posati and M. L. Orr, *Composition of foods—Dairy and egg products—Raw, processed, prepared*, Agriculture Handbook No. 8-1 (Washington, D.C.: U.S. Government Printing Office, 1976), p. 123.

tassium, sodium, and zinc), nine vitamins (ascorbic acid, thiamin, riboflavin, niacin, pantothenic acid, vitamin B_6, folacin, vitamin B_{12}, and vitamin A), individual fatty acids, total fatty acids, cholesterol, total phytosterols, and 18 amino acids. Nutrient values are expressed as the amount present in the edible portion of 100 grams, common household measures, and 1 pound of food as purchased.

So much data have accumulated that the most sophisticated tables are maintained and updated by computer. Two well-known computer-stored "nutrient data bases" are the Extended Table of Nutrient Values (ETNV) of the International Dietary Information Foundation, Inc., and the Nutrient Data Bank (NBD) of the Nutrient Data Research Center of the U.S. Department of Agriculture.

Dietary Standards

The RDAs, Recommended Dietary Allowances, which we introduced in Chapter 1 and have referred to throughout the text, are issued in the form of a table (see Appendix A) showing desirable average amounts of energy and many nutrients to be consumed. The energy levels have been estimated to meet the average needs of population groups of healthy individuals; the nutrient levels should meet *or exceed* the needs of virtually all healthy persons.

The RDAs are not intended for use by consumers, nor are they goals for individual dietary intakes. Rather, they are standards against which nutrient intakes can be compared. They are used to evaluate the nutrient content of population food supplies, of foods provided in government-sponsored or other feeding programs, and for related purposes.

Many observers have called attention to shortcomings of the RDAs. It has been suggested that they should be more applicable and understandable to consumers; that requirements should also be expressed in terms of nutrient density (that is, per 100 kcal); and that additional nutrients now known to be essential should be included. Still others complain that the RDAs do not consider the role of such nutrient-related factors as fiber and cholesterol, and therefore do not define "acceptable" levels of intake.

Perhaps a more important concern is that the RDAs by definition encourage a tendency to think in terms of getting "enough" of a nutrient, even though for energy and some nutrients (protein for example) a majority of Americans are apparently consuming a "nutrient excess." Nevertheless, the RDAs represent the best estimate we have at present to evaluate nutritional status and to plan food supplies for population groups. Continued research and reinterpretation of data can be expected to refine further the nutrient allowances and to clarify the appropriate uses of the RDAs.

Tools for the Consumer

Although the RDAs were designed for professional use, you do not have to be a professional nutritionist to learn to use them. As a nutrition student, you have an advantage. You will probably use the RDAs in conjunction with food composition tables to estimate your own nutrient intake, and you will probably have little difficulty doing it. But most consumers need a more accessible and easy-to-use guide to menu planning. Several consumer-oriented assessment systems have been designed to fill specific needs.

BASIC FOOD GROUPS. Most students are aware of the "Basic Food Groups" (see Figure 10–3, page 352). This food guide was developed in consideration of the nutrient content of foods in different broad groups; key nutrients were identified as those which should be monitored. The assumption was that if a few "index" nutrients were considered, the other 40-odd nutrients necessary for health would naturally accompany them when a variety of foods was consumed. A second assumption was that the simpler the system, the more likely it is to be accepted and used, especially by children and poorly educated segments of the population. For this reason, the food guide promoted by the USDA is presently based on five groups: milk, meat, vegetables and fruits, breads and cereals, and other foods. In the past there were more food groups. In research studies, intake is frequently evaluated using this same concept but with a greater number to overcome the limitations of using only five categories.

The *milk group*, providing high-quality protein, riboflavin, calcium, and, when fortified, vitamin D, includes all types of milk used in beverages; in natural and processed cheese, yogurt, ice cream and ice milk; in commercial soups; and in puddings. Products from the milk group supply about 75 percent of the calcium, over 35 percent of the riboflavin (vitamin B_2), and more than 20 percent of the protein available in the average American diet. Two servings are recommended for adults.

The *meat group*, noted for its high-quality protein, B vitamins, iron, and other trace elements, includes meats (beef, veal, pork, lamb, wild game), fish, shellfish, poultry, eggs, meat alternatives (dry beans, peas, lentils, peanut butter), and nuts. Two servings from this group, each equivalent to two ounces of meat, are recommended for most adults and children; pregnant women should choose three. Foods in the meat group supply over 50 percent of the protein, over 40 percent of the iron, and over 50 percent of the niacin in our diet. Since different foods from this group provide different percentages of these nutrients (see Table 10–3, page 354), choices must be made carefully. Legumes contain no vitamin B_{12}, but they are fairly rich sources of folacin. Meats, on the other hand, are good sources of B_{12} but poor sources of folacin. Food guides often recommend certain choice combinations, because protein bioavailability depends on the presence of complementary amino acids that are not found together in a single nonmeat "meat group" food, and other considerations (for example, vitamin B_{12} content) must be made as well. Again, diversity is the watchword.

The *vegetable and fruit group* includes fresh, canned, frozen, and dried fruits and vegetables (except for dried beans and peas, which are considered legumes; see meat group). Although corn is listed as a vegetable, it is also found in the grain group (corn grits and cornmeal). Fruits and vegetables supply over 90 percent of the vitamin C and almost 50 percent of the vitamin A in our diet, as well as significant amounts of other vitamins and minerals. Four fruit or vegetable servings are recommended each day.

The *bread and cereals group*, also called the *grain group*, includes breads, breakfast cereals, grits, noodles, pastas, barley, buckwheat, corn, oats, rice, rye, wheat, and all other related products. These foods supply about 40 percent of the thiamin and 30 percent of the iron (all of which is nonheme) and niacin in a typical American diet. Four daily servings are recommended.

Some common food items are missing from these groups: fats, such as butter, oil, and margarine; and honey, sugar, jam, jelly, and candy. An *other* category has been established for these items, as well as for desserts, condiments, and beverages. Intakes should be adjusted to energy needs.

One shortcoming of the Basic Food Group plan is that food portions may not necessarily coincide with standard "servings." Few home-prepared hamburgers, for example, are a uniform 2-ounce size, the quantity defined as one serving. In addition, some foods clearly belonging to basic food groups actually have minimal nutritional value. Beets and applesauce are often cited as examples. Finally, only a few nutrients—the key or index nutrients—from the approximately 45 essential nutrients are specifically identified. Although different combinations of a variety of foods within each group can provide all the other nutrients, there is no guarantee that people will know which combinations to choose or what amounts constitute a full serving.

Computer evaluation of 20 menus derived from the Basic Food Groups demonstrated that daily intakes met or surpassed current RDAs for only 8 of the 17 nutrients tested and provided 60 percent or less of the RDA levels for vitamin E, vitamin B_6, magnesium, zinc, and iron. Adding foods from an "other" category

FIGURE 10-3 *Outline of the Basic Food Group Plan.*

	MINIMUM AMOUNT RECOMMENDED DAILY	
Food group	*Number of servings*	*Approximate size of serving for people age 7 and older*
Breads and cereal products, enriched or whole grain	4	1 slice bread 1 cup flaked cereal ½ – ⅔ cup cooked cereal 1 muffin or roll 1 pancake ½ hamburger bun

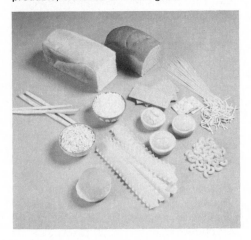

Meat and meat alternates

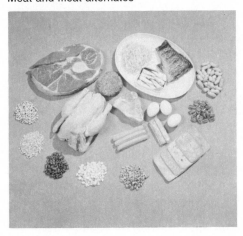

The equivalent of 4 ounces cooked meat* (not counting fat or bone)

* The equivalent of 4 ounces of cooked meat can be obtained from meat or from various combinations of the following, each of which is equivalent to 1 ounce of meat:

    1 egg
    1 ounce of nuts
    2 tablespoons peanut butter
    ½ cup cooked dried legumes (such as baked beans)
    1 ounce of cheese (if not counted in milk group)
    ¼ cup of cottage cheese (if not counted in milk group)

Source: T. J. Runyon, *Nutrition for Today* (New York: Harper & Row, 1976), p. 124.

Food group	Number of servings	Approximate size of serving for people age 7 and older
Milk and milk products	2 (age 18 and up) 4 (age 11 to 18) 2 (age 7 to 10)	1 cup milk or light cream 1 ½ ounce hard cheese 2 cups ice cream 1 ⅓ cups cottage cheese

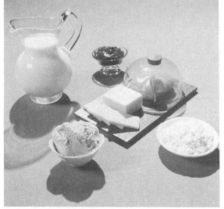

Vegetables and fruits

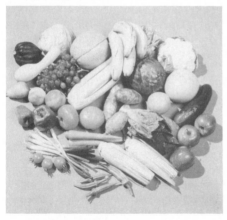

		If whole, 1 medium If raw, ⅔ to 1 cup If cooked or juice, ½ cup
a. Dark green and deep yellow vegetables and fruits	a. 1 every other day	
b. Good vitamin C sources	b. 1 good *or*	
c. Fair vitamin C sources	c. 2 fair	
d. Other fruits and vegetables	d. Variable; to total of 4	

TABLE 10-3. *Percentage Contribution of Food Groups to Nutrients Available for Consumption in the Average U.S. Diet*

Food Group	Energy	Protein	Fat	Carbo-hydrate	Calcium	Phosphorus	Iron
Milk	11.1	22.0	12.5	6.7	74.6	35.0	2.5
Meat	24.9	52.8	40.6	2.3	9.1	39.6	41.9
Meat, poultry, fish	20.0	42.6	34.1	0.1	4.0	28.5	30.9
Eggs	1.8	4.8	2.7	0.1	2.2	5.0	4.7
Legumes and nuts	3.1	5.4	3.8	2.1	2.9	6.1	6.3
Fruit and Vegetable	8.6	7.0	0.9	17.3	9.6	10.9	18.8
Citrus fruits	0.9	0.5	0.1	2.0	1.0	0.7	0.8
Other fruits	2.1	0.6	0.3	4.6	1.2	1.1	3.3
Dark green/dark yellow vegetables	0.2	0.4	trace	0.5	1.5	0.6	1.5
Other vegetables[a]	5.4	5.5	0.5	10.2	5.9	8.5	13.2
Grain	19.2	17.6	1.3	34.7	3.4	12.2	27.9
Other[b]	36.1	0.6	44.5	39.0	3.4	2.3	9.0

[a] Includes potatoes and tomatoes.
[b] Includes fats, oils, sugars.

primarily to increase vitamin E content with intake of fats and oils helped somewhat, but the menus still failed to meet many RDAs. This is not necessarily a problem, because RDAs are overestimates of nutrient needs for most people. But modification of the Basic Food Groups has been suggested to emphasize those nutrients most underrepresented. One proposed method will simply increase portion sizes of foods from the meat and fruit and vegetable groups as well as add fats and oils. Despite shortcomings, however, the basic food groups are the easiest tool developed to date for use by the general public and are particularly useful in demonstrating desirable food intakes to children, the elderly, and population groups at high risk of nutritional deficiency—those sectors it is most important to reach.

EXCHANGE LISTS. Exchange lists, introduced in 1950 for persons with diabetes mellitus, also present foods in various groups. These lists have become popular for planning fat-restricted, low-cholesterol, and weight-reduction diets as well. They contain food suggestions in specified portions in six different categories: milk, vegetables, fruit, bread (including cereals and starchy vegetables), meat, and fat.

The exchange lists were revised in 1976 to reflect changes in knowledge and philosophy, stressing foods of low cholesterol and low fat content with lower energy values. The milk exchange group became based on nonfat milk; the meat group was subdivided into high-, medium-, and low-fat meats and their equivalents. Thus, the exchange lists emphasize kilocalories, nutrients, and low-fat foods.

Each of the six exchange lists contains foods of similar energy and nutrient content, with emphasis on carbohydrate, fat, protein, and energy values. (See Appendix G.) A good deal of flexibility in meal planning can be built in. Depending on the needs of an individual, diets can be worked out providing for daily consumption of, for example, two milk exchanges, two vegetable exchanges, three fuit exchanges, five bread/cereal exchanges, six medium-fat meat exchanges, and three fat exchanges. Such a plan will provide approximately 1,250 kilocalories. An individual who prefers to drink 1 cup of whole milk instead of skim milk must eliminate two fat exchanges from the daily meal plan under this system.

Magnesium	Vitamin A	Thiamin	Riboflavin	Niacin	Vitamin B$_6$	Vitamin B$_{12}$	Ascorbic acid
21.7	13.0	8.6	39.0	1.4	10.6	20.1	3.9
27.2	27.9	33.2	30.6	52.1	53.5	78.4	1.1
14.1	22.4	25.9	24.3	45.2	47.4	70.5	1.1
1.2	5.5	2.0	4.5	0.1	1.8	0	0
11.9	trace	5.3	1.8	6.8	4.3	0	trace
25.9	48.3	16.4	8.7	15.0	26.7	0	91.4
2.3	1.6	2.7	0.5	0.8	1.2	0	27.4
3.9	5.5	1.7	1.5	1.6	5.6	0	11.6
2.0	20.2	0.8	1.0	0.6	1.7	0	8.8
17.7	21.0	11.2	5.7	12.0	18.2	0	43.6
17.9		41.6	21.0	27.9	8.9	1.5	0
7.3	10.5	0.1	1.6	3.5	0.1	0	3.6

Source: Adapted from *National Food Review*, USDA, Washington, D.C., 1978.

Exchange lists were designed for patients in consultation with a dietitian or other health professional. Without guidance on how to use them for individual needs, they are not particularly useful. Further, because they focus on energy, fat, protein, and carbohydrate, meals based on these lists may not provide adequate amounts of other essential nutrients. In nutrition education programs using the exchange lists, the vitamin A and vitamin C content of fruits and vegetables is stressed, and food sources of other vitamins and minerals are pointed out as well. The importance of making diversified choices within each group is also explained.

Another drawback is that exchange lists do not include many foods that are popular with particular ethnic groups or "combination" or commercially available foods that are difficult to assign correctly to a single exchange list. However, some food companies and fast-food restaurants publish information about the "exchange list" value of their products. Another aspect of this system is that the amount listed for an "exchange" is not always equivalent to what is commonly considered a "serving"; meats are listed in 1-ounce amounts, for instance. These shortcomings can be overcome by professional consultation and client education. The exchange list is particularly useful for its intended purposes of planning diets for individuals with special needs, and it has been found generally easier to live with on a long-term basis than other diet plans.

NUTRITION LABELING.   Food manufacturers have striven for years to produce easy-to-follow directions for preparation of their products that can be understood even by children and uneducated adults. Nutrition labels on many food packages represent the government's and the food industry's current efforts to assist consumers in planning nutritious meals. But, as many consumer groups have indicated, nutrition labels are not as easily understood as manufacturers' package directions.

One area of consumer confusion is a misunderstanding of the U.S. Recommended Daily Allowances (U.S. RDAs), which form the standard for a part of nutritional labeling policy. U.S. RDAs are dietary standards derived from tables of RDAs (Recommended Dietary Allowances) published by the Food and Nutrition

Board in 1968. The U.S. RDAs replace the "minimum daily requirements" that were formerly used on the labels of mineral and vitamin preparations, breakfast cereals, and some other products. Because they are derived from the RDAs, they too provide a margin of safety for the typical consumer. In order to simplify nutritional labeling as much as possible, four tables of U.S. RDAs were developed. The most familiar is that which is used for adults and children over four years of age (Table 10–4). The U.S. RDA for a given nutrient is the highest RDA of that nutrient for children and adults, excluding pregnant and lactating women; thus, with a few exceptions, the RDA for 18-year-old males became the U.S. RDA. For most individuals, allowances are even higher than the RDAs; this fact should be considered when comparing dietary intake to the U.S. RDAs.

Other U.S. RDA tables are for infants, children under four years of age, and pregnant and lactating women (Appendix C); these figures appear on the labels of foods for these special groups.

Figure 10–4 shows examples of food labels, giving both ingredient and nutrition information. The former is required on all manufactured food products, unless these products have a so-called standard of identity (that is, they conform to standard "recipes" that indicate specific levels of mandatory ingredients), such as mayonnaise. Ingredients must be listed on the label in order of decreasing weight in the product. Nutritional labeling, on the other hand, is mandatory for (1) products for which a nutritional claim is made ("low-calorie," "low-salt," "vitamin-fortified," "nutritious"), (2) products that have been fortified (a nutrient not normally present in a food is added, such as vitamin D to milk), or (3) products that have

TABLE 10-4. *U.S. Recommended Daily Allowances for Adults and Children over 4 Years of Age*

	Nutrients	U.S. RDA
Must	Protein	65 g[a]
be	Vitamin A	5000 IU
listed	Vitamin C (ascorbic acid)	60.0 mg
on	Thiamin (vitamin B_1)	1.5 mg
label	Riboflavin (vitamin B_2)	1.7 mg
	Niacin	10.0 mg
	Calcium	1.0 g
	Iron	18.0 mg
May	Vitamin D	400 IU
be	Vitamin E	30 IU
listed	Vitamin B_6	2.0 mg
on	Folacin (folic acid)	0.4 mg
label	Vitamin B_{12}	6.0 μg
	Phosphorus	1.0 g
	Iodine	150 μg
	Magnesium	400 mg
	Zinc	15 mg
	Copper	2.0 mg
	Biotin	0.3 mg
	Pantothenic acid	10.0 mg

[a] For proteins with a Protein Efficiency Ratio (PER) less than that of casein (<2.5), the U.S. RDA is 65 g. For foods providing high-quality protein such as meat, fish, poultry, eggs, and milk (PER ≥ 2.5), the U.S. RDA is 45 g. Proteins with a PER less than 20% that of casein may not be expressed on the label as a percent of U.S. RDA.
Source: *Federal Register 38* (13), January 19, 1973.

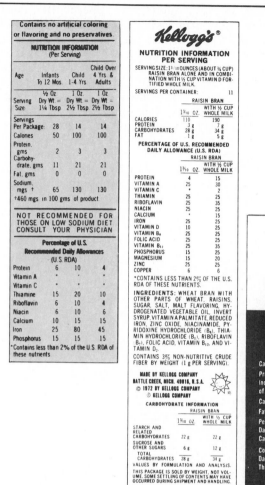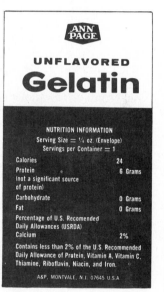

FIGURE 10-4 *Nutrition Information on Food Labels.*

been enriched (in which nutrients are added to replace those lost during processing, such as thiamin, riboflavin, niacin, and iron to wheat flour). Nutritional labeling is optional for other products.

At the present time, federal law requires that when nutritional labeling is used, the following information must be provided in a specific order: serving size; servings per container; and energy, protein, carbohydrate, and fat content per serving. And in July 1986, sodium content will be required. In addition, nutrient values for protein, vitamin A, vitamin C, thiamin, riboflavin, niacin, calcium, and iron expressed as percentages of the U.S. RDA are required. Additional information for vitamin D, vitamin E, vitamin B_6, folacin, vitamin B_{12}, phosphorus, iodine, magnesium, zinc, copper, biotin, and pantothenic acid can also be provided, but it is not mandatory. Manufacturers may also include information about saturated and unsaturated fat content and cholesterol.

An additional comment must be made about the U.S. RDA for protein. Because quantitative requirements for dietary protein are dependent on the quality of the protein (a reflection of its amino acid content), three different standards exist. The U.S. RDA for a high-quality protein such as provided by milk, meat, poultry, or eggs is 45 grams. However, for proteins (both singly and in a food combination) of lesser quality, the U.S. RDA is 65 grams. The effect of the difference is that *more* of a lesser-quality protein must be consumed to achieve the same "level" of the standard as a high-quality protein. An example should serve to clarify this point: Although two eggs and 1 cup of lima beans both have 13 grams of protein, consumption of these foods by themselves will provide 29 percent and 20 percent of the U.S. RDA for protein, respectively (Table 10–5). It should also be noted that unflavored gelatin (two envelopes contain 12 grams of protein) is of such low-protein quality that the package label states parenthetically, "not a significant source of protein." A nutrient present at less than 2 percent of the U.S. RDA per serving is so identified either by an asterisk or a statement to that effect.

Nutrition information panels can provide a relatively easy way for consumers to learn which foods are good sources of particular nutrients, which foods provide the most nutrients for the money spent, and which provide the most nutrients in relation to the energy content. Nutrition labeling is required only on manufactured food products as stated earlier. However, in order to provide the consumer with some information, the meat industry has developed information on average nutrient content of various cuts of meat. Called Nutri-facts, these data are displayed above the case containing a particular cut of meat.

INDEX OF NUTRITIONAL QUALITY.   In an attempt to provide a definition of a "nutritious food" that would be of value to both consumers and professionals alike, nutritionists at Utah State University developed the **Index of Nutritional Quality (INQ).**

Intuitively, we know that the nutritional quality of a food or combination of foods is a function of its nutrient content; what is perhaps not so obvious is that a value judgment of whether a food is nutritious should also consider the nutrient needs of an individual and the food's contribution to total energy intake. The INQ attempts to relate these important variables.

When individual food choices are limited either in quantity or variety, perhaps for health or economic reasons, it becomes increasingly important to select foods that provide an adequate intake of essential nutrients. The INQ was developed to identify foods that have a beneficial nutrient:energy ratio, relative to a standard. When originally introduced, the standard used was the U.S. RDA, but refinement of the INQ concept has led the research group to prefer a standard energy level (1,000 or 2,000 kcal) as the energy reference point. The INQ is defined as follows:

$$INQ = \frac{\text{Amount of nutrient in food/kcal of food}}{\text{Allowance for nutrient/kcal allowance}}$$

TABLE 10-5. *Protein Quality*

High-quality Protein	Lower-quality Protein
2 eggs	1 c lima beans
13 g protein	13 g protein
U.S. RDA = 45 g	U.S. RDA = 65 g
% U.S. RDA = 13 ÷ 45 = 29%	% U.S. RDA = 13 ÷ 65 = 20%

TABLE 10-6. *Standards Used for INQ Determination*

2,000 kcal	16 mg iron
50 g protein	3,000 mg sodium
4,000 IU vitamin A	5,000 mg potassium
60 mg vitamin C	350 mg cholesterol
1.2 mg riboflavin	78 g total fat
900 mg calcium	

Source: R. G. Hansen and B. W. Wyse, Using the INQ to evaluate foods, *Nutrition News*, 42(1):2, 1979. Courtesy National Dairy Council.

The reference values for adults currently used for some nutrients are listed in Table 10–6.

The INQ for *each* nutrient in a food or food combination can be determined. For example, the calcium INQ for whole milk can be calculated from the preceding formula. Although the figures in the numerator are those for 1 cup of milk, the calcium INQ will remain constant regardless of the amount of milk consumed.

$$INQ_{calcium} = \frac{290 \text{ mg calcium}/160 \text{ kcal}}{900 \text{ mg calcium}/2,000 \text{ kcal}} = 4.0$$

Rearrangement of the INQ formula results in a simplified equation:

$$INQ = \frac{\% \text{ standard of nutrient in food}}{\% \text{ standard of energy in food}}$$

$$INQ_{calcium} = \frac{290 \text{ mg calcium}/900 \text{ mg calcium}}{160 \text{ kcal}/2,000 \text{ kcal}} = \frac{0.32}{0.08} = 4.0$$

Stated in this way, it becomes apparent that 1 cup of milk provides 32 percent of the calcium allowance and 8 percent of the energy allowance; based on total adult requirements, therefore, milk supplies four times as much calcium as energy. An INQ equal to 1.0 or more for any nutrient indicates that the food has a beneficial nutrient:energy ratio for that particular nutrient.

The previous example shows that milk is a good source of calcium relative to energy. An examination of Table 10–7 reveals that milk has several nutrient INQs greater than 1.0 and also provides more than 30 percent of the dietary standard for

TABLE 10-7. *INQ: Comparison of Milk and Chocolate Candy Bar*

	MILK		CHOCOLATE CANDY BAR	
	INQ	% Standard	INQ	% Standard
Energy	1.0	8.0	1.0	7.4
Protein	2.0	16.0	0.6	4.4
Calcium	4.0	32.0	0.9	7.2
Iron	0.09	0.75	0.26	1.9
Vitamin A	0.95	7.6	0.3	2.0
Thiamin	1.16	9.3	0.003	0.02
Riboflavin	4.1	32.9	1.12	8.3
Vitamin C	0.48	3.8	0.0	0.0

Source: Adapted from R. G. Hansen and B. W. Wyse. Using the INQ to evaluate foods, *Nutrition News*, 42(1):2, 1979. Courtesy National Dairy Council.

two nutrients. In comparison, a chocolate candy bar, because it is energy-dense, generally has lower INQ values and contributes less to nutrient requirements (% standard).

INQs for all nutrients in a single food, meal, or total diet can be determined. The nutritional quality of foods can also be shown in a type of bar graph (see Table 10–8). In this example, protein, vitamin C, riboflavin, calcium, and iron are present in a favorable ratio to the energy content of the meal. Other meals consumed during the day should include foods to increase nutrient intakes to 100 percent of the standard and compare favorably with the energy standard, as shown by the length of the energy bar.

The two parameters—INQ and the percent standard—provide useful information in selecting nutritious foods. Individuals who wish to reduce their energy intake while maintaining an adequate nutrient intake should plan their meals to meet their desired level of energy consumption *and* choose foods with most or all of the nutrient INQs equal to or greater than 1.0.

Consumer Responsibility

Tools exist to aid professionals in evaluating the nutritional status of individuals and population subgroups. But there is a great deal of nutritional ignorance and misinformation in the general public. The best protection for any consumer, until nutrition education and labeling catch up with public need, is selection of a varied diet, rich in foods such as fruits, vegetables, grains, fish, meats or meat substitutes, and milk. Because no one food provides *all* the nutrients needed by the human body, selections of diverse foods from each of the major categories will help to meet daily needs for even the least-known nutrients. "Good" and "bad" foods cannot be absolutely defined. The *combination* of foods, in appropriate amounts, makes the difference.

TABLE 10-8. *INQs for Meal of Bread (B), Cheese (C), and Strawberries (S)*[a]

Nutrient	Amount	INQ	%Std	0	25%	50%
Energy[b]	295.0 kcal	1.00	14	BBBBBCCCCSS		
Protein	12.8 g	1.74	26	BBBBBBBBCC *CCCCCCCCSS		
Vitamin A	456.2 IU	0.77	12	CCCCCCCSS *		
Vitamin C	87.9 mg	11.93	176	SSSSSSSSSSS *SSSSSSSSSSSSSSSSSSSSSSSSS → (176%)		
Riboflavin	0.3 mg	1.78	27	BBBBBCCCCC *CCCSSSSSSS		
Calcium	287.0 mg	2.16	32	BBBBCCCCCC *CCCCCCCCCCCCSSS		
Iron	3.0 mg	1.12	17	BBBBBCSSSS *SS		
Sodium	456.0 mg	0.77	11	BBBBBCCCC *		
Potassium	362.0 mg	0.61	8	BBSSSSS *		
Cholesterol	29.0 mg	0.66	8	CCCCCCC *		
Fat	11.3 g	0.98	14	BBCCCCCCCC *		

* Indicates the 1.0 INQ point on each nutrient bar.
[a] 1 slice white enriched bread, 1 slice whole-wheat bread, 1 ounce cheddar cheese, and ⅔ cup strawberries. Each letter represents the relative contribution of that food to the nutrient bar.
[b] Energy bar: Nutrient bars should meet or exceed this in length. The bars for cholesterol and fat, however, should not exceed the length of the energy bar.
Source: Adapted from R. G. Hansen and B. W. Wyse, Using the INQ to evaluate foods, *Nutrition News,* 42(1):2, 1979. Courtesy National Dairy Council.

SUMMARY

Malnutrition has been implicated in chronic, debilitating diseases and in common subclinical symptoms of impaired mental and physical performance. In our society today, the problem is most often not lack of food but improper balance of energy and key nutrients in the diet.

Standardized assessment methods are used to identify nutritional deficiencies in individuals and in population groups. The four major categories of testing are *anthropometric* assessment, measurements of body size and body composition which include height, weight, and skinfold thickness; *clinical* assessment, a survey of visible, physical signs that relate to long-term disease processes; *biochemical* assessment, analysis of the chemical composition of body fluids and tissues, commonly emphasizing blood and urine testing; and *dietary* assessment, records of the foods consumed over a particular period of time.

Although each of these tools can be used alone, they provide the most useful data when used together, as has been done in nutrition surveys and in assessment of the hospitalized patient. *Food composition tables* provide a great deal of information about individual foods, and they are widely used by professionals for meal planning and other purposes. The *Recommended Dietary Allowance* (RDA) tables are also used by professionals for meal planning and for evaluation of nutrient intakes.

Because food composition tables and RDAs are too complex for the average consumer, several simplified tools have been developed. Among these are the basic food groupings, exchange lists, and the Index of Nutritional Quality (INQ).

More useful information for consumers is provided by nutrition labeling on many food packages; present federal regulations require that manufacturers indicate the number of kilocalories; grams of carbohydrate, protein, fat, and sodium in a single serving; and also the content of selected nutrients as a percentage of the U.S. RDA when they make a nutritional claim for their product. Until nutrition education and labeling catch up with public needs, the consumer's best protection against nutritional deficiencies and excess is selection of a varied diet, in amounts appropriate to achieve or maintain optimal body weight.

BIBLIOGRAPHY

ABRAHAM, S., F.W. LOWENSTEIN AND C.L. JOHNSON. Preliminary findings of the first health and nutrition survey. United States, 1971–1972: Dietary intake and biochemical findings. DHEW Publication No. (HRA) 74-1219-1, January 1974.

ALLEN, L.H. Functional indicators of nutritional status of the whole individual or the community. *Clinical Nutrition* 3: 169–175, 1984.

American Medical Association. The nutritive quality of processed foods: General Policies for nutrient additions. *Nutrition Reviews* 40:93–96, 1982.

BAKER, J.P., A.S. DETSKY, D.E. WESSON, S.L. WOLMAN, S. STEWART, J. WHITEWELL, B. LANGER AND K.N. JEJEEBHOY. Nutritional Assessment: A comparison of clinical judgment and objective measurements. *The New England Journal of Medicine* 306;969–972, 1982.

BEATON, F.H. Uses and limits of the use of the Recommended Dietary Allowances for evaluating dietary intake data. *American Journal of Clinical Nutrition* 41:155–164, 1985.

BEITMAN, R.G., S.S. FROST AND J.L.A. ROTH. Oral manifestations of gastrointestinal disease. *Digestive Diseases and Sciences* 26;741–747, 1981.

BUTTERWORTH, C.E. The skeleton in the hospital closet. *Nutrition Today* 9(2):4, 1979.

Center for Disease Control. *Ten-State Nutrition Survey In the United States, 1968–1970.* Highlights, DHEW Publication No. (HSM) 72-8134, Atlanta, GA: Health Services and Mental Health Administration, 1972.

CHUMLEA, W.C., A.F. ROCHE, AND D. MUKHER-JEE. *Nutritional Assessment of the Elderly through Anthropometry.* Columbus, OH: Ross Laboratories, 1984.

Committee for the Revision of the Dietary Standard for Canada. *Recommended Nutrient Intakes for Canadians.* Bureau of Nutritional Sciences, Food Directorate, Health Protection Branch, Department of National Health and Welfare, Ottawa, 1983.

CZAJKA-NARINS, D.M. Nutrition, in *Clinical Chemistry,* N. Tietz, ed., Philadelphia, PA: W.B. Saunders, 1986.

EVANS, H.K. AND D.J. GINES. Dietary recall method comparison for hospitalized elderly subjects. *Journal of the American Dietetic Association* 85:202–205, 1985.

FALKNER, F. Monitoring growth. In *Nutrition Needs and Assessment of Normal Growth.* M. Gracey and F. Falkner, eds. New York: Nestle Nutrition, Vevey-Raven Press, 1985.

FRISANCHO, A.R. New standards of weight and body composition by frame size and height for assessment of nutritional status of adults and the elderly. *American Journal of Clinical Nutrition* 40: 808–819, 1984.

————, AND P.N. FLEGEL. Elbow breadth as a measure of frame size for U.S. males and females. *American Journal of Clinical Nutrition* 37:311–314, 1983.

GARN, S.M., F.A. LARKIN AND P.E. COLE. The real problem with 1-day records. *American Journal of Clinical Nutrition* 31:11–14, 1978.

GARN, S.M., S.D. PESICK, V.M. HAWTHORNE. The bony chest breadth as a frame size standard in nutritional assessment. *American Journal of Clinical Nutrition* 37:315–318, 1983.

GEBHARDT, S.E., R. CUTRUFELLI, AND R.H. MATTHES. *Composition of Foods—Baby Foods—Raw, Processed, Prepared.* USDA Agriculture Handbook No. 8-3. Washington, DC: U.S. Government Printing Office, 1978.

GRANT, J.P. Nutritional assessment in clinical practice. *Nutrition in Clinical Practice* 1:3–11, 1986.

————, P. B. CUSTER, AND J. THURLOW. Current techniques of nutritional assessment. *Surgical Clinical of North America* 61:437–463, 1981.

GUTHRIE, H.A. AND J.C. SCHEER. An evaluation of the basic four food guide. *Journal of Nutritional Education* 13:46–49, 1981.

HABICHT, J.P. Some characteristics of indicators of nutritional status for use in screening and surveillance. *American Journal of Clinical Nutrition* 33:531–535, 1980.

HANSEN, R.G. AND B.W. WYSE. Expression of nutrient allowances per 1000 kilocalories. *Journal of the American Dietetic Association* 76:223–227, 1980.

HEPBURN, F.N. The USDA national nutrient data bank. *American Journal of Clinical Nutrition* 35(5 Suppl): 1297–1301, 1982.

HIMES J.H. Appropriateness of parent-specific status adjustment for U.S. black children. *Journal of National Medical Association* 76:55–57, 1984.

JENKINS, R.M. AND H.A. GUTHRIE. Identification of index nutrients for dietary assessment. *Journal of Nutrition Education* 16:15–18, 1984.

KERR, G.R., E.S. LEE, M. LAM, R.J. LORIMER, E. TANDALL, R.N. FORTHOFER, M.A. DAVIS AND S.M. MAGNETTI. Relationships between dietary and biochemical measures of nutritional status in HANES 1 data. *American Journal Clinical Nutrition* 35:294–308, 1982.

KIEFER, N.C. Less than meets the eye. *Nutrition Today* July/August, 1983, pp.18–26.

KOHRS, M.B., C. KAPICA-CYBORSKI, AND D.M. CZAJKA-NARINS. Iron and chromium nutriture of the elderly. Vol. XVIII—Annual Conference on Trace Substances in Environmental Health. University of Missouri—Columbia, Missouri, 1984.

KOHRS, M.B. AND D.M. CZAJKA-NARINS. Assessment of nutritional status of the elderly. In *Nutrition, Aging and Health.* E. Young, ed. New York: Alan Liss Co., 1985.

KOPLAN, J.P., J.L. ANNEST, P.M. LAYDE, AND G.L. RUBIN. Nutrient intake and supplementation in the United States (NHANES II). *American Journal of Public Health* 76:287, 1986.

LLEWELLYN-JONES, D. AND S. ABRAHAM. *British Medical Journal,* June 14, 1984.

LIGHT, L. AND F.J. CRONIN. Food Guidance revistied. *Journal of Nutrition Eucation* 13:57–62, 1981.

LOWENSTEIN, F.W. Preliminary clinical and anthropometric findings from the first Health and Nutrition Examination Survey, USA, 1971–1972. *American Journal of Clinical Nutrition* 29:918, 1976.

MADDEN, J.P., S.J. GOODMAN, AND H.A. GUTHRIE. Validity of the 24-hour recall: Analysis of data obtained from elderly subjects. *Journal of the American Dietetic Association* 68:143, 1976.

MARSH, A.C., M.K. MOSS, AND E.W. MURPHY. *Composition of foods—Spices and herbs—Raw, Processed Prepared.* USDA Agriculture Handbook No. 8-2. Washington, DC: U.S. Government Printing Office, 1977.

McMasters, V. History of food composition tables of the world. *Journal of the American Dietetic Association* 43:442, 1963.

Mertz, W. and J.L. Kelsay. Rationale and design of the Beltsville one-year dietary intake study. *American Journal of Clinical Nutrition* 40: 1323–1326, 1984.

Morgan, R.W., M. Jain, A.B. Miller, N.W. Chol, V. Matthews, L. Munan, J.D. Burch, J. Feather, G.R. Howe and A. Kelley. A comparison of dietary methods in epidemiologic studies. *American Journal of Epidemiology* 107(6):488, 1978.

National Center for Health Statistics. *NCHS growth charts, 1976.* Monthly Vital Statistics Report. Vol. 25, No. 3, Supplement (HRA) 76-1120. Rockville, MD: Health Resources Administration, 1976.

National Dairy Council. The food group approach to good eating. *Diary Council Digest* 52;31–35, 1981.

National Nutrition Consortium, Inc., with R. M. Deutsch. *Nutritional labeling—How it can work for you.* Bethesda, MD: The National Nutrition Consortium, Inc., 1975.

National Research Council, Committee on Food Consumption Patterns, Food and Nutrition Board. *Assessing Changing Food Consumption Patterns,* Washington, DC: National Academy Press, 1981.

Olson, J.A. New approaches to methods for the assessment of nutritional status of the individual. *American Journal of Clinical Nutrition* 35:1166–1168, 1982.

Pao, E.M. and S.J. Mickle. Problem nutrients in the United States. *Food Technology* 35(9):58–79, 1981.

Parizkova, J. Physical activity related to nutrition as a factor of variability of body composition. In *Food, Nutrition and Evolution—Food as an Environmental Factor In the Genesis of Human Variability,* D.N. Walcher and N. Kretchmer, eds. New York: Masson Publishing USA, pp. 133–141, 1981.

Pennington, J.A.T. and H.N. Church. *Bowes and Church's Food Values of Portions Commonly Used* 14th ed. Philadelphia, PA: J.B. Lippincott Co., 1985.

Pilch, S.M., and F.R. Senti. Analysis of zinc data from the Second National Health and Nutrition Examination Survey (NHANES II). *Journal of Nutrition* 115:1393, 1985.

Posati, L.P. and M.L. Orr. *Composition of Foods–Dairy and Egg Products—Raw, Processed, Prepared.* USDA Agriculture Handbook No. 8-1, Washington DC: U.S. Government Printing Office, 1976.

Roche, A.F. Growth assessment in abnormal children. *Kidney International* 14:369–377, 1978.

Ross Conference on Medical Research. *Nutritional Assessment—Present Status, Future Direction, and Prospects.* Columbus, OH: Ross Laboratories, 1981.

Schneider, H.A., C.E. Anderson and D.B. Coursin, eds. *Nutritional Support of Medical Practice.* New York: Harper & Row, 1983.

Schucker, R.E. Alternative approaches to classic food consumption measurement methods: Telephone interviewing and market data bases. *American Journal of Clinical Nutrition* 35(5 Suppl.):1306–1309, 1982.

Senti, F.R. and S.M. Pilch. Analysis of folate data from the Second National Health and Nutrition Examination Survey (NHANES II). *Journal of Nutrition* 115:1398, 1985.

Solomons, N.W. and L.H. Allen. The functional assessment of nutritional status: Principles, practice and potential. *Nutrition Reviews* 42:33–50, 1983.

Sorenson, A.W., B.W. Wyse, A.J. Wittwer and R.G. Hansen. An index of nutritional quality for a balanced diet. *Journal of the American Dietetic Association* 68:236, 1976.

Stoudt, H.W. The anthropometry of the elderly. *Human Factors* 23:29–37, 1981.

Swan, P.B. Food consumption by individuals in the United States: Two major studies. *Annual Review of Nutrition* 3:413–432, 1983.

Those new height and weight tables. *Nutrition Today* July–August, 1983, pp. 16–17.

Tietz, N.W. ed. *Clinical Guide to Laboratory Tests.* Philadelphia, PA: W.B. Saunders, 1983.

———, ed. *Textbook of Clilnical Chemistry.* Philadelphia, PA: W.B. Saunders, 1986.

U.S. Department of Health, Education, and Welfare. *Dietary Intake Findings United States, 1971–1974,* DHEW Publication No. (HRA) 77–1647. Washington, DC: U.S. DHEW, 1977.

U.S. Department of Health and Human Services. *Nutritional Screening of Children: A Manual for Screening and Followup,* DHHS Publication No. (HSA) 81–5114. Rockville, MD: USDHHS.

Watt, B.K. and E.W. Murphy. Tables of food composition; Scope and needed research. *Food Technology* 24:674, 1970.

WEIGLEY, E.S. Average? Ideal? Desirable? A brief overview of height-weight tables in the United States. *Journal of American Dietetic Association* 84:417–423, 1984.

WEINSIER, R.L. AND C.E. BUTTERWORTH. *Handbook of Clinical Nutrition.* St. Louis, MO: C.V. Mosby, Co., 1981.

What is an exchange? *Journal of the American Dietetic Association* 69:609, 1976.

WHITE, P.L. AND N. SELVY, eds. Malnutrition Determinants and Consequences. *Current Topics in Nutrition and Disease, Vol. 10.* New York: Alan R. Liss, 1984.

WRETLIND, A. Standards for nutritional adequacy of the diet: European and WHO/FAO viewpoints. *American Journal of Clinical Nutrition* 36:366–375, 1982.

YOUNG, C.M. Dietary Methodology. In *Assessing Food Consumption Patterns,* Committee on Food Consumption Patterns, Food and Nutrition Board, National Research Council. Washington, DC: National Academy of Sciences Press, pp. 89–118, 1981.

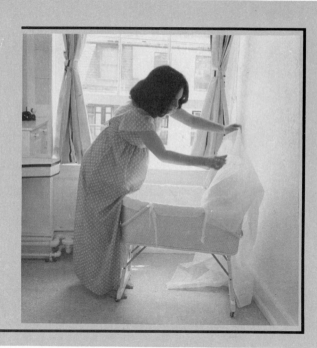

Chapter 11

NUTRITION IN PREGNANCY AND LACTATION

Growing from one single cell to a complex organism with millions of cells in just 40 weeks is quite a feat, but every human being has done it. What makes that extraordinary development possible is the nutritional bond between a mother and her unborn child.

Good nutrition maintains the optimal health of the mother-to-be, ensures that her nutrient stores are not depleted by the demands of the fetus, and provides for the needs of the growing fetus. Our discussion begins with an account of fetal development and of the stages of human pregnancy, including the postpregnancy period of milk production (lactation). Against this physiological background, we will examine the various nutrition-related concerns for the health and well-being of both baby-to-be and mother-to-be, including the ways in which the nutritional needs of pregnant and lactating women differ from those of nonpregnant and nonlactating women and the translation of the nutritional needs of this period into food intake patterns.

PREGNANCY

In previous chapters we have explained how foods taken into the body provide the raw materials for growth, structure, function, and regulation of the internal environment. This close interrelationship is probably most apparent during pregnancy and lactation. Between conception and birth, the single cell that is a fertilized egg must grow and develop into a full-sized 3 to 3.5 kilogram (6.5 to 7.5 lb) human being, capable of surviving in the outside world. Never again will growth and development proceed so rapidly. So the developing fetus requires significant amounts of energy and nutrients that must be provided by the mother.

Prenatal Development

There are three distinct prenatal developmental stages. The first, *blastogenesis*, occupies the first two weeks following fertilization. The fertilized egg (zygote) immediately divides into two cells, each of which then divides into two more, and so on. The zygote soon becomes a cell-lined hollow sphere, the *blastula*. While cell division is taking place, cell enlargement does not occur because there is as yet no source of nourishment for the zygote, which remains the same overall size as the original ovum despite the rapid division of cells. As the cells continue to divide, two layers are distinguished. The inner cell mass will become the *embryo*, and the outer "feeding" layer, or *trophoblast*, will differentiate to form the *placenta*. At this point the blastula becomes attached to the wall of the uterus. The trophoblast penetrates the uterine lining and absorbs material from the lining to provide the first nourishment for the new organism.

Meanwhile the inner cell mass is separating into two spherical forms, separated by a thin cellular disc. This disc will become the embryo itself; one of the spheres becomes a yolk sac (which in humans does not contain yolk) and the other becomes a fluid-filled sac, the amnion, which will provide a protective environment as well as nourishment for the embryo.

In the *embryonic stage* the embryonic disc begins to differentiate into three types of cells, the *germinal layers*. The *ectoderm*, or outermost layer of cells, will form the brain, nervous system, hair, skin, and sensory organs. The *mesoderm*, or

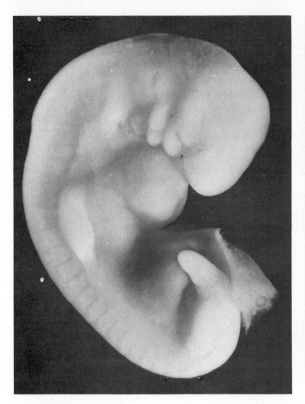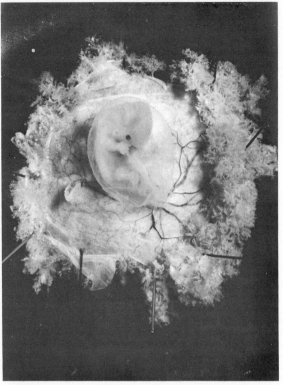

Embryo at four weeks. Tiny "buds" and indentations are the only suggestions of arms, legs, ears, and eyes that will develop in the next few weeks.
Carnegie Institution

Embryo at seven weeks surrounded by amniotic sac and placenta. Arms, hands, eyes, and ears have taken definite shape.
Carnegie Institution

middle layer, will provide the body's supporting structures—bone; muscle; connective tissue; and parts of the cardiovascular, excretory, and reproductive systems. The innermost layer, or *endoderm*, will form the lining of the respiratory, urinary, and digestive tracts. Sixty days (eight weeks) after fertilization the embryonic stage is completed, and many components of the skeleton, brain, eyes, ears, heart, and lungs are fully formed (see Table 11–1).

With the start of the third month, the embryo is considered a *fetus*. The *fetal stage* of development, which continues until birth, is a time of rapid growth. The specialized cells continue to divide and now also begin to grow in size. What at 8 weeks had been a tiny embryo weighing only 6 grams by 24 weeks has grown to about 30 centimeters and 640 grams. At the time of birth, the fetus will measure around 50 centimeters and weigh about 3,250 grams.

The information that guides this dramatic progression from blastocyst to newborn baby is programmed in the genetic material carried by the egg and the sperm. Apparently there is a different genetic timetable for the development of each body system, and each is vulnerable to nutritional insult. Each system—muscular, skeletal, circulatory, and so on—develops at its own particular rate. Research on laboratory animals, for example, indicates that severe restriction of maternal protein intake during a critical period of nervous system development causes the offspring's brain to have fewer than the normal number of cells. The same short-term nutri-

TABLE 11-1. *Development of Systems in the Embryo*

System	Chronology	
Dental	4–6 months:	Hard tissue of primary teeth
Nervous	0–9 months:	Increased number of brain cells
		Survival reflexes present at birth
Muscles	5–6 weeks:	Development of nerve attachments to muscles
	8 weeks:	Involuntary muscles function
	16 weeks:	Muscle movement can be felt
Skin	4 months:	0.5% fat
	5 months:	6% fat
	birth:	15% fat
Eyes	7 weeks:	Nerves, eyelids, lens
	10 weeks:	Eyelids fused shut
	7–8 months:	Eyes open but not mature, even at birth
Ears	4–8 weeks:	Structure develops into final form
	16 weeks:	Assumes typical appearance
Cardiovascular	6 weeks:	First fetal organ (heart) completed
	2 months:	Circulation developed
Respiratory	6 weeks:	Trachea, bronchi, lung buds
	12 weeks:	Lungs take shape, fluid inhaled
Digestive	8 weeks:	Lip fusion
	12 weeks:	Palate fusion
	5 months:	Production of bile, digestive juices
Excretory	7 weeks:	Bladder and urethra separate
	16 weeks:	Kidneys assume final form
Reproductive	6 weeks:	Gonads first appear
	7–9 weeks:	Gonads differentiate
Skeletal	2–8 weeks:	Skeleton formation
	12 weeks:	Bone begins to replace cartilage

tional deficiency that might affect the growth of the nervous system may have little effect on another body system that is not at a critical stage.

Nutrient needs throughout the embryonic stage are so infinitesimal that only severe malnutrition on the part of the mother could have a significant effect. Fetal nutrient requirements, in contrast, increase during pregnancy and are greatest during the last trimester, when expansion of both the size and the number of cells is greatest.

When severe nutritional deficiencies continue throughout the pregnancy, every body system is in some way affected. In various studies, pregnant animals placed on extremely restricted diets have produced offspring of low birth weight, reduced brain cell number and head size, and proportionate reductions in the size of various body organs. Nutrition is not, however, the only influence on fetal development. The potentially harmful effects of drugs such as Thalidomide or illnesses such as German measles are also keyed to developmental stages of specific systems.

It would be unethical to perform deprivation experiments on pregnant women. Specific data for nutritional needs in human pregnancy have accumulated as a result of studies involving natural and/or accidental disruptions to a population's food supply. The consequences of the food shortages of wartime Europe, for example, have been analyzed. Acute famines occurred in Leningrad in 1942 and in Holland during the winter of 1944–1945. The resulting data corroborate the results of animal studies: Severe nutritional deficits early in the prenatal existence increase fetal mortality rates and affect physiological development; in the later months of pregnancy the primary effect is significantly to decrease overall growth and birth weight. Similarly, autopsies of stillborn infants in the United States have shown that those from low-income families were smaller in overall size and had smaller livers, adrenal glands, and other organs than those from higher-income and presumably better-nourished families.

We must recognize, of course, that maternal nutrition is not the only factor in low birth weight. Other factors, including age under 17 or over 35 years, smoking, heavy drug or alcohol use, and certain infections, may be more common in low-income women and may therefore be responsible for the low birth weight of their infants.

The Placenta

The placenta or afterbirth, which is delivered along with the baby, has always been readily available for study. Microscopic examination of placental tissues has shown that infants who experienced prenatal growth failure, or are from low-income populations, had placentas of smaller size and fewer cells than those who were better nourished.

During blastogenesis and after, the embryo and placenta develop simultaneously. After implantation in the uterine wall, part of the embryonic mesoderm attaches as a lining to the trophoblast to become the *chorion* (see Figure 11–1). The chorion sends numerous projections into the uterine lining, and from these develop the network of blood vessels that constitutes the fetal part of the placenta. These chorionic villi function in much the same way as the intestinal villi, providing the extensive surface area needed for nutrient transfer. While the embryonic portion of the placenta is being formed, the mother's body is responding. Glands and blood vessels within the uterine lining develop, and muscle fibers increase in size and strength.

Exchanges of nutrients and wastes take place in the placenta as they do in the gastrointestinal tract: by passive transport, facilitated diffusion, and active transport across placental membranes. Oxygen and nutrients pass from the mother to the

FIGURE 11-1   *Intrauterine Environment of the Fetus.*

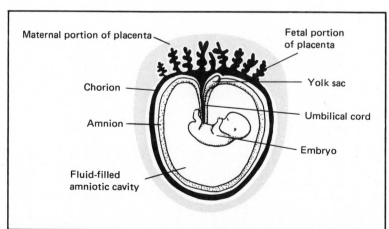

fetus; carbon dioxide and metabolic wastes pass in the opposite direction, to be eliminated by the mother's body. What makes these transfers so complex is the involvement of two separate blood supplies—one from the mother and the other from the fetus.

There is no exchange of blood between the two, only an exchange of nutrients from one blood compartment to another. Maternal hemoglobin levels are vital to maintain the oxygen exchange system. Because 1.34 milliliters of oxygen are carried by each gram of hemoglobin, it is important for the mother to avoid iron deficiency, which would depress her hemoglobin levels and could possibly reduce the supply of oxygen available to her developing child.

Water and the fat-soluble vitamins diffuse to the fetal circulation. Amino acids, glucose, the water-soluble vitamins, and such minerals as calcium, sodium, and iron are actively transported. The placental membranes have at any one time a limited carrying capacity for actively transported materials, and it is possible that excessive intakes of water-soluble vitamins (such as ascorbic acid) on the part of the mother may compete with transport of essential amino acids and impair growth and development. Placental membranes also ensure that nutrients needed by the fetus in higher concentrations than the mother requires will not rush back into the mother's bloodstream.

With one exception, protein molecules do not cross the placenta, since they are too large to penetrate the cells of the placental villi. The fetus must synthesize its own proteins from the amino acids it receives from the maternal circulation. The exception is a specific maternal antibody which is structurally able to penetrate and which provides important resistance to infection that lasts until six or more months after birth.

In addition to serving as the conduit for these exchanges, the placenta supplements the mother's hormone production, becoming the primary source of progesterone and estrogen and the sole source of several hormones normally produced only during gestation: human chorionic gonadotrophin (HCG), human placental lactogen (HPL), human chorionic somatomammotrophin (HCS), and human chorionic thyrotropin (HCT). Although much of this hormone production is stimulated by biochemical precursors produced by the fetus, the gestational hormones act primarily to regulate the mother's pregnancy and postpartum progress.

Maternal Hormones and Tissues

The normal physiological adjustment process of pregnancy causes a number of changes in the mother's body, many of which are mediated by hormones. The more than 30 hormones secreted during gestation include some that are present only during that time and others, normally present, whose rates of secretion are altered. They are proteins or steroids that are synthesized from amino acid and cholesterol precursors in endocrine glands throughout the body. Those hormones with the most far-reaching effects are progesterone and estrogen, both of which are present in increased supply.

Progesterone, which acts on smooth muscle tissue to produce relaxation, allows the uterus to expand as the fetus grows. Gastrointestinal muscles relax as well, slowing intestinal motility, with the obvious benefit to the fetus of additional absorption time and consequent increases in serum nutrient levels. Unfortunately, maternal constipation is often a side effect.

Progesterone also enhances fat storage, especially in the back, thighs, and abdomen, with smaller amounts deposited in mammary tissue. Generally increased fat storage throughout the body is not only physically protective of the fetus but also provides a potential energy reserve. Progesterone also heightens respiratory sensitivity, leading to hyperventilation, thus increasing the energy and oxygen supply available to the fetus and increasing the capacity to expire carbon dioxide.

Estrogen aids in expanding the uterus. By acting on components of connective tissue, it causes these tissues to become flexible enough to accommodate the shifts of bones and organs as they are displaced by the growing fetus and makes possible dilation at birth. But this same biochemical reaction also enhances fluid retention in connective tissue, which is common in pregnancy. At the same time, progesterone has a sodium-depleting effect. The combined results alter electrolyte and fluid balance to a considerable extent. However, unless water retention is associated with hypertension and proteinuria (protein in the urine), there is no cause for concern. Normal fluid retention in pregnancy may even provide some benefits.

Other hormones have strictly metabolic effects. Thyroxine production is increased and, by a complex series of reactions, results in increasing maternal appetite as well as speeding the rate of breathing to provide additional oxygen for energy production from ingested food. As pregnancy progresses, the action of insulin becomes less efficient. Normally this is not a problem, but in a diabetic or prediabetic mother, the output of insulin may be so low that glucose metabolism is impaired, with potentially serious effects for both fetus and mother. Cortisone, which is involved in the maintenance of blood glucose levels by stimulating gluconeogenesis from amino acids, is produced in greater amounts during the final days of pregnancy in response to increased estrogen production.

Other changes during pregnancy involve both blood volume and composition and kidney function. Expansion of maternal blood volume facilitates the transport of nutrients and metabolic wastes between mother and fetus. The highest plasma volume is reached at 34 to 36 weeks, when the mother's body contains 50 percent more plasma than when fertilization took place. As a result of this increase, the *concentrations* of many constituents in the blood (protein, water-soluble vitamins, minerals) are somewhat diminished. Kidney function is altered to accommodate the greater blood volume and increased amount of waste products. More blood flows through the kidneys, and the glomerular filtration rate is increased. There is, however, no related increase in the reabsorptive capacity of the kidney tubules, and as a result, substantial quantities of some water-soluble nutrients are flushed out of the mother's body along with normal metabolic wastes.

NUTRITION AND SUCCESSFUL PREGNANCY

Over the years the nutritional beliefs transmitted to pregnant women have been just as much a matter of fashion as the clothing they were expected to wear. The fetus was long believed to draw all the sustenance it needed from the mother's body. The concept of the fetus as a "parasite" was, in fact, prominent in obstetrical textbooks and practice during the early part of this century, despite the lack of any supporting scientific evidence. Pregnant women were also credited with the instinct to choose to eat the foods required by the fetus even if the items of choice were lobster salad, pickles, or watermelon (none of which, of course, is specifically beneficial).

Most persistent was the advice to "eat for two." Considering the increased hor-

Perspective On

PREGNANCY IN ADOLESCENCE

Of the 10 million teenaged girls in the United States between ages 15 and 19 years, 1.1 million become pregnant each year, 38 percent of these pregnancies end by induced abortion and 13 percent terminate because of spontaneous abortion (miscarriage). Of those that go to delivery over 40 percent are born to unmarried adolescents. In addition, approximately 30,000 girls under age 15 become pregnant each year.

Fetal morbidity and mortality and the risk of pregnancy complications are increased for mothers who are still in their teens. Low birth weight is increased two times if the mother is less than 15 years of age as compared to mothers in their twenties, 1.5 times if the mother is aged 15 to 17 years, and 1.3 times if the mother is 18 to 19 years old. Of babies born to mothers under 15, 6 percent of all firstborns die in the first year of life. This rate is 2.4 times higher than for infants born to mothers in their early twenties. Those that survive are from two to four times more likely to have neurological defects than babies born to women aged 20 to 24. According to some studies, the infants born to teenagers have lower scores on intelligence testing and are less responsive, less expressive, and have lower self-esteem. Other studies report no differences.

Not all the problems are in the infant part of this dyad. Maternal mortality as compared to those in their twenties is 13 percent higher for the 15 to 19 years old group and 2.5 times higher for girls under 15 years of age. Further, the rate of pregnancy-induced hypertension was 40 percent in 13-year-olds, dropping to 16.1 percent in 16-year-olds.

The social disabilities of teenage parenthood are equally dramatic. If the young parents do marry during the pregnancy, there is an estimated 50 percent chance that the marriage will end in divorce. Two-thirds of teenage mothers do not finish high school; the potential earning capacity of the young mother (and father) is sharply reduced; a cycle of dependence on public assistance may be perpetuated or begun; the baby is likely to have poor medical care, poor emotional care, and/or spend years in a public institution or a succession of foster homes.

The single leading contributor to this host of medical and social problems is the age of the mother at conception. During most of the teen years, the girl's physiological, educational, and social development are still incomplete. Although physical growth and sexual maturation proceed at varied rates in different individuals, it is generally true that growth is not completed until four years after menarche (onset of menstruation) in the adolescent girl. Today, menarche occurs at about 12½ years of age on average, earlier than in previous generations; the younger the teenager is at conception, the greater is the risk of damage to both her and her infant. Girls who become pregnant during this developmental period are at biological risk because their bodies are still anatomically and physiologically immature. During this period of rapid growth, the young woman's own body requires increased amounts of nutrients and energy. If pregnancy occurs at this time, fetal nutrient needs are met to whatever extent is possible at the expense of the young mother.

monal output, the increasing demands for nutrients and energy, the need for more oxygen, and the physical demands on the mother's body, this advice does carry a certain logic. Then the fashion shifted, at least in the United States, as the national preoccupation with slimness led to greater concern for the mother's postnatal figure than for her pregnancy needs. Now, as fitness and health have become popular concerns, the pendulum appears to be swinging back to an emphasis on nutritional plenty. This time, however, science rather than fashion is being cited as evidence.

What is the reality? For a considerable part of its uterine life, the embryo/fetus

Complicating these factors, the pregnant teenager is more likely to be a member of a lower socioeconomic group, having a history of suboptimal nutritional status and inadequate medical care.

Even more damaging, the vast majority of such pregnancies are neither planned nor desired. In many cases, the fact of pregnancy is denied for several months until even abortion is not a viable alternative. During this denial period, most probably the worried teenager restricts her food intake, in the hopes that she will not become heavier. With typical teenage concern for fashion and figure, she may fight the increasing pangs of hunger in efforts to maintain her slender curves. By the time her pregnancy can no longer be hidden and she is at last seen by an obstetrician, it may be too late to offset the damage to her health and to the development of her child.

Problems are not, however, inevitable for the pregnant teenager. Those who receive adequate prenatal medical attention do not, as a group, have any greater incidence of complications than do older pregnant women. However, 15 to 20 percent of pregnant teenagers receive no prenatal care until the third trimester. Twenty percent of teens 18 to 19 years old receive no first trimester care; for teens 15 to 17 years old this rises to 50 percent and teens less than 15 years old reaches about 67 percent.

Unfortunately, the penalties for not obtaining medical care fall more heavily upon the newborn children than upon their teenage mothers. The postnatal environment of an infant whose birth was unplanned, unwanted, and financially disastrous is unlikely to improve the prognosis for overcoming any initial medical handicaps. Those who survive the first year of life are not likely to thrive in the typical environment of unstable family life, unemployment, and welfare dependence that often follows teenage pregnancy.

Prevention of the undesired problem of teenage pregnancy is obviously preferable to perpetuation of the cycle of socioeconomic problems. Education for responsible sexuality and increased availability of contraceptives and abortion are proposed as answers. But sex education courses in the schools meet with resistance in many communities and are greeted with snickers by many students. And this high-risk age group has proved unwilling to accept birth control procedures for a variety of reasons (Zelnick and Kanter, 1977). For the present, then, provision of early medical care and attention to nutritional needs represent the best hopes for teenage mothers and their babies. The pregnant teenager must be encouraged to eat balanced, regular meals, to achieve an adequate weight gain (25 to 27 pounds) and take vitamin and mineral supplements when indicated. Health care professionals should pay special attention to ensure that these young patients follow the dietary advice they receive and make appropriate adjustments if resistance is encountered. Certain patterns suggest nutritive problems. These include: abuse or avoidance of foods, excessive weight gain or weight loss during pregnancy, psychological or economic problems, or unhealthful lifestyle.

is extremely small, and its requirements equally so. Thus, fetal development in the earliest months of pregnancy has relatively little nutritional impact on the mother. But during the growth months of pregnancy, and especially the last trimester, the mother's nutritional requirements are indeed increased. The mother's prepregnancy nutritional status has a great impact on the fetus from the moment of conception on. Women who start pregnancy with a long history of good nutrition are more likely to maintain good health and to bear healthy babies.

The desired outcome of pregnancy is a healthy and well-developed baby born with minimal difficulty to a healthy mother. Repeated studies over many years have shown that the best available measures of desirable outcome include weight at birth, fetal mortality, and maternal and infant mortality and morbidity. Consistently, babies with low birth weight (under 2,500 grams, or about 5½ pounds) have a higher mortality rate and a greater number of physical and mental handicaps than newborns of normal weight. Many studies have been done to define the maternal factors that influence the outcome of pregnancy and to examine the effects of nutritional supplementation.

Maternal Nutrition

In the United States, maternal mortality (9.2 per 100,000 live births in 1980) is largely traceable to toxemia, abortion, hemorrhage, and infection—conditions often preventable through good prenatal care. Table 11–2 shows that although U.S. maternal mortality rates are low, they are not the lowest in the Western world; there is still much that can be done to improve pregnancy outcomes, especially in particular U.S. population groups. In contrast to the average maternal mortality given above, when categorized by race, the rate for whites is 6.7 per 100,000 live births, 21.5 for blacks, and 19.8 for all others. Rates may be even higher among subgroups, for example for blacks in lower socioeconomic groups. A "natural experiment" provided by wartime conditions in England in the 1940s gave evidence of a direct association between maternal nutrition and infant viability. Food rationing policies gave priority to pregnant and lactating women, thus improving the quality of their diets. Although there were no changes in other factors such as prenatal care or maternal age, the rate of stillbirths fell dramatically. Additional evidence was obtained due to a six-month famine that occurred in Holland during the war. In the latter case, there was an increase in the rate for stillbirths conceived during the famine.

TABLE 11-2. *Maternal Mortality Rates in Selected Countries, 1975*

Country	Deaths per 100,000 Live Births
Philippines	125.0
Brazil	92.1
Guatemala	90.9
Chile	74.9
Panama	72.7
Costa Rica	24.2
West Germany (Federal Republic)	20.6
Japan	20.5
Norway	11.8
Poland	11.7
England and Wales	10.7
United States	9.2
Netherlands	8.8
Sweden	8.2
Puerto Rico	8.2
Austria	7.7
Australia	7.7
Switzerland	5.4
Israel	5.3
Denmark	1.7

Source: United Nations, Department of International Economic and Social Affairs, *Demographic yearbook 1984,* (New York: United Nations, 1986), pp. 360–363.

Duration of pregnancy is the single most critical factor in determining birth weight. Maternal nutritional status as indicated by height and prepregnancy weight (long-term status) and weight gain during pregnancy (immediate status) are also very important. These nutritional factors interact, so that four situations must be examined to determine the effects of each parameter: (1) underweight before pregnancy and low pregnancy weight gain, (2) underweight before pregnancy and high pregnancy weight gain, (3) overweight before pregnancy and low pregnancy weight gain and (4) overweight before pregnancy and high pregnancy weight gain. Increasing weight gain during pregnancy results in a larger infant no matter what the prepregnancy weight. The greatest differences in birth weight are usually between infants born to mothers who are underweight and gain little and those who are overweight and gain a lot (groups 1 and 4). Interestingly in one study, children of mothers who gained in the midrange during pregnancy scored higher on a nonverbal test of cognitive ability at age 5 than those whose mothers gained more or less.

These and other studies make it overwhelmingly clear that maternal nutrition is a major factor in pregnancy outcome as determined by birth weight. Other interrelated factors (the mother's age; the number of previous pregnancies; her socioeconomic status and race; and the extent to which she smokes, drinks alcoholic beverages, and/or uses drugs) are also important. The precise role of any particular factor is difficult to determine, and more research is needed.

Nutritional Supplementation

Determining the relative importance of any one factor is complicated by the fact that, overall, the physiological efficiency of human reproduction is very high. Current evidence contradicts the concept that the fetus is protected by the mother when her nutritional status is poor. Data from the Dutch famine revealed that infant birth weight decreased 10 percent, while most mothers lost less than 3 percent of their initial weight. This may be nature's way of ensuring species survival. If the mother became so depleted that she could not nurse the infant, both might not survive.

A number of studies have sought to determine the effect of nutritional supplementation on pregnancy. Early studies of vitamin and mineral supplements resulted in equivocal findings and have been criticized for incomplete evaluation of the nutritional status of the mothers both before and during pregnancy. More recent studies have attempted to consider this important factor.

In Guatemala, a preindustrialized country in which women typically gain an average of 15 pounds during pregnancy and where low birth weight is a significant problem, the typical diet during pregnancy provides 40 grams of protein and 1,500 kilocalories per day. Although this protein:energy ratio is adequate, the total energy intake is not. To study the effects of nutritional intervention, investigators provided one group of women with a supplement containing both protein and calories. Another group received a supplement providing calories but no protein. Both supplements contained vitamins and minerals.

The data indicated that as the supplemental energy intake increased, infant birth weights increased and fewer babies with low birth weight were delivered. Furthermore, the increased birth weights were associated with proportional increases in placental weight, suggesting that the benefit of improved maternal nutrition may be due in whole or in part to its effect on the size of the placenta. The amount, and not the type, of supplement may have influenced these results. At a given level of energy intake, it did not matter whether protein was included in the supplement.

These findings suggest that energy and not protein is the limiting factor in diets consumed by pregnant Guatemalan women.

Results of this study and others from developing nations are applicable to high-risk mothers in industrialized nations as well. In a Montreal study, dietary counseling and supplements to meet individualized needs were provided for more than 1,500 low-income pregnant women, all of whom had been at nutritional risk prior to pregnancy. The incidence of low birth weight among infants born to these women decreased to the national average and was lower than in the surrounding area, and the rate of complications was lower than in the surrounding area as well. Maternal weight gain was shown to be directly related to infant birth weight, and those women who received nutritional assistance for longer periods tended to gain more weight and have fewer low birth weight infants than those who were involved in the program for a shorter period of time.

In another study, pregnant California women were provided with three levels of supplementation: One group received a high-protein, high-energy, vitamin-and-mineral-containing beverage; a second group received a lower-protein and lower-energy version of the same beverage; and a control group received only the vitamin and mineral supplementation. None of the three levels of supplementation appeared to have any significant effects on the subsequent birth weights of infants delivered by these women. Even before supplementation, however, the majority of these women were getting from 66 to 100 percent of the recommended dietary allowances for kilocalories and protein and thus would show minimal effects of supplementation.

Supplementation apparently has no demonstrable effect on the pregnancy outcomes of otherwise adequately fed women. But evidence from a number of studies indicates that for women who are poorly nourished in their earlier years and enter pregnancy without nutrient reserves, dietary supplementation can be crucial to the outcome of the pregnancy. Pregnant teenagers who may not have completed their own growth and who may or may not be consuming an adequate diet pose a special problem (See Perspective: Adolescent Pregnancy).

In 1970, the Committee on Maternal Nutrition summarized the findings of a number of studies and issued a report which included a recommendation that special dietary review and counseling be available to all pregnant women, with special attention to those who enter pregnancy with poor dietary habits and in an undernourished state. In 1973, the Special Supplementary Food Program for Women, Infants, and Children (WIC) was started. WIC grew from a $40 million dollar pilot program in 1973 to a $1 billion dollar program in 1983. Many problems have been encountered and its worth has been questioned. However, the role of nutrition in pregnancy has been firmly established by two publications, the NRC *Guidelines for Nutrition Services in Perinatal Care* and *Standards for Obstetric-Gynecologic Services*.

NUTRITIONAL CONSIDERATIONS DURING PREGNANCY

The fetus requires nutrients for all the major metabolic processes involved in energy production, cell and tissue growth, and maintenance of structures and function. It will, to a certain extent, deplete maternal nutrient stores if necessary to supplement what is provided by the mother's food intake. The demands placed on maternal organs, and normal maintenance of the mother's health, must also be considered. Each nutrient has a role in pregnancy, but some play a more obvious role than others. Although experimentally derived data for specific physiological requirements are generally lacking, recommended dietary allowances are set higher for most nutrients during pregnancy (Table 11-3).

Energy

As any mother will tell you, pregnancy is hard work. In addition to the demands made on her system by increased basal metabolism, for almost half of her pregnancy a woman must carry around the equivalent of a small hiking pack balanced quite firmly across her midsection. The energy cost of lugging this ever-increasing extra weight, and adjusting metabolic function accordingly, has been estimated at 80,000 kilocalories over nine months. This averages out to about 300 extra kilocalories per day, a rather small amount. This additional energy is not needed equally throughout the course of pregnancy; requirements generally increase as pregnancy progresses.

Unlike previous estimates, current energy allowances do not assume that physical activity of the mother decreases near term. One study reports, in fact, that modern American women, who normally lead relatively sedentary lives, do not alter their activity appreciably during the last trimester, and thus do not "save" calories. However, a woman who remains physically active will have to adjust her energy intake accordingly, perhaps to a level of 45 kilocalories per kilogram of pregnant body weight, consuming 2,500 to 2,600 kilocalories daily in the last ten weeks.

The advisability of rigorous physical activity during pregnancy has been questioned. There were no differences in duration of labor, Apgar score, or fetal weight in 12 women who participated in an aerobics class during the second and third trimester compared to 8 control women who did not. These results are in agreement

TABLE 11-3. Comparison of RDAs in Nonpregnant, Pregnant, and Lactating Women

Nutrients	Nonpregnant Adult	Pregnant	Lactating
Energy (kcal)	2,000	+300 = 2,300	+500 = 2,500
Protein (g)	44	+30 = 74	+20 = 64
Vitamin A (RE; IU)	800; 4,000	1,000; 5,000	1,200; 6,000
Vitamin D (μg)	5	10	10
Vitamin E (mg αT.E.)	8	10	11
Vitamin C (mg)	60	80	100
Folacin (μg)	400	800	500
Niacin (mg N.E.)	13	15	18
Riboflavin (mg)	1.2	1.5	1.7
Thiamin (mg)	1.0	1.4	1.5
Vitamin B_6 (mg)	2.0	2.6	2.5
Vitamin B_{12} (μg)	3.0	4.0	4.0
Calcium (mg)	800	1,200	1,200
Phosphorus (mg)	800	1,200	1,200
Iodine (μg)	150	.75	200
Iron (mg)	18	18+	18+
Magnesium (mg)	300	450	450
Zinc (mg)	15	20	25

Source: Food and Nutrition Board, National Research Council, *Recommended dietary allowances*, 9th ed. (Washington, D.C.: National Academy of Sciences, 1979).

with earlier studies. Experienced clinicians believe that women who have an established moderate exercise program should continue it during pregnancy. Not all pregnant women should exercise during pregnancy: women with pregnancy-induced hypertension or a history of spontaneous abortions for example, should regulate their physical activity. Contact sports, high altitude climbing, and so on should probably not be considered.

Many women do not increase energy *intake* gradually. Instead, they maintain a constant level of energy consumption that is higher than necessary during the first trimester and less than recommended levels during the third trimester. Maternal fat stores deposited during the period of excessive intake early in the pregnancy provide a resource to be drawn on during the later weeks, and especially during lactation. Approximately 3,500 grams of adipose tissue, representing 30,000 kilocalories, are deposited in the mother's body during pregnancy. In chronically undernourished populations, much less, if any, fat is deposited. Those women who enter pregnancy in an underweight condition should pay particular attention to increasing energy intake levels by at least the recommended 300 kilocalories per day to replenish their body stores of energy.

Closely tied to recommendations for energy intake is medical opinion about optimal weight gain during pregnancy. In the late nineteenth century, when modern surgical techniques were not yet available, weight limitation was generally advised, especially for women whose pelvic cages were small (and whose babies today would

Women who have an established moderate exercise program should continue during pregnancy. WHO Photo

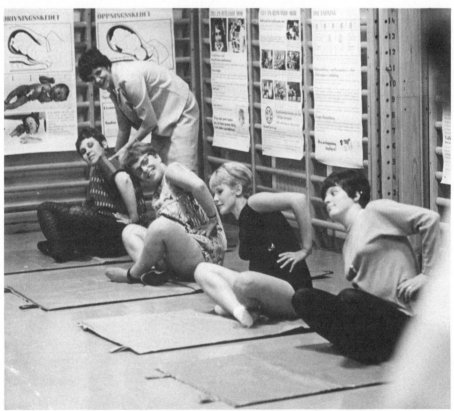

be delivered by cesarean section). A fluid-restricted, low-carbohydrate, high-protein diet was prescribed to produce infants small enough to deliver easily. This remained standard practice well into the twentieth century, despite a lack of scientific verification for its value. Weight control in pregnancy is, even today, a subject of confusion, often influenced by antiquated notions.

Weight gain of three and even four times the weight of the newborn baby is both *normal* and *desirable*. The baby accounts for about a *third to half* of the total normal weight gain during pregnancy, and most of the baby's growth in size occurs in the last trimester.

As Figure 11–2 shows, the growth of the uterus and expansion of the blood supply account for most of the weight gain during the first trimester (13 weeks) of pregnancy. The recommended weight gain over this period is approximately 1 to 2 kilograms (2 to 4.5 lb). In one study, some women said they gained four times this amount. In the second and third trimester weight gain should average 0.35 to 0.4 kilograms (0.8 to 0.9 lb) per week, much of it accounted for by growth of the placenta, uterus, and breasts and increased maternal body fluid volume. In this middle part of the pregnancy the mother's appetite and weight gain will be greatest. However, the baby's weight does not become a major component of the maternal weight gain until the third trimester. By the time of delivery, the new mother can expect to have gained *at least* 10–13 kg (22 to 27 pounds), with first-time (primapara) or young mothers gaining somewhat more than multiparous and older women. On average, daily food intake should provide a minimum of 36 kilocalories per kilogram of pregnant body weight, or about 16 kilocalories per pound. The pattern of weight gain, however, is more significant than the total amount added. A sudden leveling off or marked increase in maternal weight may indicate a problem.

FIGURE 11-2   Components of Weight Gain During Pregnancy.

Source: R. M. Pitkin, Nutritional support in obstetrics and gynecology, *Clinical Obstetrics and Gynecology* 19(3):489, 1976.

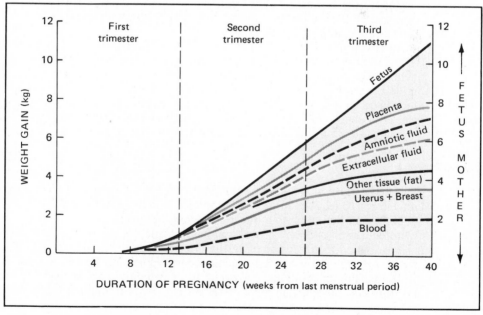

Warnings against excessive weight gain during pregnancy have been aimed in particular at preventing the development of **pregnancy-induced hypertension (PIH)**, previously called eclampsia. However, such warnings have failed to distinguish between added weight because of normal tissue growth and that resulting from excessive fluid accumulation. There is no evidence to associate weight gain per se with PIH, the quality and the pattern of gain are important.

Women who are obese before becoming pregnant do face increased risks of some complications, particularly hypertension and diabetes mellitus. Even for them, however, energy-restricted food intakes are not advisable during pregnancy. Overweight women often try to restrict their weight gain during pregnancy, hoping to lose weight at the end of the nine months. But the potential interference with fetal development makes this unwise. Weight gains of less than 6 kg (15 pounds) are associated with higher perinatal mortality. Obese women should, however, be careful to guard against excessive gain during pregnancy, and they should take the opportunity to improve their eating habits, by eliminating empty-calorie foods and consuming foods with high nutrient density, as well as increasing their physical activity. Accumulation of excessive adipose tissue should be avoided. A total weight gain of 7–10 kg (16–24 pounds) may be recommended for some obese women.

Individual energy needs can be calculated by allowing approximately 40 kcal kg pregnant body weight (about 18 kcal lb). Appetite and weight gain are the best indicators that caloric needs are being met. An energy-restricted diet quite frequently reduces the intake of nutrients necessary for fetal well-being. During short-term fasts, including an overnight fast, blood glucose and insulin concentrations drop more in the pregnant woman and ketone acids increase more rapidly than in nonpregnant women. In addition, a calorie-restricted diet carries the risk of catabolizing body protein stores and necessary fat stores, which would result in ketonemia of longer duration. This maternal condition has been correlated with mental retardation in the offspring of affected mothers. As some consolation for the figure-conscious, the high levels of progesterone that promote storage of added fat during pregnancy decrease rapidly after birth, and even more rapidly in lactating mothers. Most women have a dramatic postpartum weight loss and should be back to their prepregnant weights in a few months.

Underweight women have different problems, especially if their low body weight is associated with overall low nutrient intake. Because underweight women frequently have babies with low birth weight, nutritional supplementation, counseling, and careful supervision during pregnancy are necessary. Underweight individuals should eat sufficient amounts of carefully selected nutritious foods to meet both energy and nutrient needs. A slightly higher than average weight gain, 12–15 kg (28–36 lbs), has been recommended for these individuals.

Protein

A normal pattern of weight gain during pregnancy indicates only that overall energy intake is adequate but not that specific nutrient requirements are being met. In the United States, protein intake is seldom a problem.

Protein serves as the structural building material for synthesis of protein molecules; cells; and tissues in the fetus, the placenta, and the mother herself. The recommended protein allowance for nonpregnant women is 44 grams per day. There is little demand for additional protein in the early months of pregnancy. By the second trimester, however, an extra 30 grams per day is recommended. That is the equivalent of 4 ounces of meat or fish or 4 glasses of milk. Planning for increased protein needs of strict vegetarians requires careful consideration of complementary protein sources (see Chapter 4).

Vitamins

Because of their role in energy production, thiamin, riboflavin, and niacin are important components of diet during pregnancy. Thiamin is a coenzyme necessary in the last step of the metabolic pathway by which glucose is converted to pyruvic acid and then to acetyl CoA. Riboflavin and niacin are components of the coenzymes flavin adenine dinucleotide (FAD) and niacin adenine dinucleotide (NAD), which produce energy by controlling the transfer of hydrogen atoms through the electron transport system. Severe deficiencies of these three B vitamins during pregnancy cause fetal death, low birth weight, and congenital malformations in laboratory animals; comparable findings have not, however, been observed in humans.

Pyridoxine (vitamin B_6) and folic acid are needed for protein synthesis, and thus for fetal development and growth; folacin and vitamin B_{12} are involved in synthesis of red blood cells; and vitamin C is essential for the development of collagen, the important connective tissue protein. The coenzyme roles and other functions of these water-soluble vitamins were described in Chapter 7, and food sources of each were listed there as well. Recommended dietary allowances for all these are increased during pregnancy, as shown in Table 11–3.

Although increases for most are moderate, the recommendation for folacin doubles to 800 micrograms per day. This reflects the importance of this vitamin in DNA and RNA synthesis, not only for red blood cell formation but for the rapid growth of fetal and placental cells as well. For cells to divide, DNA must replicate itself, transmitting the identical genetic information to the new cell. Folacin is involved in almost every aspect of the process. Dietary sources of folacin are few and unreliable. Leafy, green vegetables, the best source, may lose up to 80 percent of their vitamin content during storage and cooking. As many as 60 percent of pregnant women studied have low serum folate levels, although few of them show deficiency symptoms. Pregnancy hormones may interfere with folacin absorption and thus account for the prevalence of low serum concentrations. The relationship of folate deficiency with the incidence of neural tube defects is unresolved. Since the consequences of major deficiency could be serious, however, the National Research Council recommends oral supplements to provide 200 to 400 micrograms daily in the last half of pregnancy.

Supplementation with vitamin B_{12} should be considered by strict vegetarian women who become pregnant. As discussed in Chapter 7, there is a potential problem of severe deficiency among the nursing infants of such mothers. Early treatment of affected infants will reverse infant symptoms, but if the mother's diet is supplemented during pregnancy and lactation, the problem is avoided altogether.

Folacin, vitamin B_{12}, and for nonmilk drinkers, vitamin D are the only vitamins for which supplementation should be considered. Although the allowance for ascorbic acid is increased during pregnancy because of fetal needs, supplementation is not desirable, and the recommended amount can easily be provided by ordinary foods. Overdosage in pregnancy may cause infantile "rebound" scurvy. High vitamin C levels during gestation may cause fetal adaptation in the form of rapid catabolism of the excess. When the infant's ascorbic acid supply is decreased after birth, the high catabolic rate is still maintained, at least temporarily, and so the normally necessary quantity of the vitamin is not retained by the newborn. Since there is no proof of advantageous effects of high levels of vitamin C that would justify this risk to the infant, megadoses during pregnancy are definitely not advised.

The fat-soluble vitamins A, D, E, and K are also essential components of the diet of the pregnant woman. Vitamin A is necessary for the development of skin and epithelial tissue lining internal organs, and vitamin D is required for the healthy development of bones and teeth. Vitamin E helps to protect cell membranes, and Vitamin K is important for the blood-clotting process. Because these are present in maternal body stores and can easily be provided in diet, supplementation is usually unnecessary. It is, in fact, ill-advised, particularly for women who drink vitamin D-fortified milk. Excesses of vitamins A and D have produced symptoms in laboratory animals. An infant born to a mother who consumed 150,000 IU of Vitamin A from days 19 through 40 was born with multiple deformities. Excess vitamin D may actually produce rebound hypercalcemia in the newborn and should be avoided. There is no evidence that fetuses (or their mothers) benefit from supplemental vitamin E; vitamin K is routinely administered to newborn infants.

Vitamins ingested in excess of physiological need serve no useful purpose. Therapeutic doses of any substance are not warranted unless medically prescribed. Self-dosing with an excess of vitamins is no different from self-dosing with aspirin, tranquilizers, or any other substance. In pregnancy, as at any other time, a well-balanced diet is the best protection against nutrient deficiencies.

Minerals

Table 11–3 indicates increases in the recommended allowances for the minerals calcium, phosphorus, iodine, iron, magnesium, and zinc. Other trace minerals such as chromium and copper are important in reproduction, but needs for them in human pregnancy have not been evaluated. They can be provided by consuming a diversified diet.

CALCIUM. Calcium is a vital structural component of the fetal skeleton, which will contain an average of about 28 g (1 ounce) of calcium at birth. Most skeletal calcification takes place in the third trimester, but the calcium RDA for pregnant women has been set at a constant 1,200 milligrams per day, the amount found in 1 quart of milk. Milk products such as yogurt, cheese, and ice cream contain lesser amounts, but meals can be planned to meet the recommendation from a balance of milk and milk products. Women who do not or cannot consume milk or milk products must rely on other sources. Since calcium present in plant sources may not be absorbed efficiently, strict vegetarians may require supplementation. If milk intake is clearly adequate, calcium supplementation is not necessary.

PHOSPHORUS. Phosphorus activates glucose and glycogen so that they can produce energy, aids in the transformation of many B vitamins to coenzymes, and is necessary for skeletal growth and growth of all cells. The naturally high levels of phosphorus in animal protein foods, dairy products, and snack items, ensure an adequate phosphorus supply in almost every diet to meet the RDA of 1,200 milligrams during pregnancy.

IODINE. As a component of thyroid hormone, iodine is essential for the regulation of basal metabolism. The RDA for iodine is easily supplied by the use of iodized salt. Women who avoid iodized salt must rely on other sources.

IRON. Unfortunately, iron requirements are not as easily met. Iron is a major raw material for maintaining red blood cell synthesis in both the mother and the fetus. About 290 milligrams (mg) of iron are required for additional hemoglobin as the mother's blood volume expands. Another 134 mg are stored in the placenta, and a final 246 mg goes to the blood and body stores of the fetus. This can be a significant drain on the mother's iron stores; even when they are adequate at conception, iron utilization increases dramatically. Some help comes from the gastrointestinal system, where slowed motility and other changes increases iron absorption from its usual 10 percent to approximately 30 percent of dietary intake. Also, about 120 mg of iron which would ordinarily be lost in menstruation is conserved during pregnancy.

Still, the mother often comes up short—short of iron and short of breath. Her reduced hemoglobin concentration means that her body must increase its cardiac output to meet its oxygen needs and those of the fetus. So much extra cardiac work is physiologically fatiguing, and in extreme instances of severe iron deficiency, reduced hemoglobin levels can lead to cardiac arrest or death should she hemorrhage during delivery.

As pointed out in Chapter 8, the normal iron requirements of women are not easy to satisfy even with an otherwise nutritionally balanced diet. Organ meats, some shellfish, and prune juice are the only iron-rich foods. Foods normally consumed in the typical American diet contain only 6 mg of iron per 1,000 kilocalories. To meet even the RDA for nonpregnant women (18 mg), 3,000 kilocalories would have to be consumed—an unrealistically high figure. And because most women have minimal iron stores and run the risk of developing anemia, the RDA during pregnancy is greater than 18 mg. Therefore, iron supplementation during pregnancy is routinely prescribed. The provision of 30 to 60 mg of iron per day (usually as 150 to 300 mg of ferrous sulfate) is recommended throughout pregnancy and for several months following delivery.

ZINC. Zinc deficiency has been shown to be highly tetratogenic in rats and results in abnormal brain development and behavior in zinc deficient non-human primates. As discussed in Chapter 8, zinc is a structural component of several very important enzymes, including carbonic anhydrase which helps regulate acid-base balance. It is also a cofactor for many other enzymes. Epidemiological data support a relationship between poor pregnancy outcome and zinc deficiency. Zinc supplementation of women with low serum zinc concentrations has been reported to reduce the number of complications during pregnancy. Zinc-deficient pregnant monkeys developed a microcytic anemia and decreased immune function. The recommended dietary allowance of 20 mg is difficult to meet if the diet does not contain some animal protein.

SODIUM. Although there is no RDA for sodium, recommended intakes of this mineral during pregnancy have been a source of controversy. Previous knowledge suggested that pregnancy is accompanied by sodium retention, associated with fluid accumulation, hypertension, and resultant toxemia. Therefore, sodium was frequently restricted. However, recent research indicates that pregnancy is a salt-*losing* condition that may result in decreased body fluid volume and subsequent constriction of blood vessels if sodium is not provided in adequate amounts by the diet. Proponents of this theory suggest that salt intake should be *increased* during pregnancy. Pregnant women are currently advised to salt their food "to taste," to trust the body's normal renal mechanisms to maintain the optimal sodium level, and not to restrict dietary salt.

OTHER MINERALS.   At the present time, copper deficiency during human pregnancy has only been demonstrated in an unusual case of a woman treated with penicillamine during her pregnancy. Penicillamine reacts with several minerals and causes them to be excreted from the body. Under normal circumstances, copper deficiency is not a problem. While all other minerals are needed, the role of deficiencies of these minerals in human pregnancy has not been identified.

FLUID.   Finally, pregnant women should maintain adequate fluid balance by consuming six to eight glasses of beverages per day. Diuretics should not be used, since they deplete the body of fluid, sodium, and frequently potassium.

FOOD PATTERNS DURING PREGNANCY

Many women have a significant change in their eating habits even before their first prenatal visit to a physician. Often a sudden aversion to usual early-morning favorites, such as coffee or bacon, is the first inkling of pregnancy. By the time that aversion had been translated into actual nausea or vomiting (the familiar "morning sickness"), the diagnosis was established, and the newly expectant mother was well on her way to new eating patterns. Typically, with little to eat in the morning, women reach lunch time with a ravenous appetite that is still strong at the dinner hour. The result is likely to be increased energy intake and excess weight gain in early pregnancy.

Women who may have a problem regulating weight gain could add protein from relatively low-calorie foods such as chicken and fish rather than the higher-calorie meat choices. Other good sources of protein include eggs, skim milk, and cheese. Women who are strict vegetarians should include daily an additional serving of a complementary protein combination, such as legumes and rice, or peanut butter and whole-grain bread, to assure supplies of the essential amino acids. Foods with high complex-carbohydrate content, such as bread, cereal, rice, and noodles, provide 2 or more grams of protein per serving; potatoes and many other vegetables are also moderate protein sources. Table 11–4 lists the foods that are recommended during pregnancy to meet the nutritional demands of both mother and infant.

Cravings and Aversions

Many pregnant women experience a strong change in food likes and dislikes. Many women who regularly consumed coffee and/or alcoholic beverages before becoming pregnant find that these have little appeal during pregnancy. The number of women citing nausea or loss of a "taste" for the beverage as the reason for their aversion outweigh the number who reduce intakes out of concern for their health or that of the fetus.

Cravings for food are also frequent and are often reported for ice cream, chocolate, and other candies; sweetened baked goods; and fruit juices. Fried meats and poultry, vegetables, and foods with oregano-seasoned sauces were the most common aversions in one study.

Cravings in pregnancy are hypothesized to be a response to the increased need of the mother; the number of women reporting an increased desire for ice cream and milk would seem to support this. However, although many women increase their

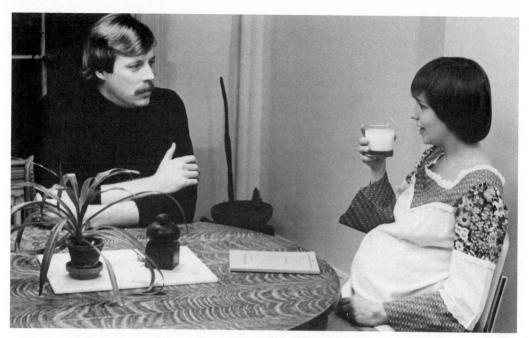

Many women experience a significant change in eating habits resulting in excess weight gain in early pregnancy. But in the final weeks, when appetite decreases just as fetal nutrient and energy needs sharply increase, the fat deposits of early pregnancy provide a "cushion" for the baby.

Suzanne Szasz/Photo Researchers

intake of milk and ice cream, others do not *crave* these, and a few even develop aversions to them.

Food aversions may have a biochemical basis and develop in reaction to substances released by the fetus. Research to confirm these hypotheses remains to be done. Many women will simply say, "Coffee didn't smell good any more" or "I just lost my appetite for steak." With all the other physiological changes taking place

TABLE 11-4. *Foods Needed During Pregnancy*

Food	Daily amount
Milk	1 qt (or equivalent)
Eggs	1–2
Meat	2 servings
Cheese	1–2 servings, additional snacks
Grains, whole, enriched	4–5 slices or servings
Legumes, nuts	1–2 servings a week
Green and yellow fruits, vegetables	1–2 servings
Citrus fruit	2
Additional vitamin C foods	Frequently, as desired
Other vegetables and fruits	1–2 servings
Butter, fortified margarine	2 tbsp (or as needed)
Other foods: grains, fruits, vegetables, other proteins	As needed for energy and added vitamins and minerals
Fluid	6–8 glasses (including milk)

Source: Adapted from S. Williams, *Handbook of maternal and infant nutrition* (Berkeley, Calif.: SRW Productions, 1976).

during these eventful nine months, it is little wonder that a woman's senses of smell and taste are altered as well.

Cravings for nonfood items during pregnancy have also been described. The intentional consumption of nonfood items, **pica**, has been documented since ancient times. It is found throughout the world among males and females, nonpregnant and pregnant, and may involve the consumption of ice, various clay and earth substances, soot, wax, and even shoe polish.

Mineral imbalance has been suggested as a cause of pica. However, studies have shown that pica may be practiced by individuals who are not nutritionally deprived. Another suggestion is that clay or starch consumption may reduce nausea. The consumption of clay, laundry starch, and similar materials by American black women, especially during pregnancy, is a well-known phenomenon. Whatever factors may be involved, there is a large cultural, traditional component to the development of this habit.

Special Nutritional Concerns

For the vast majority of women, pregnancy is medically uneventful. Although there are certain predictable and inevitable discomforts, severe problems are rare in women who receive good prenatal care and who have a history of nutritional health. Too many women still do not receive adequate prenatal care, however, and many others who regularly see a physician neglect to follow nutritional advice even when it is given. At greatest risk for complications are women who are under 15 years of age; are under- or overweight; have had three pregnancies within three years; have a history of poor obstetrical performance; are economically deprived; are heavy smokers, drinkers, or drug takers; or have a chronic systemic disease such as diabetes or hypertension and require a special therapeutic diet.

NUTRITIONAL ANEMIAS. Anemia, a significant decrease in hemoglobin and red blood cells, is the most common example of a specific nutrient deficiency. It is diagnosed by blood tests that measure the concentration of hemoglobin and the volume (size) and number of red blood cells. Normal values for hemoglobin in healthy young women average 13 to 14 g/dl. Because of the increased plasma volume that occurs during pregnancy, a "physiological anemia" develops, in which a hemoglobin level of 11 g/dl is considered acceptable. A value lower than this indicates true anemia in pregnancy.

Anemia may be due to nutrient deficiencies (iron, protein, vitamin B_6, vitamin B_{12}, or folic acid) or to medical or hereditary conditions. Symptoms include fatigue, weakness, loss of appetite, edema, and shortness of breath. Extreme cases pose the risk of maternal and fetal mortality.

Iron deficiency accounts for more than 75 percent of the anemias which develop during pregnancy, and folic acid deficiency accounts for much of the rest. Anemias due to both causes can easily be treated, and even more easily avoided, through adequate intake of appropriate foods and/or supplements. Again, prior nutritional status influences the probability of anemia.

PREGNANCY TOXEMIAS. *Toxemia* (preeclampsia and eclampsia) is a term that describes a potentially life-threatening condition occurring in a small percentage of pregnant women, usually after the twentieth week of pregnancy. The most important symptoms of preeclampsia are sudden onset of hypertension, proteinuria, and generalized edema leading to dramatic weight gain. Dizziness, headache, visual disturbances, nausea, and vomiting may also be present. When this constellation of symptoms is complicated by convulsions, eclampsia is diagnosed.

By definition, the word *toxemia* means "blood toxins," but despite significant amounts of research, no such toxins have been identified. It was once thought, for example, that sodium was the culprit because of its effects of fluid retention. The typical antidote—diuresis—unfortunately caused even more deleterious effects than the original problem. Another theory held that excess weight gain was at fault, and energy-restricted diets were recommended. However, most studies do not support this hypothesis.

Other theories have been proposed, but as yet none has been proven. Because in the United States toxemia is most prevalent in low-income, nonwhite populations known to receive poor diets and poor medical care and to enter pregnancy in a debilitated state, the presently accepted approach to preventing toxemia is comprehensive prenatal care, including education about a balanced diet adequate in all nutrients and energy content. Prenatal nutritional counseling, supplementation if needed, guidance in dealing with life stresses, and careful monitoring of pregnancy through weigh-ins and blood tests should be provided for all pregnant women, especially those from high-risk populations. Sudden weight gain, signaling edema, calls for immediate intervention. Fortunately, most cases of preeclampsia do not result in eclampsia. Because of the medical risks to both mother and infant, hospitalization and bed rest are required for eclampsia, and delivery by cesarean section is usually indicated.

GASTROINTESTINAL DISTURBANCES.   About two-thirds of pregnant women feel nauseous on arising, even before their first menstrual period is missed. Despite some assertions to the contrary, there are clear physiological reasons for this "morning sickness," related primarily to the hormonal changes of early pregnancy. Anxiety and poor dietary habits may also contribute. In some cases, morning sickness is not confined to the morning but may recur throughout the day. The best treatment is small, frequent meals consisting of dry, easily digested, high-energy foods. Avoiding highly spiced and fatty foods at mealtime also seems to help. Drinking liquids before or after, rather than with, meals is often helpful as well. The problem usually disappears by the end of the first trimester. When it does not, or when severe persistent vomiting develops, hospitalization for intravenous feeding may be necessary to prevent dehydration. Fortunately, this is quite rare.

Gastrointestinal problems of one kind or another are almost universal among pregnant women. Among them are constipation because of decreased intestinal motility and as a side effect of iron supplements in some women, as well as heartburn and abnormal fullness caused by the pressure of the enlarging uterus crowding against the stomach. All these ailments are amenable to nutritional correction. Increased intake of fluid, dietary fiber, and "natural" laxatives such as prunes and figs will do much to relieve constipation. Smaller and more frequent meals and thorough chewing will mitigate other problems. Such casual remedies as baking soda, "candy-type" antacids, and the entire gamut of nonprescription medications often resorted to for pain, tension, and sleeplessness should be avoided, as should laxative preparations in general.

Other Considerations

The Thalidomide tragedy of the early 1960s awakened many physicians and patients to the risks of medication in pregnancy. Thalidomide, a widely used hypnotic (sleep-producing) agent, was given to ease the insomnia of early pregnancy. Unfortunately, this was very bad timing; Thalidomide impaired the development of fetal limbs that were forming at that precise period.

MEDICATION.   Even common aspirin may cause fetal damage. The same medications that may be harmless at other times may have deleterious effects on the absorption, metabolism, placental transfer, and fetal utilization of nutrients when taken during pregnancy. (Look at the labels on many over-the-counter preparations. You will be surprised to see how many say "Not recommended for use by women who are or may be pregnant.") In fact, *no* medication should be taken by the pregnant woman without prescription. Pregnant women should, furthermore, question their physicians about medications given them. Often, however, the woman herself asks for "something so I can sleep" or "just a temporary prescription until my headaches go away." This practice should be avoided; the potential risks are too great.

CAFFEINE.   Caffeine is probably the most popular and most readily available drug in the world. It occurs not only in coffee but also in tea, chocolate, cola drinks, and many over-the-counter medications. Caffeine crosses the placenta, and researchers are still exploring its possible effects on the fetus. Epidemiological studies were frequently inconclusive. The best and most recent studies indicate that moderate caffeine intake has no deleterious effects on fetal development.

PSYCHOACTIVE (MOOD-ALTERING) SUBSTANCES.   Although there are few available data on the effects of marijuana in pregnancy, any type of smoking can increase blood carbon monoxide levels and possibly impair fetal oxygen supplies. We cannot, on the basis of present evidence, be certain that marijuana does not have long-term effects on the smoker or her babies. The active ingredient in marijuana is able to cross the placenta, and reports that chronic long-term marijuana use in young adult men produces breast enlargement, and lowered plasma testosterone levels suggest that marijuana may produce hormonal changes in the developing fetus as well. The subsequent effects are as yet unknown, but they may in fact be significant.

In addition, marijuana is known to affect the appetite, which may interfere with optimal food intake during pregnancy. Finally, marijuana smoke contains a pharmacological agent—tetrahydrocannabinol, the active isomer of *cannabis*, which is used medically as a sedative and analgesic. Its effects on the central nervous system are well known to users: euphoria, hallucinations, and other mental changes. How many of those effects, and unwanted side effects, may be due to unknown additives or fillers in any particular marijuana supply cannot be evaluated.

The fetal effects of heroin are well known. Heroin addicts deliver babies with low birth weight who are themselves addicted and must go through painful withdrawal immediately after birth when their "regular supply" is cut off. Addicted mothers, moreover, are not likely to obtain prenatal medical care or to be conscious of the nutritional content of their diets. The combined risks to the innocent newborn are hard to exaggerate.

ALCOHOL.   Recent studies indicate that as little as 1 ounce of alcohol per day may increase the risks of stillbirth, low birth weight, physical malformations, poor sucking ability, and numerous medical complications in the postnatal period. Damage to the fetus seems to be correlated both with the amount of alcohol intake and with how effectively the mother's body metabolizes and excretes that alcohol. Thus, it is possible that risks may be higher for some moderate drinkers than for some heavier drinkers.

Studies on known alcoholics indicate that total alcohol consumption may not be as important as the maximum concentrations that may be reached during critical periods of infant development. When these "binge levels" do impinge on critical periods, Fetal Alcohol Syndrome (FAS) can result. It is expressed in widespread neuropathologic malformations in the newborn, caused by failure of fetal brain cells to migrate to their proper location. The current incidence of FAS makes it the third leading cause of birth defects associated with mental retardation and the only one of these leading causes that is preventable. Animal studies suggest that daily consumption of more than 3 ounces may put the infant at risk for FAS. It is not known, however, if the pregnant woman should give up social drinking altogether during nine months; perhaps moderation is the key. In 1981, the Surgeon General advised pregnant women to not drink alcoholic beverages. The American Medical Association and the National Institute on Alcohol Abuse and Alcoholism make the same recommendations.

SMOKING. Numerous studies have indicated that women who smoke have a higher rate of spontaneous abortion and babies with low birth weight than do non-smokers, along with a greater likelihood of complications during labor and delivery, which is often premature. The more a woman smokes, the smaller her baby is likely to be, and those babies may never catch up in growth. Some of them don't have the chance—babies of smokers are more likely to die at birth or during the first year of life. The infants of women who smoke less than a pack a day have a 20 percent greater risk of mortality in the first month of life, and the infants of women who smoke more than a pack a day have a 35 percent greater risk. Children whose mothers smoke are more likely to have neurological defects, be hyperactive, and to have psychological and learning difficulties.

Although many of the ill effects due to smoking have been blamed on its major pharmacological component, nicotine—well known to be a nervous system stimulant at smoking dosages—the risks of smoking during pregnancy appear to be more closely related to the carbon monoxide present in cigarette smoke. The oxygen-carrying capacity of both maternal and fetal blood supplies is diminished because carbon monoxide replaces oxygen in the mother's blood, thus reducing the oxygen supply to her growing fetus. Some research indicates that compensation may occur in fetal red cells; postnatal hemoglobin and hematocrit levels in 10,399 neonates were found to be significantly higher for babies born to smokers than to non-smokers. Nevertheless, this compensation is not enough to prevent the fetal abnormalities that are so frequently reported.

In addition to the effects on blood oxygenation, the fetal malnutrition associated with cigarette smoking may be partially mediated by abnormal nutrient metabolism. Clinical and epidemiological studies have established that carbohydrate and protein metabolism may be impaired in heavy smokers and that plasma levels of ascorbic acid and vitamins B_{12} and B_6 are decreased as well. These data have clear implications for pregnant women.

LACTATION

The nine months of pregnancy are the prelude not only to childbirth but also to the nutritionally important period of lactation. The umbilical cord may be cut, but the nurturing bond between mother and child is not severed. A new system is ready to take over: the lactating breast.

Physiology

Many of the physiological changes occurring in the mother during pregnancy are preparation for lactation. During the first and second trimester, terminal tubules connected to the mammary milk ducts proliferate and group together to form what are known as *lobules*, or *acinar structures*, in which milk will be produced (see Figure 11-3). Whether the breast is large or small, it will contain from 15 to 20 of these ducts, which connect the milk-producing centers to the nipples from which milk will be released. This is all the "equipment" that is required for successful nursing. Neither breast size nor shape has any influence on the ability of women to nurse. Almost all women who want to breastfeed can do so. In the next chapter we will examine the effects of breastfeeding on infants; our concern in this chapter is the development of the capability for lactation.

Microscopic studies of breast tissue have shown that the milk is produced in secretory (alveolar) cells which synthesize lactose, the predominant carbohydrate in milk. Progesterone, the primary pregnancy hormone, inhibits lactose production, thereby preventing significant milk accumulation during pregnancy. After birth, however, progesterone levels fall; levels of prolactin, the lactation hormone, rise; and the mammary alveolar cells go into full operation (see Figure 11-4). Prolactin is released by the hypothalamus in response to suckling by the infant. Suckling also stimulates production of oxytocin from the posterior pituitary gland. Circulation of oxytocin causes the musclelike cells in the breast to contract, which propels milk through the ducts for release through the nipple.

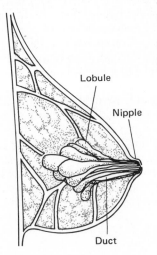

Lobule

Nipple

Duct

FIGURE 11-3 *Development of the Mammary Gland During Pregnancy.*

Source: Adapted from F. L. Strand, *Physiology: A Regulatory Systems Approach* (New York: Macmillan, 1978), p. 536.

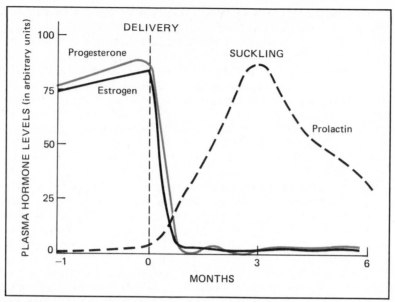

FIGURE 11-4   *Hormone Production Before and After Delivery.*

Source: Adapted from F. L. Strand, *Physiology: A Regulatory Systems Approach* (New York: Macmillan, 1978), p. 537.

In addition to lactose, three major milk proteins are synthesized by the alveolar cells: α-lactalbumin, β-lactalbumin, and casein. Most of the amino acids contained in these proteins are taken up directly from the mother's plasma, although some of the nonessential amino acids are synthesized in the alveolar cells. Full lactation does not occur instantly at birth. For the first few days colostrom is secreted. Colostrom has slightly different concentrations of several nutrients than are present in mature milk.

Nutritional Considerations

When she starts to nurse, the new mother has about 2 to 4 kilograms (about 4.5 to 9 lb) of new fat stores deposited during pregnancy, which serve as a kind of back-up energy supply. These fat stores may be mobilized to provide approximately 200 to 300 kcal per day for about three months. It has been calculated that because human breast milk contains approximately 70 kcal/100 ml, and maternal efficiency in converting stored energy to milk energy is at least 80 percent, the mother will need approximately 90 additional kcal for every 100 ml of milk she must produce. Thus, for 850 ml of milk, the average amount produced each day after lactation is established, the nursing mother needs nearly 800 kcal above her normal daily requirements. With 200 to 300 kcal available from existing fat stores, at least for the first three months, that will mean an additional 500 kcal per day that must be provided by the diet, or 200 kcal more than during pregnancy (see Table 11–3). If lactation continues beyond three months, energy intake must be increased by an additional 200 to 300 kcal per day.

A mother who does not nurse will not need this additional energy intake, and she will have to lose the accumulated adipose tissue as well. As the women resumes her prepregnancy eating pattern and normal—or probably increased—activity following childbirth, extra fat stores will gradually be lost.

Because the alveolar cells synthesize milk protein and also utilize some protein from maternal plasma, the RDA for protein is 20 grams higher for lactating women (see Table 11–3). Since there is no lack of protein in the diet of most Americans, there is little concern about protein deficiency in lactating women in the United States. Even in countries where protein-energy malnutrition is common, however, protein levels in milk are not reduced, although total milk volume may be greatly diminished. The protein content of human milk remains remarkably constant despite the variations in maternal food intakes, leading to the conclusion that the essential amino acids are supplied from maternal stores if they are lacking in the mother's diet.

Breast milk also contains significant amounts of fat, mostly in the form of triglycerides but also including small amounts of phospholipids, cholesterol, and free fatty acids. The levels of all lipids except fatty acids in breast milk appear to be independent of levels in the maternal bloodstream. Like carbohydrate and protein, the lipid content of breast milk is maintained even at the expense of maternal stores.

Breast milk also contains fat-soluble vitamins A and E and small amounts of vitamin D and calcium, iron, copper, fluoride, and other minerals. Addition of fat-soluble vitamins to the mother's diet during lactation does not appear to increase their levels in breast milk. In contrast, concentration of water-soluble vitamins and of some trace minerals reflect maternal intake. In particular, breast milk content of ascorbic acid, thiamin, and riboflavin most closely reflects intake levels; pantothenic acid, pyridoxine (vitamin B_6), biotin, folic acid, and vitamin B_{12} concentrations also relate to the mothers' dietary intake. The implications for cigarette smokers should be remembered. Excessive intakes of these nutrients are not advantageous and may even be damaging.

Food Patterns

Milk production is very efficient. Even in mothers in relatively poor nutritional status, the milk produced is of sufficiently high quality to support a growing infant. For all the major and many of the minor nutrients, maternal stores can be utilized. The breast milk content of calcium averages 250 to 350 milligrams daily, even when maternal intake is deficient. Although beneficial for the infant, significant amounts of the mother's skeletal calcium are mobilized to provide this level. To prevent their own stores of vital nutrients from being depleted, and to ensure that sufficient amounts of vitamins and trace minerals are available for milk production, nursing mothers require a plentiful, well-balanced diet.

Exactly what should be in that diet, however, is a matter of some debate. There is little specific, well-documented information to guide nursing mothers in sound diet planning, and physicians' recommendations vary widely. Some routinely prescribe nutritional supplements. Others recommend avoidance of chocolate and spicy foods but suggest consumption of large quantities of fluids, including beer and wine.

Some general guidelines have been established, however. The quality of the diet should be similar to that consumed during pregnancy, with additional energy intake to maintain lactation. At least 1 quart of vitamin D-fortified milk, or its equivalent, should be consumed every day, either as a beverage or incorporated into other foods; vitamin D will increase maternal utilization of calcium and phospho-

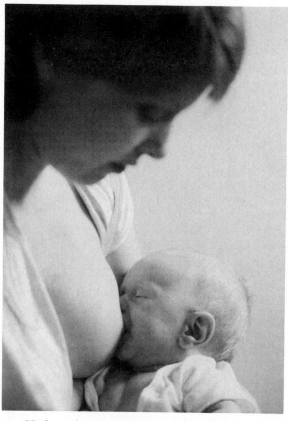

A mother who maintains her own good nutrition will maximize the quality and quantity of her milk to meet her baby's needs.

Michael Stratford

rus. High-quality protein and liberal amounts of fruits, vegetables, and grain products will ensure adequate provision of essential amino acids, vitamins, and minerals. Fluid intake is important; nursing women should consume 2 to 3 quarts of fluid per day. Supplementation practices should parallel those necessary during pregnancy, especially for strict vegetarians. Iron supplementation should be continued for several months for all women to replenish maternal iron reserves, which are usually depleted during pregnancy.

Scientific data may be scanty, but nursing mothers have been providing nutritional foundations for their young since mammals appeared on earth some 200 million years ago. The biological innovation has been a success, and the limited number of studies that have been conducted demonstrate the effectiveness of the mechanism by which infant food is produced and delivered.

Some concerns derive from today's living patterns, and they will be discussed in the next chapter. For example, there is evidence that mothers' high alcohol consumption can affect nursing infants. Many compounds (drug, nutrient, contaminants, etc.) circulating in maternal blood will appear in breast milk at concentrations which may or may not be the same as in maternal blood. The possibility of contamination of breast milk when the mother is exposed to environmental pollutants such as DDT and polychlorinated biphenyls (PCBs) has also generated some controversy. Although DDT can no longer be used and PCB levels are decreasing because of federal regulations, they may be present in the water and food supply in some areas where they were once heavily used. Women living in such areas who desire to nurse should consult their state agricultural department and county medical society for advice.

The nursing mother needs no special foods and need avoid no foods. Increased *amounts* of food are needed, however, to provide the energy, protein, calcium, and other nutrients that must be used for the infant's milk supply and the iron to replenish the mother's own depleted reserves. Energy intake should be monitored by the mother's weight status; as the baby grows older and is gradually weaned to other foods, less milk will be taken, and the amount of energy the mother needs will decline. Unless the mother decreases her own energy intake, she will have an undesirable weight gain.

Most women who want to nurse the baby can do so, but the life style of contemporary American communities does not always make this natural process easy. Many women have found that a support system, such as that offered by the international La Leche League or by other women who have nursed their babies, helps them to cope with any psychological and life style problems.

SUMMARY

The complex growth and development process known as pregnancy requires significant amounts of nutrients and energy. Starting with the early developmental stages of blastogenesis and embryonic maturation, nutritional factors can influence the precisely programmed progression from zygote to fully formed infant. The placenta, which develops simultaneously with the embryo, serves as the transfer mechanism for conveying vital nutrients and oxygen from mother to growing fetus. If placental development is impaired, as it may be in the case of various abnormalities including maternal protein-energy malnutrition, the fetus will receive less nourishment, leading to possible fetal malnutrition, low birth weight, and subsequent morbidity or mortality.

The placenta is also the primary source of progesterone and estrogen and the unique source of several other hormones. These hormones act primarily on the mother to increase the flexibility of muscle and connective tissue, to increase fluid retention and fat storage, and to expand blood volume. Other physiological adaptations influence kidney function and intestinal motility.

Although these and other physiological changes increase the demand for nutrients and oxygen, no radical dietary changes are required in pregnancy. If a woman is well nourished before pregnancy, she is likely to remain well nourished during pregnancy. A balanced diet, including 1 quart of milk daily, is recommended, with an additional allowance of 300 kilocalories per day. Iron and folate, which are seriously depleted by the demand for increased hemoglobin as the blood volume expands and fetal development proceeds, probably should be provided in the form of supplements. Women who are lactose-intolerant may need a calcium supplement; those who are strict vegetarians should have vitamin B_{12} supplementation and pay particular attention to consumption of complementary protein foods.

Women who enter pregnancy without dietary reserves and have a history of poor nutrition should have nutritional consultation, proper diet, and additional supplementation as necessary; such women are at greatest risk of developing complications during delivering babies with low birth weight.

The most important indicator of adequate fetal growth is maternal weight gain. A pregnancy weight gain of 22 to 27 pounds is both normal and desirable. In the early weeks, weight gain is slow and accounted for mostly by uterine growth and expanded blood volume. During the second trimester, weight gain should average about 1 pound per week, much of it going to the placenta, uterus, and breasts. When the fetus increases its growth in the last trimester, this constant weight gain should continue, even if the mother's appetite and food consumption decrease. Even if a woman is obese, this same pattern and amount of weight gain should be followed to ensure adequate supplies of nutrients and energy for herself and for proper fetal growth.

Despite attention to dietary requirements, several nutrition-related complications of pregnancy may occur. Anemia, which causes fatigue, anorexia, edema, and shortness of breath, can be corrected by appropriate dietary supplementation. Pregnancy-induced hypertension is another complication, most frequently seen in low-income populations known to have poor diet as well as poor medical attention. Although the exact cause and best prevention of pregnancy-induced hypertension is not known, a nutritionally balanced and adequate diet may aid in prevention. Other common but less serious medical concerns of pregnancy include "morning sickness," constipation, and heartburn. In all these conditions, simple diet modifications usually prove effective. Drugs may be prescribed, but the pregnant woman should never attempt casual self-medication. Medications and other substances—including alcoholic beverages and smoking—may have injurious effects on absorption, metabolism, placental transfer, and fetal utilization of nutrients and on the development of the fetus.

Nutrient needs during lactation are similar to those of pregnancy, but with additional caloric requirements. Even in a malnourished woman, the quality of milk is quite good but at the expense of her own meager nutrient stores. Quantity of milk may be limiting. However, a mother who maintains her own good nutrition will help to maximize the quality and quantity of her milk to meet her baby's needs. Iron supplements should be continued after delivery to replenish maternal reserves.

Additional attention to nutritional needs is required during pregnancy and lactation for certain high-risk groups, including very young (teenage) mothers, diabetics, hypertensives, and others with chronic or genetically transmitted disorders.

BIBLIOGRAPHY

ADAMS, S.O., G.D. BARR, and R.L. HUENEMANN. Effect of nutritional supplementation in pregnancy. I. Outcome of pregnancy. *Journal of the American Dietetic Association* 72:144, 1978.

ADAMS, S.O., R.L. HUENEMANN, W.H. BRUVOLD, and G.E. BARR. Effect of nutritional supplementation in pregnancy. II. Effect on diet. *Journal of the American Dietetic Association* 73:630, 1978.

ASHE, J.R., F.A. SCHOFIELD, and M.R. GRAM. The retention of calcium, iron, phosphorus, and magnesium during pregnancy: The adequacy of prenatal diets with and without supplementation. *American Journal of Clinical Nutrition* 32:286, 1979.

ATKINSON, S.A., M.H. BRYAN, and G.H. ANDERSON. Human milk: Difference in nitrogen concentration in milk from mothers of premature infants. *Journal of Pediatrics* 93:67–69, 1978.

ATKINSON, S.A., G.H. ANDERSON and M.H. BRYAN. Human milk: Comparison of the nitrogen composition in milk from mothers of premature and full-term infants. *American Journal of Clinical Nutrition* 33:811–815, 1980.

BAUMAN, D.E., and M.C. NEVILLE. Symposium on nutritional and physiological factors affecting lactation. *Federation Proceedings* 43:2430–2453, 1984.

BURKE, B.S., V.A. BEAL, S.B. KIRKWOOD, and H.C. STUART. The influence of nutrition during pregnancy upon the condition of the infant at birth. *Journal of Nutrition* 25:569, 1943.

BURKE, B.S., B.B. HARDING, and H.C. STUART. Nutrition studies during pregnancy. IV. Relation of protein content of mother's diet during pregnancy to birth length, birth weight, and condition of infant at birth. *Journal of Pediatrics* 23:506, 1943.

CHOPRA, J.G. Effect of steroid contraceptives on lactation. *American Journal of Clinical Nutrition* 25:1202, 1972.

Committee on Maternal Nutrition, Food and Nutrition Board, National Research Council. *Maternal Nutrition and the Course of Pregnancy.* Washington, DC: National Academy of Sciences, 1970.

Committee on Nutrition of the Mother and Preschool child. Food and Nutrition Board, National Research Council. *Laboratory Indices of Nutrition Status in Pregnancy*. Washington, DC: National Academy of Sciences, 1978.

CZAJKA-NARINS, D.M., and E. JUNG. Maternal anthropometric measurements in relation to infant measurements. *Nutrition Research* 6:3, 1986.

DUSDIEKER, L.B., B.M. BOOTH, P.J. STUMBO, and J.M. EICHENBERGER. Effect of supplemental fluids on human milk production. *Journal of Pediatrics* 106:207–211, 1985.

FAIRWEATHER, D.V.I. Nausea and vomiting during pregnancy. In R.M. Wynn ed., *Obstetrics and Gynecology Annual*, New York: Appleton-Century-Crofts, 1978.

FINLEY, D.A., B. LONNERDAL, K.G. DEWEY, and L.D. GRIVETTI. Inorganic constituents of breast milk from vegetarian and nonvegetarian women: relationships with each other and with organic constitutents. *Journal of Nutrition* 115:722–781, 1985.

Food and Nutrition Board, National Research Council. *Recommended Dietary Allowances*, 9th ed. Washington, DC: National Academy of Sciences, 1980. Food and Nutrition Boad, National Research Council. *Alternative dietary practices and nutritional abuses in pregnancy, summary report*. Washington, DC: National Academy of Sciences, 1982.

GROSS, S.J., R.J. DAVID, L. BAUMAN, and R.M. TOMARELLI. Nutritional composition of milk produced by mothers delivering preterm. *Journal of Pediatrics* 96:641–644, 1980.

HANSON, J.W., K.L. JONES, and W.D. SMITH. Fetal alcohol syndrome: Experience with 41 patients. *Journal of the American Medical Association* 235;1458, 1976.

HARRIS, W.S., W.E. CONNER, and S. LINDSEY. Will dietary w-3 fatty acids change the composition of human milk? *American Journal of Clinical Nutrition* 40:780–785, 1984.

HARRISON, R.D., and B.MANTILLA-PLATA. Prenatal toxicity, maternal distribution and placental transfer of tetrahydrocannabinol. *Journal of Pharmacology and Experimental Therapeutics* 180:446, 1972.

HOOK, E.B. Dietary cravings and aversions during pregnancy. *American Journal of Clinical Nutrition* 31:1355, 1978.

KING, J.C., and S. CHARLET. Current concepts in nutrition—Pregnant women and premature infants. *Journal of Nutrition Education* 10(4):158, 1978.

LAMMI-KEEFE, C.J., and R.G. JENSEN. Fat-soluble vitamins in breast milk. *Nutrition Reviews* 42;365–371, 1984.

LECHTIG, A., H. DELGADO, R. LASKY, C. YAR-BROUGH, R.E. KLEIN, J.P. HABICHT, and M. BEHAR. Maternal nutrition and fetal growth in developing countries. *American Journal of Diseases of Childhood* 129:553, 1975.

MCANARNEY, E.R. Adolescent pregnancy—A national priority. *American Journal of Diseases of Children*. 132(2):125, 1978.

MCCLAIN, P.E., J. METCOFF, W.M. CROSBY, and J.P. COSTILOE. Relationship of maternal amino acid profiles at 25 weeks of gestation to fetal growth. *American Journal of Clinical Nutrition* 31:401, 1978.

MARKESTAD, T., L. AKSNES, M. ULSTEIN, and D. AARSKOG. 25-Hydroxyvitamin D and 1, 25-dihydroxyvitamin D of D_2 and D_3 origin in maternal and umbilical cord serum after vitamin D_2 supplementation in human pregnancy. *American Journal of Clinical Nutrition* 40:1057–1063, 1984.

MELLIES, M.J., T.T. ISHIKAWA, P. GARTSIDE, K. BURTON, J. MACGEE, K. ALLEN, P.M. STEINER, D. BRADY, and C.J. CLARK. Effects of varying maternal dietary cholesterol and phytosterol in lactating women and their infants. *American Journal of Clinical Nutrition* 31:1347, 1978.

MORA, J.O., B. DEPAREDES, M. WAGNER, L. DENAVARRO, J. SUESCU, N. CHRISTIANSEN, and M.G. HERRERA. Nutritional supplementation and the outcome of pregnancy. *American Journal of Clinical Nutrition* 32:455, 1979.

NAEYE, R.L., M.M. DIENER, and W.S. DELLINGER. Urban poverty: Effects on prenatal nutrition. *Science* 166:1026, 1969.

NAGY, L.E., and J.C. KING. Energy expenditure of pregnant women at rest or walking self-paced. *American Journal of Clinical Nutrition* 38:369–376, 1983.

OGRA, P.L., and H.L. GREENE. Human milk and breast feeding: An update on the state of the art. *Pediatric Research* 16:266–271, 1982.

OUELLETTE, E.M., H.L. ROSETT, N.P. ROSMAN, and L. WEINER. Adverse effects on offspring of maternal alcohol use during pregnancy. *New England Journal of Medicine* 297(10):528, 1977.

PERSAUD, T.V.N., A.E. CHUDLEY, and R.G. SKALKO. *Basic Concepts In Teratology*. New York: Liss Publishing, 1985.

PIKE, R.L., and D.S. GURSKY. Further evidence of deleterious effects produced by sodium restriction during pregnancy. *American Journal of Clinical Nutrition* 23:883, 1970.

PITKIN, R.M. Nutritional support in obstetrics and gynecology. *Clinical Obstetrics and Gynecology* 19(3):489, 1976.

PLATZKER, A.C.D., C.D. LEW, and D. STEWART. Drug "administration" via breast milk. *Hospital Practice*, September, 1980, pp 111–122.

POTTER, J.M., and P.J. NESTEL. The effects of dietary fatty acids and cholesterol on the milk lipids of lactating women and the plasma cholesterol of breast-fed infants. *American Journal of Clinical Nutrition* 40:1050–1056, 1984.

SALMENPERA, L. Vitamin C nutrition during prolonged lactation: Optimal in infants while marginal in some mothers. *American Journal of Clinical Nutrition* 40:1050–1056, 1984.

SCHEAB, E.B., and M.L. AXELSON. Dietary changes of pregnant women: Compulsions and modifications. *Ecol. Food Nutr.* 14:143–154, 1984.

SINGLETON, N.C., H. LEWIS, and J.J. PARKER. The diet of pregnant teen agers. *Journal of Home Economics* 68:43, 1976.

SPECKER, B.L., R.C. TSANG, and B.W. HOLLIS. Effect of race and diet on human milk vitamin D and 24-hydroxyvitamin D. *American Journal of Diseases of Childhood* 139:1134–1137, 1985.

SUSSER, M. Prenatal nutrition, birthweight and psychological development: An overview of experiments, quasi-experiments, and natural experiments in the past decade. *American Journal of Clinical Nutrition* 34(Supp.4), 784–803, 1981.

Task Force on Nutrition. *Assessment of Maternal Nutrition*. Chicago: American College of Obstetricians and Gynecologists, 1978.

U.S. Department of Health and Human Services. *Breastfeeding and Human Lactation*. DHHS Publ. No. HRS-D-MC 84-2, 1984.

VIR, S.C., A.H.G. LOVE, W. THOMPSON. Riboflavin status during pregnancy. *American Journal of Clinical Nutrition* 34:2699–2705, 1981.

World Health Organization. *Contemporary Patterns of Breastfeeding*. Geneva: 1981.

WORTHINGTON, B.S., H. VERMEERSCH, and S.R. WILLIAMS, eds. *Nutrition in Pregnancy and Lactation*. 2nd ed. St. Louis: C.V. Mosby, 1985.

YOUNG, H.B., A.E. BUCKLEY, B. HAMZA, and C. MANDARANO. Milk and lactation: Some social and developmental correlates among 1,000 infants. *Pediatrics* 69:169–175, 1982.

Chapter 12

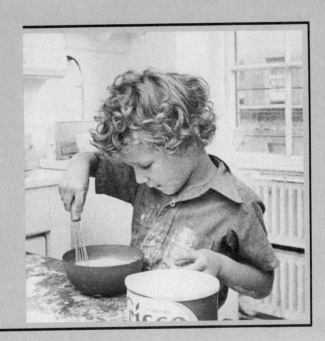

NUTRITION IN THE GROWING YEARS

In its declaration proclaiming 1979 as the International Year of the Child, the United Nations stated as its first principle, "The child must be given the means requisite for its normal development, both materially and spiritually," and as its second, "The child that is hungry must be fed." Developmental patterns established in childhood may influence both health and achievement during all the years that follow. The role of food in growth and development, from infancy (0 to 12 months) through childhood (1 to 12 years) to adolescence (13 to 19 years), is the focus of this chapter.

Growth—the accumulation of tissue—and development—the maturation, regulation, and integration of the systems of the total internal environment—are two separate but closely related processes. Their interrelationship is a complex blend of genetics and environment. Only with proper support from the external environment—food, shelter, nurturing—can the body's internal physiological program unfold in the orderly manner predetermined by the genes.

For the fetus, whose external environment is limited to the confines of the mother's uterus, growth and development depend largely on the nutrient supply available from the mother. At birth the interplay between external and internal environments becomes more complex, as the infant's external world suddenly expands. Food now begins to function not only as raw material for physiological growth and development but also as a stimulus for the sociocultural development that is equally vital to human functioning.

INFANT NUTRITION (0 TO 12 MONTHS)

The growth processes begun during gestation continue at a rapid rate in the first year of life. The most obvious indication of this rapid growth is weight gain. By age four or five months, birth weight is doubled; by about fourteen months it is tripled. With respect to this rapidity of growth, infancy is an extension of prenatal life. But in other respects, it is quite different. The newborn can no longer depend on its mother's body for oxygen, temperature control, and the removal of waste products. As a free-living being, it must learn to adapt to changes in the external environment. The mother plays a strong role in this adaptation, providing warmth, protection, cuddling, and most important to physical survival, food.

Probably no aspect of postnatal care has been scrutinized more closely than food and infant feeding practices. Current opinions on breast- versus bottle-feeding, when to introduce solid foods, desirable weight gain during infancy, and many other nutritional issues are based as much on changing social values, environmental issues, and economic conditions as on scientific knowledge. Each of these will be examined from the perspective of the healthy newborn, one for whom the outcome of pregnancy was normal birth weight and normal medical status.

Growth and Development

Growth is an increase in total cell number (hyperplasia), in cell size (hypertrophy), or in both. The rate and timing of each of these processes is controlled by heredity, hormonal action, and environmental impact. All these interact to produce identifiable patterns of growth.

PATTERNS OF GROWTH.   Growth in body length is most rapid in the early months. Using birth length as a reference, the infant's length increases 20 percent by three months of age, 50 percent by one year, and 75 percent by two years. Somewhere around age two, the child reaches 50 percent of average adult male height. If growth continued at this rapid rate, kindergarten children would be of adult size. Instead, the growth rate decreases steadily throughout the early years, reaching a plateau at age five that will last until the growth spurt of adolescence.

Changes in body composition and differential growth patterns of various body tissues are also apparent during these years. The proportion of body fat, which accounts for only about 12 percent of body weight at birth, doubles by one year of age. Body water decreases from 75 percent of body weight at birth to about 60 percent at age one year.

Brain growth is also most rapid in the early months; by one year brain growth is about 70 percent complete. Nutritional deprivation during this critical period is associated with decreased head circumference, brain weight, and brain protein content, factors that may impair intellectual functioning throughout later life. The relationship is uncertain, however, because people who are severely malnourished in early life are often also subjected to many other unfavorable conditions, such as lack of educational opportunities.

Growth phases of various body parts create the characteristic body proportions identified with infancy, childhood, and adolescence. Relative head size decreases during the infant's first year, when growth occurs mainly in the trunk (spinal column). By age 12 months, the trunk has reached approximately 60 percent of its final adult size. From then until adolescence, leg growth makes the most impressive gains, creating the typical appearance of the gangly preteenager. Trunk length increases during the adolescent growth spurt, thus balancing body proportions.

ASSESSMENT OF GROWTH.   Growth during infancy is so rapid that most mothers don't need a scale to tell them that the baby is thriving. Nevertheless, periodic measurement of weight, height, and head circumference is recommended to ensure that an infant's growth is following a normal progression. The National Center for Health Statistics has developed growth charts for infants and children that take into account the wide variability in physical growth of children of differing genetic, ethnic, and socioeconomic populations. These NCHS measures have replaced earlier standards that did not reflect the wide diversity of the contemporary U.S. population.

Figures 12–1 and 12–2 show the NCHS percentile measures for length and weight of male and female infants from birth to 36 months. Using these charts, a pediatrician can plot the appropriate values for each measure periodically, at the time of every checkup. Measurements between the 25th and 75th percentiles are generally interpreted as normal. More important, however, is consistency of development within a narrower percentile range. An infant who had been in the 95th percentile for both length and weight in the first three months of life might be suspected of having health problems if at six months weight was in the 70th percentile and length was still in the higher percentile.

The typical well-baby examination should include length and weight measurements, a thorough clinical examination, a review of the infant's skin tone and general appearance, a discussion of what the infant is presently eating and, if appropriate, advice for feeding during the next period. Measurements of head circumference are sometimes taken, and the National Center for Health Statistics provides a standardized graph of these as well. Generally, growth charts are best

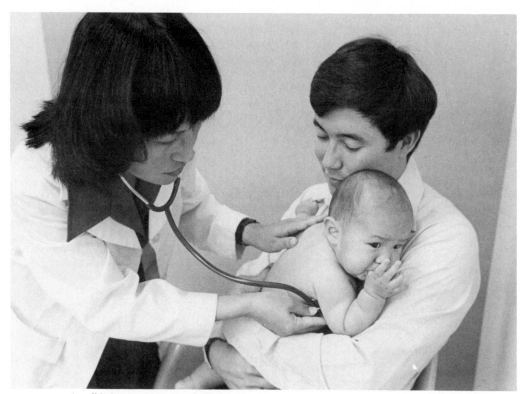

A well-baby examination includes length and weight measurements along with a thorough clinical examination.

Elizabeth Crews/Stock, Boston

used for screening, not as diagnostic tools. Although in most cases they provide reassurance that the child is growing normally, they are also helpful in identifying children whose rate of maturation is abnormal, perhaps as a result of under- or overnutrition.

Because of the high incidence of iron deficiency anemia in infants, iron status should be routinely checked by means of hematocrit and hemoglobin tests at one year of age. Monitoring of serum cholesterol has also been recommended for early identification of children who may be predisposed to elevated serum cholesterol concentrations. Because of studies suggesting that low-cholesterol diets can reduce serum levels even in very young children and possibly prevent later vascular and coronary problems, early identification of children at risk may be important.

Nutrient Requirements

While food is widely accepted as the most important determinant of infant growth and development, there is little consensus about the kinds and amount of food that are optimal. Precise information on actual need is available only for a few nutrients and very little is actually known about the needs for others. In estimating recommended levels for the first year of life, the Food and Nutrition Board relied on the traditional view that breast milk from well-nourished women is the biologically

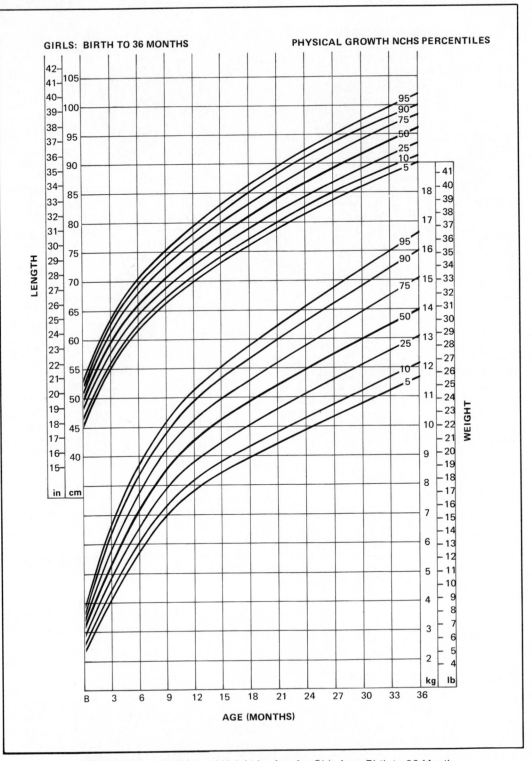

FIGURE 12-1 *Weight and Height by Age for Girls from Birth to 36 Months.*

Source: Adapted from National Center for Health Statistics, *NCHS growth charts, 1976*, Monthly Vital Statistics Report, Vol. 25, No. 3 Supp. (HRA) 7S-1120 (Rockville, Maryland: Health Resources Administration, June, 1976). Data from the Fels Research Institute, Yellow Springs, Ohio. © 1976 Ross Laboratories.

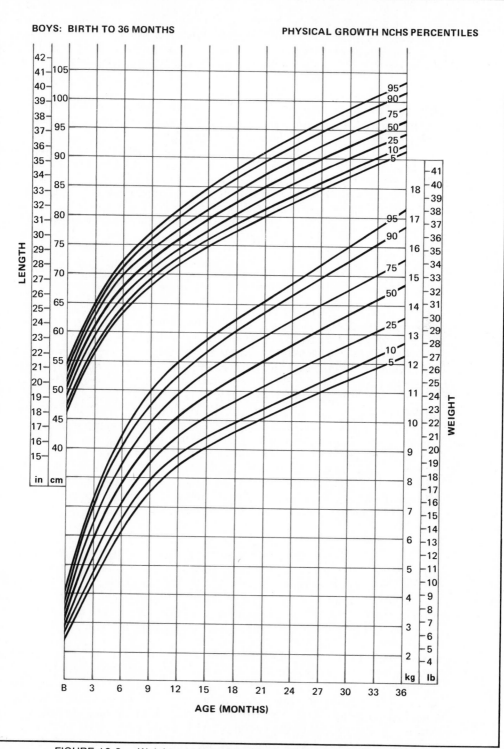

FIGURE 12-2   *Weight and Height by Age for Boys from Birth to 36 Months.*

Source: Adapted from National Center for Health Statistics, *NCHS growth charts, 1976*, Monthly Vital Statistics Report, Vol. 25, No. 3, Supp. (HRA) 76-1120 (Rockville, Maryland: Health Resources Administration, June 1976). Data from the Fels Research Institute, Yellow Springs, Ohio. © 1976 Ross Laboratories.

correct standard for infant nourishment. Infant RDAs assume that human milk supplies protein, energy, minerals, vitamins, and fluid in the amounts and proportions best suited for optimal development and that prepared formulas and food supplements should come as close as possible to duplicating these nutrient proportions.

ENERGY. Breast milk provides approximately 7 percent of kilocalories from protein, 55 percent from fat, and 38 percent from carbohydrate. Most commercially prepared formulas closely match these figures.

Because infants have a high rate of heat loss due to their relatively large body surface area, their energy requirements for basal metabolism are quite high, approximating 55 kcal/kg. Another 35 kcal/kg is required for growth and 10 to 25 kcal/kg for activity, yielding a total daily energy requirement of 115 kcal/kg (48 kcal/lb) during the first six months of life. When this figure is compared with the 35 kcal/kg recommended for adults, the high metabolic needs of infants become apparent. During the first few months of life, all energy intake can be provided by human milk or formula. In the second six months of life, the energy requirement as a function of body weight gradually decreases to approximately 105 kcal/kg, and solid food supplies an increasing proportion.

PROTEIN. The protein required for rapid muscular and skeletal growth accounts for the recommendations of 2.2 g/kg body weight for the first six months of life, and 2.0 g/kg during the second half of the first year. This compares with 0.8 g/kg recommended for adults. To facilitate comparisons between individual nutrients and prepared formulas, nutrient allowances for infants are sometimes expressed in terms of energy intake, rather than per unit of body weight. Human milk provides about 1.5 grams of protein for every 100 kilocalories and is adequate for full-term infants. Formulas should contain a minimum of 1.8 grams of protein per 100 kilocalories. (This figure assumes that the proteins in prepared formulas provide the essential amino acids required for protein synthesis.)

Protein intakes of less than 6 percent of energy intakes are considered inadequate for optimal brain growth and general development. Excessive protein intakes (levels higher than 16 percent of energy intakes) should be avoided as well, because this quantity may overwhelm the ability of the infant's kidneys to excrete the excess nitrogen; it is in any case an inefficient and expensive way of providing energy.

FAT. Fat is a significant source of energy in an infant's diet; it is a vehicle for essential fatty acids and the fat-soluble vitamins and contributes to the feeling of satiety through which the infant regulates appetite. There is no RDA for fat, but the Food and Nutrition Board recommends that at least 15 percent of kilocalories be supplied by easily digested fats, with 4 to 5 percent of total energy intake provided in the form of linoleic acid, an essential fatty acid which is a precursor of prostaglandins (regulatory substances found throughout the body).

CARBOHYDRATES. Carbohydrate provides the remainder of energy intake, accounting for 35 to 65 percent of total kilocalories. Lactose, the natural sugar in both human and cow's milk, facilitates calcium absorption and is a source of galactose. Galactose is a component of myelin in nerve fibers and of connective tissue, cartilage, and bone. Other carbohydrates (glucose, sucrose, fructose) may be used in infant formulas, and galactose is then synthesized from glucose in the liver.

Vitamins and minerals. RDAs for vitamins and minerals are listed in Table 12-1. Concentrations of water soluble vitamins are higher in the blood of the neonate than in the mother; vitamins A and E and beta-carotene are lower. Human milk from an adequately-fed mother or commercially prepared formulas will supply all the needed vitamins and minerals for the infant, with the exception of fluoride and iron. Breast-fed infants, those who consume ready-to-feed formula made with non-fluoridated water, and those whose formulas are prepared at home with non-fluoridated water should receive supplemental fluoride. Iron needs increase at about 4 to 5 months of age when fetal stores run out. Iron-enriched infant cereals provide bioavailable iron to meet the needs of the infant.

Fluid. The infant's high metabolic rate leads to the production of significant quantities of metabolic wastes, such as urea, which require water for excretion. During the first year of life, an infant needs about 120 to 160 ml/kg of fluid each

TABLE 12-1. RDAs for Infants

Nutrient	0–6 mo.	6–12 mo.
Energy, kcal/kg.	115	105
Protein, g/kg	2.2	2.0
Fat	—	—
Vitamin A, RE	420	400
Vitamin D, μg	10	10
Vitamin E, mg αT.E.[b]	3	4
Vitamin K, μg	12	10–20
Vitamin C, mg	35	35
Folacin, μg	30	45
Niacin, mg	6	8
Riboflavin, mg	0.4	0.6
Thiamin, mg	0.3	0.5
Vitamin B_6, mg	0.3	0.6
Vitamin B_{12}, μg	0.5	1.5
Biotin, μg[c]	35	50
Choline	—	—
Inositol	—	—
Calcium, mg	360	540
Phosphorus, mg	240	360
Iodine, μg	40	50
Iron, mg	10	15
Magnesium, mg	50	70
Zinc, mg	3	5
Copper, mg[c]	0.5–0.7	0.7–1.0
Manganese, mg[c]	0.5–0.7	0.7–1.0
Sodium, mg[c]	115–350	250–750
Potassium, mg[c]	350–925	425–1275
Chloride, mg[c]	275–700	400–1200

Source: Food and Nutrition Board, National Academy of Sciences, Recommended daily dietary allowances, revised 1979 (Washington, D.C.: National Research Council, 1979).
[b] Formulas containing vegetable oils should contain 0.7 IU of vitamin E/g linoleic acid.
[c] Estimated safe and adequate daily dietary intakes, Food and Nutrition Board, 1979.

day. The amount of human or cow's milk needed to supply an infant's recommended daily nutrient and energy intake would also supply 150 to 200 ml/kg of fluid, which is more than sufficient except when fluid losses are very high, as when vomiting or diarrhea occur or when sweating is profuse, as during hot weather.

FEEDING PRACTICES

For obvious ethical reasons, the nursery rarely serves as a laboratory. Thus, relatively few data exist to support one feeding practice over another, although observations throughout the years have resulted in a more informed basis for particular recommendations. Perhaps the central issue has been the relative benefits of human versus formula feeding, an area colored by culture and technology.

Traditionally, infant nutrition was considered to be solely the mother's concern. In certain societies, however, nursing an infant was considered inappropriate for women of upper socioeconomic classes. Also, some women could not supply human milk for their babies because of illness or death. In these situations, another woman could be hired as a wet nurse, but the outcome was often uncertain. Many wet nurses came from low socioeconomic backgrounds and carried diseases, which they transmitted to the nursing infants. Similarly uncertain results were associated with feeding milk from cows, goats, or donkeys. Occasionally broths were tried. In all such cases, prognosis for the infant was quite poor.

Thus, it is not surprising that until the beginning of the twentieth century, almost all women nursed their infants. By that time, the rudimentary chemical analyses of human milk (first attempted in the mid-1800s) had become sophisticated enough to permit production of synthetic formulas for infant feeding. These new products had obvious appeal to better-educated women, who were not hard to convince that formula feeding represented a modern, scientific advance over the primitive human breast. Bottle-feeding, like other fashions, was widely written about in magazines and rapidly adopted by women throughout the country.

Breast-Feeding

The past two decades have seen a reversal, with better-educated women leading the way back to breast-feeding on the basis of its being more "natural" and because of scientific support for its greater nutritional and health-promoting value. But in today's world, there are definite impediments to wide acceptance of breast-feeding. For one thing, this natural practice is embarrassing to many segments of the population. In a commentary on breast-feeding, the American Academy of Pediatrics remarked on the curious contradiction of a society that tolerates all degrees of sexual explicitness in movies, books, and other media but continues to relegate the normal act of breast-feeding to the privacy of closed doors and drawn shades.

NUTRITIONAL CONSIDERATIONS. Human milk was designed for consumption by human infants, and under normal conditions it is best suited to their nutritional needs. Most commercially available formulas simulate mother's milk by modifying the cow's milk on which they are based. Cow's milk differs in a number of ways from human milk, particularly in the amount and relative concentrations of the various proteins and in the bioavailability of minerals (see Table 12–2).

TABLE 12-2. *Average Composition of Mature Human Milk and Whole Cow's Milk (nutrients and energy content per liter)*

	Mature Human Milk	Whole Cow's Milk
Water, ml	910	906
Energy, kcal (kJ)	690	660
Carbohydrate, g	68	49
Protein, g	9	35
Lipid, g	40	38
Calcium, mg	241	340
Chloride, mg	400	103
Magnesium, mg	38	41
Phosphorus, mg	150	96
Potassium, mg	530	156
Sodium, mg	160	50
Copper, μg	60	30
Iron, mg	0.56	0.3
Zinc, mg	4	0.5
Ascorbic acid, μg	44	0.97
Thiamin, μg	150	0.04
Riboflavin, μg	380	0.17
Niacin, mg	1.7	0.09
Pyridoxine μg	130	0.04
Folacin, μg	41	84.6
Vitamin B_{12}, μg	0.5	0.37
Vitamin A, (IU)	1898	32(130)

Source: Adapted from P. L. Pipes, *Nutrition in Infancy and Childhood*, (St. Louis, MO: C.V. Mosby, 1985) pp. 90–91.

ENERGY AND CARBOHYDRATE CONTENT.   Lactose concentration of human milk may be important in controlling the volume of milk produced. Cow's milk and human milk have approximately the same energy content, about 70 kilocalories per 100 milliliters. However, this energy level is achieved with different proportions of its components, with more carbohydrate (lactose) in human milk and more protein in cow's milk.

PROTEIN.   Human milk provides approximately 0.9 gm protein per 100 ml; cow's milk, 3.5 gm per 100 ml. Approximately 25 percent of the total nitrogen in human milk is nonprotein nitrogen. Therefore, if protein is calculated from nitrogen, values are a little higher. Qualitative differences exist as well. Sixty percent of the protein in human milk is whey (lactalbumin); the rest is casein. In cow's milk, the distribution is 18 and 82 percent, respectively. Digestibility of milk protein is affected by this ratio; milk protein containing large amounts of casein forms a tough, hard-to-digest curd after exposure to hydrochloric acid in the stomach. The amino acid contents of the two milks also differ; cow's milk contains a higher methionine:cystine ratio. This appears to be significant in the feeding of premature infants, who may be less able to metabolize methionine. Human milk, particularly colostrum the early milk, contains enzymes and immunological proteins that are important to the infant.

FAT.   Although the lipid content of human and cow's milk is similar, human milk lipids are better absorbed, with about 95 percent of the fat in human milk retained, compared to only 61 percent of the fat from cow's milk. Human milk contains more unsaturated fatty acids; in addition, palmitate is found primarily in the 2-position of the glycerol molecule, which favors the absorption of monoglycerides. The replacement of butterfat with vegetable oils has significantly improved lipid absorption from commercial formulas and also decreased their cholesterol and saturated fatty acid content.

Controversy exists over whether this reduction in cholesterol is indeed advantageous. Some studies indicate that dietary cholesterol may be important to nerve tissue formation and bile salt synthesis in the infant. Studies of laboratory animals show that ingestion of cholesterol by newborns may increase production of enzymes that more efficiently metabolize cholesterol, subsequently contributing to lowered serum levels. Additional research is needed to evaluate the effects of manipulating dietary cholesterol during the neonatal period on serum cholesterol levels in later life.

TRACE MINERALS AND VITAMINS.   Recent research has focused on the micronutrient content of breast milk. Trace minerals and vitamins appear in variable amounts in human milk, a reflection at least in part of maternal intakes. Concentrations of water-soluble vitamins are more likely to reflect maternal intake. Maternal supplementation has been shown to result in increased concentrations in the milk. The amount of biologically active vitamin D and vitamin K is low while concentrations of vitamins A and E are adequate.

Human milk has lower concentrations of some of the major minerals than cow's milk, but has adequate amounts to meet the needs of the developing infant. The total mineral content of human milk is fairly constant, although there is a general trend for some minerals to decrease in the course of lactation. As knowledge of the vitamin and trace mineral content of breast milk increases, it will facilitate the estimation of requirements for these micronutrients and the addition of appropriate amounts to commercial formulas. New information about the interrelationships and bioavailability of trace minerals, with applications to nutritional science in general, will also be derived from increased understanding of the components of breast milk.

Both human and cow's milk have similar, but low, iron content. However, data suggest that the iron in human milk is better absorbed than the iron in pasteurized cow's milk. In the first three months of life, absorption may exceed 50 percent in contrast to only 10 percent absorption from cow's milk, and 4 percent from iron-fortified formula. Zinc is also more bioavailable from human milk than from cow's milk.

How long human milk meets the daily iron requirements of exclusively breast-fed, full-term infants is a matter of debate. Infants are being breast-fed for longer periods of time and the effect of solid foods on iron absorption is not clear. Therefore, iron supplements are routinely prescribed for almost all infants, unless they are fed an iron-fortified formula.

IMMUNOLOGICAL PROPERTIES.   Human milk helps protect newborns from infectious disease. Two iron-containing proteins found in breast milk, lactoferrin and transferrin, have antibacterial properties. Cow's milk contains a much smaller amount of lactoferrin, and its antibacterial effect is destroyed during processing. The presence of these agents may be one of the reasons for the immunological properties that have been attributed to breast milk. Unlike cow's milk formulas, breast milk also contains leukocytes, antibody-secreting cells, and antibodies to some intestinal microorganisms. Recent research has focused on defining the mechanisms that might explain the clinical observation that breast-fed infants, especially in developing countries, suffer from fewer infections and allergies than bottle-fed infants.

OTHER CONSIDERATIONS.   Breast milk has a lower concentration of electrolytes than cow's milk, and the low solute load is apparently better suited to the immature kidney function of human infants. The higher sodium concentration of cow's milk can strain the capacity of the infant's kidneys to excrete sodium, resulting in hypernatremia (excess sodium in the blood).

Economic and psychological factors are often cited as advantages of breast-feeding. Breast-feeding is less expensive than formula-feeding. The cost of any prepared formula for infant feeding generally exceeds the cost of human milk, and those costs increase with the conveniences built into the manufacturer's package. Formula prepared at home from evaporated milk, corn syrup, and water is less expensive than formula but does not meet recommendations for vitamin C and iron. The psychological value of breast-feeding is not easy to measure quantitatively. There is no experimental evidence to substantiate differences in psychological or physical development in infants related to their mode of feeding. Warmth, contact, and gentleness can be achieved with bottle-feeding as much as with breast-feeding.

Under some circumstances women should not breast-feed their infants. Infectious diseases such as active pulmonary tuberculosis, which might be transmitted to the infant, are a contraindication to breast-feeding. Other chronic diseases, however, including heart disease, diabetes, hepatitis, and nephrosis, do not automatically rule out breast-feeding, particularly if the mother has been under medical control during a successful pregnancy. However, conditions that are being treated with anticoagulants, certain antibiotics, thyroid gland suppressants, radioactive compounds, anticancer drugs, and even large quantities of aspirin make nursing unwise, since these drugs are likely to appear in the breast milk in harmful quantities. Combined estrogen-progesterone contraceptive pills do not inhibit lactation as long as they are not used in the immediate post-partum period.

Indiscriminate drug use is definitely not advised for nursing mothers. The high morbidity and mortality of babies born to narcotic-addicted mothers is related both to withdrawal symptoms and to frequent prematurity, respiratory distress, and generally poor pre- and postnatal care. Although nursing was once recommended as the best way of treating withdrawal symptoms in addicted infants, many addicts use more than one substance that might appear in the milk, further damaging the newborn. Tobacco and alcohol abuse, in particular, have been shown to complicate problems in such infants. In normal infants born to nonaddicted mothers, however, moderate maternal use of alcohol and nicotine (cigarettes) has not proved to be a reason for avoiding breast-feeding.

Unintentional exposure to environmental pollutants has caused concern for nursing mothers. Several incidents have been reported in which polychorinated biphenyls (PCBs), inhaled in industrial settings or consumed with contaminated cooking oil or other foods, were stored in maternal adipose tissue and later excreted in the fat of breast milk. Fortunately these incidents are rare, and there appear to be no significant effects of this exposure in breast-fed infants. Some pediatricians recommend that the milk of women who may have been exposed to this pollutant be monitored to determine PCB levels.

Bottle-Feeding

Most commercially prepared formulas contain cow's milk modified in several ways to make it more suitable for human infants. Protein and solute contents are reduced; carbohydrate levels are increased with the addition of sucrose, lactose, or oligosaccharides; vegetable oils are substituted for butter fat; and vitamins and minerals are added. The energy density of the finished product is about 670 kilocalories per liter (20 kcal/oz). This scientifically formulated mixture is then evaporated and canned or dried, to be reconstituted at home. It is important that instructions for dilution be followed precisely. To meet the needs of modern mobility, formulas are now available in ready-to-feed bottles; only a sterile nipple cap need be attached.

Home-prepared formula can also be made from a base of canned evaporated (not sweetened condensed) milk, to which boiled (sterile) water and corn syrup are added; proportions should be recommended by a pediatrician.

Simulated formulas are available and especially important in the management of infants with digestive defects or allergies.

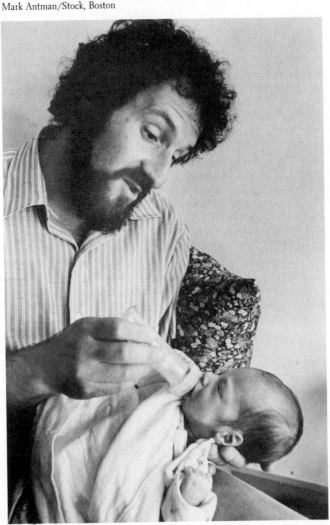

Commercial formulas have also been developed for babies with special problems such as metabolic disorders, allergy to cow's milk protein, or lactose intolerance. Some of these special formulas are made with soy protein. Simulated formulas are important in the management of infants and children with inherited digestive defects and allergies; they are also used by parents who want their formula-fed babies to follow a vegetarian diet.

Current Recommendations

Although it is generally agreed that nutritional adequacy can be attained with either breast- or formula-feeding, the American Academy of Pediatrics and many nutritionists still conclude that breast is best. Ideally, breast milk should be the major source of nutrients for the first five to six months of an infant's life to ensure proper growth and development. Human milk is assumed to be best able to meet the needs of the human species and that most nursing mothers produce it in the quantity required by the infant.

There is no way to tell if a baby at the breast has taken 3 ounces, 6 ounces, or more. But this is an advantage, not a disadvantage. There is no evidence that 8 fluid ounces (standard bottle size) at every feeding is the ideal amount for every infant. Many mothers typically persist in presenting a bottle until it is emptied, although the baby might not actually need that much. Mother's who bottle feed should allow the infant to gauge its own intake. Most infants regulate quite well. However, even a few breast-fed infants will overeat if given the opportunity. One group of women was asked to increase their milk supply by pumping their breasts after her infant had fed. A few infants responded to the increased supply by increasing their intake while most still only took what they needed. These data suggest that some young infants do not regulate their intake in response to caloric need as well as others.

An infant's requirement for milk changes with age, growth, and intake of other foods. When milk provides the only source of energy and nutrients, average daily needs increase from 18 ounces before one month of age to 21 ounces from one to two months, 24 ounces from two to three months, and 30 ounces from three to six months. It then decreases to 28 ounces from six to nine months when other sources of nourishment are added to the infant diet. Breast-fed babies can easily make these adjustments: It is less likely that bottle-feeding mothers will permit their baby's changing appetite to be the sole guide of how much formula is consumed.

Almost every woman who wants to nurse is physiologically and psychologically able to produce sufficient milk to satisfy the nutritional needs of her newborn infant. Women do require instruction and encouragement in learning how to breast-feed and, as breast-feeding is becoming more popular, health professionals and self-help groups are doing much to dispel mistaken ideas that small-breasted, nervous, or working mothers should not attempt to breast-feed. Breast-feeding a premature infant is possible and should be decided in individual situations.

Vitamin and Mineral Supplementation

Nutritionists believe that breast milk and modern commercial formulas come quite close to meeting all the nutrient requirements of infancy. Nevertheless, almost every new mother carrying home her tiny infant also carries a small bottle of vitamin drops. Most pediatricians recommend these vitamin preparations and most mothers use them, not because they have been proved necessary, but because they have not yet been proved unnecessary.

SUPPLEMENTS FOR BREAST-FED INFANTS. For the first three months of life, breast milk contains adequate amounts of all nutrients except fluorine and vitamin D. Some research suggested that breast milk supplied sufficient quantities of vitamin D in a water-soluble form. More recent data question the biological importance of this form. Nursing infants should receive vitamin D supplements (10 μg daily), especially if they are not regularly exposed to sunlight. Fluoride must be provided as well, even when the mother is drinking from a fluoridated water supply, because this mineral is inadequately transferred to her milk. Although breast milk provides only a small amount of iron, 50 percent—a relatively high proportion—is absorbed; in combination with stores of the mineral laid down in fetal life, this should be sufficient up to three or four months of age. However, some pediatricians recommend a daily supplement, preferably in the form of ferrous sulfate. Other supplements should be considered if the mother's diet is poor or unbalanced. Infants nursed by strict vegetarian mothers may be at risk of vitamin B_{12} deficiency and should receive supplementation.

SUPPLEMENTS FOR BOTTLE-FED INFANTS. Most commercial formulas contain nutrients needed by the infant, including iron, zinc, vitamin C, and vitamin D. For this reason, mothers who feed formula must be cautioned *against* additional supplements. Of course, if the particular baby has special needs, then the pediatrician may prescribe supplementation.

The fluoride content of formulas reflects the water supply used to prepare or dilute the product. Commercial formulas are prepared with nonfluoridated water, therefore bottle-fed infants should be given fluoride supplementation.

Most commercial formulas contain ascorbic acid in amounts sufficient to withstand heat processing. However, if evaporated milk formula is being prepared in the home, vitamin C supplements should be given. Because young babies are sometimes allergic to orange juice, it is not usually introduced for several months, and then in dilute form and small amounts. For this reason, supplemental ascorbic acid is generally given until orange juice has been added to the diet in sufficient quantity. All the juices processed specifically for infants are fortified with ascorbic acid or have naturally high concentrations of ascorbic acid and any of these (apple juice, cherry juice mixtures, and others) can therefore be used as a source of vitamin C.

Solid Foods

As the popularity of breast-feeding has waxed and waned, so too has the accepted wisdom concerning when to introduce solid foods.

TIMING. An infant requires solid foods when milk or formula can no longer provide the nutrients and energy necessary for optimal growth and development. A century ago, it was customary to wait until the second year of life to wean a baby from breast to solids. By the 1960s the pendulum had swung to the other extreme, and infants were commonly receiving cereal at 2 to 3 days of age and meat and vegetable combinations at 17 days. Among factors responsible for this shift were the increasing availability of commercially prepared infant foods and the popular belief that early introduction of solid foods was related somehow to better and earlier maturation and development. Most recently, solids (sometimes called *beikost*) are being introduced between 4 and 6 months of age. This timing is now considered best both from a developmental point of view and on the basis of physiological and nutritional needs.

DEVELOPMENT. Babies are not able to initiate voluntary swallowing movements until they are about 16 weeks of age. Earlier than that, swallowing is merely the final component of the sucking reflex. Thus, any solid foods introduced before that time will automatically be pushed out of the baby's mouth. This is known as the extrusion reflex. Also, in the earliest months the infant has little ability to communicate feelings about eating. Sometime during the fourth month, however, the infant becomes able not only to draw in its upper lip to keep foods inside the mouth but also to lean forward to express eagerness to eat or turn aside to signal that "enough is enough." Nutritionists believe that earlier introduction of solids runs counter to developmental patterns and may lead to overfeeding of an infant who cannot handle, but also cannot refuse, what is put into its mouth.

Physiological correlates of these developmental signs generally support this timing. The enzymes necessary for digesting complex carbohydrates are not present until the second or third month of age, and kidneys do not function efficiently until the end of the second month. The best way to tell when a baby is ready for the introduction of solid foods is to pay attention to signals given by the baby. The first appearance of drooling indicates increased salivary production. The appearance of new facial expressions, especially in the mouth area, indicates maturation of oral musculature. The most significant sign of a baby's readiness for new foods is hunger; when the baby takes 26 to 30 ounces of milk from the bottle in 24 hours, nurses voraciously and tries to get more after each feeding, or seems hungry after shorter intervals, an alert parent might sense that the time is right to introduce solid foods.

When solid foods are offered before the baby is ready to accept them, a negative pattern of interaction between infant and parent may be established, with negative ramifications for the acceptance of food at a later date. Many parents attempt to add solids in the early months in the belief that hunger is preventing the baby from sleeping through the night. But the ability to sleep for longer periods is developmentally independent of the need for sources of food in addition to milk.

Some parents go to the other extreme and delay the introduction of solid foods past the age of six months in the belief that milk is the only food a baby needs. This practice tends to be associated with breast-feeding. But because of the growing appetite of the older baby, the excessive amounts of milk consumed will prevent development of an appetite for foods that are better sources of nutrients, such as iron, needed by the middle of the first year. Also, the breast-fed infant needs some protein-rich foods by this age.

CHOOSING SOLID FOODS. A wide variety of prepared foods is waiting to tempt a baby's appetite—iron-fortified cereals in dry form to be mixed with formula or milk; jars of egg yolks, meats, strained vegetables, meat-and-vegetable combinations, fruit-and-cereal combinations, cottage cheese, puddings, and more. Generally, cooked cereal is the recommended first food. Its advantage is that it can be mixed with formula or milk to any desired consistency; typically 1 teaspoon of dried cereal mixed with 1 tablespoon of fluid should be offered by spoon before giving bottle or breast to a hungry baby.

A baby will usually look surprised at this new event, but parents should not interpret a baby's puzzled reaction as a negative response. If the first feeding of cereal is not readily accepted—and often it is not—they should try again the next day and the next, always when the baby is hungry. Soon the cereal will be received eagerly; very few mothers report problems, physiological or otherwise, with acceptance of cereals. After a while, less milk can be used in proportion to dry cereal.

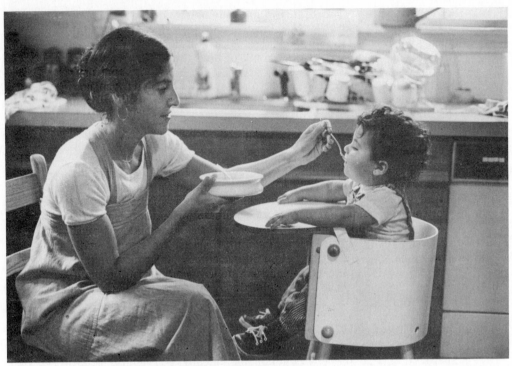

An infant requires solid foods when milk or formula can no longer provide the nutrients and energy necessary for optimal growth and development.

Stock, Boston

Once a baby has acquired the knack of eating, other foods can be tried. Usually, fruit purees are added next, then strained vegetables, vegetable-and-meat combinations, egg yolks, and strained meats.

Newborns apparently do not have a preference for the taste of salt. Despite this, salt and monosodium glutamate were routinely added in the past to commercial infant foods, probably to appeal to the tastes of parents.

Later, oversweetening was frowned on as well. Many baby fruits and desserts today are prepared with only enough sugar to counteract the natural tartness of the fruit. New formulations of baby foods do contain some additives that were not present in earlier years, such as ascorbic acid in applesauce and other fruits to prevent darkening of the fruit. Modified starch is also added to some items to improve their texture. The USDA publishes a handbook that reflects some of these changes in the composition of baby foods.

Some parents prefer to prepare their own baby foods. This practice is acceptable if sanitary conditions are maintained for all utensils and equipment. Wooden cutting boards should not be used; only fresh and unblemished produce should be purchased; leftovers should be refrigerated or frozen promptly. Homemade baby food should be prepared for the infant before salt is added; sugar should be used sparingly. Honey should not be used in food prepared for infants under one year of age.

Whenever possible the baby should be fed at the same time as, and in the same room with, the other members of the family. Eating is a social experience, and the pleasure of family intimacy at mealtime enhances appetite and establishes a wholesome pattern for the future. In this setting the infant learns to welcome both new foods and new social relationships. In the second half of the first year, some finger foods can be added—a crust of bread, pieces of chicken meat, boneless fish, carrot sticks, cubes of boiled potato. The baby should be encouraged to explore new tastes, and textures, even at the risk of some messiness. The goal is a child who enjoys food.

Special Concerns in Infant Feeding

Not all feeding problems are of social origin. A baby who refuses foods or appears uncomfortable after eating may be suffering from a physiological problem. In very young infants, bloating, abdominal pains, and similar symptoms are often interpreted as signs of lactose malabsorption. Studies indicate that true lactose malabsorption is quite rare in infancy even in ethnic groups previously thought to have hereditary lactase deficiency. Food allergies, however, are not so rare and can produce similar symptoms.

ALLERGIES. Milk allergy often causes an allergic reaction in infants, largely because milk is their primary food. There may be sensitivity not to lactose but to one of the three milk proteins: lactalbumin, lactoglobulin, and casein. Lactalbumin is the most frequent culprit. When solid foods are introduced—especially egg, wheat, citrus fruit, and fish—susceptible infants may have allergic reactions. The best treatment is to avoid the offending foods. Only one new food should be introduced at a time; if there is any reaction, it will be easy to identify the cause. In a family with a history of allergies, new foods should be introduced especially slowly and with caution. Rice and oats are less allergic than wheat and so are advisable choices as the first solid food for babies. Banana, either mashed or in dry form mixed with a little formula, is also a good early food.

LOW AND HIGH BIRTH WEIGHT INFANTS. The basal metabolic rate of infants with low birth weight is lower than that of full-term infants during the first week of life, but it reaches and exceeds the full-term's level by the second week. Thus, daily energy requirements in proportion to body weight are higher for infants with low birth weight. At the same time their stomachs are smaller than normal for their age

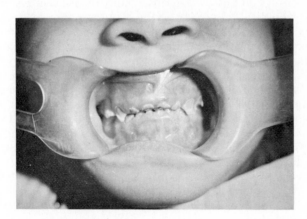

With the lips held back by a plastic device, the damage of "nursing bottle syndrome" can be clearly seen. Characteristically, there is extensive damage to the upper front teeth while the lower front teeth are unaffected.

Dr. Marvin H. Berman

and can hold less food at a time. They should receive more frequent feedings (every three hours or more often) to meet their high energy needs, and they may need more concentrated formulas to supply their energy and protein requirements.

At the other end of the scale, infants with high birth weight or those who gain excess weight in early infancy may also require nutritional monitoring. All infants put down a great deal of fat in the first year making identification of those who will become fat children difficult. The type of milk fed to infants and the early or late introduction of solid foods may not be significant factors in overweight in childhood.

VEGETARIANISM. Infants nursed by strict vegetarian mothers may have special problems. Concerns for iron and vitamin B_{12} status should not be taken lightly. Severe deficiencies have been reported, but generally can be prevented with good maternal counseling. Reports of profound protein-energy malnutrition have come from vegetarian communities where breast-fed infants were weaned early and fed an extremely low-energy diet, such as home-prepared soya milk with no foods of animal origin and no vitamin supplementation. Retarded physical development, anemia, rickets, osteoporosis, and other severe deficiency symptoms have resulted.

Nutritional Status of American Infants

Few studies have been broad-based enough to provide adequate data for an accurate, overall appraisal of the nutritional status of American infants. A Preschool Nutrition Survey, 1968 to 1970, studied about 3,400 children age 1 to 6 years and was designed to provide an overview of nutritional status for that age group. At about the same time, the Ten-State Nutrition Survey was being carried out to determine the extent of malnutrition in the United States, and it focused primarily on adults in poverty and near-poverty communities. Some 3,700 children under 6 years of age were included in the TSNS. The National Health and Nutrition Examination Surveys (NHANES I, II, and planned III) are more representative of the general population and included about 1,500 (NHANES I) and 4,000 (NHANES II) children between 6 months and 6 years of age. Designed to monitor nutritional status of a representative sample of the national population these surveys produce a sizable body of data and document changes in nutritional status with time. Smaller, more local surveys can also provide valuable information about specific populations in certain areas.

Generally, these surveys do not indicate major nutrient deficiencies in young American children. More than 30 percent of the infants in the TSNS, however, had iron and vitamin C intakes less than two-thirds of the RDA for those nutrients, and anemia was identified in many. Anemia has consistently been identified in more limited studies as well.

Other than widespread iron deficiency, few severe nutritional problems were found. It was apparent, though, that deficiencies were more prevalent among lower socioeconomic segments of the population. Evidence that early deficiencies may cause later abnormalities in physical and mental functioning has spurred programs to alleviate malnutrition in the young. The Women, Infants, and Children Supplemental Food Program (WIC) in particular has increased food-buying power for mothers and their young children.

The mother is usually the final arbiter about what, when, and how much an infant will be fed. She needs information, and considerable support, in making these decisions. Current recommendations for feeding normal infants reflect present knowledge. As research continues, the long-term consequences of early feeding practices will emerge. This is an important goal, for a good start in the early years is the best guarantee of physical and mental health in all the growth stages that follow.

NUTRITION DURING CHILDHOOD

At one year of age, the child bears little resemblance to the infant at one month. At the brink of the second year, birth weight has almost tripled and length has increased by 50 percent or more. The child has developed a full crop of hair and 6 to 12 teeth. In addition to this visible physical progress, there has been significant behavioral, emotional, and social maturation. The child can sit, stand, and perhaps walk and speak a few words, recognize family members and other familiar faces, and charm them all with a ready smile. The typical one-year-old has achieved a transition from breast milk or formula to solid food and whole milk and has joined the rest of the family at the dining table.

The attitudes toward food and eating that evolve in the preschool years will last throughout life. Although the child's food needs are a reflection of a changing internal environment, the eating habits and food preferences that develop are influenced by the external environment.

Childhood Growth Patterns

In comparison with the rapid growth of the first 12 months, the rate of growth decreases considerably during the childhood years. Between 2 and 10 years of age, the average height increment is about 2 to 4 inches per year, compared to the 9 or 10 inches typically added in the first year. Weight is gained at a proportionately slower rate as well. Whereas most infants gain about 12 to 14 pounds during the first year, toddlers and older children typically gain only 4 to 8 pounds each year. (Figures 12–3 and 12–4 depict normal growth patterns during childhood and adolescence.)

The easily visible signs of growth provided by height and weight measures reflect underlying changes in the accumulation of muscle tissue, skeletal growth, and deposition of fat. The rate of fat deposition decreases from age one to the onset of puberty. At six months of age, infants have about 30 percent body fat, higher for most individuals than they will achieve until late in life. While obese adults were taller and heavier as two-year-olds, we cannot say that tall and heavy two-year-olds will be obese as adults.

Records of height and weight are important indicators of general health in children and of nutritional health in particular. Although the effects of deprivation on weight gain are readily apparent, linear growth can also be affected by severe undernutrition. Systemic diseases that disrupt absorption, digestion, and metabolism, as well as general undernutrition, can interfere with physical growth. An accurately maintained growth record for every child is important because when abnormal signs are recognized early enough, deficits may be halted and even reversed.

There is apparently a developmental period in which "catch-up" growth, within genetically predetermined limits, is possible. In Europe during and after World

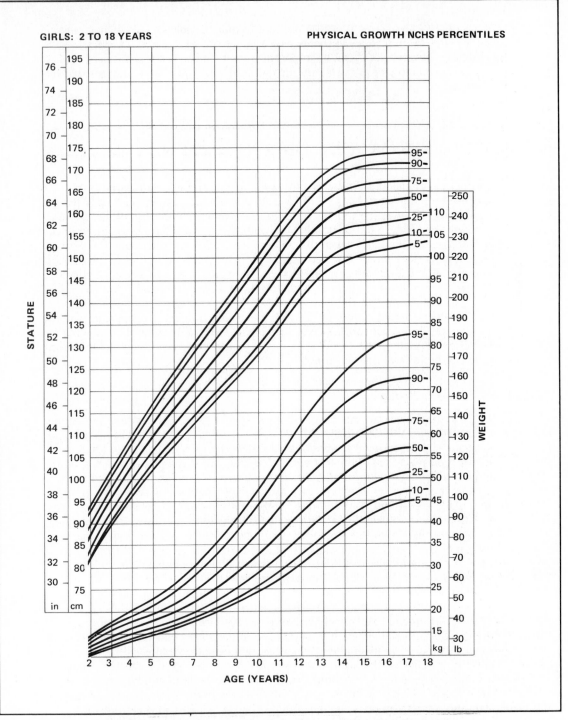

FIGURE 12-3   *Weight and Height by Age for Girls from 2 to 18 Years.*

Source: Adapted from National Center for Health Statistics, *NCHS growth charts,* 1976. Monthly Vital Statistics Report, Vol. 25, No. 3 Supp. (HRA) 76-1120 (Rockville, Maryland: Health Resources Administration, June 1976). © 1976 Ross Laboratories.

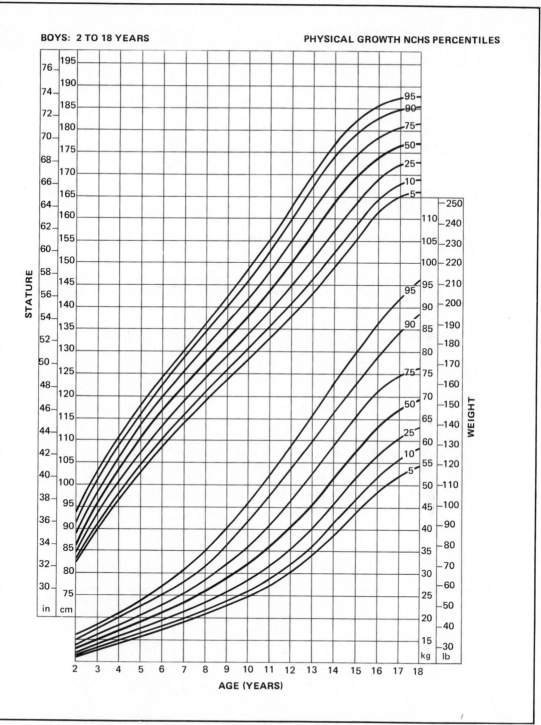

BOYS: 2 TO 18 YEARS   **PHYSICAL GROWTH NCHS PERCENTILES**

FIGURE 12-4   *Weight and Height by Age for Boys from 2 to 18 Years.*

Source: Adapted from National Center for Health Statistics, *NCHS growth charts, 1976*, Monthly Vital Statistics Report, Vol. 25, No. 3, Supp. (HRA) 76-1120 (Rockville, Maryland: Health Resources Administration, June, 1976). © Ross Laboratories.

War II, average heights of young children and adolescents were generally lower than those of the prewar generation, as a result of wartime food shortages. Dietary supplements of milk or high-energy foods given to selected groups of undernourished children produced increases in height, weight, and skeletal maturity significantly greater than those of children whose diets were not supplemented.

Similar growth spurts attributable to dietary improvements have been reported even in racial groups whose members had once been considered to be genetically small. In Japan, for example, children born since World War II are significantly taller than children of the prewar period; the increment has been ascribed to their greater intake of animal protein, although increased consumption of animal-derived foods presumably increased the energy content of their diets as well. Dietary protein would be "spared" from use for energy production, and the amino acids could be used more efficiently for growth.

Nutritional Needs During Childhood

When nutrient and energy needs of children are expressed per pound or kilogram of body weight, they are actually lower than those of infants. However, because children are larger, their total or absolute nutritional needs are of course increased. Table 12–3 shows the RDAs for children of different ages.

ENERGY. Energy needs in childhood, as in other stages of the life cycle, vary according to individual body size and composition, rate of growth, and physical activity. The amount of energy required just for growth in the first 12 months of life is so great that although toddlers and children are markedly more active than infants, their total energy needs in proportion to body weight are actually less. Thus the recommended energy allowance for a child from ages 1 through 10 is only 85 to 100 kilocalories per kilogram compared to 105 to 115 kilocalories per kilogram of body weight during the first 12 months. Individual energy requirements, of course, must take into account the variation in physical activity from one child to the next. Observations of height, weight, and general physical appearance are the best indicators of how well a given child's energy intake is matched to needs. Tendencies toward obesity or to extreme underweight can and should be monitored and corrected promptly.

TABLE 12-3. RDAs for Children

Age years	Weight kg	lb	Height cm	in	Energy kcal	Protein gm	Vitamin A (µg RE)	Vitamin D (µg)	Vitamin E Activity (mg α T.E.)
							FAT-SOLUBLE VITAMINS		
1–3	13	29	90	35	1,300	23	400	10	5
4–6	20	44	112	44	1,700	30	500	10	6
7–10	28	62	132	55	2,400	34	700	10	7

Source: Food and Nutrition Board, National Academy of Sciences, *Recommended daily dietary allowances,* revised 1979 (Washington, D.C.: National Research Council, 1979).

PROTEIN. Protein can provide energy, but its primary function is to supply the amino acids necessary for growth. As with the RDA for energy, the recommended daily protein intake for children also decreases in proportion to body weight while increasing in absolute quantity. During the years from 1 to 10, 1.8 to 1.2 grams per kilogram of body weight is recommended; this compares with 2.0 to 2.2 grams per kilogram during the first year.

This recommendation assumes that foods with high-quality proteins (milk, meat, eggs, dairy products, or combinations that provide complementary proteins) will be consumed to provide essential amino acids. Because amino acids will be used as a source of energy when total energy intake is insufficient, they will not be available for protein synthesis if the overall diet is inadequate. On the other hand, consumption in excess of this recommendation is economically wasteful as well as nutritionally unnecessary.

CARBOHYDRATE AND FAT. There are no RDAs for carbohydrate and fat for any age group. Both nutrients provide energy, and fats are important as sources of essential fatty acids. From 30 to 40 percent of energy intake should be provided as dietary lipid, with 2 to 5 percent in the form of essential fatty acids. These percentages are usually met through consumption of whole milk, meat, margarine or butter, mayonnaise, salad dressing, peanut butter, cheese, and other common foods. If there is too little fat in the diet, there will be a risk of essential fatty acid deficiency. Too much fat, on the other hand, will limit the child's appetite for other foods and might contribute to obesity.

Well-publicized findings that excess fat consumption in early life may play a role in later development of coronary heart disease have caused some parents to question the need for so much fat, especially from high-cholesterol foods, in children's diets. This concern has led nutritionists and pediatricians to recommend that consumption of foods high in cholesterol and with excessive quantities of fat be limited for children in families with a history of cardiovascular disease or hyperlipidemia. But there is little or no evidence of benefit in restricting lipid intake for healthy children. Misplaced concern about high-cholesterol foods, particularly eggs, may cause parents to limit intake of otherwise excellent foods. Especially for children with finicky food habits, eggs can be an important source of complete protein as well as of many other nutrients.

In the United States, carbohydrates supply about 40 to 50 percent of children's

WATER-SOLUBLE VITAMINS							MINERALS					
Vitamin C	Folacin	Niacin	Riboflavin	Thiamin	Vitamin B_6	Vitamin B_{12}	Calcium	Phosphorus	Iodine	Iron	Magnesium	Zinc
(mg)	μg	mg	mg	mg	mg	μg	mg	mg	μg	mg	mg	mg
45	100	9	0.8	0.7	0.9	2.0	800	800	70	15	150	10
45	200	11	1.0	0.9	1.3	2.5	800	800	90	10	200	10
45	300	16	1.4	1.2	1.6	3.0	800	800	120	10	250	10

energy needs. Although the Food and Nutrition Board has not established an RDA for carbohydrate, a minimum of 50 to 100 grams per day (200 to 400 kcal) has been suggested. The greatest part of carbohydrate intake should be in the form of complex carbohydrates and sugars found in bananas, apples, raisins, and other fruits. Carbohydrates in the form of sucrose in candy bars and soft drinks should be consumed in moderation. The excess energy provided by these foods may contribute to obesity, and the simple sugars to dental caries. In addition, these foods limit a child's appetite for other, more nutritious, foods.

VITAMINS AND MINERALS. Active, growing children require a full complement of vitamins and minerals. Although a diversified diet usually meets these needs, supplements may be useful and even necessary when food intake is limited by illness or quirky food habits or if specific deficiencies have been diagnosed.

Many of the vitamins and minerals are necessary for skeletal and tissue growth, and thus are especially important for growing children. Vitamin D is of particular importance for bone growth and development. Children whose exposure to sunlight is limited should receive 10 μg of this vitamin per day, the amount contained in a quart of fortified milk. Cod-liver oil and other supplements providing vitamins D and A are no longer considered necessary. Because these vitamins are fat-soluble, excesses tend to accumulate in adipose tissue and may build up to toxic levels. Vitamin D supplementation is advisable for healthy children only if they get no sunshine and drink little or no milk, and it should not exceed 10 μg per day.

DEVELOPMENT OF FOOD BEHAVIORS

After the first cry that fills the newborn's lungs with air, the next cry is likely to be a plaintive call for food. The way in which parents meet these early, instinctive demands sets the stage for permanent eating patterns and develops the desirable motivation we know as appetite.

There is a vast difference between hunger—the unpleasant sensation of stomach pain, weakness, and general irritability—and appetite—the pleasurable anticipation that food will both assuage hunger and delight the senses. All healthy infants and children show hunger; the fact that all do not appear to show appetite is the point of our discussion. The earliest feeding experiences are associated with comfort, contentment, and the pleasure of interpersonal closeness between mother and child. These associations are gradually extended to all other individuals who may provide food—father, relatives, babysitters, friends—and to the entire feeding environment—the chair in which the mother sits for feeding, the bottle, even the towel used for burping. Before long, the infant responds to the sight of a bottle being filled or the mother preparing food, and begins to cry. Such responses to food cues are the first signs of a developing appetite, the first signs that the infant understands the purpose of eating.

Influence of Parents and Home

Infants typically make their first chewing movements, even before a tooth has erupted, at about six months of age. Those who are given small pieces of hard toast or a similar food soon master the art of chewing. The same is true for every develop-

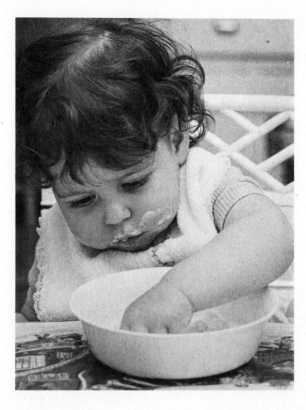

Children learn to enjoy food when they are allowed to feed themselves.

Erika Stone/Photo Researchers

mental ability. As soon as a child is able to pick up small pieces of food, to poke at and explore new foods, to hold a cup or a spoon and help in the feeding process, appropriate foods and utensils should be provided. By taking advantage of skills as they appear, parents can encourage the behaviors necessary for lifelong enjoyment of food and good nutrition.

Toddlers are often in a naturally negative stage just when they should be introduced to new foods. They say "No-no" even though that is not what they really mean. This negativism is a universal stage of development, necessary for children to separate themselves psychologically and develop the independence required for the next stages of maturation. But parents tend to respond to what the child says, not to the underlying meanings. The more the child resists, the more anxious the parent becomes, and the more likely the child is to continue resisting. This pattern of stress and resistance creates unhappy mealtimes and poor eaters, setting a destructive pattern for years to come.

With a seat at the family dining table comes a child's-eye view of not only what parents, siblings, and guests are eating, but also their attitudes about it. Adult conversation may have a strong effect. If, as one commentator has said, the purpose of grown-ups at the table is simply to make sure that the children eat, the children will learn early that they can get more attention by *not* eating. Negative comments about food from other family members can also have an impact, and so can special treatment accorded to another member of the family. If a father refuses to eat something, his children are not likely to want that food either. One wise mother served spinach and cucumbers—foods her husband would not accept—to her chil-

Perspective On

NUTRITION AND BEHAVIOR

Until recently, brain function was thought to be independent of day-to-day metabolic changes. Brain accounts for 20 to 30 percent of the body's resting metabolic rate, but only 2 percent of adult body weight. The brain depends on a continuous supply of oxygen and its major energy source is glucose. The supply of other nutrients is regulated by the blood-brain barrier. Severe malnutrition has long been recognized as producing permanent alterations in cell development and function of the brain. In 1971, Fernstrom and Wurtman demonstrated that under certain conditions in animals, the concentration of serotonin, a brain neurotransmitter, was affected by the protein-to-carbohydrate ratio of a meal. Diet can alter brain function directly, by fluctutations in concentrations of nutrients delivered to the brain, or indirectly, by influencing afferent nerve signals. The role of diet is neurotransmitter synthesis and membrane function has been the subject of many research studies. Carbohydrate meals relative to protein meals have a calming effect. In one study elderly participants were shown to be more sensitive than younger adults to the differential effects. Caffeine, in single low doses equivalent to that in coffee, tea, or cola beverages beneficially affect human performance and self-reported mood state.

HYPERACTIVITY.   Short attention span, easy distractibility, impulsiveness, restlessness—all are characteristic of the hyperactive child. But a high level of physical activity is not by itself a sure sign of hyperactivity. Unless very specific criteria are used, many children are diagnosed incorrectly.

The confusion over what actually constitutes hyperactivity has affected the validity of claims regarding effectiveness of treatment as well as incidence and possible causes. Since the 1950s, the usual treatment has been medication with stimulants, such as amphetamines, which paradoxically, have a calming, rather than stimulating, effect on some hyperactive children. Stimulating drugs have some undesirable side effects, in particular, appetite depression which can retard growth in children.

In the 1970s, Feingold, an allergist, reported dramatic improvement in behavior of many hyperkinetic children treated with special additive-free diets. According to Feingold, a variety of food components—artificial colors and flavorings, preservatives, and naturally occurring salicylates, which cause allergic reactions in sensitive people—were the cause of hyperactivity in children. In addition, he claimed that even minute amounts of such substances could make a calmed child regress. Many parents, encouraged by these results, voluntarily modified their children's diets according to his recommendations and many saw improvement. The claims could not be evaluated because the children were not definitely diagnosed as hyperactive and results were not necessarily due to dietary changes. Critics of Feingold's diet point out that he has provided only anecdotal evidence for his hypothesis. They suggest that heightened family concern and involvement with the child could account for any observed improvements.

In fact, researchers have not found significant changes when testing children under rigorous

dren only on nights when their father was not home in time for dinner, and both children have enjoyed those foods ever since. Each excessive discussion about food—Do you like the chicken? Have some more salad. Wait 'til you taste the potatoes!—can diminish a child's appetite. So can an overfilled plate.

Parents may be unable to avoid negative influences brought into the home by well-meaning babysitters or grandparents. The sitter who must get every last morsel into the child, and devises distracting entertainments while pushing a spoon into an unwilling mouth, has contributed to mealtime havoc in many homes. A grandpar-

and controlled conditions, which included no one knowing when the child was getting additives. In one study, most parents and teachers of children diagnosed as hyperactive could not detect behavioral differences when these children consumed additive-free or control diets. Even more striking, no increase in hyperactivity was apparent when the children were deliberately given foods containing artificial colors. A few children exhibited a transient response to large intakes of food colors, but this number is far less than claimed in most anecdotal studies.

A different kind of question has arisen concerning the nutritional adequacy of the special diets. Omitting foods which naturally contain salicylates also reduces the consumption of ascorbic acid. Further and possibly more serious, there is the possibility of low total intake resulting in an energy deficit which in turn can result in growth depression, an undesirable effect.

SUGAR. Sugar has been suggested as a cause of hyperactivity, juvenile deliquency, aggression, and even criminal behavior. These behaviors have been attributed to "hypoglycemia" caused by eating large amounts of foods high in sugar. Essential reactive hypoglycemia is a rare medical condition characterized by anxiety, weakness, irritability, lightheadedness, palpitations, and sweating, and it must be diagnosed by laboratory tests. Most of the concern about sugar and criminal behavior results from anecdotal information or inadequately designed studies, not from well designed studies acceptable to journals with adequate scientific standards.

In one study, the investigator compared the number of disciplinary actions recorded each day for 34 boys and compared this with the number in the records of 24 different boys after a dietary change was made. One of the dietary modifications was replacing sugar on the table with honey. There was also no strict control over access to sugar from other sources, such as parents sending packages of food to their children.

In another series of studies, adult males who were habitually violent and frequently under the influence of alcohol were studied. Although oral glucose tolerance tests were done on these individuals, no specific symptoms of hypoglycemia were reported by them. Further, the role of long-term alcohol consumption on sugar metabolism was not acknowledged.

MEGAVITAMIN THERAPY. In contrast to the supposed adverse effects of high amounts of sugar on behavior, large doses of vitamins and minerals have been suggested as beneficial. Several well designed studies failed to support improvement in patients with schizophrenia who were treated with megavitamin therapy.

Clearly, additional research is needed to define the effects of foods and food constituents on behavior. Scientists from several disciplines, including medicine, nutrition, and the behavioral sciences, must work together to ensure that studies are well designed and well controlled. The interested student should read "Diet and Behavior: A Multidisciplinary Evaluation" a special issue of *Nutrition Reviews* published in April 1986.

ent who says "eat your fish because it's good for you" can undo many happy hours of eating fish because it tastes good.

Outside Influences: School and Friends

As more mothers join the work force, the care and feeding of many young children is left to others. This situation often contributes to good nutritional practices. Because child-care centers, and the preschools and kindergartens that serve meals, are usually licensed by agencies that mandate sound mealtime patterns and provide some foods, the child whose nutrition is marginal may for the first time be introduced to well-balanced meals and a diversified diet.

In many preschool and early elementary school programs, children have an opportunity to become involved in the preparation and serving of their own meals. A class field trip to a local market to buy ingredients for vegetable soup, and then a morning spent preparing them and watching the simmering pot, may create interest in foods. The activity provided in school may help the child to work up an appetite and by lunchtime be hungry enough to eat whatever is put on the plate. Eating with other children, perhaps singing or playing a game at the table while waiting for the next course, is an enjoyable social experience that enhances appetite.

But some children who have acquired excellent attitudes at home may learn undesirable foods habits by watching their peers. It may take only one small voice saying "yeccch" to the green beans to turn a former bean lover against them. No parents can prevent such influences; they can only hope that the positive atmosphere of the home will be strong enough to counteract any damage done by other children's poor dining habits.

As the child gets older and moves up through elementary grades, increasing influence is wielded by peers. More independent now of parents, children have some money in their pockets to use at the corner candy store or the school vending machine. Nutritional quality is not guaranteed by the availability of feeding programs in the schools or even by a balanced brown-bag lunch brought from home. Children seldom eat everything on their lunch trays, and many a mother would be distressed to find that the shiny red apple she packed was traded to another child for a gooey caramel bar.

Influence of Mass Media

Parental vigilance is no match for the television set and its continual messages to "enjoy chocolatey this" or "try some finger-licking that." Almost all homes in the United States have at least one television set, and today's children spend more time in their preschool years watching television than they will spend in the classroom during four years of college. Over 20 percent of those viewing hours are spent watching commercials. And of those commercials, at least 40 percent mention food—a figure that is as high as 70 percent in the hours when children are watching. According to Federal Trade Commission studies and parental observations, much of this advertising is for presweetened cereals, candy, and fast-food products served at local "family" restaurants.

The young child is often unable to separate commercial messages from the regular program; preschoolers attend just as closely and receptively to commercial messages as to entertainment segments. Parents have been quick to realize this and have formed groups such as Action for Children's Television (ACT), which has pressured the Federal Communications Commission and the Federal Trade Commission to limit commercial interruptions during children's prime viewing hours.

In the mid-1970s, the National Advertising Board restricted by about 20 percent the amount of commercial time permitted during children's programs. Many television stations voluntarily limited this time even further. In addition, companies were prohibited from using stars to endorse food products and from advertising "kiddy vitamins" during children's shows.

By definition, the mass media comprise print as well as audio and visual materials that reach large numbers of people to provide information and entertainment.

Magazines for children, radio, billboards and other forms of public placards, and even package design carry advertising messages relating to food. We cannot isolate a child from society, even if it were desirable to do so. The child must interact with other children and learn to live as well as possible in the world as it is. Parents can monitor their children's television watching, but more important, they can refuse to give in to pressure to buy every food or snack that is advertised.

Encouraging Good Food Habits

Positive patterns cannot be legislated; they must begin in the home during the formative years and be reinforced daily. A relaxed atmosphere at mealtime gives children a chance to develop at their own rate.

Few parents realize how little food a young child actually needs. A child of average size and normal rate of development can manage only about 1 tablespoon of each type of food served at each meal for each year of his or her age. In other words, a two-year-old could be expected to consume 2 tablespoons of meat, 2 tablespoons of vegetables, and 2 tablespoons of fruit, in addition to regular servings of milk and juice. The total food served at one meal to a two-year-old should be just 6 tablespoons, or about ⅓ cup—far less than most two-year-olds are urged to eat. Using this standard, parents may realize that their "poor" eaters are actually excellent eaters, and perhaps that their "good" eaters have become overeaters. Children should be offered small servings for other reasons as well. A heaped-up plate is overwhelming and often reduces appetite. Second helpings can be freely offered, allowing the child to ask for more.

Children have their likes and dislikes just as adults do, and these should be respected. Trying to force a food a child dislikes will only stiffen the opposition and turn what is probably a temporary matter of taste into a permanent aversion. If a variety of foods is available, there should be no problem about providing nutritionally valid substitutes. A child who does not care for lettuce and tomatoes may welcome raw carrots and celery. Pineapple juice may be more acceptable than orange juice, melon preferred to grapefruit, and rice chosen over potatoes.

Even good eaters go on occasional food jags, refusing some former favorites and limiting their diet to one or two foods at each meal. When parents respond with understanding—and some ingenuity—the child's erratic eating is likely to be of short duration and little nutritional significance. For a child who will eat only desserts, the ingenious parent may fix egg custards or fruit purees. When a substitute is available, a child learns to try more foods because there is always something familiar to eat if a new food doesn't work out. Sometimes a child will even say, "I think I'll like it next time," or give another clue about food readiness to an alert parent.

Children's tastes change, often with amazing rapidity. The child who consumes nothing but hamburger at the age of 4 discovers chicken at 4½. Children's tastes may seem inconsistent: The child who cannot look at a cooked green pea on a plate may devour a bowl full of them raw. And something that might not be touched at dinnertime may appear very appetizing during a half-hour alone in the kitchen with father or mother while dinner is being prepared. This is a good time to introduce new foods: "Mommy and Daddy are going to have this; would you like to try some?"

Some children will eat only "breakfast" foods—for breakfast, lunch, and dinner. But this need not be a problem. Eggs and toast can be offered at any meal, perhaps with a slice of meat or a raw vegetable on the side. Only culture dictates that chicken is for dinner and cereals for breakfast. A cereal can be served as a side dish at dinner—cornmeal or farina are good choices, palatable with margarine or, for the more sophisticated tastes of the rest of the family, any tomato- or meat-based sauce.

An important tactic is to introduce new foods at the beginning of the meal, when the child is hungry. Hunger may win out over prejudice, and a new dish is added to the repertoire. An older child may be allowed to help plan menus; even a kindergartener can understand the basic food groups and be shown how they are used to plan the dishes that appear on the family table.

As in so many other areas, parents must steer carefully between extremes when it comes to the development of food behaviors in their children. On the one hand they must set reasonable limits on a child's intake, while on the other, they must encourage the development of self-control. They must teach the importance of eating a variety of foods, but they must respect the child's integrity and right to have likes and dislikes. They must teach table manners, while recognizing the slow development of those skills that make manners possible. And through it all they must keep the atmosphere at the dining table pleasant, even when stressful situations arise. This is as important as any other recommendation: Eating is supposed to be enjoyable for children . . . and for their parents, too.

NUTRITION IN CHILDHOOD

Foods for Children

Foods generally enjoyed by preschoolers include cereals, breads, crackers, crunchy raw vegetables, meats that are easy to chew, fruits, and sweet baked goods such as cookies. Many children will accept any meat that comes with a bone for a "handle," whereas others will eat only hamburger. Generally, because children are not yet comfortable with utensils, they are happy with finger foods. Raw vegetables—garden-fresh green beans, carrots, cucumbers, and red or green peppers cut in small pieces or "sticks"—are usually welcome. The attractive colors of raw vegetables and their crunchy texture make them more appealing than most cooked vegetables.

Mild tastes also tend to please young palates. Foods are usually preferred without sauces, gravies, or strong seasonings. And most children like to see their food arranged neatly and in separate "categories" on the plate—woe to the parent who inadvertently slips a green pea into the mashed potatoes!

Children often go through phases of extreme fussiness about their food and the way it is presented. They may eat a sandwich only if it is cut into two rectangles, but not into triangles; they may not eat anything green; they may decide that two different foods cannot occupy the same plate. A parent's best recourse when these food-related compulsions appear is to take them lightly; in all probability they will go away if no fuss is made. But a parent should avoid encouraging such behaviors and even try gently to discourage them. The favorite plate may be in the dishwasher at lunchtime one day; the sandwich can be accidentally cut on the diagonal and peanut butter will still taste the same; green food can be served appetizingly to the rest of the family, and the child will see that nothing happens to those who consume it. A sense of humor at such times goes a long way, too.

The introduction of new foods should not be anticipated with dread, even if such ventures were unsuccessful in the past. Young preschoolers may be more accepting of new foods than are four- and five-year-olds: Apparently children as well as adults get more set in their ways as they get older, even in the earliest years. Because new foods will appear throughout life, they should be presented regularly to young children, even to those who have seldom accepted them previously. There's always a first time.

Parents should not expect a child to eat a full portion of anything new. Usually several experimental tastes over a period of weeks are needed before a normal portion will be accepted. If a food is rejected, a parent should wait a few weeks and try again. One mother introduces new foods to her children by saying "I have only enough to give you a little taste, but if you like it I'll make more the next time." Usually by the third taste the children are hooked.

Meals should be served at regular times. This provides a necessary order in children's lives; helps their "biological clocks" to function effectively; and will also help establish regular work, sleep, and bowel habits. Children should be allowed to become hungry for their meals. Snacks are so widely available today that many children never learn to feel hunger, although they may develop fine appetites for filling snack foods such as soft drinks, potato chips, and candy. Snacks in themselves are not harmful, and they may help a small stomach hold out until dinner time—even adults need a coffee break—but snacks substantial enough to impair eating at regular meals should be avoided. Nuts, fruits, juices, and cheese provide valuable nutrients and can be served in moderation.

Special Concerns

Of particular concern to nutritionists today are children whose food intake patterns may result in illness or obesity, not only in the growing years but later as well. An abundance of food and an increasingly sedentary life style have made obesity all too common among children as well as adults. And the proliferation among young adults of alternate eating patterns, specifically of vegetarian diets with varying degrees of limitation, is affecting the health status of increasing numbers of young children.

OBESITY. Although it is not certain that childhood obesity produces adult obesity, there is enough evidence to suggest a correlation. Evidence from a two decade follow-up of fatness in early childhood suggests 74 percent of obese children will be less than obese as adults. Approximately 26 percent were still obese as adults, nearly twice the expected number. Childhood obesity can be difficult for parents to recognize. A plump infant or toddler is more appealing to most people than a thin, wiry one. In fact, parents of thin children are more likely to be concerned about their health than are parents of heavier children. But what appears to be cute baby fat may be the beginning of a persistent obesity problem.

Children of obese parents tend to be obese too, and those of thin parents tend to be thin. Two obese parents have a 73 chance of having an obese offspring, one obese and one lean parent a 43 percent chance, and two lean parents only a 9 percent chance. Strong correlations exist in body weight and body fatness of identical twins. While more evidence for the role of genetics in body size has accumulated, there is still a role for environment in the development of the problem. Obese children, like obese adults, are less physically active than the nonobese; family life style may be a factor in this as well.

There are apparently certain critical periods for the development of obesity. In late infancy and early childhood, when growth rate diminishes and energy requirements decrease, parents may continue to "push" foods, starting a pattern of over-feeding. Again, at about six years of age children start school and their physical activities become limited at the same time as new eating schedules and "social snacking" begin. And finally, just before puberty, many children get heavier before they grow taller and may decrease their physical activity even further; at the same time, social snacking becomes an important activity. Often, however, children who gain weight disproportionately at this time will assume more pleasing body proportions as their linear growth catches up.

Whenever obesity develops, the strategy is the same: less energy intake and more energy expenditure. For children, however, the goal is not drastic weight *loss* but *maintenance* of the weight level to allow linear growth and normal body development as the child gains in height. Because childhood is a time of active physiological growth, intake should not be less than 1,200 to 1,400 kilocalories per day, to ensure an adequate supply of all essential nutrients.

This may mean a change in a child's meal and snack patterns, but a change may benefit the entire family. For most children, the substitution of fruit for cake, candy, or soft drinks and of raw or cooked green or crunchy vegetables for some of the starchy foods will suffice. Lower-fat meats are also advised; broiled chicken and lean roasted meats should replace fried chicken and hamburgers several times a week. Skim milk can be substituted for whole milk after two years of age. At the same time, a few "special occasion" foods should be permitted, so the dieting child does not feel too deprived. Then when pizza, birthday cake, or an ice-cream sundae have been eaten, the following day's meals should be adjusted accordingly.

Weight-control programs and diet clinics have been developed for children. These group approaches introduce young people to new eating patterns and behavior changes that can help them to control food intake. Often these groups encourage other family members to join their children, on the premise that family eating patterns are the most significant contributor to childhood obesity. Social and psychological family problems should receive appropriate counseling and other supportive services.

VEGETARIANISM. The popularity of alternative life styles is reflected in nontraditional food patterns, the most popular of which is vegetarianism. Unfortunately, there has been a corresponding increase in nutrition-related problems affecting children consuming vegetarian diets.

A strict vegetarian diet, excluding eggs, milk, and other dairy products, may not provide necessary levels of energy, vitamin D, vitamin B_{12}, calcium, iron, or high-quality protein required during the growth years. Rickets has been seen among children in macrobiotic vegetarian families, and dietary intake records have documented marginal consumption of calcium and phosphorus as well as of vitamin D. Growth retardation in vegetarian children may result from insufficient intake of the essential amino acids needed for protein synthesis, as well as of energy. Breast-fed infants of vegetarian mothers develop at the average rate until about six months of age, but when other foods are introduced they may grow more slowly than children of the same age on omnivorous diets. Although some catch-up growth may be possible, apparently there is a period when growth in the young child is particularly vulnerable to nutrient deficits.

Vegetarian parents should be particularly attentive to regular health examinations for their children and to careful diet planning. A variety of different legumes; grains; nuts; oil seeds; green, leafy vegetables; and fruits can provide adequate energy, protein, most B vitamins, and most other vitamins and minerals. Iron and vitamin B_{12} supplementation, however (the latter from fortified soybean milk or other products) is advised. Unfortunately some adults belong to groups that advocate extremely restrictive diets and avoid medical services; concern for their children is growing.

Dental Health

Dental health begins with good maternal nutrition during pregnancy, continues with proper diet in infancy, and includes regular oral hygiene practices (brushing and flossing) and dental check-ups throughout childhood and adulthood.

DENTAL CARIES. Some people, no matter what their diet or dental habits, have teeth that are relatively resistant to damage. But most people are more or less vulnerable to tooth decay. Three major factors contribute to the development of dental caries. The host is a tooth made susceptible by genetic and environmental factors including prenatal nutrition. The agent is the colony of oral bacteria, the mass of microbes that inhabit the mouth and cling to the surface of teeth. The environment, consisting of conditions inside the mouth, is provided by dietary substrates that support bacterial growth and metabolism and also by saliva, which helps to protect teeth from dental decay. The gelatinous plaque formed by colonies of oral bacteria keeps these organisms in close proximity to the tooth surface and prevents the cleansing and buffering action of saliva. In addition, bacteria produce a sticky polysaccharide (dextran) from ingested carbohydrate, which further increases plaque adherence to the teeth.

The carious process begins when the bacteria metabolize glucose (derived from ingested carbohydrate and dextran) to lactic and other acids. These acids demineralize the teeth, starting with the enamel and proceeding inward toward the dentin. Because this inner layer is softer, the process is accelerated and bacteria invade the pulp. The all too familiar cavity, and sometimes toothache, is the result of this invasive bacterial infection.

PREVENTION. Although dental caries are a complex and multifactorial disease, preventive measures can be directed against each of the three factors in its development. Teeth can be made less susceptible to dental decay by treatment with fluoride—provided in drinking water, toothpaste, supplements, and dental treatment. The noteworthy decline in prevalence of dental caries in many countries, including the United States, has been attributed to the beneficial effects of fluoride. Control of oral bacteria and improvement of the oral environment can be accomplished by reducing the frequency of intake of fermentable carbohydrates (sugars and starches), particularly those which stick to the teeth. Since research has shown that many foods are potentially cariogenic, a regular and conscientious oral hygiene program will help to control plaque accumulation and enamel demineralization. A young child should be started on an oral hygiene program. Baby teeth, while lost eventually, should be well maintained to establish habits that will last a lifetime. Young children should be initially assisted by an adult, but they will quickly learn the process.

Nutritional Status of American Children

The Preschool Nutrition Survey, the Ten-State Nutrition Survey, and HANES studies indicate that nutritional status of children at all ages is generally good but that children at the lower end of the socioeconomic spectrum tend to have poorer intakes of several nutrients than children from middle- and upper-income families and tend to be of smaller stature as well. Obesity and low iron and calcium intakes were the most prevalent nutrition-related problems; the incidence of obesity tended to correlate with higher family income. Suboptimal vitamin A intakes were found particularly in Hispanic and black children; more than one-tenth of all children had low vitamin C intakes; and anemia was found in from 7 to 12 percent of all children in these studies. Protein intakes, on the other hand, were consistently from 50 to 100 percent higher than RDAs.

Large numbers of young children—from 25 to 40 percent of preschoolers, according to these surveys—receive vitamin and mineral supplements. In a study of second- and sixth-grade children it was found that without dietary supplements, iron, calcium, vitamin A, thiamin, and niacin intakes would have been unsatisfactory in significant numbers of children; fewer had to rely on supplements for ascorbic acid and riboflavin. Older children and girls were less likely to consume adequate levels of nutrients. Calcium intake of nearly half of the children was below the RDA; and for those whose intakes met or exceeded the RDA, their midmorning milk at school contributed a sizable proportion. These results would seem at first sight to make supplementation generally advisable. However, the best way to ensure adequate intake of all nutrients, including those which are *not* contained

With a seat at the family dining table comes a child's eye view of what parents are eating and their attitudes about food.
John Isaac/United Nations Photo

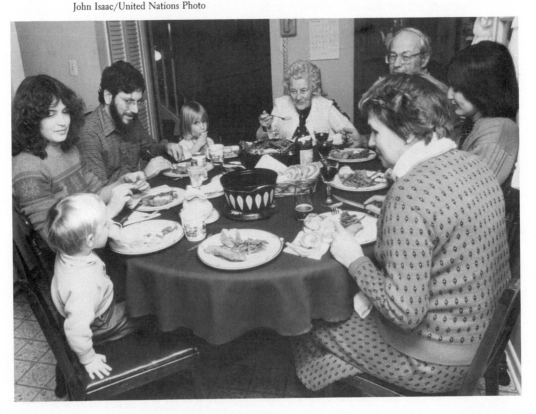

in dietary supplements, is to encourage consumption of a variety of nutritious foods.

A study of young children with iron-deficiency anemia has identified a number of related social and environmental factors. In comparison with a group of controls, anemic children were more likely to be the youngest in their family, have more siblings, drink more milk, and have been introduced to commercial baby foods at a later age; their mothers were more likely to be separated or divorced, be dissatisfied with the child's food habits and general abilities, and spend less money on food for each person in the household. Some of these factors may help to identify children who may be at risk.

Sound nutritional practices in childhood will produce adults who enjoy meals, who consume nutritionally adequate diets that are neither excessive nor scanty, who do not "use" food for emotional blackmail or other manipulative purposes— and who will bring up *their* children to have positive food attitudes also.

NUTRITION DURING ADOLESCENCE

In the continuum from infancy through adulthood, the beginning of a new stage of development is seldom clearly defined. Whereas infancy obviously starts at birth, the boundaries between infancy and childhood, and between childhood and adolescence, are not at all distinct. But although adolescence has neither a clear beginning nor a clear end, the physiological events of this period are very distinctive indeed. It is a critical period of rapid development—but in most children there is a lack of synchronization among the physical, emotional, and social aspects of that development. Although the preschool and school years are recognized as being extremely important influences on the personality and behavioral traits of the mature adult, further important modifications, coming increasingly from the world outside the home and family, are made during the adolescent years.

Teenagers are neither children nor adults, and this time can be a difficult one for them as well as for their parents and teachers. Both parents and children recognize the need for, and want, increased independence for the growing young person. Yet each too often sends out confused signals to the other, leading to varying degrees of conflict. There are many areas of parent-child disagreement—cars, dating, hours, dress, study habits, and sometimes food. As teenagers try to differentiate themselves from parental beliefs and to keep up with their peer group, their dietary habits often change. At the same time, their rapidly growing bodies require even more nutritional support than during the childhood years.

Normal Growth and Development

Of all the changes that occur during adolescence, the most obvious are increased stature, altered body composition, and sexual maturation. The rate of growth during adolescence is second only to that of early infancy. But whereas development in the first year of life is relatively predictable for all infants, the rate and timing of development in adolescents is highly individual. Although both female and male infants have the same developmental patterns, female and male adolescents have markedly different rates and patterns of development. A prepubertal growth spurt is characteristic only of human beings. Adolescents in developing countries do not have a marked growth spurt, possibly because of nutritional deprivation. Growth patterns in adolescence are shown in Figures 12–5 and 12–6.

HEIGHT.   The adolescent growth spurt for most girls occurs before the teen years and prior to menarche (the onset of menstruation). Even during grade-school years, girls are often taller than boys, a situation that continues until around age 14 or 15, when boys catch up and rapidly exceed the height of their female schoolmates. Girls who have a particularly large and early growth spurt also reach puberty at an early age. They do not, however, necessarily grow taller than later-maturing contemporaries. Once reproductive capacity is achieved by adolescent girls, the rate of growth slows dramatically.

In males the secondary sexual characteristics appear at the onset of the growth spurt. Male growth continues far longer than is generally believed; from 17 to 28 years, boys grow about 2.3 centimeters, compared with 1.2 centimeters for girls. This prolonged growth period has implications for the nutritional requirements of young adults, although admittedly the growth rate is modest compared to growth at the peak of the adolescent growth spurt.

WEIGHT.   The adolescent growth spurt is related to increases in both cell number and cell size, which are paralleled by significant weight gains. Girls progress earlier than boys in this area as well. During the preadolescent years, girls store fat and may gain significant weight—as much as 10 pounds in a single prepubertal year. And because weight gain precedes the increase in height, preteens are frequently chubby. But girls who have not previously been overweight normally regain more slender proportions at the time their growth spurt begins. Boys may not lose

FIGURE 12-5   *Growth-Patterns—Height.*
Mean height attained by U.S. youths 6–18 years of age by quarter-year age groups.
Source: National Center for Health Statistics, *Height and weight of youths 12–17 years, United States 1966-70.* Vital and Health Statistics, Series 11, No. 124. USDHEW Pub. No. (HSM) 73-1606 (Washington, D.C.: U.S. Government Printing Office, 1973).

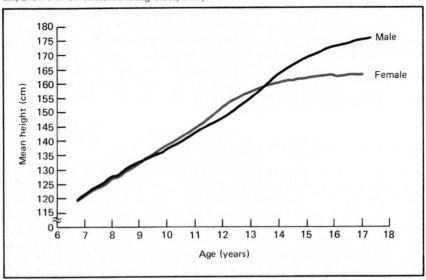

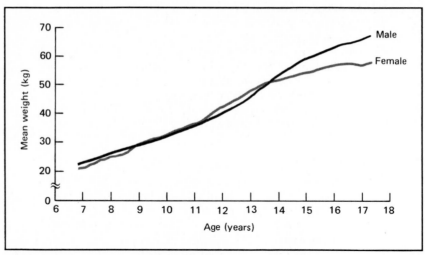

FIGURE 12-6   *Growth Patterns—Weight.*

Mean weight attained by U.S. youths 6-18 years of age by quarter-year age groups.

Source: National Center for Health Statistics. *Height and weight of youths 12-17 years, United States 1966–70.* Vital and Health Statistics Series 11, No. 124, USDHEW Pub. No. (HSM) 73-1606 (Washington, D.C.: U.S. Government Printing Office, 1973).

prepubertal fat until the time of their greatest linear growth and after; loss of body fat at that time is probably related to the increased levels of testosterone and the coordinate development of upper-body musculature.

BODY COMPOSITION.   Just as the timing of height and weight spurts differs in males and females, so does their body composition, which is markedly influenced by hormones. In girls, body fat increases and is deposited particularly in the hips and breast tissues. Boys have a greater lean body mass, with greater muscular and skeletal development. Percent of body fat in boys stays the same or actually decreases during adolescence.

SEXUAL MATURATION.   The hormonal changes that cause fat deposition in females and increased lean body mass in males are also responsible for maturation of the reproductive systems of both sexes. Menarche in girls is an obvious sign of sexual maturation, although ovulation generally does not occur with regularity until one or two years later. Hormonal changes also trigger the development of secondary sex characteristics, such as the growth of pubic and body hair and the voice change and growth of facial hair in males.

Because chronological age is not the best indicator of maturation, secondary sex characteristics are used as an index of development, and they form the basis of the sex-maturity ratings (SMR). In girls the quantity and pattern of pubic hair and the development of breasts are key indicators; in boys the growth of the penis and testes and the development of pubic hair are used. A five-point scale has been developed, with SMR 1 representing the prepubertal stage, SMR 2 indicating the first visible signs of change, SMR 3 and 4 being intermediate stages of development, and SMR 5 representing adult maturation. Other developmental events can be correlated with these stages: In girls, peak growth velocity occurs at SMR 2 and menarche usually occurs at SMR 4, although it may occur at SMR 3. In boys, peak growth velocity occurs at SMR 3 and is followed by the growth of facial and body hair in SMR 4; chest hair usually does not develop until after SMR 5.

In industrial nations the onset of puberty has for more than a century been occurring at earlier ages, and this is often attributed to improved nutrition; some would include improved control of infectious diseases as well. Evidence suggests that the onset of menses in girls takes place only after a certain body weight and proportion of body fat has been attained. Thus, any factor that retards growth and prevents normal fat storage—not only undernutrition but also chronic or repeated infections and overly strenuous physical exertion—could delay puberty in girls.

Nutritional Requirements

Because of individual variation in adolescent growth and development, the problems of establishing RDAs for this age group are greater than for any other. The RDAs are presently categorized by age and sex to reflect *average* adolescent growth patterns (see Table 12–4). Use of SMRs to estimate nutrient allowances for teenagers has been suggested. This would be more accurate than standards based on chronological age, but in practical terms little would be gained and some convenience would be lost. Another suggestion is that RDA tables should differentiate energy and nutrient needs by sex from the ages of 8 or 9, because of the increase in growth rate that starts before 11 years of age in most girls today.

ENERGY.   The demand for energy closely parallels the velocity of growth. In girls, growth velocity peaks between age 11 and 14 and then declines, whereas boys' growth velocity—and therefore energy requirements—are highest in the mid- and late teen years. Adolescents' natural appetites increase markedly to accompany these growth spurts—and parents are usually surprised to find their 12-year-old

TABLE 12-4. *RDAs for Adolescents*

	11–14 YEARS		15–18 YEARS		19–22 YEARS	
	M	F	M	F	M	F
Energy (kcal)	2,700	2,200	2,800	2,100	2,900	2,100
(MJ)	11.3	9.2	11.8	8.8	12.2	8.8
Protein (g)	45	46	56	46	56	44
Vitamin A (RE)	1,000	800	1,000	800	1,000	800
Vitamin D (μg)	10	10	10	10	7.5	7.5
Vitamin E (mg αT.E.)	8	8	10	8	10	8
Vitamin C (mg)	50	50	60	60	60	60
Folacin (μg)	400	400	400	400	400	400
Niacin (mg)	18	15	18	14	19	14
Riboflavin (mg)	1.6	1.3	1.7	1.3	1.7	1.3
Thiamin (mg)	1.4	1.1	1.4	1.1	1.5	1.1
Vitamin B_6 (mg)	1.8	1.8	2.0	2.0	2.2	2.0
Vitamin B_{12} (μg)	3.0	3.0	3.0	3.0	3.0	3.0
Calcium (mg)	1,200	1,200	1,200	1,200	800	800
Phosphorus (mg)	1,200	1,200	1,200	1,200	800	800
Iodine (μg)	150	150	150	150	150	150
Iron (mg)	18	18	18	18	10	18
Magnesium (mg)	350	300	400	300	350	300
Zinc (mg)	15	15	15	15	15	15

Source: Food and Nutrition Board, National Academy of Sciences, *Recommended daily dietary allowances*, revised 1979 (Washington, D.C.: National Research Council, 1979).

daughter consuming as much or more food than they do. Typically, energy expenditure is also increased, so that what may seem to be overeating is actually necessary.

PROTEIN.   Accurate experimental data on which to base protein recommendations do not exist for adolescents, and the estimates shown in the table are extrapolated from the needs of infants, taking growth velocity and body weight into account. Protein requirements for girls are highest in the years from 15 to 18 and then decrease as growth rate declines. Adolescent males require additional protein to promote the growth of skeletal and muscle tissue; their needs remain higher than those of women throughout the adult years.

VITAMINS AND MINERALS.   There are few experimental data to support specific recommendations, but the rapid rate of development and growth during the adolescent years is itself evidence of increased need for the micronutrients. Calcium and phosphorus allowances are increased by 50 percent for both boys and girls during the periods of maximum growth to provide for rapid bone development; recommended intakes then decrease to adult levels.

Increases in blood volume and muscle mass during adolescence and the onset of menstruation in girls account for the higher iron requirements in these years. The allowance for both girls and boys is 18 milligrams per day; after 18 years of age, the RDA for males decreases to the adult level of 10 milligrams per day.

ADOLESCENT EATING PATTERNS

Just as growth and appetites peak, psychological and social pressures dramatically alter the adolescent's response to food. The growing desire for independence, peer acceptance, and socializing may conflict with increased physiological needs for more food and more sleep.

Casual eating, caused by the erratic work and social schedules of young people, is characteristic of these years. School activities that differ from day to day, athletic training and events, part-time jobs, and the haphazard demands of an active social life may all interfere with normal mealtimes. In early adolescence, eating patterns are likely to be regular because these children still spend most mealtimes at school or at home, and they are under closer parental supervision. But by the mid-teens, adolescents increasingly are somewhere other than home at mealtimes, and availability tends to determine their food choices. When hunger strikes it's easy to get a soft drink and a packet of cookies from a vending machine or to join the crowd for pizza or a burger and fries.

Although the influence of peers is significant, a survey of nearly 400 college freshmen showed that it is modified by individual preferences as well as by the influence of family food patterns. Those whose mothers had prepared breakfast for them during childhood continued to follow regular breakfast and lunch habits away from home. Changes in food selections made by these students were attributed to the difficulty in obtaining the kinds of foods, such as fruit and cheese, that were readily available in the home.

In the teen years, snacking is a way of life and may account for as much as a third of total energy and nutrient intake; for some teens it may represent an even

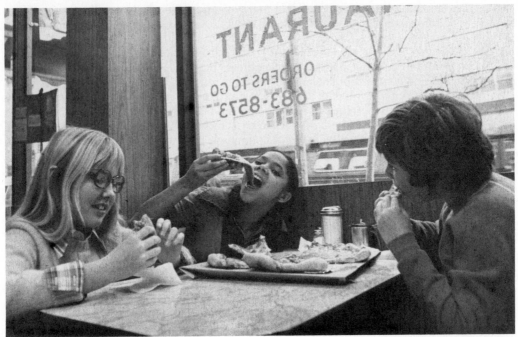

As teenagers differentiate themselves from parental beliefs, and keep up with their peer group, their dietary habits often change.
Ed Lettau/Photo Researchers

greater proportion. Depending on the choice of snack foods, individual nutrients may be in short supply. The nutrient value of the usual snack choices is highly variable. Soft drinks and candy, although readily available, provide energy but few if any nutrients. Fresh fruits and vegetables are least likely to be consumed as snacks because they are usually least likely to be at hand when an imperative hunger pang is felt.

Teenagers have always been interested in their appearance, particularly at this time of rapid body change. In their desire to conform to cultural ideals of the tall, broad-shouldered male and the slim but buxom female, teenagers often fluctuate between skimping and gorging. But adolescent self-image can be wildly inaccurate: 70 percent of girls in one study thought they were too fat, although only about 15 percent were actually overweight. Of the males surveyed, 59 percent thought they were too thin, although only 25 percent were really underweight. Skipping meals to be skinny or because of lack of time is common. Breakfast and lunch are the meals usually skipped. Omitting nutritious foods such as bread and milk can be detrimental to overall health in the teen years.

Adolescent rebelliousness, peer pressure, and a new-found interest in health may actually lead to a greater emphasis on nutrition in the home. Many young people are using food as one means of asserting independence, and they have introduced new food patterns such as vegetarianism, use of organically grown foods, or adherence to kosher dietary laws into the home. As long as a wide enough variety of food items is consumed to meet the adolescent's increased nutrient and energy needs, alternate food patterns do not pose any problem.

Recently consuming "health" foods such as freshly prepared vegetable juices, salads, and yogurt has become socially acceptable for teenagers. Students are requesting such foods from their school cafeterias, and in some instances food service managers have invited student participation in menu planning. Teenagers have also become involved in the political and social issues affecting food supply; ecological concerns on a world and community level are reflected in greater attention to the quality of what is consumed by the individual. Curiosity about nutrition and their own bodies is also characteristic of today's adolescents, and it affords an opportunity for nutrition education.

Recommendations for Good Nutrition

Teenagers should consume at least four servings of milk or milk products (cheese, ice cream, yogurt, puddings), two servings of meat-group foods (meat, fish, poultry, eggs, legumes), and four servings each from the fruits and vegetables and grain groups. Since surveys indicate that adolescents' diets are typically low in calcium, ascorbic acid, and vitamin A, a special effort should be made to include foods containing these nutrients in the daily meal plan. Girls should pay particular attention to including good sources of iron in their diets.

Increased portion sizes and second helpings at regular family meals will meet teenagers' increased nutrient requirements and their increased energy needs as well. Breakfast should not be skipped; the high nutrient content of breakfast foods and the energy provided by this meal are needed for the day's activities. Teenagers should be reminded that a cheese or peanut butter sandwich or dinner leftovers are perfectly acceptable breakfast foods. Girls are most likely to skip breakfast in a misguided attempt to control their weight; they often end up snacking more as a result.

Snacks can be counted on to provide additional energy, but they should not replace foods that contribute significant nutrients as well. The availability of nutritious snacks in the family refrigerator and pantry—fruits and juices, cheese and crackers, ice cream, milk, yogurt, peanut butter, raw vegetables, whole-grain cereals—will increase the probability that at least some snacks will be nutritionally valuable. For young people who make it a practice to select such items, consuming a soft drink shouldn't be guilt-provoking.

Special Concerns

Superimposed on the increased physiological demands for energy and nutrients for the adolescent body are the many external pressures of teenage life. Because of social pressures and erratic physical development, eating patterns may not be adjusted to actual nutrient needs. Changes in physical activity may significantly increase or decrease energy needs. Both girls and boys are subject to peer pressures to participate in alcohol and drug use, which may impair food intake and nutrient metabolism.

ENERGY BALANCE.   About 30 percent of teenagers are overweight, although only about 15 percent are actually obese. Teenage obesity is often a continuation of a childhood pattern. But adolescent obesity also characteristically develops in the years from 10 to 14. If the body fat deposited in early adolescence is not dissipated during the growth spurt that follows, the teenager will have to work hard to lose it. Otherwise an overweight future is very likely because those who remain overweight at the end of adolescence tend to be overweight throughout adult life.

Adolescent obesity may also result from dramatically lowered activity levels, especially for girls. Boys, who are generally more active, tend to lose stored adipose tissue more readily. Also, because of their greater energy requirements over a longer period of time, a moderate deficit in energy consumption will be reflected more rapidly in changed body build. But many overweight teenagers, too embarrassed to participate in sports, lose an opportunity not only to lose weight but to enhance their social lives as well. The increasing opportunity for today's young women to participate in active sports is beneficial and far more effective in weight control than crash diets and skipping meals. Habits of physical activity developed during adolescence carry over into the adult years, a further benefit.

For the overweight teenager of either sex, moderate decreases in energy intakes, while maintaining nutrient levels, can usually be achieved by reducing the number of snacks, desserts, and second portions. An occasional "treat" should be allowed to avoid strong feelings of deprivation and to provide for social activities. Denying the urge to socialize at the local pizzeria may be even more difficult than denying the urge for pizza itself. Regular meals, instead of skipping meals, will discourage binging. Fruit snacks and salad bar lunches will also help. Diet groups especially for teenagers have been formed in many communities and schools; these groups may be particularly helpful to some at this socially conscious time of life.

At the opposite end of the energy spectrum is anorexia nervosa. Teenage girls are particularly prone to this syndrome of self-imposed starvation; those who succumb to it require medical, nutritional, and psychological support. Many teenagers also use excessive exercise or vomiting as a method of weight control (see Bulimia, Chapter 5).

ALCOHOL AND DRUG USE. An increasing number of teenagers have been using mood-changing substances in the past few decades. Widespread use of drugs is a relatively recent phenomenon, which seems to have peaked in the mid-1970s. Since then, however, alcohol use among adolescents has been increasing. Many drugs affect the biochemical mechanisms and physiological systems involved in nutrient metabolism, and they may alter appetite and influence food intakes as well. Alcoholic beverages contain significant amounts of energy and will contribute to weight gain if consumed regularly; because they contain few nutrients, overall nutritional status will be compromised if they replace nutritious foods.

For the increasing numbers of girls still in the growing years who are taking oral contraceptives, there is concern as well. Effects on nutrient metabolism of adult women have been noted, and it seems likely that younger women would be even more strongly affected.

ACNE. Skin problems, a particular trial of adolescents, are popularly ascribed to dietary causes. Nutrition often does play a role, but not the role it is popularly assigned. There is, for example, no evidence that fatty foods such as chocolate, fried chicken, and french fried potatoes or acid foods such as pickles and vinegar cause acne. A derivative of vitamin A has a beneficial effect in cases of severe acne; this compound, retinoic acid, is available only by prescription. Large doses of vitamin A are not an effective substitute. Moreover, large doses of vitamin A are dangerous.

DENTAL HEALTH. Adolescents' dental hygiene is often complicated by orthodontic appliances. Braces and other hardware that appear almost indigenous to the teenage mouth interfere with tooth brushing and may contribute to decay, especially if the wearer consumes sticky foods that adhere to the appliances and remain in contact with the tooth surface. For this reason, and because of possible damage to the wires, orthodontists advise against chewing gum and eating caramels and similar foods and stress the importance of regular and thorough oral hygiene.

PREGNANCY. The demands of pregnancy at a time of unfinished growth and increased nutrient requirements for the mother create serious competition between her needs and those of her growing baby. Combined with the typically inadequate medical supervision and poor dietary habits of those girls most at risk of incurring pregnancy, this almost ensures a poor outcome for both mother and infant. Nutritional guidance, medical supervision, counseling, and continued schooling should all be available for the pregnant teenager.

Nutritional Status of American Teenagers

Data from national and local surveys indicate that adolescents have a high prevalence of "unsatisfactory" nutritional status. In a relatively affluent Iowa population the iron intake of girls was inadequate, and both boys and girls often skipped breakfast and rarely ate green vegetables. But vitamin A, riboflavin, and calcium intakes from the generous consumption of dairy products were good in this group.

Generally, adolescents consistently fall below RDA levels in their intake of calcium, vitamin A, vitamin C, and iron, with these deficiencies being accentuated in girls. Boys tend to come closer to RDA levels simply because of the greater amount of food they consume to meet appetite demands and energy needs. Girls, whose energy needs are less, frequently diet and decrease their total food and nutrient in-

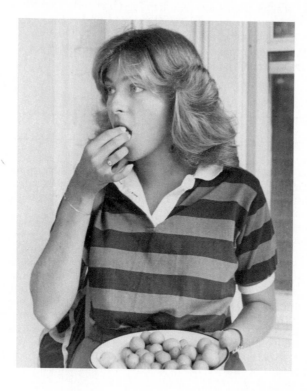

The availability of nutritious snacks, such as fresh fruits and vegetables, will increase the probability that at least some snacks will be nutritionally valuable.

David A. Strickler/Monkmeyer Press

takes even more. Too often, energy-rich and nutrient-poor foods are chosen instead of more nutritious items. Soft drinks, coffee, tea, and alcoholic beverages may replace milk and juice consumption. Milk drinking diminishes in the teen years because it has a "kid's food" image, and it may also be a particular problem for those with lactose intolerance. But ice cream, yogurt, and cheese are nutritious substitutes, and milk itself can be consumed in moderate amounts even by those who are lactose intolerant. Although surveys in the United States indicate that some nutrients are in short supply in teenage diets, the major concerns are obesity, iron deficiency, anorexia nervosa, dental caries, and pregnancy.

Attention should focus on defining more realistically the nutrient requirements of this age group. Nutrition education at school and for the family will give individuals the information they need to monitor and improve their own food intakes. Whether they do or not, however, depends on their degree of motivation.

Adult condemnation of the sometimes quirky food habits of teenagers will fall on deaf ears. Mere repetition of the basic food groups and advice from teachers or parents to eat "because it's good for you" are just plain boring to most adolescents, who have been hearing it all since kindergarten—or think they have. But teens are a potentially receptive audience for nutrition information presented in a factual, interesting, and nonpatronizing way. Teens want the facts. They want to know how their bodies work and what their bodies need. They are concerned about their health, their appearance, and their performance in school and in athletic events. They will respond to information that can be put to use *now*.

Participating in learning activities in the classroom, sharing responsibilities for meal planning and preparation in the home, involvement in nutrition-related projects at school and in the community—all these are approaches through which young people can be reached and their food habits influenced. True learning comes with self-discovery. Given the information they need and want, teens will have their own reasons for incorporating it into their daily lives. This is a period of energy, enthusiasm, and intellectual discovery; it is an opportunity for sound nutritional education that must not be lost.

SUMMARY

From the moment of birth an individual becomes dependent on the external environment for food, shelter, and nurturing. Food does more than provide nutrients needed for physical growth; it is part of the environment that fosters social, emotional, and behavioral development.

Growth during infancy (birth to 12 months) is very rapid—birth weight almost triples and height increases by 9 or 10 inches. Although there is wide agreement that food is an important determinant of growth and development, actual feeding practices have been the subject of controversy—and changes of fashion—over the years. Most experts now agree that the average infant can be adequately nourished by either human milk or formula, but the American Academy of Pediatrics has endorsed breast-feeding for normal infants.

Breast milk confers several advantages over commercial formulas, including immunological protection. Most commercially available formulas are based on cow's milk that is modified to approximate the composition of human milk. The use of unmodified cow's milk, whether whole or skim, is not appropriate. Young infants require supplementation with vitamin D, iron, and fluoride, unless these are provided in formulas.

The optimal time for introducing solid foods is now considered to be four to six months of age, when babies become able to initiate swallowing. Solid foods should be introduced gradually. Diversity in nutrients, tastes, and textures at this early time will be a positive influence on food preferences in later life.

Growth during childhood (1 to 12 years) is much less rapid than in infancy, averaging 2 to 4 inches and 4 to 8 pounds per year for most of this period. Height and weight records are important indicators of health and may provide the earliest signs of undernutrition, disease, or overnutrition.

Nutritional requirements during childhood reflect growth rate and physical activity. In relation to body weight they are proportionately less than during the first year of life.

Eating behaviors and food preferences are influenced by the school environment, by friends, and by the mass media. Children are better able to withstand adverse influences if appropriate eating habits are developed at home and reinforced daily. Children should not be forced to "finish everything" or to eat foods they initially reject. A relaxed mealtime atmosphere and tolerance of the child's changing tastes are important.

The growth rate during adolescence (13 to 19 years) is second only to that during infancy. The most obvious changes are increased stature, change of body composition, and sexual maturation. But unlike the relatively predictable growth of infants, the rate and timing of adolescent growth and development are highly variable.

Nutritional requirements for adolescents are as variable as their growth patterns and closely parallel the latter. Adolescents tend to have casual attitudes toward eating and are greatly influenced by peers. The major concerns during teen years are obesity, iron deficiency, anorexia nervosa, dental caries, and pregnancy.

BIBLIOGRAPHY

AAS KJELL. Antigens in food. *Nutrition Reviews* 42;85–91, 1984.

American Academy of Pediatrics. Breast-feeding. *Pediatrics* 62(4): 591, 1978.

ANDERSON, G.H., W.M. LOVEBERG, H. LUBIN, D. MORRIS, AND R.E. OLSON, eds. *Nutrition Review Supplement: Diet and Behavior.* Vol. 44, April 1986.

ATKINS, F.M. The Basics of immediate hypersensitivity reactions to foods. *Nutrition Reviews* 41:229–234, 1983.

BEHAR, D., J.L. RAPOPORT, A.J. ADAMS, C.J. BERG, AND M. CORNBLATH. Sugar challenge testing with children considered behaviorally "sugar reactive." *Nutrition and Behavior* 1:277, 1984.

BERKOWITZ, R.I., W.S. AGRAS, A.F. KORNER, H.C. KRAEMER, AND C.H. ZEANAH. Physical activity and adiposity: A longitudinal study from birth to childhood. *Journal of Pediatrics* 106:734–738, 1985.

BRADY, M.S., K.A. RICKARD, J.A. ERNST, R.L. SCHREINER, AND J.A. LEMONS. Formulas and human milk for premature infants: A review and update. *Journal of the American Dietetic Association* 81:547–552, 1982.

BRECHIN, S.J.G. The etiology of low birthweight and its economic impact in developing countries. *Ecology of Food and Nutrition* 14:325–335, 1984.

BROWN, R. et al. Iron status of adolescent female athletes. *Journal of Adolescent Health Care* 6:349, 1985.

BURT, J.V., AND A.A. HERTZLER. Parental influence on the child's food preference. *Journal of Nutrition Education* 10(3):127, 1978.

CALIENDO, M.A., D. SANJUR, J. WRIGHT, AND G. CUMMINGS. Nutritional status of preschool children. *Journal of the American Dietetic Association* 71:20, 1977.

CASEY, C.E., P.A. WALRAVENS, AND K.M. HAMBIDGE. Availability of zinc: Loading test with human milk, cow's milk, and infant formulas. *Pediatrics* 68:394–396, 1981.

Committee on Nutrition, American Academy of Pediatrics. Toward a prudent diet for children. *Pediatrics* 71:78–80, 1983.

CONNERS, C.K., AND A.G. BLOUIN. Nutritional effects on behavior of children. *Journal of Psychiatric Research* 17:193–198, 1982/83.

CONNERS, C.K., C.H. GOYETTE, D.A. SOUTHWICK, J.M. LEES, AND P.A. ANDRULONIS. Food additives and hyperkinesis: A controlled double-blind experiment. *Pediatrics* 58:154, 1976.

COWART, B.J. Development of taste perception in humans: Sensitivity and preference throughout the life span. *Psychological Bulletin* 90:43–73, 1981.

CRAYTON, J.W. Immunologically mediated behavioral reactions to foods. *Food Technology* 40:153–157, 1986.

CZAJKA-NARINS, D.M., T.B. HADDY, D.J. KALLEN. Nutrition and social correlates in iron deficiency anemia. *American Journal of Clinical Nutrition* 31:955, 1978.

Diet, Nutrition, and Oral Health. *Journal of the American Dental Association* 109:20–32, 1984.

DIETZ, W.H., AND R. HARTUNG. Changes in height velocity of obese preadolescents during weight reduction. *American Journal of Diseases of Children* 139:705, 1985.

DOBBING, J. Infant nutrition and later achievement. *American Journal of Clinical Nutrition* 41:477–484, 1985.

Doing more with less: Innovative ideas for reducing costs in the school nutrition programs. Washington, DC: Food Research and Action Center, 1983.

DRISKELL, J.A. AND S.W. MOAK. Plasma pyrodoxal phosphate concentrations and coenzyme stimulation of erythrocyte alanine aminotransferase activities of white and black adolescent girls. *American Journal of Clinical Nutrition* 43:599, 1986.

DUGDALE, E.E. Infant feeding—an unfinished debate. *Ecology of Food Nutrition* 12:71–74, 1982.

DWYER, J. Diets of children and adolescents that meet the dietary goals. *American Journal of Diseases of Children* 134:1073–1080, 1980.

————. Nutritional requirements of adolescence. *Nutrition Reviews* 39:56–72, 1981.

DWYER, J.T., W.H. DIETZ, JR., G. HASS, AND R. SUSKIND. Risk of nutritional rickets among vegetarian children. *American Journal of Diseases of Children* 133:134, 1979.

EPSTEIN, L.H., AND R.R. WING. Reanalysis of weight changes in behavior modification and nutrition education for childhood obesity. *Journal of Pediatric Psychology* 8:97–100, 1983.

FEINGOLD, B.F. *Why Your Child Is Hyperactive.* New York: Random House, 1974.

FISHER, M.C., AND P.A. LaCHANCE. Nutrition evaluation of published weight-reducing diets. *Journal of the American Dietetic Association* 85:450–454, 1985.

FOMON, S.J. *Infant Nutrition*, 2nd ed. Philadelphia: Saunders, 1974.

Food and Nutrition Board, National Research Council. *Recommended Dietary Allowances.* Washington, DC: National Academy of Sciences, 10th, ed., 1985.

FOUCARD T. Development aspects of food sensitivity in childhood. *Nutrition Reviews* 42:98–104, 1984.

FRICKER, H.S., AND S. SEGAL. Narcotic addiction, pregnancy, and the newborn. *American Journal of Diseases of Children* 132:360, 1978.

FRISH, R. Weight at menarche: Similarity for well-nourished and undernourished girls at differing ages, and evidence for historical constancy. *Pediatrics* 50:445, 1972.

GARN, S.M., AND B. WAGNER. The adolescent growth of the skeletal mass and its implications to mineral requirements. In F. Heald, ed. *Adolescent Nutrition and Growth.* New York: Meredith Corp., 1969.

GILLESPIE, A. Assessing snacking behavior in children. *Ecology of Food Nutrition* 13:167–172, 1983.

GRAY, G.E. AND L.K. GRAY. Diet and juvenile deliquency. *Nutrition Today*, pp. 14–22, 1983.

GROSS, M.D. Effect of sucrose on hyperkinetic children. *Pediatrics* 74:876–891, 1984.

GUSTAFSON, B.E., C. QUENSEL, L. LANKE, et al. Vipeholm dental caries study. *Acta Odontologica Scandinavia* 11:232, 1954.

HARPER, A.E., AND D.A. GANS. Claims of antisocial behavior from consumption of sugar: An assessment. *Food Technology* 40:142–149, 1986.

HAGER, A. Nutritional problems in adolescents—obesity. *Nutrition Reviews* 39:89–95, 1981.

HANES, S., J. VERMEERSCH, AND S. GALE. The national evaluation of school nutrition programs: Program impact on dietary intake. *American Journal of Clinical Nutrition* 40:390–413, 1984.

HARLEY, J.P., R.S. RAY, L. TOMASI, P.L. EICHMAN, C.G. MATTHEWS, R. CHUN, C.S. CLEELAND, AND E. TRAISMAN. Hyperkinesis and food additives: Testing the Feingold hypothesis. *Pediatrics* 61:818, 1978.

HEIMENDINGER, J., N. LAIRD, J.E. AUSTIN, P. TIMMER, AND S. GERSHOFF. The effects of the WIC program on the growth of infants. *American Journal of Clinical Nutrition* 40:1250–1257, 1984.

HODGES, R.E. Vitamin and mineral requirements in adolescence. In *Nutrient Requirements in Adolescence*, J.I. McKigney and H.N. Munro, eds. Cambridge, MA: M.I.T. Press, 1976.

HUSE, D.M., AND A.R. LUCAS. Dietary patterns in anorexia nervosa. *American Journal of Clinical Nutrition* 40:251–254, 1984.

JELLIFFE, D.B., AND F.P. JELLIFFE. The volume and composition of human milk in poorly nourished communities: A review. *American Journal of Clinical Nutrition* 31:492, 1978.

JUNG, E., AND D.M. CZAJKA-NARINS. Birth weight doubling and tripling times: An updated look at the effects of birth weight, sex, race and type of feeding. *American Journal of Clinical Nutrition* 42:182, 1985.

KARE, M.R., AND G.K. BEAUCHAMP. The role of taste in the infant diet. *American Journal of Clinical Nutrition* 41:418–422, 1985.

KIRSKEY, A., J.A. ERNST, J.L. ROEPKE, AND T.L. TSAI. Influence of mineral intake and use of oral contraceptives before pregnancy on the mineral content of human colostrum and of mature milk. *American Journal of Clinical Nutrition* 32:30, 1979.

KLESGES, R.C., J.M. MALOTT, P.F. BOSCHEE, AND J.M. WEBER. The effects of parental influences on children's food intake, physical activity and relative weight. *International Journal of Eating Disorders* 5:335, 1986.

KRIEGER, I. *Pediatric Disorders of Feeding, Nutrition, and Metabolism.* New York: John Wiley and Sons, 1982.

KRUESI, M.J.P. Carbohydrate intake and children's behavior. *Food Technology* 40:150–152, 1986.

KUCZMARSKI, R.J., E.R. BREWER, F.J. CRONIN, B. DENNIS, K. GRAVES, AND S. HAYNES. Food choices among white adolescents: The lipid research clinics prevalence study. *Pediatric Research* 20:309, 1986.

KULIN, H.E., N. BWIBO, D. MUTIE, AND S.J. SANTNER. Gonadotrophin excretion during puberty in malnourished children. *Journal of Pediatrics* 105:325–328, 1984.

LEBOW, M.D. *Child Obesity: A New Frontier of Beahvior Therapy.* New York: Springer, 1984.

LEVY, Y., A. ZEHARIA, M. GRUNEBAUM, M. NITZAN, AND R. STEINHERZ. Copper deficiency in infants fed cow milk. *Journal of Pediatrics* 106:786–788, 1985.

LIPTON, M.A., AND J.P. MAYO. Diet and Hyperkinesis—an update. *Journal of the American Dietetic Association* 83:132–134, 1983.

LOWENBERG, M.E. The development of food patterns in young children. In *Nutrition in Infancy and Childhood*, 3rd ed. P. Pipes, ed., St. Louis, MO: C.V. Mosby, 1985.

MCKIGNEY, J.I., AND J.N. MUNRO, eds. *Nutrient Requirements in Adolescence.* Cambridge, MA: M.I.T. Press, 1976.

MALLER, O., AND J.A. DESOR. Effect of taste in ingestion by human newborns. In *Oral Sensation and Perception*, J.F. Bosma, ed. USDHEW publication No. (NIH) 73–546, Bethesda, MD: USDHEW, 1973.

MALLICK, M. Health hazards of obesity and weight control in children: A review of the literature. *American Journal of Public Health* 73:78–82, 1983.

MILLER, S.A. Social policy issues in the introduction of food to infants: Limitations of government. *American Journal of Clinical Nutrition* 41:502–507, 1985.

MUELLER, J.F. Current dietary recommendations for adolescents. in *Nutrient Requirements in Adolescence*, J.I. McKigney and H.N. Munro, eds. Cambridge, MA: M.I.T. Press, 1976.

OWEN, G.M. et al. A study of nutritional status of preschool children in the United States, 1968–1970. *Pediatrics Supplement* 53:597, 1974.

OUNSTED, M., V.A. MOAR, AND A. SCOTT. Children of deviant birthweight: The influence of genetic and other factors on size at seven years. *Acta Paediatrica Scandinavica* 74:707, 1985.

OWEN, G.M., P.J. GARRY, AND E.M. HOOPER. Feeding and growth of infants. *Nutrition Research* 4:727, 1984.

PIPES, P. *Nutrition in Infancy and Childhood.* 3rd ed. St. Louis, MO: C.V. Mosby, 1985.

POPKIN, B.M., R.E. BILSBORROW, AND J.S. AKIN. Breast-feeding patterns in low-income countries. *Science* 218:1088–1093, 1982.

PUGLIESE, H.T., F. LIFSCHITZ, G. GRAD, P. FORT, AND M. MARKS-KATZ. Fear of Obesity: A Cause of Short Stature and Delayed Puberty. *New England Journal of Medicine* 309:513–518, 1983.

ROWE, J.D., ROWE, E. HORAK, R. SPACKMAN, R. SALTZMANN, S. ROBINSON, A. PHILLIPS, AND J. RAYE. Hypophosphatemia and hypercalciuria in small premature infants fed human milk: Evidence for inadquate dietary phosphorus. *Journal of Pediatircs* 104:112–117, 1985.

RUMSEY, J.M, AND J.L. RAPOPORT. Assessing behavioral and cognitive effects of diet in pediatric populations. In R.J. Wurtman and J.J. Wurtman, eds. *Nutrition and the Brain*, Vol. 6, New York: Raven Press, 1983.

SAARINEN, U.M., M.A. SHMES, AND P.R. DALLMAN. Iron absorption in infants: High bioavailability of breast milk iron as indicated by the extrinsic tag method of iron absorption and by the concentration of serum ferritin. *Journal of Pediatrics* 91:36, 1977.

SAVAGE, R.L. Drugs and breast milk. *Journal of Human Nutrition* 31:459, 1977.

SCHLEIMER, K. Anorexia nervosa. *Nutrition Reviews* 39:99–103, 1981.

SHULL, M.W., R.B. REED, I. VALADIAN, R. PALOMBO, H. THORNE, AND J.T. DWYER. Velocities of growth in vegetarian preschool children. *Pediatrics* 60:410, 1977.

SPADY, D.W. Total daily energy expenditure of healthy, free ranging school children. *American Journal of Clinical Nutrition* 33:766–775, 1980.

STEKEL, A., ed. *Iron Nutrition in Infancy and Childhood.* New York: Raven Press, 1984.

STORZ, N.S., AND W.H. GREENE. Body weight, body image, and perception of fad diets in adolescent girls. *Journal of Nutrition Education* 15:15–18, 1983.

TANNER, J.M. *Growth at Adolescence*, 2nd ed. Oxford: Blackwell Scientific Publications, 1962.

TYRALA, E.E. Zinc and copper balances in preterm infants. *Pediatrics* 77:513–517, 1986.

U.S. Department of Health, Education, and Welfare. NCHS Growth Curves for Children, Birth-18 Years United States (DHEW Publication NO. (PHS) 78–1650). Hyattsville, MD: National Center for Health Statistics, 1977.

VENTERS, M., AND R. MULLIS. Family-oriented nutrition education and preschool obesity. *Journal of Nutritional Education* 16:159–161, 1984.

WARD, S., D. LEVINSON, AND D. WACKMAN. Children's attention to television commercials. In *Television and Social Behavior, Vol. 4: Television in Day-to-Day Life: Patterns of Use*, E.E. Rubinstein, G.A. Coinstock, and J.P. Murray, eds. Washington, DC: U.S. Government Printing Office, 1972.

WORSLEY, A., P.A. BAGHURST, A.J. WORSLEY, AND W.COONAN. Nice good food and us: a study of children's food beliefs. *Journal of Food and Nutrition* 40:35–41, 1983.

WORSLEY, A., P. BAGHURST, A.J. WORSLEY, W. COONAN, AND M. PETERS. Australian ten year olds' perceptions of food: 1. Sex differences. *Ecology of Food Nutrition* 15:231–246, 1984.

WORTHINGTON, B.S. AND L.E. TAYLOR. Guidance for lactating mothers. In *Nutrition in Pregnancy and Lactation*, 3rd ed. B.S. Worthington, J. Vermeersch, and S.R. Williams, eds. St. Louis, MO: C.V. Mosby, 1985.

WORTHINGTON-ROBERTS, B. Nutrition and maternal health. *Nutrition Today* Nov./Dec. 1984 p. 6.

YEUNG, D.L., M.D. PENNELL, M. LEUNG, AND J. HALL. The effects of 2% milk intake in infant nutrition. *Nutrition Research* 2:651, 1982.

Chapter 13

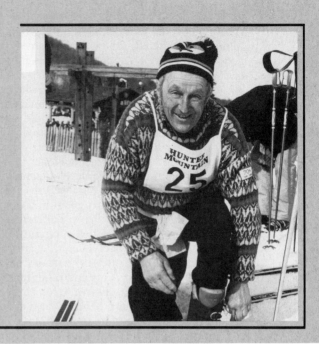

THE ADULT YEARS

447

Adulthood is the most creative, productive, and active stage of life. New responsibilities are assumed; a new generation is conceived and nurtured; and the ideas, goods, and services that contribute to national growth and the well-being of society are produced.

To divide the adult years into three stages—early, middle, and elderly—is somewhat false and arbitrary. No one landmark birthday separates early adulthood from the middle years or maturity from old age. In our youth-oriented society, this stereotyping tends to promote a biased point of view. Most of us will become middle-aged and then elderly, and this should be ample motivation to change our attitudes toward the older generation.

Aging is continuous with development, and in this sense can be said to begin at conception. Although physical growth is generally complete by early adulthood, the body's tissues and cells remain in a dynamic state. Aging does not proceed at the same rate in all individuals. Differences in heredity, environment, and health care can cause wide disparities in physical condition and health status between individuals of the same age. There is a greater probability that older adults will be afflicted with chronic diseases that may cause discomfort and eventually result in death. But chronic ailments and other factors contributing to increased morbidity and mortality often appear in the fourth decade of life—hardly "old age," as anyone over thirty can attest. Most of these factors minimally alter the lifestyle of individuals unless they become severe.

Gerontology, a field of study that effectively began in the late 1950s and expanded rapidly in the 1970s, explores the psychosocial, physiological, economic, and medical aspects of aging. The rapid recent development of this field is related to the increasing numbers of people surviving into the seventh, eighth, and ninth decades of life. There are in the United States some 27 million people over 65 years of age and more than 10 million age 75 and over, representing 11.3 and 4.4 percent of the total population respectively (see Table 13-1). The Bureau of the Census has projected that by 2050, there will be approximately 70 million people over age 65, representing 21.7 percent of the total population. The most rapidly growing segment of the population is the 85 and over group, which will increase from 1 percent of the total population in 1980 to a projected 5.2 percent in 2050 or about 17 million. The sex ratio increases rapidly with age. In 1983 there were 241 women for every 100 men in the 85 and over age group.

These projections challenge us as a nation to find new measures to ensure the quality of life for older adults. They challenge us to revise the stereotypical thinking of the past, when the truly old were few and often infirm. We can no longer perceive all older adults as impoverished, sickly, helpless, and ineffective. There are certainly many who conform to this description, but as more people live longer and healthier lives, the inactive and incapacitated elderly become an ever-smaller proportion of the total which at present is only about 5 percent. The needs of the

TABLE 13-1. *Population of Older Adults in the United States, 1980–2050*

	POPULATION IN MILLIONS				PERCENT OF TOTAL POPULATION			
	1980	*2000*	*2025*	*2050*	*1980*	*2000*	*2025*	*2050*
65 and over	27	37	60	68	11.3	13.1	19.5	21.7
75 and over	10	19	28	30	4.4	6.5	8.5	9.1
85 and over	2	5	9	17	1.0	1.9	2.8	5.2

Sources: G.A. Leveille and P.F. Cloutier. Role of the food industry in meeting the nutritional needs of the elderly. *Food Technology* 40:82, February 1986.

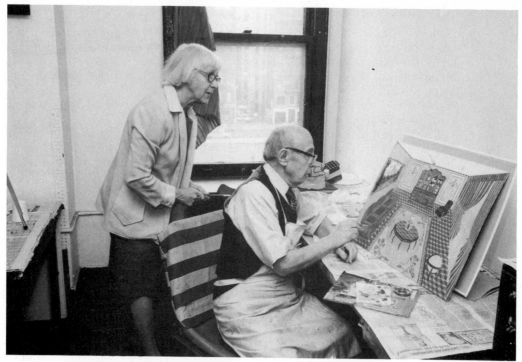

Nutritional status does have a great deal to do with the quality of life. Individuals who are well nourished feel healthier, have more energy, and are usually better able to withstand the stresses of life.

Ken Karp, Sirovich Senior Center

helpless elderly must be met, as must the needs of the helpless of all ages. But an increasing number of today's older adults are financially comfortable, healthy, and physically and economically active.

Our concern in this chapter is with the nutrition-related health problems and the nutritional status of adults of all ages, with particular attention to the special nutritional needs of people of older age. Throughout life, cells remain active, producing energy and metabolic products to sustain the whole organism. Metabolism may slow down, but it does not cease. Nourishment is therefore needed until the end of life.

THE AGING PROCESS

Although aging takes place throughout life, the physiological processes of adulthood are different from those of the growing years. Once physical growth has ceased and reproductive capacity has been attained, the catabolic rate (cell breakdown) slightly exceeds the anabolic rate (cell growth), except during pregnancy and lactation. As a result of this new equilibrium, there is a gradual decrease in the number of cells in the body.

Theories of Aging

All body structures are made of molecules and all body functions depend on molecules. Yet only in the last 20 years have theories of aging been developed that take molecular changes in the body into account. Earlier theories were predicated on observations of the external evidence of aging, such as stooped gait, gray hair, and wrinkled skin. Today's theories attempt to explain these observations in terms of events taking place at the cellular and molecular levels, ascribing the causes of aging to environmental or genetic conditions.

Environmental theorists use a "wear and tear" approach: The accumulation of external and physiological stress eventually wears out the body and its tissues. Some believe that exposure to naturally occurring radiation produces cumulative tissue damage that is ultimately fatal. Radiation causes mutations that result in cell abnormalities, ultimately damaging DNA and impeding protein synthesis so that the cell deteriorates before it can replicate or be repaired. Because cellular repair mechanisms are quite efficient, however, this theory is not widely accepted.

A related theory centers on "free radicals," highly reactive compounds produced intracellularly by cosmic radiation. Free radicals induce peroxidation of unsaturated fatty acids, thereby affecting cell membranes and damaging vital cell structures such as mitochondria and the endoplasmic reticulum. Those who promote the free radical theory of aging tend to believe that vitamin E can protect against lipid peroxidation by free radicals. Others recommend ascorbic acid and selenium as antioxidants. Whether this chain of events is the cause of aging, and whether vitamin E or any other nutrient can affect it, is subject to much debate, although it is clear that free radical formation and related cell pathology are real events in the aging body.

A predominant genetic theory postulates a biological "time clock" that puts a natural limit to the number of times a cell can replicate itself. According to another genetic view of aging, there may be losses of the information coded into the DNA and RNA. This may cause defective or insufficient amounts of enzymes to be produced during protein synthesis, resulting in various kinds of cell dysfunction. Other effects of changes in nucleic acids have also been suggested, among them that the body's immunologic capacity progressively decreases with advancing age. Lacking this protection, the autoimmune reactions of the body increase, and the body virtually attacks itself.

A variation of the "time clock" theory focuses on collagen, the most abundant body protein and a major constituent of connective tissue, found throughout the body. Progressive cross-linking between collagen molecules apparently is responsible for the loss of flexibility of muscle fibers (resulting in body stiffness) and the decreased efficiency of cardiac muscle contraction. Although collagen cross-linkage does occur in the aging process, the extent to which it is a cause of aging is unclear.

Extensive research is needed to clarify all these theories and others. Probably no single reason for aging will be found and no way will be found to reverse or halt its effects. The aging process is complex. It is also, despite the claims of fad-diet promoters and cosmetic and drug companies, irreversible. To foster any hope of increasing an individual's life span through use of any food, nutrient, or other substance, taken internally or applied externally, is irresponsible.

Nutrition and Longevity

Because the nutrients contained in food are metabolized into body components and structures to hypothesize that nutritional factors play a direct and decisive role in longevity is tempting. However, there is no concrete evidence that any one food or nutrient will guarantee extra years. But nutritional status does have a great deal to do with the quality of life and may indeed have an effect on its length.

Individuals who are well nourished feel healthier, have more vigor, and are usually better able to withstand physiological and psychological stresses than are those on nutritionally poor diets. There also appears to be a relationship between long-term energy intake and longevity in animals. Years ago it was demonstrated that rats had a longer life span when their energy intakes were severely restricted from early life. Lean and chronically undernourished rats live longer. Although these results support the observations that human obesity is associated with a shortened life, the severe experimental conditions used in these studies cannot be imposed on humans. Thus, direct application of these research findings to humans is not warranted.

Excessive intakes of some nutrients as well as some nonnutrient substances have been implicated in decreasing life span by contributing to serious illnesses. Excess sodium appears to play a part in promoting hypertension in susceptible people, and a high-fat diet may contribute to coronary heart disease and certain types of cancer. Relatively few of the many food additives on the market have been found to be harmful. But much more research is needed to clarify the relationship of individual foods and nutrients to disease and longevity.

Physiological Changes During the Life Span

The *causes* of aging may be unknown, but all individuals experience gradually decreased and/or altered function of various physiological systems throughout their lives. The degree and rate of change vary from one individual to the next due to genetic potential and/or lifestyle, including dietary intake, but ultimately every human who lives long enough will experience some of these body changes.

Skin changes are among the most obvious. Changes in the molecular structure of collagen and in the activity of sebaceous glands under the skin can cause the skin to become increasingly dry and wrinkled and can produce warts and tumors. Bruise marks on the skin indicate that underlying blood vessel walls have become fragile.

Changes in bones, muscles, ligaments, and joints are responsible for body stiffness and stooped posture. There is some shrinkage in height because of shrinkage in cartilaginous material between the bones of the spinal column. Those structural changes can affect other systems: When the body is compressed and stooped, respiration becomes more labored; weakened abdominal and pelvic muscles contribute to difficulties in urination and defecation.

Alterations in the nervous system may be reflected in tremors or changed facial expressions. Reflexes are slowed, and it may take a longer time to change position or recover balance. Short-term memory may be less efficient. Personality changes such as increased passivity, fear of anything new and unusual, possessiveness, and depression may have a physiological as well as psychological component. Changes in the blood supply to the brain as well as changes in the nervous system are at least partly responsible for these and other effects.

Efficiency of renal function also decreases with age, even when there is no diagnosed renal disease. This in turn alters the electrolyte and water balance in the body, which depends on highly intricate kidney functions to reabsorb water and sodium, filter out wastes, and maintain the delicate balance of body fluids.

In the cardiovascular system, several age related changes occur. These include a slight hypertrophy of the left ventricle. In spite of this increase, the pumping ability of the heart is reduced as the strength of contraction is diminished. There is also a reduction in the ability of the heart to respond to stress. Decreased output and increased circulatory time have the effect of delivering nutrients to the cells less efficiently.

Many people find one or more of their sensory organs becoming less sensitive; sight, hearing, smell, touch, and taste may all be impaired, although not equally in all individuals. Lessened taste acuity is due to a reduction in the number of taste buds as well as to neurological changes. Diminished salivation may cause an increase in dental caries and difficulty in swallowing.

Decreased secretion of hydrochloric acid, pepsin, and intrinsic factor by stomach cells will impair the efficiency of digestion and absorption, particularly of protein and vitamin B_{12}. Changes in digestive glands often affect the absorption of calcium, lactose, and the fat-soluble vitamins. There is a slowing down of the reflex muscular movements that propel nutrients and wastes through the digestive tract. Digestion and absorption become less efficient. While this is not as important for well absorbed nutrients, it is potentially more critical for those absorbed with lower efficiency such as the trace minerals. Constipation because of slowed colonic motility is a common complaint.

Among other frequent metabolic changes are the decreases in glucose tolerance and in the basal metabolic rate. The latter change is due to the fact that since lean body mass decreases by 10 to 15 percent after the age of 50, less energy is needed to maintain the smaller lean body mass. This lowers energy requirements. All these changes may be exacerbated when disease is imposed on the aging process.

Changes in the reproductive systems are experienced by both men and women; loss of the ability to reproduce takes place earlier—usually in the late 40s or early 50s—and is more obvious in women than are corresponding changes in men. Although their physical responsiveness gradually alters, men have been able to father children even in their late 70s. In women the menopause is not physiologically associated with a loss of sexual interest or capacity, nor is it necessarily accompanied by distressing symptoms. Only 15 to 25 percent of women consult physicians because of discomfort and difficulties at this time.

Although none of these changes happens overnight, and indeed many people never have them, they can adversely affect nutritional status in various ways. Individuals who are not able to breathe deeply or move easily, or whose vision, smell, or taste is impaired, are likely to have a loss of appetite. Lack of exercise also impairs digestion. Shopping and food preparation become burdensome for those who are unable to move about readily or who have difficulty reading signs and labels. Disturbed enzyme production and renal dysfunction affect nutrient metabolism.

The cumulative deficits of body function in older age are increasingly apparent because more and more people are living longer. Average life expectancy at birth for the population as a whole is expected to reach 80 years before the year 2000. Figure 13-1 shows the increase in life expectancy for males and females since 1930.

The generally steady increase in longevity over the years is largely due to the conquest of the communicable diseases that formerly proved fatal. Hygienic measures, immunizations, and antibiotics have virtually removed this category of diseases from the leading causes of death during the twentieth century. Today, heart disease, cancer, and cerebrovascular diseases account for more than two-thirds of all deaths; less than 3 percent were caused by influenza and pneumonia, formerly significant causes of death.

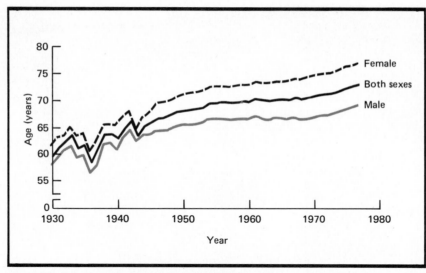

FIGURE 13-1   *Life Expectancy by Sex, 1930–1977.*

Source: National Center for Health Statistics, Final mortality statistics, 1977. *Monthly Vital Statistics Report*, USDHEW Pub. No. (PHS) 79-1120, Vol. 28, No. 1, Supplement, May 11, 1979.

NUTRITIONAL REQUIREMENTS FOR ADULTS

Younger adults as well as older ones may have medical problems that interfere with food intake and utilization and thus alter their nutrient requirements. Gall bladder disease often strikes people in their 30s; ulcers, hiatus hernia, and other chronic conditions of the gastrointestinal tract may cause adults to be concerned over what and when they eat. These and other conditions require medication that in turn may alter metabolism of one or more nutrients.

Nutrient Needs

Because of the various physiological changes throughout adult life, nutrient requirements change as well. If an individual has consumed a well-balanced diet through the developmental years, there needn't be dramatic changes in terms of the quality or kinds of food eaten in adulthood; the same nutrients are essential at every age, because basically the same body processes are taking place.

ENERGY.   For most people, energy needs change with age. After the growth spurt of adolescence, there is a steady decline in energy requirements. As aging progresses and activity levels and the basal metabolic rate decline, energy requirements drop steadily. The total amount of food consumed should decrease accordingly. Most individuals will automatically and consciously reduce intakes at some point in every decade of life, starting in the mid- to late twenties. The exact ages

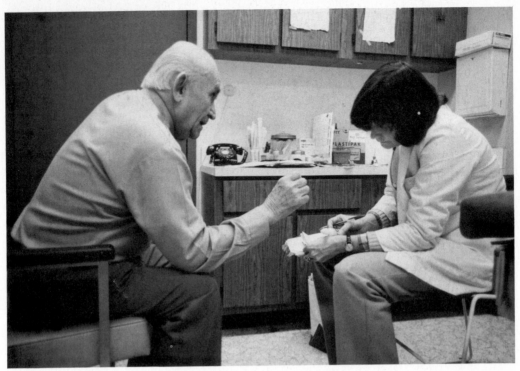

Public awareness of the role of preventive care is lessening the need for crisis intervention.
Ken Karp

and amounts involved, however, vary from one individual to the next; those who are physically active will need to consume more kilocalories than those who are less active at any age. Experts do not agree whether the elderly should weigh more than younger adults.

Although the elderly need less energy, the need for protein, vitamins, and minerals (except iron for women) does not decline with advancing years. The RDAs for energy and nutrients in adulthood are shown in Table 13–2. Remember that RDAs are designed for healthy Americans and do not provide for the special needs of individuals who are ill, under stress, or taking medication for chronic disease.

CARBOHYDRATES. Because of reduced ability to metabolize glucose, consumption of simple carbohydrates may need to be restricted to avoid placing excessive demands on the body's ability to digest and absorb sugar. In addition, excessive complex carbohydrates are important in the diet of all adults; such foods as whole-grain or enriched breads and cereals, potatoes, and dried beans should be included regularly. These foods contain B vitamins, iron, various trace minerals, and fiber and should constitute 40 to 45 percent of the total energy intake of an adult, according to the Food and Nutrition Board. High-fiber foods are of particular importance because they help to maintain intestinal function and prevent constipation. Older adults, especially those who are not so physically active, should make a concentrated effort to include high-fiber foods in their diet. Glucose intolerance, the decreased ability to handle glucose, is more prevalent in the elderly. Current research suggests a possible role for some minerals, such as chromium and zinc, in glucose metabolism. A lower intake of certain foods plus decreased ability to absorb the minerals may combine to produce less than optimal status with regard to required minerals.

FAT. Because of research linking dietary fat to high serum cholesterol levels and atherosclerosis, intake of dietary fat should be reduced to 30 to 35 percent of total energy intakes throughout the adult years. Serum cholesterol levels seem to peak in men between the ages of 50 and 59, and in women from 60 to 69. Serum triglycerides, on the other hand, increase with age for both sexes. To eliminate

TABLE 13-2. RDAs for Adults

Nutrient	MALES		FEMALES	
	23–50 yrs	51 + years[a]	23–50 years[b]	51 + years[a]
Energy (kcal)	2,700	2,400	2,000	1,800
(MJ)	11.3	10.0	8.4	7.6
Protein (gm)	56	56	44	44
Vitamin A (RE)	1,000	1,000	800	800
Vitamin D (μg)	5	5	5	5
Vitamin E (mgαTE)	10	10	8	8
Vitamin C (mg)	60	60	60	60
Folacin (μg)	400	400	400	400
Niacin (mg NE)	18	16	13	13
Riboflavin (mg)	1.6	1.4	1.2	1.2
Thiamin (mg)	1.4	1.2	1.0	1.0
Vitamin B_6 (mg)	2.2	2.2	2.0	2.0
Calcium (mg)	800	800	800	800
Phosphorus (mg)	800	800	800	800
Iodine (μg)	150	150	150	150
Iron (mg)	10	10	18	10
Magnesium (mg)	350	350	300	300
Zinc (mg)	15	15	15	15
Vitamin K (μg)[c]	70–140	70–140	70–140	70–140
Biotin (μg)[c]	100–200	100–200	100–200	100–200
Pantothenic acid (mg)[c]	4–7	4–7	4–7	4–7
Copper (mg)[c d]	2.0–3.0	2.0–3.0	2.0–3.0	2.0–3.0
Manganese (mg)[c d]	2.5–5.0	2.5–5.0	2.5–5.0	2.5–5.0
Fluoride (mg)[c d]	1.5–4.0	1.5–4.0	1.5–4.0	1.5–4.0
Chromium (mg)[c d]	0.05–0.2	0.05–0.2	0.05–0.2	0.05–0.2
Selenium (mg)[c d]	0.05–0.2	0.05–0.2	0.05–0.2	0.05–0.2
Molybdenum (mg)[c d]	0.15–0.5	0.15–0.5	0.15–0.5	0.15–0.5
Sodium (mg)[c]	1,100–3,300	1,100–3,300	1,100–3,300	1,100–3,300
Potassium (mg)[c]	1,875–5,625	1,875–5,625	1,875–5,625	1,875–5,625
Chloride (mg)[c]	1,700–5,100	1,700–5,100	1,700–5,100	1,700–5,100

[a] For age 76 and above, the energy RDA for men is 2,050 kilocalories (8.6 mJ) and for women 1,600 kilocalories (6.7 mJ).
[b] Nonpregnant, nonlactating.
[c] Estimated safe and adequate daily dietary intakes of additional selected vitamins and minerals. Because there is less information on which to base allowances, these figures are provided in the form of ranges of recommended intakes.
[d] Trace elements. Since the toxic levels for many trace elements may be only several times usual intakes, the upper levels for the trace elements given in this table should not be habitually exceeded.
Source: Food and Nutrition Board, National Research Council, *Recommended dietary allowances*, 9th ed. (Washington, D.C.: National Academy of Sciences, 1979).

foods containing cholesterol from the diets of people over age 65 is neither necessary nor advisable, because of the lack of data relating cholesterol intake and the development of heart disease in this group. Egg yolk, liver, and vitamin-D-fortified milk are excellent sources of nutrients which may otherwise be consumed in inadequate amounts if these foods are unduly restricted. Use of polyunsaturated fats in cooking and for salad dressing, avoidance of excessive use of fried foods, and trimming the visible fat from meat is advised. These changes will adequately minimize intake of saturated fats for most people. Indigestion associated with fat intake can be lessened if fat is consumed in moderate amounts at every meal rather than in large quantities at one meal.

PROTEIN.   A study of protein synthesis in infants, young adults, and elderly women, all consuming adequate diets, showed that the rate of protein synthesis declines with age, but that there is no marked variation in the efficiency of nitrogen utilization. Based on such studies, the dietary protein requirements are estimated to decline by approximately 30 percent between the ages of 20 and 75. Decreased protein synthesis and the decline of body protein mass with age, it would seem that older adults would need less protein than younger adults. However, some research has indicated otherwise. For example, in older adults who are inadequately nourished, protein intake is diverted to meet energy needs and that additional protein might retard deterioration of muscle tissue. Pending more definitive research, the RDA for protein is constant throughout the adult years (Table 13–2).

VITAMINS.   Generally, there are few experimental results on which to base requirements for the micronutrients. Recommendations are consequently based on observations indicating relatively widespread deficiencies of some vitamins and minerals.

The RDA for vitamin A is 1,000 RE for adult males and 800 RE for females. Deficiencies frequently observed in the elderly could be the result of impaired ability to absorb or store vitamin A compounds or to convert the provitamin forms to the active vitamin. Lack of dietary fat, inadequate bile secretion, use of laxatives and antibiotics, and/or pancreatic insufficiency may all interfere with vitamin A absorption. Some clinical findings that often occur in older adults—slow adaptation of the eyes to darkness, scaly skin, and some eye lesions—have responded favorably to the administration of vitamin A.

Vitamin D is especially important in older age because of its role in the metabolism of calcium needed for bone health and maintenance. Because bone decalcification is common in the later years, daily vitamin D intake of 5 micrograms of cholecalciferol—from fortified milk or a supplement—is advisable.

Because of its antioxidant properties, vitamin E has received a great deal of popular attention as a possible factor in retarding the effects of aging; as yet research has not definitely supported this role. In any case, usual intakes of the vitamin appear to be adequate for most individuals, without supplementation.

Older adults may need greater amounts of some B vitamins, especially thiamin, vitamins B_6 and B_{12}, and folic acid. Inadequate intakes of vitamin B_{12} could contribute to disorientation, fatigue, and depression among the elderly. The increased need for these vitamins may result from less efficient absorption or altered metabolism and excretion, resulting not only from physiological change but also from certain medications.

MINERALS.   Calcium absorption apparently decreases with age, contributing to osteoporosis or a reduction in the amount of bone, often resulting in fractures. Recent evidence suggests that increased dietary calcium leads to an improvement in this condition for at least some people. The importance of maintaining adequate calcium intakes throughout adult life is underscored by the present RDA of 800 milligrams. An even higher recommendation starting in early adult life can be anticipated in future revisions of the RDA. This will be based on data which relate high peak bone mass with better bone strength in the elderly. Calcium is also important for maintaining health of the oral tissues; decalcification of the jawbone may contribute to tooth loosening and periodontal disease. Adequate calcium, phosphorus, and fluoride intakes throughout life may be preventive factors.

Iron deficiency is common among the elderly, especially among those with low incomes. It may develop gradually when a diet low in iron is coupled with chronic blood loss or there is poor absorption or inadequate utilization by the body. Iron-rich foods should be included in the diets of all older adults. The Food and Nutrition Board recommends a daily dietary allowance of 10 milligrams of iron for all individuals over the age of 50. The iron requirements of women are higher during the years of menstruation, but after menopause women's need for iron is the same as that of men.

FLUID.   Adequate fluid intake will increase the efficiency of kidney and bowel function, helping to eliminate wastes and relieve constipation. To maintain fluid balance, it is suggested that individuals over 65 should consume a minimum of 2 liters of fluid daily, 50 percent of which can come from foods. The Food and Nutrition Board recommends 1 milliliter of water for each kilocalorie of food consumed for all individuals of all ages. Drinking three to five glasses of water or other liquids per day is advised.

Effects of Medication

If ours is an overfed society, as is often suggested, it is also an overmedicated one. The numbers and combinations of drugs—both prescription and nonprescription—that are taken by people of all ages, and especially by older adults, is astonishing. Drugs may interfere with the absorption, metabolism, and excretion of nutrients. Conversely, nutrients may interfere with drug action, thereby modifying the effectiveness of a prescribed dose. As more is learned about this fascinating subject, changes will undoubtedly be made in the practices of pharmacists, physicians, and nutritionists, and perhaps even of consumers themselves.

DRUG-NUTRIENT INTERACTIONS.   The significance of the interaction between medication and nutrients in any individual depends on the previous nutritional status of that person, the dose and duration of drug use, the condition for which the medication is being used, and the particular drug or drug combination being taken. In general, drugs taken for chronic disease have a greater effect because they are taken for longer periods of time than those taken for acute episodes. Older adults are more likely to be using multiple drugs on a routine basis than are younger people, and thus the possibility of creating a biologically significant interaction is increased in the later years. Undesired effects may be exacerbated by the inadequate nutritional status commonly seen in an individual who is both elderly and ill.

Even in earlier adulthood, drug-nutrient interactions may be significant. People

NUTRITION AND CANCER

Cancer is second only to heart disease as a cause of death in the United States. Epidemiological studies, which show that the incidence of a particular kind of cancer is associated with specific environmental factors, suggest that a high proportion of cancers may be induced by a variety of agents in the environment. Smoking, occupational contaminants, air and water pollutants, and certain food substances have been implicated as possible causes of cancer.

Association, however, does not prove causation; the causes of the complex diseases known as cancer are not yet definitely known. In the beginning, or initiation, stage of cancer development, the DNA of cells is changed by a virus, chemical, or other agent. As a result, the cells become capable of multiplying more rapidly than normal. However, multiplication only occurs in the second or promotion stage when triggered by an agent aptly called a promoter. From evidence currently available, dietary factors may be more important in the promotion stage than in the initiation stage. Masses of rapidly dividing cells form a firm structure known as a tumor. The tumor may be benign and remain confined to the area in which it developed. Or it may be malignant, invading surrounding tissues and releasing cells that initiate secondary tumors known as metastases throughout the body.

Among findings that suggest relationships of diet to cancer are the following:

1. In women, cancers of the breast, gall bladder, and uterus are more common in the obese.
2. In men, although not in women, cancer of the large intestine is more common in the obese.
3. Several studies have reported a higher incidence of cancer in individuals with lower vitamin A or carotene intake and a lower incidence among those with higher intakes of these nutrients.
4. Seventh Day Adventists, whose diet is largely vegetarian, have a much lower incidence of cancer than other groups.

Do these findings prove that cancer is directly caused by high calorie intakes or by milk, or that it is prevented by vegetarian diets? No, they do not; many variables other than diet could be responsible. For example, Seventh Day Adventists do not smoke or drink alcohol; these characteristics, at least as much as their dietary habits, may explain their low incidence of cancer.

Research into possible roles of diet in initiating or promoting cancer may give us more clear-cut answers than we can get from epidemiological studies alone. Evidence must come from animal experiments and human cells grown in tissue culture in the laboratory.

There are several theories regarding how cancer develops. One is the "free radical theory" which suggests that superoxide radicals and hydroygen and organic peroxides formed during metabolism cause genetic modification.

of all ages, hoping to feel better, unthinkingly down tranquilizers, amphetamines, sleeping pills, aspirin, and antihistamines—not to mention various quantities of alcohol—totally unaware that they may be upsetting their bodies' ability to absorb the very nutrients that would truly help them to feel good. Several drugs stimulate appetite which may not be a desirable result. Over-the-counter drugs may be abused because of their perceived safety.

Interactions include the following:

• Hydralazine, used for moderation of hypertension, and L-dopa, a treatment for Parkinson's disease, may cause vitamin B_6 deficiency.

Promoters have the ability to produce oxygen radicals. Antioxidants have been studied as possible modifiers of the effects of promoters. Vitamins A, C, E, and the mineral selenium are all antioxidants and have been shown to have some anticarcinogenic activity under specific conditions in animal studies. Retinoids and/or carotenoids may also act by way of the immune system. Vitamin A deficiency results in suppressed immune function in animal studies. Animal studies have also shown that ascorbic acid and vitamin E may inhibit formation of nitrosamines in the stomach and intestine. These compounds are potent carcinogens, formed when certain amine-containing substances react with the nitrites which are used to cure meats such as bacon and which occur naturally in foods. However, other studies have shown no anticancer effect of vitamins E or C, and it is therefore premature to suggest that these nutrients can prevent cancer. Epidemiologic and experimental studies support the hypothesis of a role for selenium in modifying metabolism of carcinogens and decreasing proliferation of the cancer cells. However, selenium can be toxic in high doses so ingestion of large quantities is ill advised.

For the person who already has cancer, several consequences of the disease itself or its treatment can influence nutritional status. Anorexia, or loss of appetite, is common; cachexia, or wasting, can be extreme; metabolic abnormalities including impaired absorption and utilization of nutrients such as iron can occur. Many patients report a change in taste perception in which foods seem tasteless or perhaps bitter. Some of these changes may be the direct result of the disease itself; others may be caused by the radiation and drug therapies used in treating the cancer. In either case, the cancer patient requires consultation with a nutritionist and vigorous nutritional support. Otherwise, the patient is likely to succumb not to the cancer, but to the effects of the severe and prolonged malnutrition that often accompanies the disease.

Based on our current state of knowledge, some recommendations can be made with at least reasonable assurance. Increased consumption of fiber from fruits, vegetables, and whole grains, and decreased intake of fat, are probably in order. Smoking cigarettes definitely appears to enhance the effect of other carcinogens, and should be avoided. On the other hand, roles of food additives, which have received a great deal of publicity in recent years, are not at all clear.

Consumption of a variety of foods in moderate amounts, and maintenance of appropriate body weight, are recommended. These precautions do not, however, guarantee that cancer will not develop, any more than decreasing cholesterol and salt intake is any guarantee against heart disease. In the etiology of multifactorial diseases such as these, too many unknown variables are involved. Diet is only one of many possible causes.

- Mineral oil, often used as a laxative, impairs the absorption of all fat-soluble vitamins and can have a significant effect on vitamin A and D status.
- The antibiotic Neomycin alters the body's absorptive capacity within six hours after the first dose is ingested and diminishes production of pancreatic lipase.
- Long-term diuretic therapy for cardiac failure could result in magnesium, potassium, and zinc depletion.

In addition, drugs may cause nausea, vomiting, altered taste sensations, and loss of appetite. These effects have serious implications for nutritional status.

Food and nutrients can also interfere with the action of a drug. For example, consumption of foods high in vitamin K, such as green vegetables, may counteract the effects of anticoagulant medication; because vitamin K promotes blood clotting, it works against the desired effect of the drug.

Food prevents rapid absorption of medication, which should generally be taken when the stomach is empty (unless the drug itself is a gastric irritant). Delayed drug absorption will decrease its effective dose in most circumstances. In addition, certain nutrients can influence the absorption of particular medications. Milk and milk products interfere with tetracycline absorption, for example.

As research continues to identify drug-nutrient interactions, professionals should provide (and consumers should expect) information about when to take drugs in relation to mealtimes and about food items to be included or restricted to maximize drug effectiveness without compromising nutritional status.

ORAL CONTRACEPTIVES. Few drugs are as widely and continuously used over long periods of time as are hormonal contraceptives. In the years since they were introduced, epidemiological and clinical evidence has been accumulating on their effects, including those on nutrient metabolism. But experimental data on their metabolic consequences, or the influence of nutritional status on the side effects of these contraceptives, are still scarce.

Hormonal contraceptive use raises serum levels of triglycerides, cholesterol, phospholipids, and lecithin and also increases the risk of some vascular conditions. Studies have also noted an increased risk of myocardial infarction, but it is not clear whether this is due to altered lipid metabolism or to alterations in blood-clotting factors. Contradictory effects on carbohydrate metabolism have been noted. Abnormal glucose tolerance may occur in about 10 percent of women who have taken oral contraceptives for a year or more, especially those with a family history of diabetes, who deliver infants with high birth weights, or who are obese. This condition is reversible and disappears within three months after oral contraceptive use is discontinued.

Oral contraceptive hormones appear to affect protein metabolism in much the same way as the hormonal changes of pregnancy, with a decrease in blood levels of amino acids as well as of albumin; they increase the levels of many of the proteins synthesized in the liver, and especially of carrier proteins. Alterations in protein metabolism may affect the serum concentrations or metabolism of other nutrients as well. The development of abnormal glucose tolerance may be related to alteration in tryptophan metabolism, which also affects vitamin B_6 status. Deficiency of this vitamin has been linked to the onset of depression in many women taking a combination-hormone-type of oral contraceptive; moderately large doses of the vitamin have been reported to be therapeutic. Because of possible negative impacts of large amounts of pyridoxine, however, and because not all women are equally affected, routine vitamin B_6 supplementation for all women using combined oral contraceptives has not been recommended.

Plasma levels of vitamin A, iron, and copper apparently increase in women using hormonal contraception. The increases in iron may in part be due to lessened menstrual flow and consequent reduction of hemoglobin loss. An increase in carrier proteins may also account for the greater presence of these nutrients in the circulation; for example, an increase in retinol-binding protein is associated with increased serum levels of vitamin A. Studies of the effects of oral contraceptives on ascorbic acid metabolism have produced contradictory findings.

Metabolic effects of oral contraceptives are not uniformly felt by women taking these drugs, and there are not yet enough data to assess their long-term effects. Especially lacking are data about the effects for women whose nutrient intakes are inadequate; this problem is currently being addressed by the World Health Organization by studies in India, Thailand, and Egypt.

Health Status of Adults

Good health is not merely the absence of disease but a state of physical, mental, emotional, and social well-being. Young and middle-aged adults who are relatively healthy will occasionally show the effects of chronic or acute disease, undoubtedly related to an interaction between genetic and environmental factors. The environmental factors include, among others, life style, exposure and reaction to stress, food-related behaviors, and economics. There is increasing evidence that the impact in the later years of at least some environmental factors can be modified by the behaviors and attitudes formed earlier in life. At any age, conditions of life style and personal habits that may make one unnecessarily vulnerable to physiological stress can be changed, and preventive health measures can be instituted. If habits of good health care have not been previously established, the early and middle adult years are the time to make appropriate changes.

Just as adults in the middle years plan for their financial future, so should they plan for their future health status. And today many are. More concerned than ever

Many adults regularly participate in some form of exercise to keep fit.
Jay Lurie/Black Star

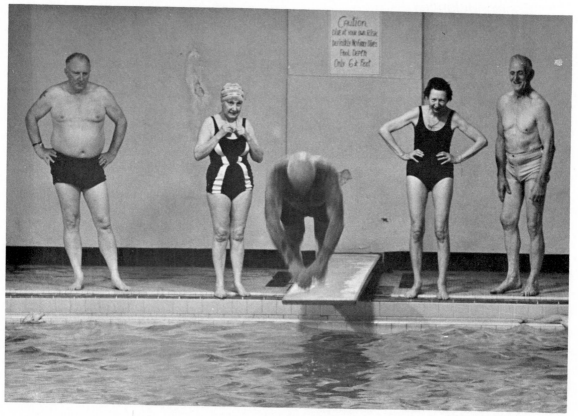

about health, today's adults are walking, jogging, swimming, playing tennis, skating, and regularly participating in other forms of exercise to keep all muscles, including heart muscle, in optimum condition. Many are cutting down on fat, excess calories, and sodium consumption in the hopes of avoiding debilitating diseases associated with later life.

The major factors hindering adequate preventive medical care for younger adults are inconvenience and economics. Programs instituted by various government agencies and the corporate world are helping to overcome these problems, by bringing clinical care into the neighborhood and the workplace and through prepaid medical insurance and memberships in health maintenance organizations (HMOs) that distribute costs broadly over the years and among large groups of people. At the same time the media have increased public awareness of the role of preventive care during earlier adulthood in lessening the need for crisis intervention later on.

NUTRITIONAL CONCERNS

Although it is beyond the scope of this text to deal with the medical and nutritional management of some of the conditions associated with aging, a summary of some widespread concerns will indicate some important problem areas.

Energy Balance

An estimated 30 to 40 percent of the adult population in the United States is moderately overweight or obese; because this third of the population is more likely to have additional health problems, there is cause for concern. Many people simply don't realize that the eating habits they enjoyed as teenagers and young adults are inappropriate in their middle years. As life becomes more sedentary; as basal metabolic rate decreases; as labor-saving devices, cocktail parties, dinner parties, and business meetings proliferate, the chances of weight gain increase immeasurably. Women whose activity levels suddenly drop, and men over 30 who are still eating as much as when they were teenagers, are particularly susceptible to development of that roll of fat around the middle.

The problem is compounded because overweight people are less likely to exercise. Like poor eating habits, the habit of not exercising is difficult to reverse. Individuals must be persuaded to reduce energy intake before it's too late and to establish an exercise routine early in life and follow it through adulthood. The evidence linking obesity to diabetes, hypertension, gall bladder disease, arteriosclerosis, and some forms of cancer is too overwhelming to be ignored.

There is also a sizeable number of older adults who are underweight. This may be related to an underlying disease process or to insufficient food intake. Anorexia nervosa has been identified in some elderly women, although it is mainly seen in younger women. Markedly underweight individuals are particularly vulnerable when illness strikes; they literally have no reserves with which to fight back, and they can become increasingly debilitated. When steady weight loss is noticed, attempts should be made to prevent further losses, identify the underlying cause, and to increase energy intakes to restore reserves. When food intake is decreased, nutrient intake is also diminished, further compromising health status.

Diabetes Mellitus

Insulin independent diabetes has been found to be highly age-dependent, doubling with every decade of life and most likely to appear during the 40s. Patients with diabetes are 17 times more prone to kidney disease than nondiabetics, 5 times more susceptible to gangrene, twice as likely to have heart disease and stroke, and 25 times more likely to become blind—the disease is now the leading cause of newly developed blindness.

Diabetes has in fact been shown to have an adverse effect on virtually all systems of the body. Because it accelerates the onset of other degenerative diseases, diabetes might be categorized as an accelerated form of aging. Maturity-onset diabetes can usually be controlled by diet, weight loss, and perhaps medication; insulin therapy is seldom necessary.

Digestive Problems

TEETH. Approximately half of the population over 65 years of age have lost all their teeth. Three-quarters of them have satisfactory dentures, leaving one-quarter without any chewing apparatus at all. Many cannot afford the cost of dentures; others may have ill-fitting appliances that are too uncomfortable to use. If dentures are uncomfortable, chewing is difficult and painful. Of the 50 percent of elderly who do have their natural teeth, a great many have periodontal disease, a chronic infection of the gums with erosion of the underlying bone, followed by loosening and ultimately loss of teeth.

These dental changes affect many older adults and may limit food intake. If soft foods must be eaten as a result of dental problems, sources of many nutrients and fiber are not consumed. The blandness and lack of texture of most soft foods lessens appetite and thus limits intake even more.

PEPTIC ULCER. Ulcers are lesions in the lining of the gastrointestinal tract. Gastric ulcers occur in the stomach, and duodenal ulcers are located in the upper part of the small intestine. The direct cause of an ulcer is an excessively acidic gastrointestinal environment. Why the acidity increases and why the normally protective mucus secretion of the stomach and duodenum are not effective in preventing this condition is not clear. Faulty dietary habits, smoking, heavy aspirin use, and excessive consumption of coffee have all been implicated although caffeine does not seem to be the culprit. So have physical and emotional stress, as well as family predisposition. No single cause has been ascertained.

Ulcers may cause gastric discomfort several hours after eating, when the stomach is empty and its excessive acid content is in direct contact with the stomach or intestinal lining. The lesion may eventually penetrate the entire mucosal wall; the result is a perforated ulcer that in turn leads to hemorrhage.

Treatment for ulcers consists of rest, antacid therapy, and regular and frequent meals; the food acts as a buffer against the acid. Meals should contain all nutrients, including moderate amounts of fat so that some food remains in the stomach for a longer period. In the past milk was thought to be the supreme buffer for stomach acid and large quantities were recommended, but this is no longer believed to be so. Sipping milk at intervals during an acute attack may alleviate distress to some extent, but consumption of large amounts is unnecessary.

A considerable body of folklore has built up concerning the diet for the ulcer sufferer. Studies indicate that most persons with chronic ulcers can eat almost anything. Black pepper, chili, horseradish, coffee, alcohol, and cola drinks are exceptions—and some can tolerate even those.

GALL BLADDER DISEASE. The gall bladder is the storage organ for bile synthesized by the liver. Most gall bladder disease is due to irritation, inflammation, and obstruction caused by the formation of gallstones. These cholesterol-containing crystals can become quite large and may necessitate the removal of the gall bladder. The incidence of gall bladder disease increases with age. Women in their 40s who are overweight seem to have a tendency toward the disease, as do an increasing number of women using oral contraceptives.

There is no evidence that cholesterol-restricted diets will decrease gallstones, but a high-fat diet does cause discomfort to persons with the disorder. A low-fat diet is therefore recommended. Once the gall bladder has been surgically removed, most individuals can resume their normal eating habits within several months. This is possible because the liver continues to synthesize bile, which is released into the upper part of the small intestine, apparently in sufficient quantity and concentration to emulsify dietary fats, aiding digestion and subsequent absorption.

INFLAMMATORY BOWEL DISEASE. Crohn's disease (regional enteritis) and ulcerative colitis occur most often in younger adults. The incidence of Crohn's disease seems to be increasing while that of ulcerative colitis is about the same. Inadequate intake or reduced absorption of total calories, iron, folate, and vitamin B_{12} may be a problem in persons with these conditions. The diet should therefore provide adequate amounts of all nutrients and be individualized to the person's tolerance.

MALABSORPTION. Lactose malabsorption, due to inadequate production of lactase, occurs most frequently among adults in the nonwhite population and in certain white ethnic groups as well. Malabsorption of vitamin B_{12} and of calcium are also associated with advancing age, possibly as consequences of lower gastric acidity. Since most absorption takes place in the small intestine, intestinal diseases or removal of part of the intestine will also compromise absorptive capacity.

DIVERTICULOSIS. Diverticulosis occurs when outpouchings (diverticula) form in the intestinal wall because of pressure. These bulging pockets may become inflamed, a condition known as *diverticulitis*, which is often accompanied by considerable pain. Serious diverticular disease may affect 5 to 10 percent of the over-60 population in the United States. Lack of dietary fiber has been implicated as a contributing factor, and increased consumption of fiber-containing complex carbohydrate foods is recommended as a preventive as well as a treatment measure.

CONSTIPATION. Constipation often results when the diet consists largely of highly processed and easy-to-chew foods and inadequate amounts of fiber-containing fruits, vegetables, whole-grain breads, and bran. Single adults, young and old, can have a problem with constipation albeit for different reasons. It can also be aggravated by the misuse of laxatives taken to relieve the condition. Moreover, a constant use of cathartics can lead to diarrhea, vomiting, fluid loss, depletion of potassium, damage to the lining of the colon, and hemorrhoids. Medication frequently taken for "acid stomach" can also interfere with normal bowel function; constipation is a frequent side effect of antacids that contain aluminum or calcium carbonate. Antihistamines, antidepressants, antispasmodics, muscle relaxants, and tranquilizers—all used frequently—can also retard bowel function.

The preferred treatment for constipation is consumption of high-fiber foods which increase the bulk of stools and reduce transit time through the gastrointestinal tract. Also recommended are generous fluid intake and exercise. If laxatives are required, those containing nonirritating ingredients such as cellulose derivatives should be selected. Laxatives should be used sparingly, and always accompanied by an 8-ounce glass of water.

Anemias

Nutritional anemia, often found in older adults, results from multiple deficiencies, usually of iron, protein, vitamin B_{12}, folacin, and/or ascorbic acid, along with reduced gastric acidity. The elderly are more often afflicted by the various anemias than are younger adults. The Ten-State Nutrition Survey found a higher incidence of iron deficiency in adults over 60 years of age, regardless of income or race, than in younger people. Iron deficiency, as measured by low serum iron, varied in HANES-II from a low incidence of 0.6 percent for black females to 15.6 percent for black males.

Older people are particularly at risk for nutritional anemias because their lower energy requirement and lower food intakes result in lower nutrient intakes as well. Folic acid deficiency and its result, megaloblastic anemia, is particularly common in the elderly because this vitamin is not widely present in food, is easily destroyed in cooking, and may be poorly absorbed.

Atherosclerosis and Coronary Heart Disease

Obesity; stress; lack of exercise; smoking; and excess dietary cholesterol, saturated fat, and sodium have all been implicated as contributors to blood vessel and coronary heart disease (CHD). Women under 50 are less likely than men to experience CHD, but after menopause, rates for women are similar to those for men of the same age. Women at younger ages are increasingly being affected as well, presumably becauses of the changed life style of many women today. As women become full participants in the work force, they are subject to the same occupation-related stresses that men have traditionally experienced. For many this is superimposed on the stresses of managing a household and guilt and conflict over responsibilities to husbands and children.

The role of cigarette smoking in the development of cardiovascular disease is being given new attention as it has been observed that women who smoke are more susceptible than nonsmokers to heart attacks and certain kinds of cerebral hemorrhages, as well as to other noncardiovascular conditions. Risk of CHD drops about six months after the person stops smoking and eventually reaches the risk of the nonsmoker. Diagnosed arteriosclerosis and heart disease respond to medication, weight loss, and nutritional management, as well as to behavioral and life style changes to reduce stress and other contributing factors.

Hypertension

Hypertension, which affects about 60 million people in the United States, has been implicated as a risk factor for coronary heart disease, stroke, and renal failure. Blacks are more susceptible to hypertension than whites (Table 13–3). Although

TABLE 13-3. *Black-White Ratio in Prevalence of Hypertension*

Age and Weight Class	Men	Women
20–39		
Underweight	2.28	2.30
Normal weight	1.69	2.47
Overweight	1.48	1.82
All weights	1.59	2.34
40–64		
Underweight	1.65	2.19
Normal weight	1.53	1.86
Overweight	1.44	1.53
All weights	1.48	1.77

Note: Ratio is rate in blacks divided by rate in whites. Hypertension is defined here as diastolic blood pressure ≥ 95 mm Hg or reporting current use of antihypertensive medication.
Source: R. Stamler, J. Stamler, W. F. Riedlinger, G. Algebra, and R. H. Roberts, Weight and blood pressure, *Journal of the American Medical Association* 240:1,607, 1978.

there is no certain evidence that nutritional factors *cause* high blood pressure, there is some evidence that blood pressure can be reduced by lowering sodium intake. The role of other minerals in hypertension is currently under active investigation. Obesity is also a contributing factor; in the 20 to 39 age group, hypertension is more prevalent among those who are overweight than in the normal-weight population. Weight loss in obese hypertensive adults, continued weight control with sound nutritional and exercise habits, reduction of sodium intake, and antihypertensive medication are effective treatments.

Bone and Joint Problems

Arthritis, osteoporosis, and osteomalacia are all common ailments of older adulthood. Arthritis, which is painful and debilitating to millions in their middle and later years, is an inflammation of the joints, and it may afflict any movable part of the skeleton. Despite many popular theories, there is no effective nutritional therapy. Weight control to minimize the burden on the joints and aspirin to relieve pain are advised. Because those with arthritis often take large doses of aspirin daily, side effects such as gastrointestinal bleeding and decreased ascorbic acid absorption are possible. Other anti-inflammatory medications, both nonsteroid and steroids, such as cortisone, are frequently used.

Osteoporosis, or decreased bone mass, is especially common in women between the ages of 40 and 60. A decrease in the calcium content of bone, accompanied by a reduction in the amount of bone, is apparently the direct cause of this disorder. Relative estrogen deficiency, physical inactivity, and perhaps inadequate calcium intake in the early and middle adult years are thought to be involved in this disorder, which weakens bones and makes them more susceptible to fracture. A diet high in calcium and vitamin D to promote calcium absorption may be effective in preventing and/or reversing bone loss.

Osteomalacia is characterized by demineralization of bone, leaving the structure vulnerable to fracture. It is most likely to affect older adults who do not drink milk or get adequate sunlight, who have conditions interfering with calcium absorption such as certain liver or kidney diseases, or who take anticonvulsant medication. Because osteomalacia is caused by a deficiency of vitamin D, supplements are necessary. Calcium supplements may also be prescribed.

FOOD PATTERNS

Food patterns in the adult years are determined by likes and dislikes, availability, life style, and other environmental factors. Consumption of a diversified diet from all food groups will maximize the probability of consuming all nutrients in adequate balance.

For most of the adult years, moderate rather than excessive amounts of food will provide energy balance without undesirable weight gain. Because obesity is associated with chronic diseases and is a major problem among the middle aged, a special effort may be needed to achieve and maintain ideal body weight through sound dietary practices and exercise.

Determinants of the foods desired, available, and consumed are more complex for many older adults. Both physiological and psychosocial factors are involved.

Physiological and Psychosocial Factors

The physiological changes of the later years may have a variety of impacts on the foods that are preferred, allowed, or available. The net effect is often lessened overall intake or lower nutrient intake.

Food loses its appeal when there is poor taste and smell perception or when bland, soft, or pureed foods are required because of illness or dental handicaps. The number of receptors for smell decreases to about 50 percent during adulthood so that the threshold for smell doubles every 20 years after age 40. The number of receptors for taste decreases less than those for smell. Elderly people are less sensitive to most taste qualities, such as bitter and spicy, and texture, such as smooth and crunchy. Eating can be less enjoyable if food is perceived as weakly flavored. Poor vision may interfere with shopping and with acquiring information about food quality and availability. In the unusual case of loss of taste because of zinc deficiency and not other causes, supplementation with 15 milligrams per day of the mineral in the form of zinc sulfate is effective. Other minerals may also play a role in taste.

Physical disabilities affecting mobility also tend to reduce the variety and quantity of the diet. Disabilities may affect the ability to feed oneself and to chew and swallow some foods. Because a limited diet is often an inadequate diet, individuals with motor disabilities are likely not to get the nutritional support to promote healing. Tea and toast may become the boring, and nonnutritious, staples of an overall inadequate diet.

Therapeutic diets prescribed for those with heart disease, diabetes, or other chronic ailments may further limit food choices and make selection and consumption of a nutritionally balanced diet even more difficult. Medication taken for these and other conditions may also interfere with nutritional status by upsetting metabolism and limiting absorption of key nutrients.

For too many of the elderly, economic, demographic, and attitudinal factors all interact to limit the quality of nutrition. Economic realities affect not only the mi-

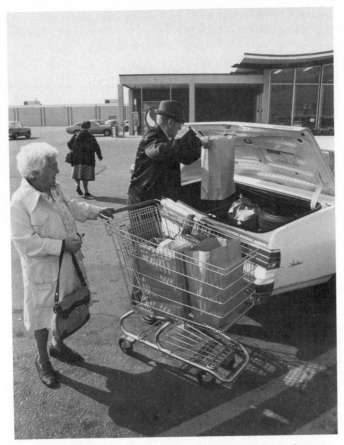

Nutrition for the elderly can often be improved most readily at the source when food is purchased. Shopping can provide exercise and recreation.
Biddle, SCP, Action

nority of the elderly who are truly poor but also the majority who are living on fixed and minimal incomes. These millions have little leeway with which to respond to rising costs. Heating and housing costs have proper claims on limited budgets. As food costs rise, the kinds and quantities of foods purchased must be restricted. It is particularly important for those on limited budgets to learn to identify relatively low-cost foods with high nutrient density.

Older adults can be active and conscientious shoppers. One study of food-buying behaviors found that when families with at least one member 65 years or older compared prices before buying, most favored merchants who offered senior citizens discounts and used advertising as a guide to purchases. Other studies have indicated that a majority of older adults do not take advantage of food stamps to which they are entitled. To many of today's elderly who are strong believers in the work ethic, food stamps carry the connotation of charity. Also, many may be intimidated by the bureaucratic procedures involved in establishing eligibility.

Loneliness may be the most important determinant of food-related behaviors in many older people. A meal to be eaten alone often does not seem worth the effort to prepare it. Older women who once cooked for a husband and family have difficulty cooking just for themselves. Older men have had little experience in cooking, and in too many instances do not have the skills or experience to prepare even the simplest meals. Analysis of HANES-I data for adults aged 65 to 74 years revealed that dietary patterns of the men were more closely associated with type of living arrangement and income than for the women. Low income men not living with a spouse were at higher risk for poor dietary intake. Canned and frozen foods become staples. Prewrapped supermarket packages of meat and produce seldom come in single or two-portion amounts, and higher prices per unit weight are charged for smaller-sized cans and frozen foods. Food purchased and prepared in larger quantities may spoil before it is eaten. Supermarkets are stocking more single-serving items, especially in metropolitan areas, but there is still an economic penalty as well as a psychological one for those who are alone.

As young people relocate to take advantage of career opportunities elsewhere, their older parents are left at home, often in changing communities in which they do not know their new neighbors or in a deteriorating part of an older city succumbing to urban blight. Fear of going out at night or of leaving the home at all may in many cases be a realistic response to an unpleasant situation. But these and other realities can produce changes in attitude and personality. For many of the solitary elderly, fear of contact with outsiders can become a phobia.

Those who own their own homes may be unable to afford necessary heating oil and maintenance costs or the moving and rental costs a new apartment would require. Others cannot move for psychological reasons—too many beloved possessions would have to be disposed of and too many memories would be reawakened. Yet remaining in the old house may contribute to a feeling of isolation and even to desolation and depression if it is strongly associated with memories of earlier, happier times.

Many older people must, for economic reasons, live in single rooms where there may not be adequate space for food storage or facilities for food preparation. They are then restricted to the purchase of nonperishable foods and perhaps a minimal amount of cooking on a hot plate. In too many communities, public transportation is inadequate or lacking. Those who cannot drive (and because of the expense of maintaining a car, faltering eyesight, and other factors, this is true of many older people) or have difficulty walking must rely on others for assistance with shopping, or they may have to patronize small neighborhood stores where the prices are higher and the selection smaller.

Loneliness, isolation, boredom, and depression all can cause lack of appetite. So can a monotonous diet because of financial limitations, ill health, or inability to shop for and prepare food. Other older adults may turn to overeating out of boredom and instead of choosing nutrient-rich products, indulge in energy-dense, nutrient-poor foods. Those who are set in their ways may have strong food preferences and prejudices and be reluctant to try anything new, no matter how beneficial it might be for them. Others, used to the food patterns of their ethnic heritage and prevented by chronic problems from consuming familiar foods, may find substitutions tasteless.

Fears of ill health also affect the eating habits of the elderly. They fall prey to claims made by health faddists and often, instead of purchasing nutritious and varied foods, purchase expensive supplemental vitamins and so-called health foods.

What is the safe level of alcohol intake? Some would say that moderate drinking is not harmful and may even be beneficial. Others might approve of moderate drinking for most adults, but caution that any alcohol at all could have adverse effects under unusual circumstances, such as during pregnancy. Still others point out that alcohol is a depressant and as such no more deserving of approval than any other drug in its class.

The very fact that the question of safety keeps arising, and the answers keep being debated, points to a high level of awareness of the potential hazards associated with the drug-nutrient called alcohol.

As a nutrient, alcohol (or ethyl alcohol, to be more precise) serves no vital specific functions in the cells. Instead, like other empty-calorie substances such as sugar, it is solely a source of energy. More than 90 percent of ingested alcohol is oxidized to carbon dioxide and water. The small proportion that is not oxidized is excreted, mostly in the urine and the expired air. During its oxidation, each gram of alcohol yields 7 kilocalories. If this energy represents excess intake over the drinker's needs, the excess is used for synthesis of body fat and stored as such.

Like any empty-calorie food, alcohol can be detrimental by contributing to weight gain and by replacing other more nutritious foods in the drinker's diet. If those were the only negative effects on nutritional status, alcohol could be criticized as much as, but no more than, candy or soda pop. In fact, alcohol has health effects in addition to its ability to provide calories without contributing essential nutrients.

Alcohol can be exceedingly destructive to every system in the body, but the digestive, neuromuscular, and endocrine systems seem to be most vulnerable. Furthermore, alcohol can apparently cause disease in every organ that it contacts directly; cancers of the mouth, tongue, esophagus, pharynx, and larynx (voicebox) are all associated with very heavy drinking. For those who both smoke and drink (and many heavy drinkers also smoke immoderately), the risk of cancer is even higher.

In the stomach and intestine, alcohol does not have to be digested, but is absorbed unchanged directly into the blood. Small amounts are absorbed from the stomach, although most is absorbed from the small intestine. This absorption, requiring as it does no prior digestion, accounts for the speedy effects of alcohol on the brain and hence on behavior.

While it is still in the digestive tract, alcohol irritates the cells lining the tract. This can cause food to be hurried through the intestine thus contributing to decreased absorption of many nutrients, particularly calcium, thiamin, folacin, vitamin B_{12}, and amino acids.

Although alcohol has access to all the body's cells once it is absorbed, the liver is the organ that suffers the greatest damage. Alcohol disrupts the liver's normal conversion of amino acids to glucose (gluconeogenesis), to the point of producing hypoglycemia in susceptible individuals; excessive fatty acid breakdown may occur as a means of compensating for impaired energy release from amino acids. Alcohol inhibits liver enzymes involved in synthesis of certain

Recommendations for the Adult Years

Consumption of a diversified diet is the best nutritional approach throughout life, including all the stages of adulthood. Problems of providing adequate diversity of foods in single-person households affect not only the elderly but also the increasing numbers of single adults living alone at all ages. Young adults are postponing marriage while they establish their careers; more people who have been married are di-

blood proteins while promoting synthesis of others. Altered lipoprotein synthesis tends to increase serum triglyceride levels, which in turn can contribute to the condition known as "fatty liver." In this condition, the fat-engorged organ becomes so abnormal that liver function fails; the vital functions performed by the complex factory known as the liver falter and gradually cease. Lack of materials needed by other organs, or intolerably high levels of substances that should be constantly removed by the liver, can lead to death due to liver failure. In some cases, liver cells have been replaced by scar tissue, a visibly detectable disorder known as cirrhosis.

Heavy alcohol consumption causes nervous system disorders, including depression. An addictive disease, alcoholism can be characterized by withdrawal symptoms, the most dramatic of which is delirium tremens. The lungs can also be affected, as seen in the shortness of breath in some heavy drinkers; the heart can show signs of abnormal function, such as irregular heartbeat. In short, every organ in the body can show the effects of the poisoning that occurs in heavy drinkers.

Why, then, do so many people continue to inflict such damage on their own bodies? The answer is unknown; although alcohol has been the drug of choice of many civilizations for thousands of years, we do not yet know why a substance can be part of the good life for many people and yet constitute the central theme of a nightmare existence for millions whose lives are ruled by alcohol.

What about the benefits of alcohol? Small to moderate amounts before a meal can stimulate appetite, promote digestion of food, provide relaxation, and become a vehicle for sociability that enhances mealtime enjoyment. These effects can, of course, be a double-edged sword; good appetite can readily become overeating, and relaxed mealtimes can turn into sessions in which neither quantity nor quality of food receive much thought.

Some studies have shown that the incidence of certain types of heart disease may actually be lower among men who drink moderately than among those who do not drink at all. This does not, of course, prove that alcohol has a protective effect on the heart. Rather, it may be that those with a relaxed personality or associated traits tend to have both characteristics coincidentally: low incidence of heart disease and high probability of drinking at least some alcohol.

The best treatment for alcohol abuse and alcoholism remains to be discovered. Research in this area has lagged, at least in part because of societal attitudes. On the one hand, drinking is condoned and even encouraged; on the other hand, the alcoholic is considered undesirable and hopeless. In average Americans of drinking age, alcoholic beverages—distilled spirits, wines, and beer—contribute somewhat over 200 kilocalories to the daily diet. It is a myth that alcohol is reserved almost exclusively for social events or special occasions; many individuals consume alcohol regularly, even daily. For an unknown but presumably substantial proportion of these apparently normal people, the most serious nutrition-related health problem facing them is not the problem of getting enough of some nutrient, but the problem of decreasing alcohol intake or even eliminating it from their lives.

vorced and living alone. At every age, a solitary meal is likely to be an unplanned, carelessly prepared, and hurriedly gobbled snack, a hasty visit to a fast-food outlet, or a sandwich brought in from a counter delicatessen.

FOOD FOR SINGLE ADULTS. Young or old, single adults should make an effort to *dine,* even when they must dine alone. A table that is set, music or a good book for company, and a planned menu even if only for one will pay off in greater enjoyment, better digestion, and improved nutrition. Even breakfast should be given this attention as a pleasant start to a busy day. Remember, a nutritious breakfast can vary from cold cereal with milk, to leftovers from dinner, to a cheese sandwich on whole-grain bread. All of these can be accompanied by fruit and beverage and provide more fiber and nutrients than a sweet roll picked up on the way to the commuter train. Prepared cereals fortified with iron are a significant source of this often limiting mineral in the diet of young women.

Developing an interest in cuisine and experimenting with herbs, spices, and new food items can create interest in food preparation even in single-portion quantities. Purchase frozen vegetables in plastic bags so you can pour out as much as you need rather than cooking a whole box and having leftovers. Double portions can be prepared and half promptly labeled and placed in the freezer as a treat for the following week. Nutrition is enhanced when social activities are planned for mealtimes; friends can be invited to dinner regularly or dinner visits between two or more people planned. Dinner in a "tablecloth" or ethnic restaurant should be a regularly scheduled treat. Frozen dinners have come a long way. While they are frequently more expensive and higher in salt than a home prepared equivalent, these dinners are a good alternate for exceptionally busy days. There are also several lines of portion-controlled dinners that contain 300 to 400 kilocalories. Eating out has become a way of life for many adults. Careful choices must be made so as not to exceed energy needs and to obtain needed fiber. Fast-food restaurants offer a variety of mainly fried items. While these foods are a legitimate part of a person's diet they should not be the mainstay. Salads and salad bars have introduced an alternative fare in both fast-food and standard restaurants, providing additional nutrients and fiber and fewer calories if you are selective with the dressings and toppings. In general, the quality of the vegetables served in restaurants has improved, but there still is a tendency to serve them swimming in butter. Some restaurants have introduced alternative meals for the health conscious diner.

IRON NEEDS.   Women who have not yet reached menopause may require iron supplementation. Intakes of less than the RDA of 18 milligrams per day are common in this group, particularly young adult women who limit food intake to stay thin.

Data from the two HANES surveys revealed percentages of abnormal values for individuals aged 65 to 74 years which ranged from 0.6 percent for serum iron to 64.4 percent for mean corpuscular hemoglobin. For hemoglobin, the percent of abnormal values in HANES-II ranged from 4.0 percent for white females to 53.4 percent for black males. There is some evidence which suggests that part of the problem in the elderly may be a decreased ability to mobilize stored iron.

RECOMMENDATIONS FOR OLDER ADULTS.   Preparation of balanced meals may be a challenge for older adults for whom economic, physiological, or other factors interfere with previous food patterns. High-quality protein, provided by foods of animal origin or complementary plant proteins, is important; vitamins and minerals from whole-grain breads and cereals, fruits, and vegetables should be included as well. Fiber from these foods is particularly beneficial in keeping the digestive tract in good working order and is as effective as most laxatives in improving chronic constipation, without their side effects.

Because bone disorders can result from lack of calcium, a special effort should be made to include good sources of calcium daily. For those who have difficulty drinking adequate quantities of milk as a beverage, consumption of cheese, ice cream, yogurt, custards, and puddings will make a good contribution. Some people avoid drinking milk because they fear the gastrointestinal distress that can result from decreased production of lactase, the enzyme that digests lactose. Even those in whom lactase deficiency has been diagnosed, however, can consume milk in moderate amounts. In addition to providing calcium, milk is a good source of protein and, if fortified, of vitamins A and D, and is thus an important component of the diet of older adults.

Fluid intake is important, too, to maintain bowel regularity and electrolyte and fluid balance. Milk, soups, cereals, and juices, as well as water, provide fluid. For most adults, soft drink consumption should be limited as should energy-dense snack foods in general: They add to energy intake without providing nutrients.

Money-saving ways to maximize nutrient intake include saving vegetable cooking liquid for use in soups and cream sauces; combining leftover vegetables in a casserole with toasted strips of cheese; and baking or poaching apples, pears, or peaches or sauteeing banana slices in margarine for dessert or snacks.

Those who are not able to consume an adequate quantity of food at three regular meals may be helped by eating four or five small meals or by snacking regularly between meals. Flagging appetites can be improved with regular exercise, such as daily walking or swimming. Meals shared with friends, either at home or in a restaurant (breakfast get-togethers are inexpensive and a pleasant break in routine), are also appetite stimulants. An effort should be made to avoid monotony by trying new foods or recipes. Meals should be eaten at regular times. The overweight should avoid snacks and all energy-dense and nutrient-scarce foods.

Nutrition for the elderly can often be improved most readily at the source—when food is purchased. Shopping can provide both exercise and recreation. Use of a shopping cart will eliminate the need to carry heavy bundles. Ways to economize on food should not be overlooked: Some supermarkets offer senior citizens discounts on one day of the week; food coupons—but only for items one normally uses—should be clipped from newspaper and magazine advertisements. Nutritional information on package labels should be consulted. Meal plans and shopping lists should be made after consulting weekly advertisements to take advantage of advertised specials—and shopping lists should be followed. Purchased foods should be stored properly and perishables used promptly.

Nutritional Status of Adults

The major nutritional problems in adults involve essential minerals. Although there are some pockets of malnutrition throughout the country, it is not as widespread, or of the same proportion, as in other parts of the world. More prevalent is undernutrition, which has been shown by surveys to affect particularly people from low-income population groups. Nutritional status of older people who live in nursing homes may differ from that of individuals in their own homes due in part to the drugs needed by many of the former.

Analysis of HANES-I data on 3,477 adults aged 65 to 74 years revealed that 12.2 percent of the men and 32.4 percent of the women lived alone. The most favorable dietary pattern was for those living with a spouse. Those who lived alone or with someone other than a spouse have less favorable dietary patterns. This and other studies suggest that older men who live alone have less adequate diets than older women who live alone. Income, as shown in other studies, also strongly influences dietary patterns although it appears to affect women less than men. Iron, calcium, zinc, chromium, folacin, vitamin A, and ascorbic acid have been reported problem nutrients based on various limited surveys of elderly populations. Nursing homes generally have a consulting dietitian, and studies have shown that foods served in nursing homes usually provide nutrients in adequate amounts provided it is eaten. There have been few studies of actual requirements, there is some difficulty in assessing nutritional status by dietary means. The RDAs for this segment of the population are therefore based on extrapolation from studies on younger adults.

LOOKING AHEAD

Life is a continuum, and the last part of the life cycle can be as rewarding as any other stage. If health is good and positive habits and a variety of interests are cultivated throughout the adult years, physical and intellectual activity can be maintained through the ninth and even tenth decade, as increasing numbers of older people are demonstrating every day. Optimal health and body function can be achieved by maintaining appropriate body weight; exercising regularly and in mod-

Life is a continuity, and the last part of the life cycle can be as rewarding as any other stage.
Action

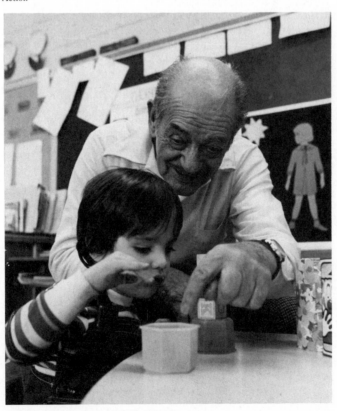

eration; eating a diversified diet in moderation; and minimizing stress by creating a balance in one's life among work, friends and family, and recreational activities.

Because how one eats affects how one's life progresses, nutrition education is important, especially for young adults. They can be reached in the work place, in their children's schools, through nutritional counseling when a new baby is born, through popular publications, and as a consequence of new interests such as travel and gourmet cookery. Public education is a new and growing career area for nutritionists who can now reach a wide public through such means as advertisements and pamphlets sponsored by food companies and supermarkets. Government-funded group-feeding programs for older adults present a particularly good opportunity for nutrition education.

Older adults can also be reached through their various social organizations and the specialized publications targeted to this group. The elderly are eager for information that can be put to practical use: ways to save money, interesting new recipes, and suggestions for adding nutrient content to their daily meals. Most important, in open-ended group sessions, they should be given the opportunity to raise questions about their own problems, so that discussion can be targeted to their needs.

As a result of the growing numbers of older people and the growing interest in all aspects of aging, more government funding has been made available for research as well as for social programs. Eventually this emphasis should lead to a satisfactory determination of actual nutrient requirements, providing more definitive data against which to assess nutritional status. These in turn will lead to more accurate and specific recommendations for food and nutrient intake, will emphasize the importance of nutrition in the later years, and will have an impact on supplementary feeding programs.

As the increased longevity of the population attests, nutritional improvements in the last century have benefited millions living and enjoying life in older age today. As more is learned, the quality of life for all members of this large and growing segment of our population can be enhanced. This research frontier is important to all of us at every age, for in the continuity of the life cycle we will be the older adults of the future.

SUMMARY

In the United States today more than 27 million people are over 65 years of age; by the year 2050 at least 70 million people will be in this age group. Aging, however, begins at conception and is continuous throughout life. Although physical growth is completed by early adulthood, the body's tissues and cells remain in a dynamic state, with catabolism slightly exceeding anabolism, resulting in a decrease in the number of cells. There are wide differences between individuals in the effects of aging.

Theories variously ascribe aging to changes in DNA produced by low-level radiation, to wear and tear that ultimately depletes cell resources, and to free radicals resulting from cosmic radiation oxidizing fatty acid components of cellular structures. A genetic explanation involves a biological "time clock" that naturally limits the number of times a cell can replicate itself; and some believe that information coded into DNA and RNA is progressively lost or altered over the years. Aging is probably multifactorial, resulting from the interaction of numerous mechanisms.

There is no concrete evidence that any one food or nutrient will increase longevity, but there is abundant evidence that the quality of nutrition throughout life is an influence on health and well-being. Obesity; excessive intakes of salt, fats, and sugar; and inadequate consumption of fiber-rich foods are all associated with chronic and severe disease conditions in the middle and later years and with higher mortality rates.

Among the many physiological changes that come with advancing years are changes in metabolism. Decreases in taste sensitivity and in the production of saliva and several digestive enzymes lead to poorer appetite and lowered efficiency of metabolism. The use of medications may also lessen nutrient absorption and impair nutrient metabolism.

A decrease in the basal metabolic rate along with generally lower levels of physical activity reduce the need for energy in the later years. Since recommendations for most nutrients remain at the same level throughout the adult years, nutrient intakes must be maintained even while energy intake is reduced. Fluid intake of 2 liters per day is also advised.

Although today's older adults are in generally better health than those of any previous generation, many are afflicted with chronic and serious disease conditions, especially toward the end of life. Among the most debilitating of these conditions are diabetes, peptic ulcers, arthritis, and osteoporosis. Various forms of cancer, atherosclerosis, coronary heart disease, and hypertension affect millions in the middle as well as later years. Those receiving treatment for any of these or other conditions should be aware that medication can interfere with nutrient utilization, and conversely, that food can decrease the effectiveness of some medications.

Especially in older age, health problems may have an adverse effect on appetite, interfere with shopping and food preparation, and make feeding oneself or chewing difficult. Economic and psychosocial factors also affect food behaviors and therefore nutritional status. Public information programs about nutrition targeted at all ages will encourage younger adults to establish positive eating and exercise habits, improve the quality of food consumed throughout life, and prepare the way for a healthy and well-nourished old age.

BIBLIOGRAPHY

ALEXANDER, M., G. EMANUEL, T. GOLIN, J.T. PINTO, AND R.S. RIVLIN. Relation of riboflavin nutriture in healthy elderly to intake of calcium and vitamin supplements: Evidence against riboflavin supplementation. *American Journal of Clinical Nutrition* 39:540, 1984.

AVIOLI, L.V. Calcium and osteoporosis. *Annual Review of Nutrition* 4:471, 1984.

BETRAND, H.A., T.T. LYND, E.J. MASORO, AND B.P. YU. Changes in adipose mass and cellularity through the adult life of rats fed *ad libitum* on a life-promoting restricted diet. *Journal of Gerontology* 35:835–872, 1980.

BOREL, M.J., R.E. RILEY, AND J.T. SNOOK. Estimation of energy expenditure and maintenance energy requirements of college-age men and women. *American Journal of Clinical Nutrition* 40:1264–1272, 1984.

CALLOWAY, D.H., AND M.S. KURZER. Menstrual cycle and protein requirements of women. *Journal of Nutrition* 112:356, 1982.

CALLOWAY, D.H., AND E. ZANNI. Energy requirements and energy expenditure of elderly men. *American Journal of Clinical Nutrition* 33:2088, 1980.

CHINN, H.I. Effects of dietary factors in skeletal integrity in adults: Calcium, phosphorous, vitamin D and protein. Bethesda, MD: Life Sciences Research Office, FASEB, 1981.

DAVIS, M.A., E. RANDELL, R.N. FORTHOFER, E.S. LEE, AND S. MARGEN. Living arrangements and dietary patterns of older adults in the United States. *Journal of Gerontology* 40:434, 1985.

EISENSTEIN, A.B. Nutritional and metabolic effects of alcohol. *Journal of the American Dietetic Association* 81:247–251, 1982.

FARKAS, M.E., AND J. DWYER. Nutrition education for alcoholic recovery homes. *Journal of Nutritional Education* 16:123–125, 1984.

Food and Nutrition Board, National Research Council. *Recommended Dietary Allowances*, 9th ed. Washington, DC: National Academy of Sciences, 1979.

GROTKOWSKI, M.L., AND L.S. SIMS. Nutritional knowledge, attitudes, and dietary practices of the elderly. *Journal of the American Dietetic Association* 72:499, 1978.

GRUCHOW, H.W., K.A. SOBOCINSKI, AND J.J. BARBORIAK. Alcohol, nutrient intake, and hypertension in U.S. adults. *Journal of the American Medical Association* 253:1567–1570, 1985.

HANSSON, P., AND P. NILSSON-EHLE. Acute effects of ethanol and its metabolites on plasma lipids and lipoprotein lipase activity. *Annals of Nutrition and Metabolism* 27:328–337, 1983.

HARTZ, A.J., AND A.A. RIMM. Natural history of obesity in 6946 women between 50 and 59 years of age. *American Journal of Public Health* 70:335–338, 1980.

HILLERS, V.N., AND L.K. MASSEY. Interrelationships of moderate and high alcohol consumption with diet and health status. *American Journal of Clinical Nutrition* 41:356–362, 1985.

HORWITZ, D.L. Diabetes and aging. *American Journal of Clinical Nutrition.* 36:803, 1982.

KOHRS, M.B., C. KAPICA-CYBORSKI, AND D. CZAJKA-NARINS. Iron and chromium nutriture in the elderly. In *XVII Conference on Trace Substances in Environmental Health*, D. Hemphill ed. University of Missouri, Columbia, MO, 1984.

LEVEILLE, G.A., AND P.F. CLOUTIER. Role of the food industry in meeting the nutritional needs of the elderly. *Food Technology* 40:82, February 1986.

LEVEILLE, P.J., R. WEINDRUCH, R.L. WALFORD, D. BOK, AND J. HORWITZ. Dietary restriction retards age-related loss of gamma crystallins in the mouse lens. *Science* 224:1247–1249, 1984.

LYNCH, S.R., C.A. FINCH, E.R. MONSEN, AND J.D. COOK. Iron status of elderly Americans. *American Journal of Clinical Nutrition* 36:1032, 1982.

McCAY, C.M., M.F. CROWELL, AND L.A. MAYNARD. The effect of retarded growth upon the length of lifespan and upon the ultimate baby size. *Journal of Nutrition* 10:63, 1935.

McDONALD, J.F., AND S. MARGEN. Wine versus ethanol in human nutrition, IV: Zinc balance. *American Journal of Clinical Nutrition* 33:1096–1102, 1980.

MARRS, D.C. Milk drinking by the elderly of three races. *Journal of the American Dietetic Association* 72:495, 1978.

MASORO, E.J., B.P. YU, H.A. BERTRAND, AND F.T. LYND. Nutritional probe of the aging process. *Federation Proceedings* 39:3178–3182, 1980.

OFFENBACHER, E.G., AND F.X. PI-SUNYER. Beneficial effect of chromium-rich yeast on glucose tolerance and blood lipids in elderly subjects. *Diabetes* 29:919–925, 1980.

REIF, A.E. The causes of cancer. *American Scientist* 69:437–447, 1981.

RIGOTTI, N.A., G.S. THOMAS, AND A. LEAF. Exercise and coronary heart disease. *Annual Review of Medicine* 34:391–412, 1983.

ROE, D.A., ed. *Diet, Nutrition, and Cancer: From Basic Research to Policy Implications.* (Vol. 9, Current Topics in Nutrition and Disease.) New York: Alan R. Liss, Inc., 1983.

ROE, D.A. *Geriatric Nutrition.* Englewood Cliffs, NJ: Prentice-Hall, 1983.

ROE, D.A. Therapeutic effects of drug-nutrient interactions in the elderly. *Journal of the American Dietetic Association* 85:174–181, 1985.

SCHNEIDER, C.L., AND D.J. NORDLUND. Prevalence of vitamin and mineral supplement use in the elderly. *Journal of Family Practice* 17:243, 1983.

SIMOPOULOS, A.P., AND T.B. VAN ITALLIE. Body weight, health, and longevity. *Annual Internal Medicine* 100:285–295, 1984.

TURNLUND, J., S. COSTA, AND S. MARGEN. Zinc, copper, and iron balance in elderly men. *American Journal of Clinical Nutrition* 34:2641, 1981.

VAN EYS, J. Nutrition and Neoplasia. *Nutrition Reviews* 40:353–359, 1982.

VIR, S.C., AND A.H.G. LOVE. Zinc and copper status of the elderly. *American Journal of Clinical Nutrition* 32:1471, 1979.

WATKIN, D.M. *Handbook of Nutrition, Health and Aging.* Park Ridge, NJ: Noyes Publications, 1983.

WATSON, R.R., ed. *CRC Handbook of Nutrition in the Aged.* Boca Raton, FL: CRC Press, 1985.

WOOD, R.D. AND W.L. HASKELL. Interrelation of physical activity and nutrition on lipid metabolism. In *Diet and Exercise: Synergism in Health Maintenance*, P.L. White and T. Mondeika, eds. Chicago: American Medical Association, pp. 39–47, 1982.

YOUNG, V.R., W.P. STEFFEE, P.B. PENCHARZ, J.C. WINTERER, AND N.S. SCRIMSHAW. Total human body protein requirements at various ages. *Nature* 253:192, 1975.

YUNG, L., I. CONTENTO, AND J.D. GUSSOW. Use of health foods by the elderly. *Journal of Nutrition Education* 16:127–131, 1984.

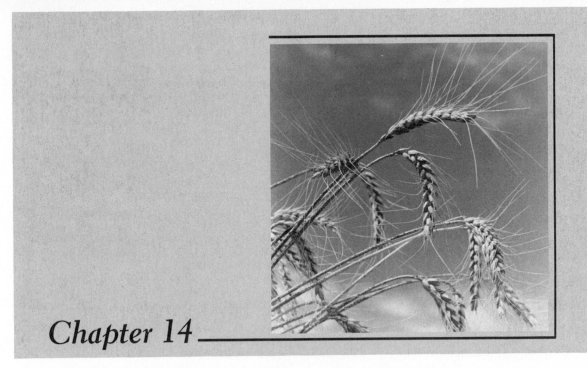

Chapter 14

THE FOOD SUPPLY: ISSUES AND PROSPECTS

478

Deciding what, where, when, and how we will eat depends on our preferences, our nutrition knowledge, our cultural background—and on the supply available to us. For most Americans today, the choice is wide and plentiful; we are limited only by our budgets. For some Americans and others, the situation is different: Food is limited in quantity and in variety, quality is poor, and knowledge of nutrition is rudimentary. So when we talk about the food supply, we need to look at various levels of issues and prospects: national and international, general and specific high-risk groups.

Nationally, today, we face issues of choice determined by changing life styles and by health and environmental concerns such as the effects of preservatives and additives, pollution of the environment, and the long-term health effects of consuming certain foods. Internationally, we face the growing problem of large-scale malnutrition and starvation in Third World areas. In this chapter we will look briefly at all these issues to give you an idea of what has happened and what is being done, as well as what ought to happen and what ought to be done. We will begin with our own situation and our changing life styles.

CHANGING SOCIAL PATTERNS

For most, America has proved to be a land of plenty beyond the wildest dreams of pilgrim and pioneer. Though malnutrition remains a pressing concern, widespread undernutrition is not a strong public health issue. This is not to say, however, that things are so perfect that every American gets enough to eat. There are pockets of hunger in this country that ought not to exist in a land that is so productive.

From the early years of our country's history, right up through a good part of the last century, most people grew their own food. Now, a mere 4 percent of the U.S. population produces not only enough food for the nation's needs but millions of tons for export as well. Mechanization, fertilizers, improvements in plant strains and in food-processing techniques and transportation—all these developments have allowed agricultural productivity to increase geometrically. American farms are the most productive in the world.

A greater variety of food items is available today than could have been imagined barely a generation ago. There are some 11,000 to 39,000 items in supermarkets, and the food industry is constantly creating new ones to tempt consumer tastes. This wide selection of foods presents a new kind of problem: *choice*. Behind every supermarket purchase lies a complex decision-making process in which convenience, economy, nutritional knowledge, individual tastes, cookery know-how, home storage capabilities, and several other factors are balanced. Shoppers are aware of these considerations, but they may be less aware of the other factors that determine what they eat—factors that they take for granted.

Urbanization and Suburbanization

As fewer people have been needed on the farm to produce our food, millions have moved to towns and cities to find work. Largely because of the increased complexity of most jobs, and the increasing number of technologically demanding jobs, we have become a nation of specialists: hematologists, computer programmers, market

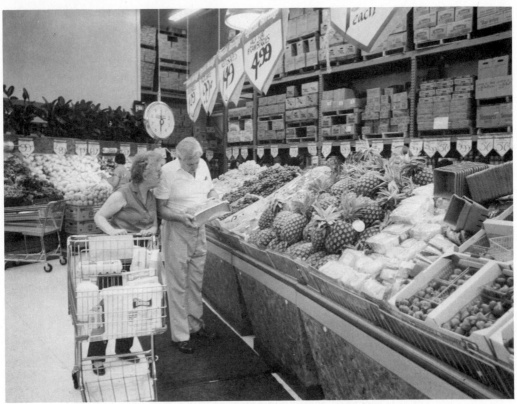

For most Americans today, varieties of foods are diverse and plentiful.
Laimute E. Druskis

researchers, educational administrators. Recent demographic movements have produced urbanization of the suburbs. "Research and Development" or "High Technology" corridors have spawned high- and low-rise office buildings and additional demand for housing closer to the workplace. People are commuting longer distances and the flow out from the city may be nearly as heavy as the flow into the city. The rural or farm population continues to decline significantly every year due to losses of family farms and the desire by some for the city life.

With increased urbanization and suburbanization there are two trends, the first at this point in time still much larger than the second. Simply prepared home-grown foods have been replaced by the store-bought variety, grown months before, hundreds or thousands of miles away, often preseasoned and precooked. Consumers now load up their station wagons at the supermarket once a week and bring everything home to the pantry and freezer, further lengthening the time as well as the physical distance between field and table.

The second trend is a boom in local "Farmers' Markets" and farm stands that generally sell local or regional produce to people who want their fruits and vegetables as fresh as possible. As part of this trend and spurred on by the rising cost of harvesting fruits and vegetables, are the pick-your-own farm stands where the cost of purchasing is less than in the supermarket. Home freezers also allow the family to preserve produce easily.

Family Structure

Some of these same economic and social forces have led to radical changes in the organization of American families. The traditional extended family—several generations living together under one roof—has never been the norm in the United States. The American family has always tended to be nuclear. But even if they did not live with their children, it was traditionally customary for grandparents to live nearby and to help in raising the grandchildren. Today it is uncommon to find grandparents living in the same neighborhood, or even in the same state, as their offspring. In this age of the car and airplane, succeeding generations tend to live farther apart.

Today, families are being started later, and are smaller, than in the previous generation. The average size of a family is 2.71 persons down from 3.33 in 1956. Increasing numbers of young men and women are electing to stay single or are postponing marriage until they are in their twenties or even thirties. The number of one- and two-member households has increased dramatically during the past decade. In 1983, persons living alone accounted for 23 percent of all households, an increase from 17.9 percent in 1970. Although the majority of families still include at least one parent with a child under 18, about a third of all families consist of *only* two persons and 20.5 percent of all children live with their mother only and 2.0 percent live with their father only. Some of these are single-parent families, some are young married couples who have postponed or decided against child rearing, and some are older couples whose adult children have moved elsewhere, even before they marry—another fairly recent social phenomenon. And 20 percent of all children now live in one-parent families, 90 percent of them with their mothers.

The postwar baby boom is over. Today women are postponing their childbearing until their education is completed and their careers are launched. Not only are women having their children later, but also they are having fewer of them. The birthrate (number of live births per thousand population) reached its lowest level a few years ago. At the other end of the human lifespan, people are living longer. This means that more older people are living *alone*, since grandparents typically make their homes away from their children. In 1983, 19.3 million people lived alone, 7.5 million males and 11.8 million females.

The trend toward smaller, isolated families directly affects the housing, energy, manufacturing, and food industries. Because of the greater number of families, more houses and apartment buildings are needed, which in turn consume more gas and fuel oil for heating. More beds and sofas, carpets and dinnerware, dishwashers and automobiles are produced and purchased. But smaller families also mean fewer people at the table, which normally means less-elaborate meals with food requiring less preparation time. Mealtimes become less personal and more routine as the nightly family get-together gives way to the TV dinner.

Today 34.8 percent of all females are employed. This shift, which has really been a social revolution, is itself due to a number of economic and social factors. Increasing numbers of single and divorced women must support themselves and their families. About 53.2 percent of all children under 18 living in families had mothers in the labor force in 1980. The constant inflation of the 1970s left many middle-income couples unable to live in the style to which they had become accustomed on only one income. The women's movement not only motivated more women to seek career satisfaction but also opened up more job opportunities for them.

Perspective On

FAST FOODS

Fast-food outlets fit comfortably into our way of life. Teenagers grab a snack on the way home from school; working mothers can bring home Colonel Sanders instead of a bag of groceries. Some restaurants offer birthday parties for children, special gimmicks for holidays, and even lotteries. And the chains have begun bringing their food to us, accepting contracts to service cafeterias in schools, factories, and even aircraft carriers. A generation of adults has already grown up on burgers and fries. Fast-food outlets will account for a quarter of all meals consumed in this country, at a price tag of $25 billion annually.

Speed and ecoonomy remain the mainstays of the fast-food business. Limited menus offer economies in purchasing, distribution, preparation, equipment, and training of personnel—economies that do make it possible to serve millions of meals at moderate cost. Bulk purchasing, assembly-line operation, centralized design and advertising, and management expertise all make the expansion of food chains possible.

As tastes become more sophisticated, though, the fast-food industry is attempting to keep up. First it was hot dogs, pizza, and "submarines" (or hoagies, grinders, or heroes, depending on locality). Then hamburgers (our way or your way), fried chicken, and fried fish became the fast foods of choice. More recently ethnic foods made their appearance, along with breakfast choices, salad bars, and soft frozen yogurt.

But how well are we eating at these places? Information about the nutritional content of fast foods is available. (Examination of Appendix Table H will allow you to compare the nutritional values of different fast-food meals.) The nutrient composition of additional items is also available in other publications and from the food chains themselves.

A typical meal at a fast-food restaurant is relatively high in energy content, with substantial contributions made by the fat in fried foods and meats and by the sweeteners in beverages commonly purchased, such as soft drinks and shakes. The most frequently eaten meal—cheesburger, fries, chocolate shake, and apple pie—contributes 1,180 kcal, with 39 percent of those kilocalories provided by fat, 50 percent by carbohydrate, and 11 percent by protein. This is obviously not a small contribution to the day's energy intake, and it may in fact be more than half of the total daily energy requirement.

Usual meals at fast food restaurants are adequate, even generous, in protein content, primarily derived from animal sources. Intakes of

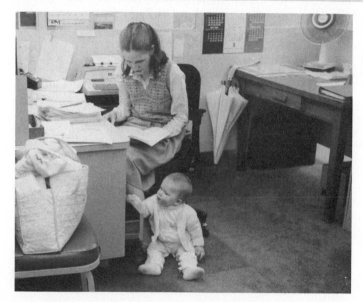

Women employed outside the home have less time for food shopping and meal preparation.
Ken Karp

niacin, thiamin, ascorbic acid, vitamin B_{12}, and vitamin D compare favorably with the RDAs, depending of course on the particular food items selected. Vitamin A content tends to be low in most fast-food meals.

Consideration of the types of foods served at most fast-food restaurants will indicate that the crude fiber content is minimal. Although measures of crude fiber content underestimate total dietary fiber (Chapter 2), the amount of undigestible material in most fast foods is undeniably low.

Data provided in the Appendix demonstrate that fast-food restaurants are not suitable choices for people who must adhere to a sodium-restricted diet. Even the mildest restriction, 2 grams of sodium per day, would be difficult to achieve at a fast-food outlet, especially when other meals eaten during the day must be considered.

Other concerns related to the popularity of fast-food establishments focus on the limited number of food selections available. Moreover, people tend to order the same meal each time they go to a given restaurant, further reducing the variety of food consumed. The introduction of "fast-food lunches" into school systems has increased the opportunity of children to consume fast foods. Because of the importance of consuming a variety of foods to provide a nutritionally balanced and adequate diet, it becomes even more necessary to incorporate additional food varieties into the total dietary plan. Salad bars provide a limited number of raw vegetables but more variety should be achieved at other meals.

Frequent consumption of fast-food meals will not aid someone with a weight problem; and the appropriate strategy in this case is not to skip other meals. Adequate diets must provide enough of the essential nutrients needed for health and well-being, and not be planned only on the basis of calories. Lower-calorie foods can be selected at a fast-food restaurant by choosing an unsweetened beverage, milk or plain water, passing up dessert (or bringing an apple along), and eating single portions. Foods eaten during the rest of the day should include milk, a serving of dark green or yellow vegetables, and fruit or fruit juice.

Choices would be more informed if the nutrient composition of fast foods were more widely available for consumers to add to their own basic nutrition knowledge. Policies concerning the display of nutrition information to customers were proposed several years ago but have not been implemented.

Women who work obviously have less time to devote to food shopping, preparation, and serving. Sales of convenience foods and appliances to save food-preparation time (food processors, slow cookers, microwave ovens, freezers) have been steadily increasing for years. Families also eat out more—over one-third of all money spent on food in the United States is spent for meals consumed away from home.

Although women are still the primary "gatekeepers" to family food patterns, increasingly the entire family has become involved in the meal-preparation process. In many families, husbands and teenagers now share the responsibility for shopping and cooking.

Culture

Wednesday is Food Day in some newspapers across the country, Thursday in others. Television takes us into the kitchens of the "Frugal Gourmet" and the great chefs of Chicago, New Orleans, or New York. It brings us information affecting our food choices on the evening news (for example, in features on the cost of feeding a family or new research relating dietary patterns to health) and in commercials. Even the introduction of a new product may be given air time.

Food has become a status symbol. Gourmet club members exchange recipes and invite one another for dinners. "Adventures in eating" clubs go on restaurant expeditions. There are gourmet magazines, cooking schools, and lavishly illustrated "coffee-table" cookbooks. A recent traveler to Marrakesh might serve Lema Ma'amrra (chicken stuffed with eggs, onions, and parsley) or couscous. A newspaper article giving recipes on how to make chocolate pudding from scratch received an unprecedented response. Where food was once only a necessity of life, it has become, for today's affluent society, a visible sign of one's education and status, and food preparation and consumption have become a source of entertainment as well as sustenance.

Economics

Poverty is one, but not the only cause of poor nutritional status. In 1981, 14 percent of the population, 31,822,000 people, had incomes below the poverty line. Poverty is not evenly distributed in the population; it ranges from 7.7 percent of suburban families to 15.2 percent for families in rural areas and 16.7 percent for families in the central city. At one point in time, poverty was most prevalent in rural areas, but the rise of agribusiness and the decline in the farm population have reduced the number of rural poor.

Comparing the shares of total family income in 1947 and 1981 shows that the wealthiest 20 percent received 43.0 percent and 41.9 percent, respectively. For the poorest 20 percent, the figure is 5 percent in both cases. In the interim, inflation has eroded buying power so that in the case of the poor staying the same, they have been losing ground. Over 60 percent of the poor in 1980 were over 65 years of age, invalids, or children. The special needs of some members of these groups further reduces their ability to obtain adequate food.

Issues: Health, Fitness, Ecology

Our national preoccupation with food has two facets. One focus is on the sociable and status aspects. The other reflects a growing concern over controversial issues relating to food and nutrition.

Substantial numbers of individuals and groups have chosen to abandon the "traditional American diet" for a variety of reasons. Some advocate new methods of food production or distribution to achieve certain public benefits. The vegetarian movement has many converts. Other people are concerned with removing from their diets—and from supermarket shelves—an item or ingredient believed to be dangerous or unhealthy. Still others are looking for "miracle" foods or nutrients.

HEALTH AND FITNESS.   Consumers have eagerly greeted "health" and "natural" foods. The FDA, concerned over accuracy of package labeling, can intervene if false information about ingredients or health benefits is given or if a product is found to be dangerous. Some items sold in "health food stores" may even be *unhealthy*. Arsenic may be found in kelp tablets; potassium chloride may cause hyperkalemia, and in fact a decade ago caused the death of an infant in Florida. Those who must limit their intake of sodium should be aware that tamari (fermented soy sauce), also sold in health food stores, can make a substantial contribution to sodium intake; 1 tablespoon of tamari contains 3 *grams* of salt.

Cholesterol, saturated fat, fiber, vitamin A are, or have also been, "health" issues. At this time many people are concerned about the relationship between dietary intake and personal health. By reading labels, the concerned consumer is able to make choices regarding foods in order to limit cholesterol or fat intake, and to increase the intake of fiber or vitamin A. Recent advertising has changed to promote a product as possibly improving your health. The claim is not that a product will guarantee your good health, but that it will help you to be healthy.

Most women and many men want to lose 5 to 10 pounds whether they need to or not. According to a recent survey, only 8 percent of the women were not at all concerned with keeping their weight down, 30 percent were extremely concerned, 32.5 percent were very concerned, and 29.5 percent were somewhat concerned. The concern with weight loss is pervasive, and the food industry has responded. High intensity sweeteners have made it possible to reduce the sugar and caloric content of many products. In this same survey, approximately 30 percent of the respondents reported increased use of diet soft drinks and 17 percent reported increased use of diet foods. Bulking agents and fibers are used to lower the caloric content of other types of foods. Calories per spoonful can also be decreased by incorporating air to increase volume, by replacing part of the oil with water in salad dressing, and by using fat replacements in other foods.

Preservatives are substances added to foods to prolong shelf life and to maintain or enhance nutritional quality. They may appear as wax on vegetables, but usually they are invisible. Foods sold in health food stores are frequently touted as being free of preservatives. But unless the store takes great care in handling, repackaging, and storing its products, contamination will set in and the food quality will deteriorate in a very short time.

ECOLOGY. Pesticides and fertilizers are used to protect or increase crop yield, which is both profitable to farmers and has made possible a plentiful supply of food at reasonable prices for consumers. Pesticides retard losses due to insects, rodents, and other wildlife. Fertilizers replace or add nutrients to the soil. Concern over environmental pollution from synthetic chemicals as suspected danger to life forms, however, has led many people to turn to foods grown without fertilizers or pesticides, given minimal or no food processing, and not preserved with "additives." Those who are extremely concerned over this issue have turned to so-called **organic foods.** This term generally refers to foods grown by methods that use plant-and-animal-derived (instead of factory-produced) fertilizers and plant rotation or mechanical rather than chemical means of averting insects and other predators. Organically raised livestock are fed only with organically raised feed and receive no dietary supplements or chemicals to accelerate growth. Three states and the Federal Trade Commission have developed legal definitions of organic agriculture.

Soil conditions markedly affect crop yields; in depleted soil, plants will not grow. Within limits, the mineral content of plants tends to parallel the mineral content of the soil. However, genetics are a far more significant factor in the nutrient composition of a plant. Whether fertilized or not, corn will never contain as much calcium as spinach. But as long as crops are grown in nutrient-rich soils, it matters little whether those nutrients are produced in a factory, a compost heap, or a manure pile. And as long as livestock receive a diet of nutrient-rich grasses, grains, and other plant products, they will not lack essential nutrients. But soils do become depleted, and nutrients must be returned to the earth, in one form or another.

The movement which began with the publication of *Silent Spring* by Rachel

Carson in 1962 is still active, but perhaps not as much in the limelight as in the 1970s. Over the past decade there have been ideological shifts in the ecologically based environmentalist movement resulting in differences of opinion regarding how the environment should be managed. Pesticides and fertilizers are needed, but types and quantity must be carefully monitored in order to maximize benefits and minimize the risk of harmful effects. Current regulations on pesticide residues in foods are based on the "tolerance principle." This assumes that all pesticides are toxic in high doses, but at low doses injury does not occur. The World Health Organization and the Food and Agricultural Organization of the United Nations have established acceptable daily intakes of pesticide residues.

SOURCES OF THE FOOD SUPPLY

A changing country and changing life styles affect not only the kinds of foods we eat but also where we get them and how we prefer to cook them. Dinner tonight in many an American home will be broiled chicken taken out of the home freezer last night to defrost; frozen green beans, bought three weeks ago; spinach, prewashed, tossed in a commercial Italian dressing; cherry pie made from canned cherries and a crust mix or selected from the frozen dessert section in the supermarket two days ago; ground coffee from a vacuum-packed can; milk from a paper carton, use-dated; sugar bought a month ago.

Agriculture: Where the Food Supply Originates

Farming today is very different from what it was in the past. Increasingly, farmers are at the mercy of events and conditions over which they have little or no control. Farmers have always had to deal with severe weather conditions and pest infestations, but the centralization of our agricultural system tends to amplify their effects. Since 1985, the number of farms has declined by nearly two-thirds.

The technological demands of high-intensity farming; the capital needed for land, supplies, and equipment; the need for adequate storage facilities; and the high cost of labor drive up farmers' costs. National and international events increasingly influence the economy quickly, with prices seeming to defy the law of supply and demand. Moreover, farmers appear not to be receiving their proportionate share of the food dollar. As the price of food skyrockets, farmers contend that the so-called "middleman" is reaping the profits and have called on the government for financial and regulatory aid.

There are no easy answers to these problems. More efficient use of land, development of new crops and animal breeds, new uses for old products, a comprehensive energy policy, and support of local agriculture and marketing systems—long ago abandoned as our cities grew—are some of the approaches that should be examined. At present we are dependent on only a handful of crops; most of the world's food comes from about twenty species. Throughout history humankind has used some 3,000 plant species. Development of species that can survive in arid lands or on marginal lands would provide an important stable food supply for many countries. Many potential food crops have been ignored, not because of any inherent inferiority, but because the crops grow in the tropics while the world's research resources are concentrated in the temperate zone. Another reason for neglect is the idea that some foods are "poor peoples crops." Peanuts and potatoes once fell into this category. Amaranth (a cereal), arracacaha (a celery-like plant), and yam beans (a legume) are among the potential crops that could be used to develop a more stable food supply for many parts of the world.

Climate and weather have always been important to agriculture. An alternative method is to grow plants hydroponically in an atmosphere in which light, temperature, and growing conditions are carefully controlled (controlled-environment agriculture). Unlike greenhouses that need to be cooled in the summer and heated in the winter, controlled environment agriculture uses only artificial light. There is no need for fertilizer because all the nutrients needed are supplied in the water; there is no need for pesticides because there are no pests. An additional benefit is spinach without residual sand. The growing conditions and the lighting system have been improved vastly and commercial production is now possible. Currently this method is used on a limited number of crops that adapt easily to the growing conditions. Corn will never be grown this way, but various leafy green vegetables such as varieties of lettuce and spinach, do very well.

Computers are also finding their way into agriculture. One system has been developed to manage cotton crops by determining the best strategy for irrigating, applying fertilizer, defoliants, and cotton-boll openers based on daily automatic weather reports. Eventually similar systems will manage other crops.

Food Processors: How Food Is Preserved

Many techniques of food preservation have been used for thousands of years. Egyptian hieroglyphs show smoking and drying foods for preservation; people who lived along the seacoast or where sugar cane was grown used salt on fish and meats and sugar on fruits and vegetables to extend the useful life of these foods. The nineteenth century brought many changes with the introduction of new technologies for canning and freezing food. Nicolas Appert won an award offered by Napoleon for technologies that would help his armies. Within fifty years, his canning process was used in most developed countries, freeing them from the seasonal availability of foods. In 1850 John Gorrie patented a device to make ice, but it was not very efficient. Only with the discovery of Freon did home refrigeration and frozen food expand as an industry. In 1940 only 30 percent of the homes in the United States had mechanical refrigerators. More recently chemical additives, preservatives, and chemically modified ingredients have resulted in longer storage and less waste. The most recent addition to the technology of food preservation is *food irradiation*. It offers advantages to the consumer that include improved sanitation of foods, extended shelf life, safe transport of produce from insect quarantine areas, replacement of some chemical fumigants, and reduction of spoilage and waste. Consumers in the United States, however, have responded negatively to irradiated produce. Many fear exposure to radiation, not understanding that the food does not become radioactive, just as you do not become radioactive when you have an x-ray. Fear that toxic products are formed during irradiation is also common, but not true. Attitude toward irradiated food is more positive in other countries.

Another new way to add to the food supply is with fabricated foods. These differ from conventional foods in that the basic components may be derived from several sources and combined with micronutrients, flavors, and colors to form a new and attractive product. You may already have tested this new process if you have had some of the "crab" and "shrimp" products that contain only 10 percent of either crab or shrimp. The rest of the product is surimi that comes from the muscle proteins of various fish that are not as desirable to the consumer. Food technology and food science respond to the consumer. Notice the proliferation of high-fiber cereals in response to the desire to add fiber to the diet.

Supermarkets, Restaurants, Institutions: How Food Gets to Us

SUPERMARKETS. Today we get our food preeminently from supermarkets which supply us with foods grown around the world. This includes both fresh and processed foods. Strawberries are grown in Mexico and even further south for consumption in the middle of winter. Some canned products come from mainland China. The variety available in supermarkets is now greater than ever. Like its forerunner, the general store, the supermarket still provides a means of socializing, a place to exchange opinions on brands, prices, and personal food choices.

There have been many changes in items available in supermarkets in the last decade. Where once there was mainly white, now rye, and egg bread, several types of whole wheat and several other varieties are frequently available, as well as are bagels and croissants. Many supermarkets now have bakeries on the premises.

Fresh produce is offered in greater variety: The average number of items offered in 1972 was 65; in 1983 the number was 173. Some larger stores may carry as many as 250 items. Mangoes, kiwi fruit, and plantains share the produce space with pineapples and carrots. Lettuce is available as Bibb, Boston, and Red, as well as the old faithful Iceberg. Fresh spinach, romaine, and endive are also available to add variety to the salad and many supermarkets now have salad bars where you buy ingredients by the pound. Fresh produce departments have replaced the meat counter as the major drawing card.

Another addition in many markets has been the bulk food section. Depending on the store a greater or smaller variety of items can be purchased. In one market the selection can be very large from dry animal food to nuts, to cookies and candy, to eight or ten dry-soup mixes, to several types of beans and lentils. In another market only ten items in total may be offered. Generic foods have also become a part of the supermarket offerings. Ethnic food, both fresh and processed, is also available.

In addition to changes within the stores themselves, supermarkets now come in various types from traditional to several levels of no-frills stores. No-frills stores may or may not offer the same range of foods as the supermarket. They frequently carry limited brand selections of basic items; customers help themselves to merchandise still in half-opened shipping cartons and pack their own groceries, saving up to 30 percent of food costs at a standard supermarket. At the other end of the spectrum is the supermarket where you can buy several types of frozen duck, gourmet prepared foods, fancy candy, crystal goblets, and even jewelry. Bulk-food stores, co-ops, convenience stores, and the various types of supermarkets each meet the need of part of the market.

Supermarkets are becoming more responsive to consumer needs and wants, offering advice from nutritionists, recipes for dieting and other special needs, and "best buy" labels. One chain offers bilingual information on nutrition; another has nutrition information leaflets to be picked up in every aisle. New kinds of supermarkets are making their appearance. Conscious of growing consumer resentment at rising prices and increased skepticism about the nutritional quality of food, retailers are seeking a more positive image. Handsome graphic design, striking colors, piped-in music, and streamlined fixtures enhance appeal and tempt customers to linger longer. Special services—custom-cut meats in freezer portions, telephone orders and delivery service, appetizer and bakery departments—build customer loyalty.

The modern technologies of preservation make many previously seasonal foods available year-round. Frequently, processed foods are less expensive than the unprocessed products and are generally of comparable nutritional value. Delays in transportation, sitting in the sun without refrigeration, bruising during shipping and handling, and other causes of damage may reduce nutrient content of freshly picked produce—unless it is purchased at or near the original source. Frozen and canned products often preserve the original nutrient content with high efficiency, because the processing is done at or near the point of origin of the produce. Nutrient losses can occur in the home kitchen if the already processed foods are cooked too long.

Prices of processed foods reflect the addition of sauces, spices, and other foods to the basic product, as well as labor and overhead. But for the shopper to whom time saved in food preparation is a paramount consideration, the prepared food even at a higher price will be preferable. Customers should be aware that processed foods still may be relatively high in salt. Some producers have decreased the salt in certain foods, but others have not. An educated customer can read the package information and make informed choices. Processed foods and whole meals now come in a greater variety and price range. Any one consumer wants different things at different times, sometimes opting for convenience, sometimes for nutrition, sometimes for taste, and sometimes for price. The supermarket is large enough to satisfy a variety of decisions.

In the debate over whether the consumer is really queen—and king—in the domain of food supply and demand, the reliance of the food industry on marketing research suggests that demand does create supply. Only one of every ten manufacturers' product ideas survives to be test-marketed by consumer panels. Only one of every ten of these test-marketed products survives for general distribution. All told, 4,000 to 5,000 food products are introduced each year; scarcely a handful are truly innovative. Those that survive a rigorous marketing trial do so because they satisfy some consumer desire.

Supermarkets are a necessary part of contemporary life. We may grow our own herbs in window boxes or back yards and raise tomatoes and vegetables for the unusual pleasure of eating a variety rarely available in the shops. But for most of the year the variety of foods, safely transported, preserved, and packaged, which supermarkets make available, cannot be duplicated.

RESTAURANTS. We also get our meals (particularly lunch) in restaurants of many kinds and price ranges, both near and far from home, during our working days, our weekend golf outing or while visiting a museum, and when we are on our vacation. Institutional cafeterias at schools, factories, and corporate offices take 5 percent of our total food expenditures (see Figure 14–1). Whether at an elegant "tablecloth" restaurant, a truck stop, or a vending machine, Americans spend over 37 percent of their food dollars eating away from home and will probably spend 45 percent by 1990. Although eating at home is still the norm, eating out is clearly part of the way we live now. For our parents and grandparents, it was a much rarer event. Today many senior citizens eat out regularly, preferring the "off" hours at a restaurant. A relatively large meal at mid-day is frequently less expensive and meets

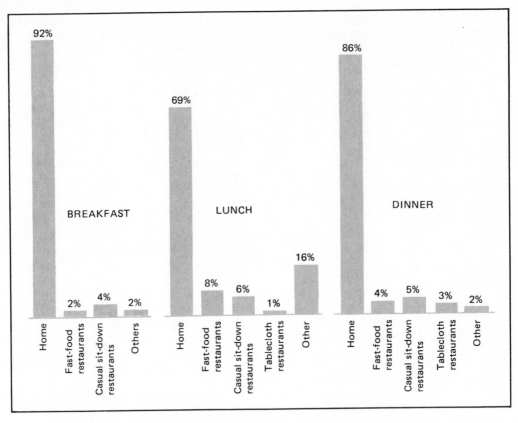

FIGURE 14-1   *Where Meals Are Eaten.*

Source: Adapted from R. E. Shaw and D. Pinto, Where's your next meal coming from?, *The Nielsen Researcher*, No. 1, 1978, pp. 5, 6.

their needs. Many other seniors go to congregate meal sites where they eat as well as have the opportunity for social interaction.

In 1982, fast-food chains accounted for 30 percent of food dollars spent eating out. More traditional eating establishments—ranging from diners and cafeterias to fancy "tablecloth" restaurants—accounted for 40 percent. Lunch is the meal most likely to be eaten out, breakfast the least likely; dinner falls in between. Almost one in three Americans eats lunch away from home—one in twelve at a fast-food restaurant. Put another way, Americans average two lunches and one dinner a week and about one breakfast every two weeks away from home.

Men eat out more frequently than women, as they have always done, but no longer by a decisive margin; men now consume 56 percent of all meals eaten away from home. The increasing number of working women, who eat out more often than do nonworking women, has narrowed the gap. Single men in the 22-to-34 age group eat nearly half of their lunches away from home, and women in that age group, close to a third. But no segment of the population is excluded from the phenomenon—all ages, all incomes, all ethnic groups, and all social strata take part.

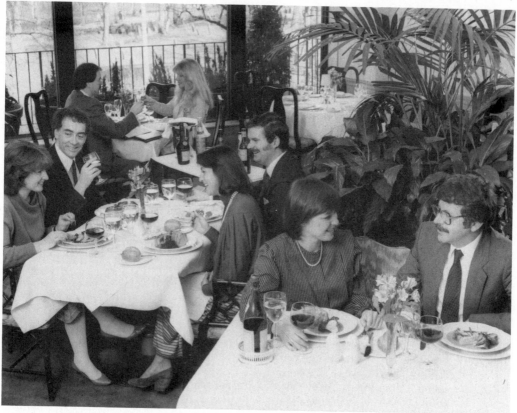

Although eating at home is still the norm, eating out is clearly a part of today's lifestyle.
Miro Vintoniv/Stock, Boston

This democratization of dining out is paralleled by the variety of foods available in restaurants. Affluence, travel, education, and the opportunities given by our mobile society to mix with people of different ethnic backgrounds have broadened American tastes for new and "foreign" foods. New immigrant groups such as the Bengali and Vietnamese begin to open restaurants in neighborhoods where they settle, widening the food experience of all diners. The rapid spread of pizza throughout the nation following World War II, and the more recent proliferation of taco and souvlaki stands and Szechwan-style Chinese restaurants, attest to our appetite for new taste experiences. Traditional restaurants have changed their menus to meet the needs of customers. In many the emphasis is on food that's fresh, light, made-to-order, lower in calories, and promotes good health. The American Heart Association and its local units have worked with restaurants advising them on foods for a healthy diet. Many offer "alternative" menus with entrees low in calories, fat, and salt. Some provide a shaker of herb seasonings as an alternative to salt. Fast-food operations now offer salads, baked potatoes, and other lighter fare. Nutrition information is now offered "on-site" at one fast-food chain;

such information has always been available but the customer needed to write to the company. For the customer who asks, many restaurants will prepare foods without butter or salt or make other changes.

INSTITUTIONS.   Food is eaten away from home not only at restaurants and fast-food chains but also in cafeterias at school and work, at museums and other tourist locations, on airplanes, in trains, and in camps. Children particularly have become accustomed to institutional meals. Today school lunches are a $4-billion-a-year industry, the fourth largest food sector in the country. Suburban sprawl, regional school systems, and integration mean that children can no longer return home for lunch. Furthermore, lunch periods are short: Even children who live nearby cannot return home for the 20-minute break allotted in some schools. Although some children still bring their lunch, most eat the food provided at school because working mothers have less time to pack lunches.

Working people generally do not go home for lunch. Some bring a bag lunch, which is money-saving but time-consuming to prepare; others buy lunch. Many company cafeterias provide excellent food at low cost to cultivate employee goodwill, save workers travel time, cut down desk time lost after lunch, and provide fringe benefits for employees with both the lowest and the highest salaries. Large, prosperous corporations have established their own eating places at their headquarters and larger branches. For smaller facilities and even around some larger ones, there are also the food trucks which sell sandwiches, chips, and beverages. Finally there are the smaller vendors who sell hot dogs or sausage sandwiches.

Increasingly, more of our meals as a nation will come from mass-feeding situations—as we spend more years in school, work for larger corporations, and have more time to travel. Also fewer foods are prepared on-site in the cafeteria of the school or workplace. Many schools receive prepared food and reheat it in microwave ovens; others may use partially prepared foods which are cooked or baked on site and still others prepare food pretty much from scratch. Corporation cafeterias are just as diverse in the types of food operations.

THE CONTENT OF TODAY'S FOODS

What's in Our Food: Addition of Nutrients

The increased consumption of fabricated and processed foods presents two separate issues. In the course of processing, foods lose some of the nutrients naturally contained in them, and so manufacturers add the very vitamins and minerals that have been removed. Terms associated with addition of nutrients in the United States are: restoration, fortification, and enrichment. Restoration means the addition to restore the original nutrient content. To fortify a food means to add nutrients in amounts sufficient to render the food a good-to-superior source of the added nutrients. This may include addition of nutrients not normally associated with the food or the addition to concentrations above that in the unprocessed food. Therefore a soft drink can be fortified with a vitamin or calcium. Vitamin D can be added to milk, and cereal can have more vitamins than the natural product. Enrichment is defined as the addition of specific amounts of selected nutrients in accordance with the standard of identity (specific recipe) as defined by the U.S. Food and Drug Administration. For regular purposes, the latter two are interchangeable.

Nutrition groups of the American Medical Association and the National Academy of Sciences/National Research Council continue to endorse the additions of nutrients to foods under the following circumstances:

1. the dietary intake of the nutrients being below the desirable level in a significant number of the population;
2. the food which has the nutrient will be consumed in an amount sufficient to make a contribution;
3. the addition will not create an imbalance of essential nutrients;
4. the nutrient is bioavailable;
5. there is little chance of excessive intake leading to toxicity.

Some consumers incorrectly assume that addition of vitamins and minerals always makes a product better. Adding more nutrients to an already adequate diet provides no extra benefit.

Food Additives: Other Direct Additives

Other direct food additives are used to maintain freshness of the food, to make the food more appealing, or to help in processing and preparation. Sugar, salt, and corn syrup are the three most frequently used additives. Together with citric acid, baking soda, vegetable colorings, mustard, and pepper, these account for more than 98 percent by weight of all food additives used.

Food can spoil: Bacteria, molds, fungi, and yeasts are ever present. Food safety will be covered in the next section, here we will only deal with the role of food additives in preventing or slowing food spoilage. Mold growth makes food look bad and certain molds produce toxins which have caused death and illness in humans. Another way food can spoil is by change in color and flavor caused by oxidation. Freshly sliced apples will turn brown as a result of oxidation but squeezing lemon juice that contains the anti-oxidant vitamin C, ascorbic acid, will keep them from turning dark.

Flavors are the largest category of food additives, numbering more than 1,700 substances. Foods containing artificial flavors must say so on the label. Raspberry yogurt means all natural raspberry flavor; raspberry flavored yogurt contains all natural raspberry flavor and other natural flavors. Artificially flavored raspberry yogurt contains all artificial flavor or a mixture of natural and artificial.

Food Safety

Microorganisms which can cause illness continue to be an important problem. The exact extent of the problem is not really known because most cases of food related gastroenteritis are not severe enough to be reported. The majority of food poisoning epidemics occur because of mishandling of food either in processing, food service, or in the home. Improper holding temperature is the most common error, but unclean hands, knives, and cutting boards can spread the organisms. Contamination in the home probably accounts for the greatest number of cases. However, outbreaks attributed to mishandling by processors are much more widespread because

Perspective On

ADDITIVES

A food additive is any substance or mixture of substances that becomes part of a food during any stage of production, processing, storage, or packaging. Additives are of two types, direct and indirect. Direct additives, of which there are approximately 2,800, are added deliberately to maintain or improve nutritional value, to maintain freshness and product quality, to help in processing or preparation, and to make foods more appealing. Some examples include sodium bicarbonate, which is added to control acidity, methyl cellulose, which imparts and maintains a desired consistency, and food coloring.

Indirect additives, of which there are some 10,000, are present in foods in trace quantities as an unintentional result of some phase of production, processing, storage, or packaging. Some of these are pesticide residues, minute amounts of drugs fed to animals, and chemical substances that migrate from plastic packaging materials.

Food additives are not a new invention. Humans have always tried to preserve their food. Salt was probably used long before recorded history to preserve meat and fish; herbs and spices have always been added to foods to enliven the taste, and often in the past to conceal evidence of spoilage.

Today's extensive use of additives accompanied the shift from an agricultural to an urbanized society. There was a need for foods that could be mass-produced, distributed over long distances, stored for considerable periods of time, and made available at reasonable prices. As merchandising shifted from the local produce market to the interstate supermarket chain, shelf storage and packaging needs became evident. And as the population expanded there was a bigger market to be reached.

Food is certainly safer now than at the turn of the century when it was almost impossible to keep things from spoiling, and when manufacturers freely used toxic pigments as food coloring. But recently people have begun to wonder if we need all those chemicals. Some have been implicated as carcinogens, and people wonder how safe others may be. How valid are these worries? What should be done?

Until 1958, the government had the authority to remove from the market foods that were obviously adulterated, spoiled, or toxic. But in 1958, the Food Additive Amendment was enacted, providing that no additive could be used until it was proved *safe*. With this and the 1960 Color Additives Amendment, the burden of proof shifted from the government to the manufacturers: The manufacturer must demonstrate the safety of an additive which is defined as "reasonable certainty" that no harm will result from the intended use of the additive. The laws empowered the FDA to regulate additives only on the basis of safety. The agency could not limit the number of additives used, approve or judge the quality of a substance, or determine whether the additive was really needed.

Some additives are not subject to testing. The Food Additives Amendment exempted two major categories from testing: Some 700 additives

of the scale of most food handling and distribution operations. Contamination of two lots of milk with salmonella resulted in thousands of cases of salmonellosis.

The federal government is responsible for safety of foods that cross state lines; state and local governments are responsible for local products. Individuals are responsible for foods they process and should make sure that foods are not mishandled. A good rule is to keep cold foods cold and hot foods hot. Microorganisms can thrive in foods kept at moderate temperatures.

"generally recognized as safe" (GRAS), had been used extensively over the years with no known harmful effects. Others had been specifically approved before 1958 by the FDA or the USDA. But increasing concern over additives has brought the GRAS substances under scrutiny. A group called the Select Committee on GRAS Substances (SCOGS) is systematically reviewing some 450 additives that are considered GRAS. In addition, FDA is reviewing the safety of 2,100 flavoring agents.

Recently sulfites have come under particular scrutiny. Adverse reactions to sulfites have been reported in a small percentage of people who have asthma and in some people who have no previous history of asthma. Over 500 complaints have been received by the FDA since 1982. Approximately 42 percent of the reactions are associated with eating at salad bars, 15 percent with consumption of wine or beer, 14 percent with packaged foods, 4 percent with grocery produce and the remaining less specifically identified. Typical reactions include difficulty in breathing, skin rash, rapid pulse, and dizziness.

The FDA has banned the use of sulfiting agents on fruits and vegetables that are intended for consumption in the raw state. In addition, food products which contain sulfiting agents as direct food additives and those which contain more than 10 ppm "incidental" sulfite must indicate their presence on the ingredient statement. These measures will alert sulfite-sensitive individuals to the presence of sulfites in foods.

A national food safety system that would encourage reasonable goals for reduction of risks in the food supply, regulate substances comprehensively taking risk levels into consideration, and permit a variety of regulatory procedures is desirable. Decision-making responsibility should incorporate the best scientific information and enlist full expression of informed public opinions (National Academy of Sciences, 1979). But it is difficult to quantify risks and benefits, particularly because they are often influenced by individual or group value judgments. Certain additives, used only for esthetic appeal, might be removed from use if consumers would accept products with an unfamiliar appearance. Most risk-benefit equations, however, are not that simple.

It is not possible to prove that a food—or anything else for that matter—is absolutely safe at all times for all people. Testing must continue and be extended. At this time, more is known about chemical additives than about the chemicals in the natural foods we eat. Moreover, consumers must recognize that very high doses of additives are used in safety testing—much higher than people can be expected to consume.

The subject of additives continues to be controversial, and investigations are continuing to determine additive safety. The best protection against potential toxic effects from any food chemical is consumption of a diversified diet, which will also help to provide an adequate intake of all essential nutrients. And consumers must choose which food qualities—appearance, convenience, storage time, or freedom from additives—are most important to them.

What We Get from Foods: Nutrients

Contrary to popular belief, energy and carbohydrate intake is lower than at the turn of the century, and we consume about as much protein as ever. But our energy is being provided more by fats, sugars, and meats, and our protein more by meat, instead of by the traditional cereals and grains. In 1910, fat and sweeteners supplied 44 percent of our calories; recently, they were providing 60 percent. The percentage of energy intake from complex carbohydrates fell from 37 to 21 during the same period. Flour and cereal products supplied about twice as much of the protein in our diets at the beginning of the century than they do now; meat, poultry, and fish now account for about 15 percent more of the protein in our diets than they once did.

ENERGY.   Our overall caloric intake from all foods (excluding liquors) declined steadily until the early 1960s, but it has risen since then and is now almost as high (3,300 kcal per day) as it was 70 years ago (3,480 kcal per person per day). Remember that these figures reflect disappearance data and, although undesirably high, do not reflect *real* individual intakes. In part they may indicate only that we are more wasteful of our foods; it has been shown that smaller households throw out more food than larger ones do, and the typical American household is shrinking, accounting for proportionally more waste.

Most of the recent increase in energy intake has come from fat, which furnishes over twice as many kilocalories per gram as protein or carbohydrates. In the 1909 to 1913 period, only 16 percent of the fat consumed came from vegetable sources; in 1982 the figure was 44 percent. Foods of animal origin, in the form of meat, eggs, milk, butter, and cheese, supply the rest.

VITAMINS AND MINERALS.   Overall, vitamin A consumption has stayed about the same over the years, although a slight decrease has been noted in recent years. Intakes of thiamin, riboflavin, niacin, and iron tend to change in parallel fashion since they are usually found in the same foods. Consumption of these nutrients slowly declined until the late 1930s and increased when bread enrichment began in the 1940s. A much greater consumption of poultry in recent years has also been a factor. Meat provides proportionally more of these nutrients than it did 50 years ago and vegetables proportionally less.

FIGURE 14-2   *Total Fat: Proportionate Contributions by Major Food Groups.*

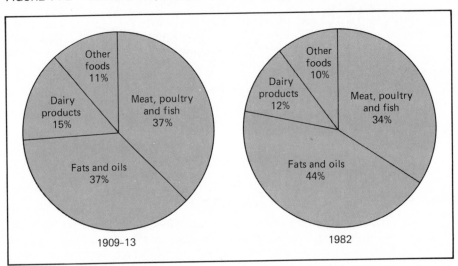

Source: R. M. Marston and S. O. Welsh, "Nutrient Content of the U.S. Food Supply, 1982," *National Food Review,* Winter 1984, p. 10.

Vitamin B$_6$ is another nutrient of which less was consumed during the Depression years. We now eat as much as in 1909 but about 15 percent more than in 1935. The flour-refining process removes much of the B$_6$ from grains, but today the vitamin is being added to several foods, including breakfast cereals and baby formulas. Throughout this century the disappearance data figures have hovered around the adult RDA of 2 milligrams of vitamin B$_6$ per adult per day.

Because we're eating more meat, we're getting about 14 percent more vitamin B$_{12}$ than 70 years ago. Animal-origin foods are the only natural source of the vitamin, but other foods such as breakfast cereals are fortified with it, so that now 1.5 percent of our intake of B$_{12}$ comes from flour and cereals. Adequate consumption of vitamin B$_{12}$ is a concern for those on strict vegetarian eating patterns.

Everybody knows that citrus fruits are rich in vitamin C, but so are vegetables, especially potatoes and tomatoes. Since improved transportation and the development of frozen juices have multiplied our consumption of citrus products, and vitamin C-fortified drinks have also increased in number and use, it's little wonder that we're getting more vitamin C than ever.

Calcium intake parallels the consumption of milk. All the pregnant mothers and babies of the post-World War II baby boom pushed milk and calcium consumption to record levels. Calcium intake has decreased in the population, particularly among women. Availability tends to be unevenly distributed among the population.

Magnesium is one nutrient of which substantially less is being consumed, perhaps because it is not normally added to fortified foods. Daily personal consumption fell from 408 milligrams in 1909–1913 to 339 milligrams in 1965, but it has stayed almost exactly the same since then. Since these figures reflect disappearance data only, it is very likely that most people are getting less magnesium than the adult RDAs of 350 milligrams for men and 300 for women. The decrease in magnesium consumption parallels the decreased consumption of breads and cereals and of coffee. Though dairy products, processed potatoes, and poultry are providing a greater proportion of dietary magnesium than formerly, there has still been an overall decrease.

Accurate figures for phosphorus intakes are not available. This mineral is a component of foods but exact quantities are not known. Total phosphorus intake has remained almost static during this century, although in earlier years a larger proportion of the mineral was provided by grains and cereals.

THE GOVERNMENT AND A NATIONAL FOOD POLICY

Nutritional concerns have prompted legislation throughout the years, but there is not yet a coordinated national nutrition policy in the United States. The growing awareness of these problems in the past two decades has, however, led to many government programs. Today many federal agencies are involved with agriculture, food, and health programs. In 1974 the National Nutrition Consortium issued guidelines for a national nutrition policy (see Table 14–1). By 1977, the results of two national nutrition surveys had been published, and a Select Committee of the U.S. Senate had issued national Dietary Goals. In 1980, *Dietary Guidelines for*

TABLE 14-1. *Goals of a National Nutrition Policy*

1. To assure an adequate wholesome food supply at reasonable cost to meet the needs of all segments of the population, this supply being available at a level consistent with the affordable life style of the era
2. To maintain food resources sufficient to meet emergency needs and to fulfill a responsible role as a nation in meeting world food needs
3. To develop a level of sound public knowledge and responsible understanding of nutrition and foods that will promote maximal nutritional health
4. To maintain a system of quality and safety control that justifies public confidence in its food supply
5. To support research and education in foods and nutrition with adequate resources and reasoned priorities to solve important current problems and to permit exploratory basic research

Source: National Nutrition Consortium, Inc., Guidelines for a national nutrition policy, *Nutrition Reviews* 32:153, 1974.

Americans was published; a slightly revised set of *Guidelines* was published in 1985 (Table 14-2 on page 503) by the U.S. Department of Agriculture and the U.S. Department of Health and Human Services.

A number of different agencies within the federal government are involved in nutrition-related research, educational, regulatory, and food-assistance programs. The Departments of Agriculture and of Health and Human Services have the major roles in formulating and carrying out national food policies; other government agencies act in specific areas. An Interagency Committee on Human Nutrition Research, with representatives from eight federal agencies, has been formed to develop priorities for research and to exchange information.

The Department of Agriculture

The Department of Agriculture (USDA) inspects meat and poultry shipped interstate and inspects animal and food plant sanitation to assure the standards of quality of the food supply. As a service to food companies, upon request it grades fruit, vegetables, bread, and dairy products. The USDA has a tradition of success in consumer education. It funds the Expanded Food and Nutrition Education Program (EFNEP), which utilizes nutrition aides, trained homemakers from the target community who demonstrate and explain nutritional precepts in home visits. Funds for EFNEP have been shaved steadily over the years.

The USDA conducts research through its Science and Education Administration. The Agricultural Research Service coordinates research at six human nutrition research centers and a regional laboratory and awards grants to other institutions. A Human Nutrition Center coordinates research projects at a number of laboratories throughout the country. The USDA also administers several food-assistance programs through its Food and Nutrition Service. These include food stamps, school food programs, and the Special Supplemental Food Program for Women, Infants, and Children (WIC).

FOOD STAMPS.   The Food Stamp Act was enacted in 1964 to enable low-income households to buy more food in greater variety. The stamps are coupons that can be used like money at the grocery stores that have been approved to accept and redeem food coupons. Those eligible for them are given an Authorization to Participate (ATP) Card each month. With the ATP Card and a Food Stamp

Identification Card, an individual can get the stamps at a bank or at another licensed outlet. Average monthly assistance was estimated at $42.67 per individual in fiscal 1983 and $39.32 in fiscal 1984. In fiscal 1982, participation averaged 21.7 million persons per month.

SPECIAL NUTRITION PROGRAMS. These programs, designed to benefit children from low-income families, include the National School Lunch Program, the Special Milk Program for Children, the School Breakfast Program, the Summer Food Service Program for Children, and the Child-Care Food Program. Under these programs, lunches and breakfasts are provided free or at reduced prices to children from low-income families as determined by local authorities. The 1946 National School Lunch Act evolved from the recognition that the economic and agricultural crisis of the 1930s had resulted in malnutrition of significant numbers of young people. At the same time, food surpluses were beginning to accumulate following World War II.

The School Lunch Program provided a nutrition program to reach all children based on tested nutritional research. A "Type A" lunch was planned to provide approximately one-third of a school-age child's RDAs for nutrients and energy.

In 1966 the Child Nutrition Act reached out to more children through a pilot School Breakfast Program and with meals for preschoolers and for poverty-area children in summer recreation and other nonschool groups. This expansion, originating in the context of the first national commitment to preschool education through Operation Head Start and the beginnings of a national day-care program, led to further expansion through a number of amendments in the 1970s. The School Breakfast Program was formally added in a 1973 amendment.

Some school children bring their lunch from home, but most eat the food provided at the school.
USDA Photo by Larry Rana

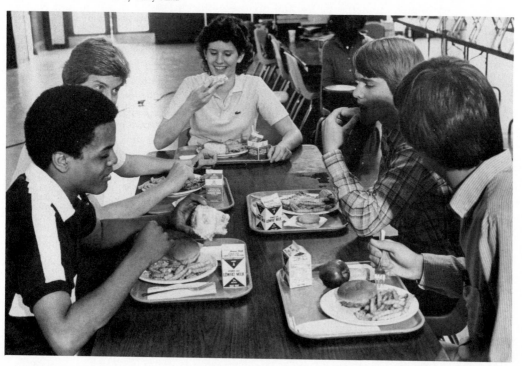

Recently the "offer versus serve" option was mandated for senior high schools and is optional for some junior high and elementary schools. This option allows five items to be offered. The student is encouraged to take all five, but the institution will be reimbursed for the meal if the student only takes three or four of the items.

WIC. The Special Supplemental Food Program for Women, Infants, and Children began as a consequence of the findings of the Ten-State Nutrition Survey and other surveys of the nutritional status of the poor between 1968 and 1970. All showed that although there was little evidence of vitamin deficiencies or severe protein-energy malnutrition, a great number of infants and children were smaller than average, and about half the children age one to two years showed a dietary deficiency of iron. It was also clear that the extent of undernourishment increased in direct proportion to the poverty of the family, and that the undernutrition was due to an overall inadequate intake and not to an inappropriate diet.

In 1972, Congress authorized a two-year pilot program to provide food supplements for low-income pregnant and lactating women, infants, and children under five years. In 1974 the program was extended and given increased funding for four more years; continued funding was provided in 1978. Grants for fiscal 1983 and 1984 were over $1 billion per year.

Funds are channeled to state health departments or comparable state agencies; to Indian tribes or groups recognized by the Department of the Interior; or to the Indian Health Service of the Department of Health and Human Services. These agencies distribute funds to participating local agencies. Food is distributed directly or by voucher, home delivery, or a combination of systems. Local agencies are directed to utilize paraprofessionals and to provide nutrition education in culturally appropriate form.

Currently there are WIC programs in 50 states, 31 Indian agencies, Puerto Rico, the Virgin Islands, Guam, and the District of Columbia providing aid to over 2½ million women, infants, and children; but an estimated 8.3 million eligible low-income individuals are not reached by the program.

EXTENSION SERVICE. The extension service is an educational agency and part of the Cooperative Extension System. Extension home economists are on the staff of the state land-grant universities and provide nutrition information to the public. Federal extension services assist the state programs. Extension workers cooperate in many community programs, including 4-H programs for children and special programs for low-income families. The Expanded Food and Nutrition Program (EFNEP) was established in 1968 to teach nutrition and solve housekeeping problems. Between 1968 and 1983, more than 2.1 million families and 5.5 million youths participated in the program.

The Department of Health and Human Services

The mission of the Department of Health and Human Services (DHHS) is to protect and advance the health and well-being of the nation's people. Several agencies within DHHS play significant roles relating to foods and nutrition.

ADMINISTRATION ON AGING. The Administration on Aging (AoA) is a branch of the Office of Human Development Services. AoA was established by the Older Americans Act of 1965 and is the principal agency charged with its implementation. The AoA, in addition to supporting research on aging and training professionals to work in this field, implements the national nutrition program for this segment of the population.

The Older Americans Act established research and demonstration nutrition projects, the results of which led to the creation of a Nutrition Program for older Americans in March 1972. Known originally as Title VII, this program provided funding for at least one meal a day, plus supportive services in a congregate setting, for persons 60 years of age and older and their spouses. Special emphasis is placed on those with the greatest social and economic need. Congregate meal programs are administered by health centers and senior citizens and church groups in the community. Their goal is to offer a social experience along with a hot meal providing one-third of the adult RDAs for key nutrients.

When problems of transportation in a number of communities prevented many older people from taking advantage of congregate meals, home delivery programs were established. Currently nutrition services are funded under Special Programs for the Aged, Title III, through formula grants to state and area agencies. States must provide some matching funds and, as with other programs, one goal is nutrition education. About 732,000 meals were served daily in the two programs at the end of fiscal 1982.

ADMINISTRATION FOR CHILDREN, YOUTH, AND FAMILIES. This administration seeks to expand and improve the range of services that promote the development of children and youth. Head Start, which provides nutritional services among others, is funded through this channel. The purpose of Head Start is to help children overcome the handicap of poverty. Families with incomes below the poverty line, or who are receiving aid to dependent children, must represent 90 percent of the total enrolled in a program; handicapped children 10 percent. Since 1965 when it was established, Head Start has served over 8 million children from low-income families.

THE U.S. PUBLIC HEALTH SERVICE. The U.S. Public Health Service (USPHS) encompasses several agencies that also have specific responsibilities in food and nutrition.

The Food and Drug Administration (FDA) has primary responsibility for protecting the safety of the American food supply. Its job is to inspect food-processing plants; to approve food additives for safety; to determine and set standards for foods made according to a standardized recipe (peanut butter or mayonnaise, for example) and to test such products to assure they meet these "standards of identity"; to obtain samples of foods after they are offered for sale, testing them for safe consumer use; and to develop regulations for food package labeling.

In 1906 public pressure forced the passage of the Pure Food and Drug Act, the basis of all subsequent safety regulations. The USDA was given responsibility for ascertaining the safety of all foods in interstate commerce and assuring that any chemical added to foods was safe and had a useful purpose. But the USDA was given only the right to inspect food-processing plants and to publish the results of its investigations of food products; it did not have the power to impose fines or penalties.

The FDA was created within the USDA in 1931 but was not effective until the passage of the Federal Food, Drug, and Cosmetic Act in 1938; this legislation gave the FDA power to fine and imprison those found guilty of misbranding and adulterating foods. The burden of proof was on the government, which has to investigate and prosecute alleged violators. The FDA and its powers were reassigned to the Department of Health, Education, and Welfare (now the DHHS) in 1953. Only meat inspection remained under the jurisdiction of the USDA.

In 1954, the Miller Pesticide Amendment, specifying maximum levels of pesticides that could remain on foods once they entered the marketplace, was added to the 1938 Food, Drug, and Cosmetic Act. The Food Additive Amendment of 1958 defined additives and for the first time placed responsibility for proving the safety and efficacy of an additive on the food industry rather than on the government. The Delaney Clause prohibiting the addition of carcinogenic substances to food was a rider attached to this act.

Another amendment, added in 1960, specified that synthetic coloring agents had to be tested and certified by the government before they could be used in foods. The Fair Package and Labeling Act of 1966 gave the FDA specific authority over the content of package labels.

The FDA has been quite visible in several areas of contemporary public concern, among them the safety of food additives and fortification of foods. It has also played a prominent role in consumer education through labeling of food products. Present regulations regarding ingredient and nutrition information on foods (except for alcoholic beverages) come from the FDA.

DIETARY GUIDELINES. In February 1980, *Nutrition and Your Health, Dietary Guidelines for Americans* was issued jointly by DHHS and USDA. The guidelines were preceded by publication of *Healthy People: A Report by the Surgeon General on the State of National Health*. In *Healthy People*, a national program of health promotion was proposed in which diet played a critical role. Although the guidelines were a mild and moderate set of proposals, their publication touched off an outcry of charges and countercharges. Part of the problem resulted from conflicting viewpoints that (1) scientific evidence was not adequate to make dietary recommendations for the general public and (2) the need of the public for realistic, reli-

FIGURE 14-3   *Graphic Nutrient Labeling.*
This is the nutrient label on a potato chip package in use by a Dutch supermarket chain.

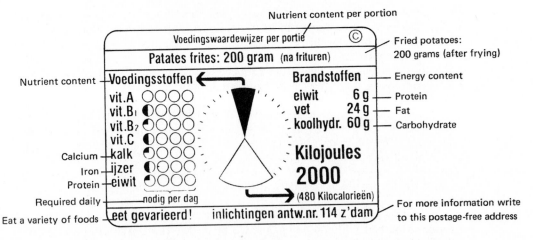

Source: H. E. Nelson, Consumer attitudes and trends. In *Plant and animal products in the U.S. food system* (Washington, D.C.: National Research Council, 1978), p. 163.

able guidance. Supporters of the guidelines state that public health policy cannot wait for complete and unequivocal verification, instead they must be developed using the best available data.

A scientific committee jointly appointed by the two departments recently reviewed the scientific literature relating to each of the seven *Dietary Guidelines* and the guidelines themselves were exhaustively discussed. Changes were minimal in the 1985 revision (Table 14-2). Some nutritionists supported combining the guidelines and changing "desirable" to "reasonable" weight, but these changes were not accepted. The Committee that produced the second edition recommended that the *Dietary Guidelines* be reviewed for scientific accuracy on a 5- to 10-year cycle to incorporate future scientific findings.

Other Government Agencies

The Federal Trade Commission (FTC) regulates food advertising and the application of antitrust laws. One of the FTC's major missions is to protect consumers from false and misleading advertising. The Bureau of Alcohol, Tobacco, and Firearms (BATF) of the Treasury Department is responsible for ingredient labeling of alcoholic beverages. BATF's responsibility for this area came about in 1972 when consumer advocates noticed that no ingredients were listed on beer cans. All foods were required to have ingredient listings, and a check of the lawbooks revealed that no exception had been made for wine, beer, and distilled spirits. Subsequently, BATF agreed to require full ingredient labeling on all alcoholic beverages.

Congress and Nutrition

Congress plays an important role in determining food and nutrition policy. It makes laws the regulatory agencies cannot make, and it appropriates—broadly— the monies they and other enforcement agencies have to spend. Congressional concerns vary. In recent years Congress has acted on saccharin. Appropriations have been provided for food stamps, feeding programs for schoolchildren and the elderly, and WIC.

Both houses of Congress are concerned with matters related to food and nutrition. Through its various committees and subcommittees Congress acquires information on which to base legislation and appropriations. Private citizens have the right and responsibility to let their senators and representatives know where they stand on issues and how they want their tax dollars spent.

Select committees are sometimes established by Congress to conduct investigations of particular topics. They cannot propose legislation, and their reports do not

---

TABLE 14-2. *Dietary Guidelines for Americans, Second Edition. Developed by the Dietary Guidelines Advisory Committee appointed by the Department of Agriculture and the Department of Health and Human Services.*

1. Eat a variety of foods
2. Maintain desirable weight
3. Avoid too much fat, saturated fat, and cholesterol
4. Eat foods with adequate starch and fiber
5. Avoid too much sugar
6. Avoid too much sodium
7. If you drink alcoholic beverages, do so in moderation

require congressional approval. The Senate Select Committee on Nutrition and Human Needs, under the leadership of then Senator George McGovern, was established in 1968 to reconcile the food and farm orientation of the Agriculture Committee with the health, welfare, and research concerns of the Labor and Public Welfare Committees. Work by this committee has been responsible for expansion of the food stamp, school lunch, summer feeding, and school breakfast programs and for establishment of the WIC program.

By 1975 the committee had become concerned over the role of overnutrition in the etiology of, particularly, coronary heart disease, obesity, cancer, and stroke. A series of hearings and expert testimony led committee members to conclude that the U.S. government should have an overall nutrition policy, so that legislation affecting agriculture, the food industry, and the public could specifically implement this policy. The result was the issuance in 1977 of the *Dietary Goals for the United States*, a report intended to provide guidelines for the development of a national nutrition policy (see Table 14–3).

TABLE 14-3. *Dietary Goals for the United States, Second Edition, December 1977*

1. To avoid overweight, consume only as much energy (calories) as is expended; if overweight, decrease energy intake and increase energy expenditure.
2. Increase the consumption of complex carbohydrates and "naturally occurring" sugars from about 28 percent to about 48 percent of energy intake.
3. Reduce the consumption of refined and other processed sugars by about 45 percent to account for about 10 percent of total energy intake.
4. Reduce overall fat consumption from approximately 40 percent to about 30 percent of energy intake.
5. Reduce saturated fat consumption to account for about 10 percent of total energy intake and balance that with polyunsaturated and monounsaturated fats, which should account for about 10 percent of energy intake each.
6. Reduce cholesterol consumption to about 300 mg per day.
7. Limit the intake of sodium by reducing the intake of salt (sodium chloride) to about 5 g per day (2 g sodium).

Source: Select Committee on Nutrition and Human Needs, U.S. Senate, *Dietary Goals for the United States*, ed 2. December 1977.

THE WORLD FOOD SUPPLY: MEETING THE PROBLEM OF UNDERNUTRITION

The results of nutrient deficiencies can be quite varied and range from minor to moderate to severe. Among the most devastating are stunted physical and mental development, nutritional deficiency diseases, decreased wound-healing ability, general tissue breakdown, impaired metabolism, and consequent increases in morbidity and mortality. Affected populations typically show decreased activity levels and impaired mental functioning, which in turn decreases their productivity and lessens the chance that they will be able to improve their own life style. Because of their rapid growth rate and concomitant need for energy and nutrients, children are particularly vulnerable to all these effects and under such conditions seldom achieve their genetic potential for physical or intellectual development.

Scope of the Problem

Various estimates of the worldwide prevalence of malnutrition suggest that from 400 to 500 million persons are affected. Malnutrition may be due to a simple lack of one or more essential nutrients, resulting in a specific deficiency disease, or to a general shortage of food. Protein and energy deficits cause listlessness, muscle wastage, growth failure, and ultimately kwashiorkor, marasmus, or—usually—combined protein-energy malnutrition (PEM).

The basic cause of undernutrition is a severe shortage of food. In developing countries, traditional methods of food production and distribution cannot provide enough food for an ever-increasing population. The result is a chronically inadequate food supply (Figure 14-4).

In some parts of the world malnutrition is an episodic event, due to a sudden and temporary but major disruption in food availability. Famine caused by warfare and drought have been the primary causes of this kind of malnutrition, producing starvation when there is simply little or no food to be had. The sudden onset of protein-energy malnutrition, with associated secondary symptoms such as infectious disease, is accompanied by a sharp and widespread increase in mortality rates. In Biafra in the late 1960s and in Cambodia in the late 1970s, civil strife led tens of thousands to flee their homes and farms, bringing food production to a halt and causing mass starvation. Today in Africa, famine in a broad belt stretching across the middle of the continent is causing malnutrition, famine, and death on an unprecedented scale. There are no signs of a turnaround, despite the efforts of international agencies and emergency groups. The African famine was a result of weather interacting with poor agricultural policy. Drought has occurred in regions of the United States that fortunately has a large enough area so that all parts of the country are not affected at the same time.

The Effects

The specific impairments seen in malnourished populations depend on the specific nutrients that are lacking in the diet.

FIGURE 14-4   *Food Production and Population for (a) Developed and (b) Developing Countries.*

Food production has increased in both developed and developing countries at a comparable, steady rate over the past two decades. The population increases in the developing countries, however, have far outstripped the increase in food production, resulting in less food per capita.

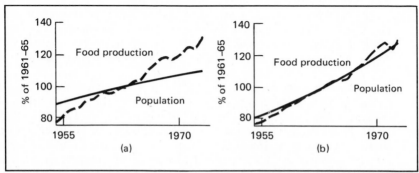

Source: M. A. Caliendo, *Nutrition and the world food crisis* (New York: Macmillan, 1979), p. 185.

PROTEIN-ENERGY MALNUTRITION.   Protein-energy malnutrition (PEM) is the most prevalent type of undernutrition in the developing countries of the world. PEM has two principal forms, kwashiorkor and marasmus. *Kwashiorkor* results from a diet in which energy intake is adequate but protein content is not. It is characterized by edema, which gives a bloated, pot-bellied appearance to its victims, usually young children who have been weaned from breast milk to an inadequate diet consisting primarily of starchy or sugary liquid gruels. These children are also likely to have depigmented skin, which looks patchy and gray, and depigmented reddish hair. Kwashiorkor is not a single deficiency problem because foods that are good sources of protein are also sources of iron, zinc, and several other micronutrients. Therefore when the diet is deficient in protein-rich foods, it is also deficient in the other nutrients. Therefore the physical signs of kwashiorkor are the sum of the physical signs of all the deficiencies.

Marasmus results from severe energy deficits caused by overall food deprivation. It is common in poverty-level infants who are not breast-fed and in children of any age who have a markedly insufficient diet. Children with marasmus appear to be all skin and bones with an aged appearance. Linear growth is compromised and the child frequently is apathetic, listless, and unable to cry. Although protein intakes may on the surface appear to be adequate, protein is diverted from its usual anabolic role to meet energy needs, and tissue wastage is the consequence.

In reality, the etiology of these two conditions is often indistinguishable because diets deficient in protein are generally characterized by insufficient energy content as well. Why one child develops kwashiorkor and another suffers from marasmus is not always clear. Research has suggested that individual differences in adaptation to nutritional stress may explain this confusing phenomenon.

Because of the overlapping causes and effects of kwashiorkor and marasmus, and because essentially the same nutritional therapy is applied for both conditions, it is more convenient to consider them as two sides of the same coin, protein-energy malnutrition. Without treatment the disease is fatal. With treatment the prognosis is good; symptoms can be reversed in a matter of months. The extent of lasting effects depends on the stage of physical development during which the deficiency occurred, the length of time and severity of the condition, and the stage of development at which therapy was instituted.

OTHER NUTRITIONAL DEFICIENCY DISEASES.   PEM is not the only nutritional deficiency disorder prevalent in developing nations. Nutritional anemias, endemic goiter, ariboflavinosis, and a variety of dental conditions are widespread. Vitamin A deficiency is a current public health problem in 75 countries and territories as evidenced by the development of nightblindness and other eye manifestations in at least 5 to 10 million children every year. Even mild vitamin A deficiency causes problems because it is associated with a rise in respiratory disease and diarrhea. Rickets afflicts many as well. Pellagra, beriberi, and scurvy are found in some areas.

NUTRITION AND INFECTION.   One of the first published reports to call international attention to the synergistic relationship between malnutrition and infection was issued by the World Health Organization in the late 1960s. Since then, many studies have concurred that undernourished children are more susceptible to infections and, conversely, that infection worsens nutritional status. Undernourished Mexican populations, for example, suffer a fatality rate from measles that is 180 times higher than in the United States. Multiple nutritional deficiencies inhibit the body's ability to produce antibodies and other mechanisms to protect against infectious disease. In animal models, deficiencies of vitamin A, zinc, and other micronutrients illustrate the importance of these micronutrients in maintaining the immune system at optimal function. Studies of malnourished hospitalized patients have also provided much data on the importance of adequate nutrition in the host-defense system, from keeping intact the skin as a barrier, to cell-mediated immunity where production of small amounts of potent chemicals is reduced.

The relationship may not be that simple, however. In one study it was found, for example, that undernourished children from one small village in India were actually less susceptible to measles infection than the better-nourished children when body weight was used as the criterion for nutritional status. Much remains to be learned about the biochemical relationship between malnutrition and susceptibility to infection.

The effect of infection on nutrition is more clear. Bacterial and vital infections deplete the body's nitrogen content. Diseases that produce vomiting, sweating, or diarrhea cause fluid, protein, energy, and general electrolyte and nutrient losses. At the same time, infection is often accompanied by loss of appetite. Furthermore, cultural traditions often dictate the use of enemas or purgative treatment for diarrhea and restrict intake to teas or weak broths, all of which reduce nutrient intake and absorption just when it is most needed.

NUTRITION AND BEHAVIOR. The apathy, irritability, and inattention so common in malnourished children have led nutritionists to postulate a direct link between dietary deficiency and behavior. This hypothesis has received strong support from many animal studies, in which malnourished rats demonstrated behavioral and learning difficulties that persisted even after refeeding and rehabilitation; these abnormalities even appeared to be transmitted to succeeding generations whose prenatal nutrient supplies were sufficient. Attempts to confirm these effects in humans are complicated by the fact that malnutrition rarely occurs in isolation from other factors known to affect behavior.

Studies have repeatedly documented associations between childhood malnutrition and lower socioeconomic status, poor housing, unemployment, broken homes, and recurrent illness. Do the frequently observed emotional or learning problems in these children result from inadequate nutrition, unstimulating environment, or a family's preoccupation with economic and/or personal problems? What are the roles of poor maternal nutrition or lack of prenatal medical care? A number of studies have demonstrated a clear association between malnutrition and retarded mental development in school-age children.

Biochemical evidence demonstrates a significant role for nutritional effects on the central nervous system. The quantity of neurotransmitter substances, the activity of brain enzymes, and even the size and composition of brain cells are adversely affected by severe malnutrition. Some of these changes depend on the timing of deprivation, since the brain is most vulnerable to nutritional insult during periods of growth. Studies of brain components in Ugandan children who died between the ages of 1 day and 15 years have found lower than normal brain weights at every age in those who were malnourished. There may be potential for catch-up growth and development, and even that central nervous system changes may be reversible at early stages.

Some studies indicate that learning problems among poorly nourished urban children in the United States and elsewhere may be deficits in performance rather than intellect and due to a variety of interacting factors. Although additional research is needed, better evidence has accumulated, not only to support the role of undernutrition and deficiencies of iron and other nutrients in behavior, but also to support other aspects of nutrition in behavior (see Perspective On: Nutrition and Behavior, page 422).

FACTORS CONTRIBUTING TO MALNUTRITION. Nutrient deficiencies do not exist in a vacuum. Lack of food to eat is related to inadequate production and distribution. Environmental factors influence the choice of diet and the availability of food and its component nutrients. These are, in turn, influenced by individual human differences in nutrient needs and utilization. Human factors affect the means of production as well. These three factors—environment, diet, and host—form an epidemiological triangle, interacting to determine the incidence of nutritional disease.

FACTORS AFFECTING FOOD PRODUCTION. Unfavorable climatic events—droughts, floods, and cold spells—can cause widespread famine, while favorable temperatures and adequate rainfall ensure a long-term abundance of crops. Generally, weather conditions are unpredictable and uncontrollable, but meteorological methods are improving and long-range predictions are aided by cameras and other instruments placed on space satellites.

Careful management of available water supplies is important not only for agriculture, but for human survival. Although three-fourths of the earth is water, only 2.5 percent of that is nonoceanic; of the limited fresh water, more than 70 percent is located in glaciers and ice caps where it is unavailable for productive purposes. Rain and snow recirculate the world's water resources and help increase local supplies, but it is estimated that only 0.007 percent of the earth's water returns as precipitation, of which two-thirds evaporates or is transpired by plants.

Overpopulation also threatens to diminish available land resources, and when land is scarce, people go hungry. Land is necessary not only for agricultural use, but for grazing, housing, energy production, and transportation. Land for these purposes is usually taken from the best growing areas, because that is where the population centers are. Moreover, cropland is constantly being lost through erosion, diversion of irrigation water to nonfarming uses, and overcultivation. As a result, expanding deserts are depriving increasing numbers of people of their means of food production and, potentially, of a means of survival; one in every seven of the world's people now lives in areas classified as arid or semiarid.

FOOD DISTRIBUTION. Like food production, distribution is influenced by environmental and human factors. If a nation is able to increase its food supply while stabilizing its population, the average amount of food available for distribution to each person then increases. This principle has worked in developed countries, where food production has increased while population growth has slowed. But in developing countries population gains have absorbed nearly all production increases.

Cultural and religious practices often limit food usage. No culture utilizes all available potential foods. In our own culture, although there is no specific religious or other taboo for most of us, insects and horseflesh are viewed with repugnance; rabbit is consumed by only a few, usually from a cultural tradition such as that of Germany, Czechoslovakia, or France where this is an accepted food item. Often foods are permitted to some members of the community, but not others. Children or pregnant women are frequently prevented from eating eggs, because "the baby will cluck like a hen" (Jamaica) or the newborn child will be female (Liberia). Even where there are no food taboos, people are generally reluctant to add new and strange items to their diet.

No matter how much food is produced, people who can't afford to buy it will remain malnourished. Although improved productivity will result in an additional purchasing power on a national, as well as an individual level, the increased mechanization needed to add to productivity may have the unwanted effect of promoting unemployment. Increased demand by developing nations drives prices up on the international market and may further deprive poorer peoples. The staggering debt of many developing countries also works against providing the population with enough to eat.

STRATEGIES FOR CHANGE

Technology can serve as a buffer against changes in weather, population, and economic conditions. Technology can make possible increased crop yields, better storage, and more efficient distribution. What technology can't do, however, is to prevent major natural disasters, stabilize political unrest, or convince individuals to select nutritionally beneficial foods. Recent decades have seen recurrent energy crises, growing Third World populations, unstable governments on every continent, and large gaps between "have" and "have not" nations and individuals.

An integrated approach combining better production, storage, and distribution with curtailed population growth, better and more available health care, and improved sanitation is needed. The goal is getting food to the people who need it, at a price they can afford. Rich nations must help poor ones. Technology must be tempered with regard for personal needs and values. Poverty is at the root of the problem of undernutrition, but political consciousness must also be raised to solve the problem. Nutrition education programs must be tailored to local customs and beliefs. Only a broad range of strategies will accomplish the far-ranging changes that are required to improve nutritional status and health for all the world's peoples (see Figure 14–5).

Increasing Food Production and Distribution

The question facing developing nations is not only *how* to increase food supplies but also *what* food supplies to increase. Everywhere, as income levels rise, people seek different food. People at the lowest socioeconomic level consume diets high in starch from rice, corn, and root crops. With higher incomes, protein-rich foods such as meat are added to the menu. Finally luxury items such as refined foods and out-of-season fruits and vegetables make their appearance. This does not necessarily mean that as income increases, the quality of the diet is better; it may improve to a point and then worsen again as quality "poor folks" foods are replaced by less nutritious luxury foods. Further, a rise in income for a nation does not always mean a rise in income for all segments of the population. In Latin America, where 8 percent of the population owns 80 percent of the land, subsistence crops decreased by 10 percent in a ten-year period while cash crops for exports increased by 27 percent. The average African is eating 20 percent less than 20 years ago while production of tea increased sixfold, sugar threefold, and coffee fourfold.

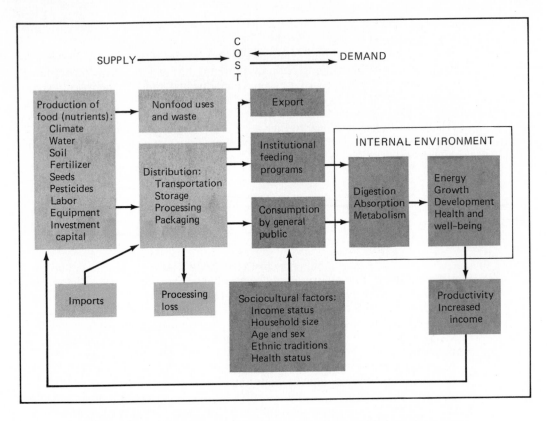

FIGURE 14-5 *Strategies and Consequences of Effective Nutrition Planning.*

Source: Adapted from J. M. Pines, A systematic approach to nutrition planning, *Professional Nutritionist,* Fall 1976, pp. 13-14.

In industrialized nations there has been considerable controversy over diets that include large amounts of meat, which are resource-expensive.

Many people believe that using grain to feed cattle is quite wasteful when that same grain could be used directly as food, contributing to world food supplies. Others argue that the grazing lands used for cattle could not be efficiently transformed into growing lands, that meat products contribute to general nutritional health and serve as "buffers" during temporary periods of bad weather and crop shortages. An in-between group suggests that we could increase our intake of grains, legumes, fruits, and vegetables and improve, not harm our health.

This is a complex question and is related to the efficiency of the so-called **food chain.** The food chain starts with the inorganic materials provided in soil—minerals, nitrogen, and water—and carbon dioxide from the atmosphere. Energized by the sun, plants synthesize sugar and starch, releasing oxygen to the air; they incorporate nitrogen and minerals into other plant materials. Plants are consumed by animals, including humans. In turn, humans consume some animals. In their life processes animals (including humans) utilize oxygen and release carbon dioxide, water, and nitrogenous wastes, which are recycled back to the beginning of the food chain. The food sources found in every environmental setting (or *ecological niche*, as environmentalists and others term it) follow this general pattern. In any given ecological niche the interactions between plants and animals may be quite complex, with important economic and nutritional implications. Large scale mechanized agriculture takes 10 kilocalories of energy to produce *one* kilocalorie of food. If the world used the U.S. system as a model for agriculture, 80 percent of the annual energy expenditure would be needed. There is enough food produced in the world to provide enough calories for everyone. However, distribution is not equitable. Our eating eggplant from Kenya, grapes from Chile, and pineapple from the Philippines has not helped the average peasant in the Third World to feed his family. Many agricultural experts now state that small-farm operators are more efficient, not less, than vast farms in the United States and elsewhere.

The goals of food-supply planners are to increase agricultural productivity and make a sufficient and nutritionally balanced diet available at a cost that can be afforded by all people. The Food and Agriculture Organization (1976) of the United Nations believes that nutrition, as an integral part of national development, must be promoted through three related strategies:

1. Plans for development should stress increased food production and more equitable distribution of income among populations, especially in rural areas.
2. Processing, marketing, and distribution of foods to all parts of a population should be improved by altering agricultural customs and patterns and the types of foods being produced.
3. Population subgroups most at risk of poor health and nutritional status should receive multifaceted intervention.

In Africa, famine in a broad belt stretching across the middle of the continent is causing malnutrition and death in spite of the efforts of international agencies and emergency groups.
United Nation/Jerry Frank

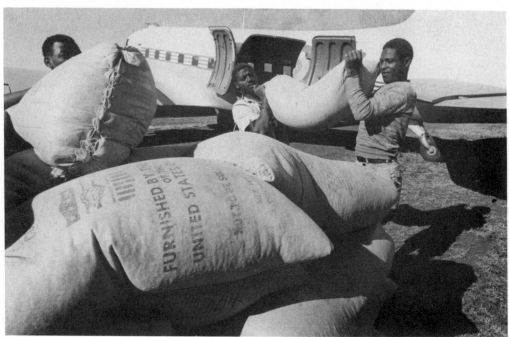

New Food Sources

Many believe that agriculture alone, even enhanced by modern technology, can never provide enough food for all the world's people. For a time, believing that protein deficits were the greatest problem, many food technologists turned to industrial synthesis of new protein foods. There was a great deal of interest in texturized vegetable protein, single cells protein, and others. Other strategies rely on fortifying foods and exploring locally available items not generally used for food.

FABRICATED FOODS. Texturized vegetable proteins (TVP) were developed from a soybean base during World War II, and soybeans were soon being incorporated into many protein foods as "extenders." Although this was a new food item for most Americans and Europeans, the Chinese and Japanese have been consuming a variety of soybean products for centuries. During the beef shortages of the 1970s, TVP became a familiar "stretcher" for hamburger meat. It has also become a popular item at vegetarian and "health bar" restaurants, served as a "steak" with mushroom sauce, for example, or as a "mock hamburger" sandwich. Texturized vegetable protein is also used to simulate other meat products as well.

Surimi is a wet-frozen concentrate of certain proteins of fish muscle that is used to fabricate seafood products. Check out the less expensive shrimp or crab products in your local supermarket, they are probably made from surimi. Surimi uses flesh of fish not considered desirable for direct consumption. There is nothing wrong with the fish except a reputation for a different taste, that is, a cultural aversion to the fish. By processing the muscle flesh and combining this with new flavors, a product is produced that is acceptable to many more people than the original fish. Flaked and formed steaks and chops are also restructured from small pieces of meat plus, in some cases, by-products and non-skeletal meats. Beef, pork, lamb, chicken, turkey, and veal have all been used, but other muscle meats could also be processed in this fashion. These products may not be directly useful to poor nations because of their cost, but they do increase the general supply of food.

REGIONAL FOODS. When a mule-train expedition of botanists discovered an extremely hardy perennial variety of corn in the remote mountainous regions of Sierra de Manantlan in Mexico, hopes were raised that it might provide genetic material to transform traditional corn into a low-cost, self-perpetuating perennial crop. At present, a substantial part of the cost of cultivating corn arises from the need to plow under old crops and sow new ones every year. The discovery of *Zea diploperennis* surprised scientists, but it was no news to Mexican natives of that region. They were accustomed to grinding the seeds of the wild variety with those of their regular corn, but only in times of hardship.

Tofu (soybean protein curd), sufu (fermented soybean protein curd), miso (fermented soy paste), and natto (fermented whole soybean), have been used in the Orient for centuries. These products have been an important source of protein in the diet, but for a long time were not considered acceptable by other cultures. This has changed rapidly since World War II with the steady penetration of various ethnic foods into the American market. Tempeh, an Indonesian food that is also soy based, is also becoming accepted in America.

FORMULATED, FORTIFIED, AND SUPPLEMENTAL FOODS. A related approach involves fortification of locally available foods. The addition of vitamins D and A to milk is a common practice in the United States; the addition of niacin to flours was in part

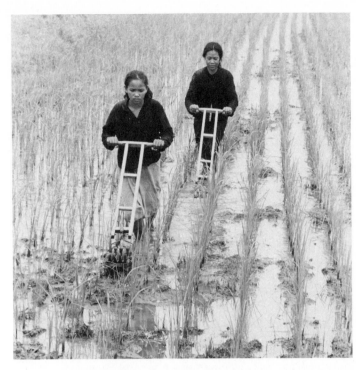

Many believe that agriculture alone, even enhanced by modern technology, can never provide enough food for all the world's people.

United Nations

responsible for the control of pellagra. Similar efforts have been tried in countries where specific vitamin and mineral deficiencies are widespread. Synthesized forms of vitamin A have been added to such foods as margarine, milk, tea leaves, cereal grains, rice, sugar, and salt in various parts of the world. Iodized salt has been introduced in areas where goiter is prevalent. Iron and thiamin are other nutrients used in fortification efforts. Foods chosen for fortification must be centrally supplied and consumed widely, especially by children and other vulnerable members of the population.

Special food products (termed *commerciogenic nutritious foods*, or CNF) have been formulated to meet local needs. Protein beverages have been among the most successful CNF products. CNF products also include milk-based foods for infants, high-protein snack foods, and enriched cereal products. Incaparina is a high-protein mixture of maize and cottonseed flour widely advertised and available throughout Latin America.

The problem with CNF products sold in local markets is that those who need them most can't afford to buy them. It has been suggested that CNF be distributed free to the poor and needy, in the same manner as foods have been distributed for many years by international agencies such as UNICEF and CARE, with an emphasis on feeding hungry children. However, the high cost of production and distribution and the lack of long-term benefit to needy nations argue against this type of supplementary feeding, except in emergency famines.

NEW ENERGY SOURCES AND APPROPRIATE TECHNOLOGY. Wood, plant matter, and animal dung are used as fuels in many parts of the world because commercial fuels and the equipment to use them are too expensive. Wood is the fuel source for cooking and warming homes used by more than one-third of the world's population. According to some estimates one-and-a-half-billion people in the Third World use wood or charcoal to meet all their basic energy needs. For another billion approximately one-half of their energy needs are met by wood and charcoal. According to one report hedges around homes and scaffolding on buildings disappeared to meet the shortage of firewood in some areas. As supplies of wood fuel diminish, more animal dung is used, thus reducing the supply of an inexpensive, widely available natural fertilizer. In India, one of the few countries to collect data, 120 million tons of wood, 50 million tons of dried dung, and 30 million tons of vegetable waste were burned each year. The relative share of the dung and vegetable waste has decreased in spite of what may appear to be large amounts. Almost 100 million hectares (one hectare equals 2.47 acres) could be fertilized with the annual dung production and could result in about one-half ton per hectare increase in produce. In many countries, forest management is concerned solely with production of industrial wood, not fuel wood. Producing fuel wood is technically simple, but socially difficult because of the inherent sociocultural complexities of most countries.

In the past, efforts were made to improve methods of extracting energy from other natural resources, using materials readily available in these lands. These efforts continue to some extent to date. A solar heater to purify water made of burned-out fluorescent tubes is the product of a research community of Colombia, where highly trained technicians devise simple, low-cost hardware and processes for developing areas. This is "appropriate technology" concentrated on small-scale, energy-efficient means that can be used at the family or village level. Results include a pedal-powered grinding machine that can process as much yucca root in a day as traditionally done by hand in two months, and a windmill, powered by breezes of as little as 5 miles an hour, to pump water for irrigation and drinking. Small-scale farm machinery and low-cost housing materials and techniques are other products of the A.T. approach.

Nutritional Anthropology

How can new foods be introduced to people whose diet, reinforced by religious practices, has been unchanged for centuries? How can nutritious products be marketed to an undernourished population too poor to purchase them? A productive approach to these and related problems is contributed by **nutritional anthropology**. This new discipline is concerned with patterns of food acquisition and consumption and the health and nutritional status of human beings within a cultural and ecological context.

Participant observation, living with the group being studied, is the basic research method of traditional anthropology. To study food behaviors, nutritional anthropologists record the kinds and amounts of foods gathered, raised, exchanged, purchased, prepared, and consumed, and they observe the human behaviors and interactions involved in these processes.

IDENTIFICATION OF FOOD SOURCES. Through this combination approach, food sources that are used by a people, and additional sources available to them, can be identified. Strategies can then be devised for taking the best advantage of the resources of an area. When one tribe was observed to have a high incidence of xerophthalmia, whereas a group sharing the same semidesert area and having similar social patterns was free of the disease, an anthropologist was consulted. The disease-free group gathered seedling shoots in the early morning, when there was just enough dampness from dew to produce them; after a few hours the seedlings with-ered. The disease-ridden tribe did not make use of this food resource, which was a source of sufficient carotene to prevent deficiency.

Analyzing the food patterns of a people to determine the nutrient content of their diet often reveals considerable wisdom in the food choices of native peoples. In Malaysia, small sun-dried fish are consumed, bones and all, twice daily, providing substantial amounts of calcium and the essential amino acids needed to complement protein in rice, the dietary staple. Similarly, the Latin American custom of soaking maize in a solution of lime (calcium carbonate) before pounding it into meal has been shown to add dietary calcium and to convert the niacin content of the corn into a biologically available form, thus acting as a pellagra preventive.

The anthropological approach also relates foodways to other aspects of daily life. The San Bushmen are hunter-gatherers of the Kalahari desert of southern Africa. Great seasonal variation in rainfall and temperatures leads to sharp fluctuations in their natural food supply. Weight losses of as much as 6 percent were observed in the dry season, and analysis of birth data indicated that this was the period of lowest fertility for San women. Birth data for a neighboring people whose diets were supplemented with cultivated food showed a more even distribution of fertility. These findings led to the hypothesis that the diminished food intake of San women in the dry season sharply reduces production of the steroid hormones that maintain fertility. The seasonal fluctuation of the natural food supply provides a natural cyclic method of population control, and introduction of supplemental food resources may contribute to an increase in birth rates.

DEVELOPING STRATEGIES FOR CHANGE. Nutritional anthropology is an offshoot of applied anthropology, which aims to use research findings to improve human living conditions. An important nutritional application lies in the development of strategies for dietary change among peoples consuming marginal or inadequate diets. In one early attempt, a multidisciplinary medical team worked with the Zulus of South Africa. In discussions, the Zulu recalled long-forgotten vegetable-eating customs of their pastoral ancestors, and this made possible the subsequent introduction of vegetable cultivation. They had a strong taboo against drinking milk from cows that did not belong to their family of origin; as a result, married women who lived with their husbands' families did not drink milk. Powdered milk, which could not be identified as coming from the cows of any family, was accepted. Over the ten-year period of this project, infant mortality dropped from 276 to 96 per thousand live births.

Health and Education Programs

Education is a slow process. Food habits are deeply embedded in cultural traditions and fulfill many needs. Changes should ideally be compatible with existing cultural traditions and not disrupt traditional values and practices. Grivetti illustrates the strength of dietary taboos and mistargeted food relief as follows. Suppose the world situation were reversed and the United States was an emerging nation with severe food shortages and Nigeria had a lot of food to help solve the shortage. Would most Americans accept termite porridge, locust bread, and beetle soup, favorite and nutritious Nigerian food specialities? Hungry people will not eat just anything offered.

Improved feeding practices by themselves can do little to improve life when infection and poor hygiene remain constant. Many of the world's people have little concept of the association between sanitation and health; the germ theory of disease is unknown to them. The period of weaning is the time when infants are most vulnerable to disease spread through poor hygiene and also the time when they are suddenly exposed to bacteria, viruses, parasites, and insects. Undernutrition, repeated bouts of infection, and "weanling diarrhea" are widespread throughout the Third World. Each year 15 million infants die of two preventable problems, poor nutrition and diarrhea. The introduction by UNICEF of oral rehydration therapy to correct the problem of dehydration from diarrhea has saved an estimated half-million lives. Correction of poor nutrition has not been as successful, but monitoring growth to detect early signs of malnutrition is becoming more widespread. Many countries are also working to improve drinking water and sewerage to eliminate the source of the problem.

GAZING INTO THE CRYSTAL BALL: PROSPECTS

Where do we go from here? What will our foodways be in the near—and not so near—future? What new fads, new concerns, new products, new food technologies, new information about diet and health, and new life styles will come along to alter our menus and meals? Each day, the world grows by approximately 190,000 people, more than two-thirds of whom are born in developing nations. About 12 percent will die in infancy, and the majority of those that live will suffer from hunger and malnutrition. Must this be so?

Making generalizations about the future is difficult. Prospects vary from country to country and region to region and from year to year. In the United States, the effects of regional disasters are buffered by the size of this country. Drought in the productive southeast resulted in tremendous loss of crops. How much more havoc would be created if this region was a whole country with no area left to pick up the slack. In spite of the fact that the general population can be protected by food production in other parts of our country, losses from large regions lower the world's food reserve.

There are some bright spots in the projection. Technology can be expected to find additional methods for processing and storing so that we can be buffered from supply changes. Technology will also find a way to keep the nutrient losses minimal during processing. More texturized, structured foods can be expected in the future; ditto more food in boxes, aseptic packaging. Hopefully there will also be a greater variety of grains, legumes, fruits, vegetables, and meats available.

For emerging nations where hunger is endemic, optimism is difficult but necessary. Multisector approaches must be used to break the pattern of unemployment and the status quo of a small segment of the population controlling 85 to 90 percent of the land and wealth. Providing an environment for all people to work and earn a living is the responsibility of the political superstructure of a country.

Consumers have an important role in defining strategies for change. There are many things individuals can do: participate in state consumer councils and other groups that are concerned with food and nutrition; become aware of the community's education programs in nutrition; learn by reading and taking courses from qualified people; write to state and federal legislators about concerns; write to food industry executives for more information about their products or to protest improper practices or poor quality. Support of local agriculture can increase the local food supply and reduce food costs. Customers' opinions can influence the kinds of foods available from retailers. It should not be assumed that Congress is influenced only by the farm lobby or the food industry; both retailers and Congress have been affected by consumer action.

Consumers have the ultimate responsibility for maintaining the quality and safety of the food supply. From the time it is purchased, throughout preparation, and until it is served, food can lose its nutritional value and become the transmitter of serious, even fatal, illness. Food safety in the home should be a key component of nutrition education for the public.

A national nutrition policy must involve all sectors of our population. We must learn to be economically self-sufficient, to be healthy, and to use our tax dollars wisely. Comprehensive policies require input from nutritional and other research. Food safety policies must involve the Food and Drug Administration, the Department of Agriculture, and the Environmental Protection Agency. Continuation of food stamps, School Food Service, WIC, and other feeding programs will improve nutritional status and knowledge for those most at risk of the consequences of under- and overnutrition. Nutrition education in schools at every level, in extension programs, and for community groups will produce a more knowledgeable and better nourished people.

Agribusiness, industrialized farming, requires flat land with no hedges or trees to allow the sowing machines, fertilizer distributors, and harvesting machines to function. With these methods, the layer of soil gets thinner. The bottom line of farming can not be only profit. A factory destroyed by poor management can be rebuilt, but the land, once destroyed, is gone. Agribusiness must not be allowed to have absolute control over the heritage of the whole population.

Pessimists fear a bleak future for world food production, although not everyone agrees with this assessment. Some state that chemical technology is crucial to eliminate both poverty and hunger. Crop losses to insects and fungi total almost half the world production. Cutting these losses would increase the food supply substantially and is certainly a good beginning commitment.

SUMMARY

For most of human existence, people's food supplies consisted only of what nature placed before them. But in today's technological society, a greater variety of food items is available than could ever before have been imagined. Among developments making this plenty possible have been genetic research, the chemical fertilization industry, new means of transportation and refrigeration, marketing techniques, and more.

Our food behaviors are shaped not only by productivity and availability but also by social and cultural influences. These include urbanization and suburbanization, changes in the family structure and the growing number of smaller household units, postponement of childbearing, increase in the number and proportion of working women of all ages, increase in mobility, inflation, energy shortages, and ethnic diversity. There is also a growing interest in food and cookery as well as a heightened awareness of health and nutrition.

Most food purchases are made in supermarkets. At the same time, more meals are being consumed outside the home, at restaurants ranging from "fast" to "fancy," and in the workplace, schools, and other institutional settings as well.

A growing concern nationwide has been in relation to the health aspects of food. People want to know what to eat to help reduce the risk of cancer and heart disease. They want to know the best diet for physical activity. They want foods with fewer calories coming from fats. Sometimes they want simple answers to complex questions. Nutritionists need to answer the questions and make recommendations based on the best scientific information available.

Over the years, nutritional concerns have changed. For a long time, undernutrition was the focus of national food programs, but in recent years there has been increased awareness of problems associated with overnutrition, a consequence of the affluent life style of most Americans. The typical diet of the population contains large amounts of energy-dense foods, fats, sugar, and salt, and may in its own way be as damaging to the human body as a vitamin-deficient diet.

Determining the nutrient content of processed foods, the value of vitamin and mineral fortification, and the potential for damage of additives requires continued research.

Government agencies concerned with food and nutrition include the Department of Agriculture (USDA), which administers the food stamp program, school lunch programs, and WIC; the Department of Health and Human Services which sponsors the Administration on Aging, the Food and Drug Administration, and the National Institutes of Health. Congress makes laws, assigns responsibilities to agencies, and appropriates the funding for many of these programs.

The U.S. Dietary Goals, proposed in 1977 by the Senate Select Committee on Nutrition and Human Needs, may have been a turning point in the role of government in determining human nutrition priorities for the nation. The second edition of the *Dietary Goals* shows that the commitment of the government is long standing.

Malnutrition, the result of imbalance between nutrient needs and nutrient intake, can be traced most often to an imbalance between the world's food production and food distribution systems and is particularly evident in economically disadvantaged nations. Nutritionists have estimated that malnutrition affects from 400 to 500 million people. Problems range from simple deficiencies of one or more essential nutrients to chronic deficiencies of protein and energy, which cause listlessness, muscle wastage, growth failure, infection, and often, death. Because of their high growth rate and increased need for nutrients, infants and children are particularly vulnerable to these problems. They typically develop kwashiorkor or marasmus, conditions characterized by impairment in growth and mental functioning.

Dealing with the causes of malnutrition requires attention to environmental factors that affect food *production* (climate, water supply, land availability, agricultural technology, economic costs, energy requirements, local customs), *distribution* (economic purchasing power, population densities, trade agreements, processing techniques, transportation systems, cultural practices), and *human* characteristics (age, sex, nutritional history, activity level, genetic inheritance, pregnancy, lactation, disease states, metabolism, psychological and cultural conditioning). Multifaceted programs that introduce new technology, new food sources, economic growth, and nutritional and health education programs, within the context of local culture and ecology, will prove most successful in improving the health and nutritional status of the people in the developing world.

BIBLIOGRAPHY

American Society for Clinical Nutrition. 1985 Public Policy Forum—The making of federal nutrition policy. *American Journal of Clinical Nutrition* 42:891–942, 1985.

Baidyai, K. N. The firewood crisis in India: A major sociocultural problem of rural communities. *International Journal of Environmental Studies* 26:279–294, 1986.

Brown, R. Organ weight in malnutrition with special reference to brain weight. *Developmental Medicine and Child Neurology* 8:512, 1966.

Brozek, J. Malnutrition and behavior: A decade of conferences. *Journal of the American Dietetic Association* 72:17, 1978.

Bruhn, C. M., H. G. Schutz, and R. Summer.

Attitude change toward food irradiation among conventional and alternative consumers. *Food Technology* 40:86–91, January 1986.

BUNCH, K. L. "Food away from home and the quality of the diet." *National Food Review*, Winter 1984, pp. 14–16.

BUREAU OF THE CENSUS. Characteristics of American children and youth: 1980. *Current Population Reports*, Series P-23, No. 114. Washington, D.C.: U.S. Dept. of Commerce, 1982.

CURRIE, L. Sources of growth. *World Development* 14:541–547, 1986.

ECKHOLM, E. Firewood crops: Shrub and tree species for energy production. National Academy of Sciences, U.S.A., 1980.

FIELD, J. O. Implementing nutrition programs: Lessons from an unheeded literature. *Annual Review of Nutrition* 5:143–172, 1985.

FOOD AND NUTRITION BOARD/NATIONAL RESEARCH COUNCIL. Recommended dietary allowances: Scientific issues and prospects for the future. *Journal of Nutrition* 116:482–488, 1986.

FUKUSHIMA, D. Fermented vegetable protein and related foods of Japan and China. *Food Reviews International* 1:149–209, 1985.

GRIVETTI, L. E. Cultural nutrition: Anthropological and geographical themes. *Annual Reviews of Nutrition* 1:47–68, 1981.

HARWOOD-JONES, J. Custodians of the planet? *World Futures* 21:231–243, 1985.

HINMAN, C. W. Potential new crops. *Scientific American* 255:33–37, July 1986.

HORTON, D. Assessing the impact of international agricultural research and development programs. *World Development* 14:453–468, 1986.

INSTITUTE OF FOOD TECHNOLOGISTS SCIENTIFIC STATUS SUMMARY. Sulfites as food ingredients. *Food Technology* 40:47, 1986.

KAHN, S. G. World hunger: An overview. *Food Technology* 35:93–98, September 1981.

KNORR, D., and A. J. SINSKEY. Biotechnology in Food production and processing. *Science* 229:1224–1229, 1985.

KORN, D. A. Ethiopia: Dilemma for the West. *The World Today* 42:6–11, 1986.

LANIER, T. C. Functional properties of surimi. *Food Technology* 40:107–114, 1986.

LAPPÉ, F. M., and J. COLLINS, with C. FOWLER. *Beyond the Myth of Scarcity.* Boston: Houghton Mifflin, 1977.

LEHMANN, P. More than you ever thought you would know about food additives. *FDA Consumer* HHS Publication No. (FDA) 82–2160.

LEMMON, H. COMAX. An expert system for cotton crop management. *Science* 233:29–33, 1986.

LEVERTON, R. M. Organic, inorganic: What they mean. In *1974 Yearbook of Agriculture.* Washington, D.C.: USDA, 1974.

LOWENBERG, M. E., and B. L. LUCAS. Feeding families and children—1776 to 1976. *Journal of the American Dietetic Association* 68:207, 1976.

MCNUTT, K. W., M. E. POWERS, and A. E. SLOAN. Food colors, flavors, and safety: A consumer viewpoint. *Food Technology* 40:72–76, 1986.

MILLER, S. A., and M. G. STEPHENSON. Scientific and public health rationale for the dietary guidelines for Americans. *American Journal of Clinical Nutrition* 42:739–745, 1985.

PEPPER, D. Determinism, idealism and the politics of environmentalism—a viewpoint. *International Journal of Environmental Studies* 26:11–19, 1985.

PINSTRUP-ANDERSON, P., and P. B. R. HAZEL. The impact of the green revolution and prospects for the future. *Food Reviews International* 1:1–15. 1985.

STANLEY, D. W. Chemical and structural determinants of texture of fabricated foods. *Food Technology* 40:65–69, March 1986.

STARE, F. J. A member of the Dietary Guidelines Revision Committee dissents. *Nutrition Today*, Jan./Feb. 1986, pp. 23–24.

STUMPF, S. E. The moral dimension of the world's food supply. *Annual Review of Nutrition* 1:1–25, 1981.

SWIENTEK, R. J. Food irradiation update. *Food Processing*, June 1985, pp. 82–90.

THUROW, L. C. Building a world-class economy. *Society*, Nov/Dec. 1984, pp 16–29.

VIETMEYER, N. D. Lesser known plants of potential use in agriculture and forestry. *Science* 232: 1379–1384, 1986.

APPENDIX

APPENDIX A

Recommended Dietary Allowances (RDA)

	Age (years)	Weight (kg)	Weight (lbs)	Height (cm	(In)	Energy needs (kcal)[b]	Protein (g)	Fat-Soluble Vitamins Vitamin A (µg RE)[c]	Vitamin D (µg)[d]	Vitamin E (mg α T.E.)[e]
Infants	0-0-0.5	6	13	60	24	kg x 115	kg x 2.2	420	10	3
	0.5-1.0	9	20	71	28	kg x 105	kg x 2.0	400	10	4
Children	1-3	13	29	90	35	1300	23	400	10	5
	4-6	20	44	112	44	1700	30	500	10	6
	7-10	28	62	132	52	2400	34	700	10	7
Males	11-14	45	99	157	62	2700	45	1000	10	8
	15-18	66	145	176	69	2800	56	1000	10	10
	19-22	70	154	177	70	2900	56	1000	7.5	10
	23-50	70	154	178	70	2700	56	1000	5	10
	51-75	70	154	178	70	2400[i]	56	1000	5	10
Females	11-14	46	101	157	62	2200	46	800	10	8
	15-18	55	120	163	64	2100	46	800	10	8
	19-22	55	120	163	64	2100	44	800	7.5	8
	23-50	55	120	163	64	2000[j]	44	800	5	8
	51-75	55	120	163	64	1800	44	800	5	8
Pregnant						+300	+30	+200	+5	+2
Lactating						+500	+20	+400	+5	+3

[a] The allowances are intended to provide for individual variations among most normal persons as they live in the United States under usual environmental stresses. Diets should be based on a variety of common foods in order to provide other nutrients for which human requirements have been less well defined.

[b] Energy allowances for children through age 18 are based on median energy intakes of children these ages followed in longitudinal growth studies. The energy allowances for younger adults are for men and women doing light work. Over age 51 the allowances re-present mean energy needs, allowing for a 2% decrease in basal (resting) metabolic rate per decade and a reduction in activity. At any age there is a variation in energy needs.

[c] Retinol equivalents, 1 Retinol equivalent = 1 µg retinol or 6 µg βcarotene.

[d] As cholecalciferol. 10 µg cholecalciferol = 400 I.U. vitamin D.

[e] α tocopherol equivalents, 1 mg d-α-tocopherol = 1α T.E.

[f] 1 N.E. (niacin equivalent) is equal to 1 mg of niacin or 60 mg of dietary tryptophan.

Estimated Safe and Adequate Daily Dietary Intakes of Additional Selected Vitamins and Minerals[a]

	Age (years)	Vitamins Vitamin K (µg)	Biotin (µg)	Pantothenic Acid (mg)	Copper (mg)	Manganese (mg)
Infants	0 - 0.5	12	35	2	0.5 - 0.7	0.5 - 0.7
	0.5 - 1	10 - 20	50	3	0.7 - 1.0	0.7 - 1.0
Children	1 - 3	15 - 30	65	3	1.0 - 1.5	1.0 - 1.5
and	4 - 6	20 - 40	85	3 - 4	1.5 - 2.0	1.5 - 2.0
Adolescents	7 - 10	30 - 60	120	4 - 5	2.0 - 2.5	2.0 - 3.0
	11+	50 - 100	100 - 200	4 - 7	2.0 - 3.0	2.5 - 5.0
Adults		70 - 140	100 - 200	4 - 7	2.0 - 3.0	2.5 - 5.0

[a] Because there is less information on which to base allowances, these figures are provided here in the form of ranges of recommended intakes.

[b] Since the toxic levels for many trace minerals may be only several times usual intakes, the upper levels for the trace minerals given in this table should not be habitually exceeded.

Water-Soluble Vitamins							Minerals					
Vitamin C (mg)	Thiamin (mg)	Riboflavin (mg)	Niacin (mg N.E.)^f	Vitamin B_6 (mg)	Folacin^g (μg)	Vitamin B_{12} (μg)^h	Calcium (mg)	Phosphorus (mg)	Magnesium (mg)	Iron (mg)	Zinc (mg)	Iodine (μg)
35	0.3	0.4	6	0.3	30	0.5	360	240	50	10	3	40
35	0.5	0.6	8	0.6	45	1.5	540	360	70	15	5	50
45	0.7	0.8	9	0.9	100	2.0	800	800	150	15	10	70
45	0.9	1.0	11	1.3	200	2.5	800	800	200	10	10	90
45	1.2	1.4	16	1.6	300	3.0	800	800	250	10	10	120
50	1.4	1.6	18	1.8	400	3.0	1200	1200	350	18	15	150
60	1.4	1.7	18	2.0	400	3.0	1200	1200	400	18	15	150
60	1.5	1.7	19	2.2	400	3.0	800	800	350	10	15	150
60	1.4	1.6	18	2.2	400	3.0	800	800	350	10	15	150
60	1.2	1.4	16	2.2	400	3.0	800	800	350	10	15	150
50	1.1	1.3	15	1.8	400	3.0	1200	1200	300	18	15	150
60	1.1	1.3	14	2.0	400	3.0	1200	1200	300	18	15	150
60	1.1	1.3	14	2.0	400	3.0	800	800	300	18	15	150
60	1.0	1.2	13	2.0	400	3.0	800	800	300	18	15	150
60	1.0	1.2	13	2.0	400	3.0	800	800	300	10	15	150
+20	+0.4	+0.3	+2	+0.6	+400	+1.0	+400	+400	+150	i	+5	+25
+40	+0.5	+0.5	+5	+0.5	+100	+1.0	+400	+400	+150	i	+10	+50

^{g} The folacin allowances refer to dietary sources as determined by *Lactobacillus casei* assay after treatment with enzymes ("conjugases") to make polyglutamyl forms of the vitamin available to the test organism.

^{h} The RDA for vitamin B_{12} in infants is based on average concentration of the vitamin in human milk. The allowances after weaning are based on energy intake (as recommended by the American Academy of Pediatrics) and consideration of other factors such as intestinal absorption.

^{i} Over age 75, 2050 kcal.

^{j} Over age 75, 1600 kcal.

^{k} The increased requirement during pregnancy cannot be met by the iron content of habitual American diets nor by the existing iron stores of many women; therefore the use of 30-60 mg of supplemental iron is recommended. Iron needs during lactation are not substantially different from those of non-pregnant women, but continued supplementation of the mother for 2-3 months after parturition is advisable in order to replenish stores depleted by pregnancy.

Source: Recommended Dietary Allowances, Revised 1979. Food and Nutrition Board, National Academy of Sciences-National Research Council, Washington, D.C.

Trace Minerals^b						
Fluoride (mg)	Chromium (mg)	Selenium (mg)	Molybdenum (mg)	Sodium (mg)	Potassium (mg)	Chloride (mg)
0.1 - 0.5	0.01 - 0.04	0.01 - 0.04	0.03 - 0.06	115 - 350	350 - 925	275 - 700
0.2 - 1.0	0.02 - 0.06	0.02 - 0.06	0.04 - 0.08	250 - 750	425 - 1275	400 - 1200
0.5 - 1.5	0.02 - 0.08	0.02 - 0.08	0.05 - 0.1	325 - 975	550 - 1650	500 - 1500
1.0 - 2.5	0.03 - 0.12	0.03 - 0.12	0.06 - 0.15	450 - 1350	775 - 2325	700 - 2100
1.5 - 2.5	0.05 - 0.2	0.05 - 0.2	0.1 - 0.3	600 - 1800	1000 - 3000	925 - 2775
1.5 - 2.5	0.05 - 0.2	0.05 - 0.2	0.15 - 0.5	900 - 2700	1525 - 4575	1400 - 4200
1.5 - 4.0	0.05 - 0.2	0.05 - 0.2	0.15 - 0.5	1100 - 3300	1875 - 5625	1700 - 5100

Source: Recommended Dietary Allowances, Revised 1979. Food and Nutrition Board, National Academy of Sciences-National Research Council, Washington, D.C.

APPENDIX B
Dietary Standards for Canada

Age (years)	Sex	Weight (kg)	Height (cm)	Energy[a] (kcal)	Pro-tein (g)	Fat soluble vitamins			Thia-min (mg)
						Vit. A (μg RE)[b]	Vit. D (μg cholecal-ciferol)[c]	Vit. E (mg α-to-copherol)	
0.0–0.5	Both	6	—	kg x 117	kg x 2.2 (2.0)[g]	400	10	3	0.3
0.5–1	Both	9	—	kg x 108	kg x 1.4	400	10	3	0.5
1-3	Both	13	90	1400	22	400	10	4	0.7
4-6	Both	19	110	1800	27	500	5	5	0.9
7-9	M	27	129	2200	33	700	2.5[j]	6	1.1
	F	27	128	2000	33	700	2.5[j]	6	1.0
10-12	M	36	144	2500	41	800	2.5[j]	7	1.2
	F	38	145	2300	40	800	2.5[j]	7	1.1
13-15	M	51	162	2800	52	1000	2.5[j]	9	1.4
	F	49	159	2200	43	800	2.5[j]	7	1.1
16-18	M	64	172	3200	54	1000	2.5[j]	10	1.6
	F	54	161	2100	43	800	2.5[j]	6	1.1
19-35	M	70	176	3000	56	1000	2.5[j]	9	1.5
	F	56	161	2100	41	800	2.5[j]	6	1.1
36-50	M	70	176	2700	56	1000	2.5[j]	8	1.4
	F	56	161	1900	41	800	2.5[j]	6	1.0
51+	M	70	176	2300[k]	56	1000	2.5[j]	8	1.4
	F	56	161	1800[k]	41	800	2.5[j]	6	1.0
Pregnant				+300[l]	+20	+100	+2.5[j]	+1	+0.2
Lactating				+500	+24	+400	+2.5[j]	+2	+0.4

Source: Canadian Council on Nutrition: *Dietary standards for Canada,* Can. Bull. Nutr. 6.1, 1964 (suppl. 1974).
[a] Recommendations assume characteristic activity pattern for each age group.
[b] One μg retinol equivalent (1 μg RE) corresponds to a biological activity in humans equal to 1 μg of retinol (3.33 IU) and 6 μg of β-carotene (10 IU).
[c] One μg cholecalciferol is equivalent to 40 IU vitamin D activity.
[d] Approximately 1 mg of niacin is derived from each 60 mg of dietary tryptophan.
[e] Recommendations are based on the estimated average daily protein intake of Canadians.
[f] Recommendation given in terms of free folate.
[g] Recommended protein allowance of 2.2 g/kg of body weight for infants age 0 to 2 mo and 2.0 g/kg of body weight for those age 3 to 5 mo. Protein recommendation for infants, 0 to 11 mo, assumes consumption of breastmilk or protein of equivalent quality.

	Water-soluble vitamins					Minerals					
Niacin[d] (mg)	Ribo-flavin (mg)	Vit. B_6[e] (mg)	Fo-late[f] (μg)	Vit. B_{12} (μg)	As-corbic acid (mg)	Ca (mg)	P (mg)	Mg (mg)	I (μg)	Fe (mg)	Zn (mg)
5	0.4	0.3	40	0.3	20[h]	500[i]	250[i]	50[i]	35[i]	7[i]	4[i]
6	0.6	0.4	60	0.3	20	500	400	50	50	7	5
9	0.8	0.8	100	0.9	20	500	500	75	70	8	5
12	1.1	1.3	100	1.5	20	500	500	100	90	9	6
14	1.3	1.6	100	1.5	30	700	700	150	110	10	7
13	1.2	1.4	100	1.5	30	700	700	150	100	10	7
17	1.5	1.8	100	3.0	30	900	900	175	130	11	8
15	1.4	1.5	100	3.0	30	1000	1000	200	120	11	9
19	1.7	2.0	200	3.0	30	1200	1200	250	140	13	10
15	1.4	1.5	200	3.0	30	800	800	250	110	14	10
21	2.0	2.0	200	3.0	30	1000	1000	300	160	14	12
14	1.3	1.5	200	3.0	30	700	700	250	110	14	11
20	1.8	2.0	200	3.0	30	800	800	300	150	10	10
14	1.3	1.5	200	3.0	30	700	700	250	110	14	9
18	1.7	2.0	200	3.0	30	800	800	300	140	10	10
13	1.2	1.5	200	3.0	30	700	700	250	100	14	9
18	1.7	2.0	200	3.0	30	800	800	300	140	10	10
13	1.2	1.5	200	3.0	30	700	700	250	100	9	9
+2	+0.3	+0.5	+50	+1.0	+20	+500	+500	+25	+15	+1[m]	+3
+7	+0.6	+0.6	+50	+0.5	+30	+500	+500	+75	+25	+1[m]	+7

[h] Considerably higher levels may be prudent for infants during the first week of life to guard against neonatal tyrosinemia.
[i] The intake of breast-fed infants may be less than the recommendation but is considered to be adequate.
[j] Most older children and adults receive enough vitamin D from irradiation but 2.5 μg daily is recommended. This recommended allowance increases to 5.0 μg daily for pregnant and lactating women and for those who are confined indoors or otherwise deprived of sunlight for extended periods.
[k] Recommended energy allowance for age 66+ years reduced to 2000 for men and 1500 for women.
[l] Increased energy allowance recommended during second and third trimesters. An increase of 100 kcal per day is recommended during first trimester.
[m] A recommended total intake of 15 mg daily during pregnancy and lactation assumes the presence of adequate stores of iron. If stores are suspected of being inadequate, additional iron as a supplement is recommended.

APPENDIX C

United States Recommended Daily Allowances (U.S. RDA)

	Adults and children 4 or more years of age[b]	Infants	Children under 4 years of age[c]	Pregnant or lactating women[c]
Nutrients which must be declared on the label (in the order below)				
Protein[d]	45 g "high quality protein"	—	—	
	65 g "proteins in general"			
Vitamin A	5000 IU	1500 IU	2500 IU	8000 IU
Vitamin C (or ascorbic acid)	60 mg	35 mg	40 mg	60 mg
Thiamin (or vitamin B_1)	1.5 mg	0.5 mg	0.7 mg	1.7 mg
Riboflavin (or vitamin B_2)	1.7 mg	0.6 mg	0.8 mg	2.0 mg
Niacin	20 mg	8 mg	9 mg	20 mg
Calcium	1.0 g	0.6 g	0.8 g	1.3 g
Iron	18 mg	15 mg	10 mg	18 mg
Nutrients which may be declared on the label (in the order below)				
Vitamin D	400 IU	400 IU	400 IU	400 IU
Vitamin E	30 IU	5 IU	10 IU	30 IU
Vitamin B_6	2.0 mg	0.4 mg	0.7 mg	2.5 mg
Folic acid (or folacin)	0.4 mg	0.1 mg	0.2 mg	0.8 mg
Vitamin B_{12}	6 µg	2 µg	3 µg	8 µg
Phosphorus	1.0 g	0.5 g	0.8 g	1.3 g
Iodine	150 µg	45 µg	70 µg	150 µg
Magnesium	400 mg	70 mg	200 mg	450 mg
Zinc	15 mg	5 mg	8 mg	15 mg
Copper[e]	2 mg	0.5 mg	1 mg	2 mg
Biotin[e]	0.3 mg	0.15 mg	0.15 mg	0.3 mg
Pantothenic acid[e]	10 mg	3 mg	5 mg	10 mg

[a] The U.S. RDA values chosen are derived from the highest value within an age category for each nutrient given in the 1968 NAS-NRC tables except for calcium and phosphorus.

[b] For use in labeling conventional foods and also for "special dietary foods."

[c] For use only with "special dietary foods."

[d] "High quality protein" is defined as having a protein efficiency ratio (PER) equal to or greater than that of casein; "proteins in general" are those with a PER less than that of casein. Total protein with a PER less than 20% that of casein are considered "not a significant source of protein" and would not be expressed on the label in terms of the U.S. RDA but only as amount per serving.

[e] There are no NAS-NRC RDAs for biotin, pantothenic acid, zinc, and copper.

APPENDIX D
Metropolitan Weight Tables for Adults 25 to 59 Years of Age[a]

Men			
HEIGHT FEET INCHES	SMALL FRAME	MEDIUM FRAME	LARGE FRAME
5 2	128–134	131–141	138–150
5 3	130–136	133–143	140–153
5 4	132–138	135–145	142–156
5 5	134–140	137–148	144–160
5 6	136–142	139–151	146–164
5 7	138–145	142–154	149–168
5 8	140–148	145–157	152–172
5 9	142–151	148–160	155–176
5 10	144–154	151–163	158–180
5 11	146–157	154–166	161–184
6 0	149–160	157–170	164–188
6 1	152–164	160–174	168–192
6 2	155–168	164–178	172–197
6 3	158–172	167–182	176–202
6 4	162–176	171–187	181–207

Women[b]			
HEIGHT FEET INCHES	SMALL FRAME	MEDIUM FRAME	LARGE FRAME
4 10	102–111	109–121	118–131
4 11	103–113	111–123	120–134
5 0	104–115	113–126	122–137
5 1	106–118	115–129	125–140
5 2	108–121	118–132	128–143
5 3	111–124	121–135	131–147
5 4	114–127	124–138	134–151
5 5	117–130	127–141	137–155
5 6	120–133	130–144	140–159
5 7	123–136	133–147	143–163
5 8	126–139	136–150	146–167
5 9	129–142	139–153	149–170
5 10	132–145	142–156	152–173
5 11	135–148	145–159	155–176
6 0	138–151	148–162	158–179

[a] Weight in pounds according to frame (in indoor clothing weighing 5 lbs. for men and 3 lbs. for women; shoes with 1″ heels).
[b] For women 18 to 24 years of age, subtract 1 pound for each year under 25.
Source: Copyright 1983 Metropolitan Life Insurance Company. Source of basic data: 1979 Build Study, Society of Actuaries and Association of Life Insurance Medical Directors of America, 1980.

APPENDIX E
Percentile Values for Triceps plus Subscapular Skinfold Measurements (in mm)

| | PERCENTILES | | | | |
	15	25	50	75	85
MEN					
20–24 years	13.0	15.0	22.0	31.0	36.1
25–34 years	15.0	19.0	26.0	35.5	41.1
35–44 years	17.5	21.0	28.0	36.0	41.0
45–54 years	17.5	21.0	28.0	37.0	42.0
55–64 years	16.5	20.0	26.0	34.1	40.1
65–74 years	16.0	19.5	26.0	34.1	38.5
WOMEN					
20–24 years	21.0	24.0	31.5	43.0	50.0
25–34 years	22.5	26.5	35.1	48.1	58.0
35–44 years	25.5	30.0	40.5	55.0	62.0
45–54 years	28.0	33.5	45.0	58.0	64.0
55–64 years	27.5	33.0	46.0	58.0	63.5
65–74 years	27.5	32.1	41.0	52.5	59.0

Data from S. Abraham, M.D. Carrol, M.F. Najjar, and R. Fulwood, *Obese and Overweight Adults in the U.S.* Department of Health and Human Services Publication 83-1680, Series 11, No. 230, 1983.

APPENDIX F
Metric Conversion Factors Commonly Used in Nutrition

Unit	Multiply by	Temperature
Length:		Fahrenheit to Centigrade (Celsius):
centimeters to inches	0.394	F° − 32° , multiply by 5/9
centimeters to meters	0.010	Centigrade (Celsius) to Fahrenheit:
foot to centimeters	30.480	Multiply C° by 9/5, add 32°
foot to meter	0.305	Examples:
inches to centimeters	2.540	32°F or 0°C (freezing temperature)
meters to inches	39.370	212°F or 100°C (boiling temperature)
meters to feet	3.281	98.6°F or 37.0°C (body temperature)
Weight:		
grams to micrograms	1 million	
grams to milligrams	1000	
grams to ounces	0.035	
grams to pounds	0.002	
kilograms to pounds	2.2	**Abbreviations commonly used in Nutrition**
ounces to grams	28.350	
pounds to kilograms	0.454	kcal = kilocalorie dl = deciliter
Volume:		kJ = kilojoule qt = quart
milliliter to fluid ounce	0.034	MJ = megajoule pt = pint
fluid ounce to milliliter	29.574	kg = kilogram c = cup
liter to quart	1.057	g = gram tbsp (T) = tablespoon
quart to liter	0.946	mg = milligram tsp (t) = teaspoon
Energy:		μg (mcg) = microgram m = meter
kilocalorie to kilojoule	4.184	lb = pound cm = centimeter
kilocalorie to megajoule	0.004	oz = ounce ft = foot
kilojoule to kilocalorie	0.239	l = liter in = inch
megajoule to kilocalorie	239	ml = milliliter

APPENDIX G
Exchange Lists for Meal Planning

Meals are planned by figuring menus to include a selection from all exchange groups that adds up to an individual's daily energy requirement in kilocalories. Consumption of some foods will use exchanges in more than one group; a glass of whole milk, for example, represents 1 milk exchange plus 2 fat exchanges. Exchange Lists are discussed in Chapter 5.

Exchange lists are groups of measured foods that have approximately the same carbohydrates, protein, fat, and energy content, and can therefore be substituted for one another.

1. Milk Exchanges
One Milk Exchange equals 12 g carbohydrate, 8 g protein, trace fat, 80 kilocalories.
One Milk Exchange is the equivalent of 1 cup skim milk.

	One Milk Exchange
Nonfat fortified milk	
Skim or nonfat milk	1 cup
Powdered (nonfat dry, before adding liquid)	⅓ cup
Canned, evaporated-skim milk	½ cup
Buttermilk made from skim milk	1 cup
Yogurt made from skim milk (plain, unflavored)	1 cup
Low-fat fortified milk	
1% fat fortified milk (plus ½ Fat Exchange)	1 cup
2% fat fortified milk (plus 1 Fat Exchange)	1 cup
Yogurt made from 2% fortified milk (plain, unflavored) (plus 1 Fat Exchange)	1 cup
Whole milk (plus 2 Fat Exchanges)	
Whole milk	1 cup
Canned, evaporated whole milk	½ cup
Buttermilk made from whole milk	1 cup
Yogurt made from whole milk (plain, unflavored)	1 cup

2. Vegetable Exchanges
One Vegetable Exchange equals 5 g carbohydrate, 2 g protein, 25 kilocalories.
One vegetable exchange is ½ cup of the following:

Asparagus	Green pepper
Bean sprouts	Greens:
Beets	Beet
Broccoli	Chard
Brussel sprouts	Collards
Cabbage	Dandelion
Carrots	Kale
Cauliflower	Mustard
Celery	Spinach
Cucumbers	Turnip
Eggplant	Mushrooms
Okra	Summer squash
Onions	Tomatoes
Rhubarb	Tomato juice
Rutabaga	Turnips
Sauerkraut	Vegetable juice cocktail
String beans, green or yellow	Zucchini

The following vegetables may be eaten in any amount:

Chicory	Lettuce
Chinese cabbage	Parsley
Endive	Radishes
Escarole	Watercress

Note: starchy vegetables are listed under *Bread Exchanges.*

3. Fruit Exchanges
One Fruit Exchange equals 10 g carbohydrate, 40 kilocalories.

	One Fruit Exchange
Apple	1 small
Apple juice	⅓ cup
Applesauce (unsweetened)	½ cup
Apricots, fresh	2 medium
Apricots, dried	4 halves
Banana	½ small
Berries	
Blackberries	½ cup
Blueberries	½ cup
Raspberries	½ cup
Strawberries	¾ cup
Cherries	10 large
Cider	⅓ cup
Dates	2
Figs, fresh	1
Figs, dried	1
Grapefruit	1
Grapefruit juice	½ cup
Grapes	12
Grape juice	¼ cup
Mango	½ small

Melons

Cantaloupe	¼ small
Honeydew	⅛ medium
Watermelon	1 cup
Nectarine	1 small
Orange	1 small
Orange juice	½ cup
Papaya	¾ cup
Peach	1 medium
Pear	1 small
Persimmon, native	1 medium
Pineapple	½ cup
Pineapple juice	⅓ cup
Plums	2 medium
Prunes	2 medium
Prune juice	¼ cup
Raisins	2 tablespoons
Tangerine	1 medium

Cranberries have negligible carbohydrate and energy content if no sugar is added.

4. Bread Exchanges

(Includes bread, cereals, starchy vegetables, and prepared foods.)
One Bread Exchange equals 15 g carbohydrate, 2 g protein, 70 kilocalories.

One Bread Exchange

Bread:

White (including French and Italian)	1 slice
Whole wheat	1 slice
Rye or pumpernickel	1 slice
Raisin	1 slice
Bagel, small	½
English muffin, small	½
Plain roll, bread	1
Frankfurter roll	½
Hamburger bun	½
Dried bread crumbs	3 tablespoons
Tortilla, 6''	1

Crackers:

Arrowroot	3
Graham, 2½'' square	2
Matzoth, 3'' x 6½''	½
Oyster	20
Pretzels, 3⅛'' long x ⅛'' diameter	25
Rye wafers, 2'' x 3½''	3
Saltines	6
Soda, 2½'' square	4

Grains and Cereals:

Bran flakes	½ cup
Other ready-to-eat-unsweetened cereal	¾ cup
Puffed cereal (unfrosted)	1 cup
Cereal (cooked)	½ cup
Grits (cooked)	½ cup
Rice or barley (cooked)	½ cup

Pasta (cooked), spaghetti, noodles, macaroni	½ cup
Popcorn (popped, no fat added)	3 cups
Cornmeal (dry)	2 tablespoons
Flour	2½ tablespoons
Wheat germ	¼ cup

Dried Beans, Peas, and Lentils:

Beans, peas, lentils (dried and cooked)	½ cup
Baked beans, no pork (canned)	¼ cup

Starchy vegetables:

Corn	⅓ cup
Corn on cob	1 small
Lima beans	½ cup
Parsnips	⅔ cup
Peas, green (fresh, canned or frozen)	½ cup
Potato, white	1 small
Potato, mashed	½ cup
Pumpkin	¾ cup
Winter squash (acorn or butternut)	½ cup
Yam or sweet potato	¼ cup

Prepared foods:

Biscuit 2'' diameter (omit 1 Fat Exchange)	1
Cornbread 2'' x 2'' x 1'' (omit 1 Fat Exchange)	1
Corn muffin, 2'' diameter (omit 1 Fat Exchange)	1
Crackers, round butter type (omit 1 Fat Exchange)	5
Muffin, plain small (omit 1 Fat Exchange)	1
Potatoes, French fried, length 2'' to 3½'' (omit 1 Fat Exchange)	8
Potato or corn chips (omit 2 Fat Exchanges)	15
Pancake, 5'' x ½'' (omit 1 Fat Exchange)	1
Waffle, 5'' x ½'' (omit 1 Fat Exchange)	1

5. Meat Exchanges

Meat Exchanges are based on lean meat. One Lean Meat Exchange equals 7 g protein, 3 g fat, 55 kilocalories.

Lean Meat	*One Lean Meat Exchange*
Beef: baby beef (very lean), chipped beef, chuck, flank steak, tenderloin, plate ribs, plate skirt steak, round (bottom, top), all cuts rump, spare ribs, tripe	1 ounce

Lamb: leg, rib, sirloin, loin (roast and chops), shank, shoulder	1 ounce
Pork: leg (whole rump, center shank), ham, smoked (center slices)	1 ounce
Veal: leg, loin, rib, shank, shoulder, cutlets	1 ounce
Poultry: meat without skin of chicken, turkey, cornish hen, guinea hen, pheasant	1 ounce
Fish:	
Any fresh or frozen	1 ounce
Canned salmon, tuna, mackerel, crab and lobster	¼ cup
Clams, oysters, scallops, shrimp	5 or 1 ounce
Sardines, drained	3
Cheeses containing less than 5 percent butterfat	1 ounce
Cottage cheese, dry and 2 percent butterfat	¼ cup
Dried beans and peas (omit 1 Bread Exchange)	½ cup

Medium-Fat Meat

One Medium-fat Meat Exchange equals 1 Lean Meat Exchange plus ½ Fat Exchange:

	One Medium-Fat Meat Exchange
Beef: ground (15 percent fat), corned beef (canned), rib eye, round (ground commercial)	1 ounce
Pork: loin (all cuts tenderloin), shoulder arm (picnic), shoulder blade, Boston butt Canadian bacon, boiled ham	1 ounce
Liver, heart, kidney, and sweetbreads	1 ounce
Cottage cheese, creamed	¼ cup
Cheese: mozzarella, ricotta, farmer's cheese, neufchatel,	1 ounce
parmesan, grated	3 tablespoons
Egg	1 large
Peanut butter (plus 2 additional Fat Exchanges)	2 tablespoons

High-fat Meat

One High Fat Meat Exchange equals 1 Lean Mean Exchange plus 1 Fat Exchange:

	One High-Fat Meat Exchange
Beef: brisket, corned beef (brisket), ground beef (more than 20 percent fat), hamburger (commercial), chuck (ground commercial), roast (rib), steaks (club and rib)	1 ounce
Lamb: breast	1 ounce
Pork: spare ribs, loin (back ribs), pork (ground), country style ham, deviled ham	1 ounce

Veal: breast	1 ounce
Poultry: capon, duck (domestic), goose	1 ounce
Cheese: cheddar types	1 ounce
Cold cuts	4½'' x ⅛'' slice
Frankfurter	1 small

6. Fat Exchanges

One Fat Exchange equals 5 g fat, 45 kilocalories.

	One Fat Exchange
Margarine, soft, tub, stick[a]	1 teaspoon
Avocado (4'' in diameter)[b]	⅛
Oil: corn, cottonseed, safflower, soy, sunflower	1 teaspoon
Oil, olive[b]	1 teaspoon
Oil, peanut[b]	1 teaspoon
Olives[b]	5 small
Almonds[b]	10 whole
Pecans[b]	2 large whole
Peanuts[b]	
Spanish	20 whole
Virginia	10 whole
Walnuts	6 small
Nuts, other[b]	6 small
Margarine, regular stick	1 teaspoon
Butter	1 teaspoon
Bacon fat	1 teaspoon
Bacon, crisp	1 strip
Cream, light	2 tablespoons
Cream, sour	2 tablespoons
Cream, heavy	1 tablespoon
Cream cheese	1 tablespoon
French dressing[c]	1 tablespoon
Italian dressing[c]	1 tablespoon
Lard	1 teaspoon
Mayonnaise[c]	1 teaspoon
Salad dressing (mayonnaise type)[c]	2 teaspoons
Salt pork	¾'' cube

[a] Made with corn, cottonseed, safflower, soy or sunflower oil only.
[b] Fat content is primarily monounsaturated.
[c] If made with corn, cottonseed, safflower, soy or sunflower oil can be used on fat-modified diet.

7. "Free" List

The following foods have negligible protein, carbohydrate, fat, and energy content:

Diet calorie-free beverage	Parsley
	Nutmeg
Coffee	Lemon
Tea	Mustard
Bouillon without fat	Chili powder
Unsweetened gelatin	Onion salt or
Unsweetened pickles	powder
Salt and pepper	Horseradish
Red pepper	Vinegar
Paprika	Mint
Garlic	Cinnamon
Celery salt	Lime

Source: Exchange Lists for Meal Planning, prepared by Committees of the American Diabetes Association, Inc., and The American Dietetic Association in cooperation with The National Institute of Arthritis, Metabolism and Digestive Diseases and the National Heart and Lung Institute, National Institutes of Health, Public Health Service, U.S. Department of Health, Education, and Welfare, 1976.

APPENDIX H
Nutrient Composition of Foods*

Food	Amount	Weight g	Water g	Energy kcal	Protein g	Fat g	Total Carbohydrate g	Calcium mg	Iron mg	Magnesium mg	Phosphorus mg	Potassium mg	Sodium mg	Vitamin C mg	Thiamin mg	Riboflavin mg	Niacin mg	Vitamin B_6 mg	Folacin μg	Total Vitamin A I.U.
Baby Foods																				
Cereal, barley, dry	1 tbsp	2.4	0.20	9	0.30	0.10	1.80	19.0	1.80	3.0	11.0	9	1	0.10	0.066	0.065	0.864	0.009	0.7	—
Mixed, dry	1 tbsp	2.4	0.20	9	0.30	0.10	1.80	18.0	1.52	2.0	9.0	10	1	0.10	0.059	0.065	0.833	0.005	1.0	—
Mixed, w/bananas, dry	1 tbsp	2.4	0.10	9	0.30	0.10	1.90	17.0	1.62	2.0	9.0	16	3	0.10	0.091	0.085	0.493	0.010	nd	3
Oatmeal, dry	1 tbsp	2.4	0.10	10	0.30	0.20	1.70	18.0	1.77	3.0	12.0	11	1	0.10	0.069	0.063	0.863	0.004	0.8	—
Rice, dry	1 tbsp	2.4	0.20	9	0.20	0.10	1.90	20.0	1.77	5.0	14.0	9	1	0.10	0.063	0.053	0.750	0.011	0.6	5
Dessert, Apple Brown Betty, strained	1 oz[a]	28.0	22.70	20	0.10	0	5.60	5.0	0.05	nd	nd	14	3	9.80	0.004	0.010	0.013	nd	0.1	5
Fruit, strained	1 oz[a]	28.0	23.70	17	0.10	0	4.50	2.0	0.06	1.0	2.0	27	4	0.70	0.005	0.003	0.041	0.010	0.9	71
Vanilla custard pudding	1 oz[a]	28.0	22.60	24	0.40	0.60	4.60	16.0	0.07	2.0	13.0	19	8	0.20	0.003	0.023	0.011	0.006	1.7	18
Dinner, beef & noodle, strained	1 oz[a]	28.0	25.10	15	0.60	0.50	2.00	3.0	0.12	2.0	8.0	13	8	0.30	0.010	0.012	0.205	0.014	1.4	233
Mixed vegetable, strained	1 oz[a]	28.0	25.20	11	0.30	0	2.70	6.0	0.09	nd	nd	34	2	0.80	0.004	0.009	0.142	nd	2.3	773
Vegetables & beef, strained	1 oz[a]	28.0	25.10	15	0.60	0.60	2.00	3.0	0.11	2.0	12.0	29	6	0.30	0.006	0.008	0.143	0.015	1.3	337
Vegetables & lamb, strained	1 oz[a]	28.0	25.10	15	0.60	0.60	2.00	3.0	0.10	2.0	14.0	27	6	0.30	0.005	0.010	0.150	0.013	1.0	566
Vegetables, noodles & chicken	1 oz[a]	28.0	24.70	18	0.60	0.70	2.20	8.0	0.10	nd	9.0	16	6	0.20	0.009	0.014	0.115	0.006	0.9	402
Fruit, applesauce, strained	1 oz[a]	28.0	25.10	12	0.10	0	3.10	1.0	0.06	1.0	2.0	20	1	10.90	0.003	0.008	0.017	0.009	0.5	5
Bananas with tapioca	1 oz[a]	28.0	23.80	16	0.10	0	4.30	1.0	0.06	3.0	2.0	25	3	4.70	0.003	0.009	0.052	0.033	1.6	12
Peaches, strained	1 oz[a]	28.0	22.70	20	0.10	0	5.40	2.0	0.07	3.0	3.0	46	2	8.90	0.003	0.009	0.173	0.004	1.1	46
Pears & pineapples	1 oz[a]	28.0	25.10	12	0.10	0	3.10	3.0	0.07	2.0	2.0	33	1	7.80	0.006	0.008	0.059	0.005	0.8	8
Juice, apple	1 fl oz	31.0	27.30	14	0	0	3.60	1.0	0.18	1.0	2.0	28	1	18.00	0.002	0.005	0.026	0.009	8.2	6
Orange	1 fl oz	31.0	27.40	14	0.20	0.10	3.20	4.0	0.05	3.0	3.0	57	0	19.40	0.014	0.009	0.074	0.017	1.6	17
Meat, beef, strained	1 oz[a]	28.0	22.90	30	3.90	1.50	0	2.0	0.42	5.0	24.0	62	23	0.60	0.003	0.040	0.808	0.040	2.9	52
Chicken, strained	1 oz[a]	28.0	22.00	37	3.90	2.20	0	18.0	0.40	4.0	27.0	40	13	0.50	0.004	0.043	0.923	0.057	0.6	38
Lamb, strained	1 oz[a]	28.0	22.80	29	4.00	1.30	0.40	2.0	0.42	4.0	27.0	58	18	0.30	0.005	0.057	0.829	0.043		24
Liver, strained	1 oz[a]	28.0	22.50	29	4.10	1.10	0.30	1.0	1.50	4.0	58.0	64	21	5.50	0.014	0.514	2.361	0.097	95.7	10,811
Egg yolks, strained	1 oz[a]	28.0	20.00	58	2.80	4.90		22.0	0.78	2.0	81.0	22	11	0.40	0.020	0.075	0.007	0.045	26.1	355
Vegetables, beans, green, strained	1 oz[a]	28.0	26.10	7	0.40	0	1.70	11.0	0.21	7.0	6.0	45	1	1.50	0.007	0.024	0.098	0.011	9.8	127
Carrots, strained	1 oz[a]	28.0	26.20	8	0.20	0	1.70	6.0	0.10	3.0	6.0	56	11	1.60	0.007	0.011	0.131	0.021	4.2	3249
Mixed, strained	1 oz[a]	28.0	25.40	11	0.30	0.10	2.30	4.0	0.09	3.0	6.0	36	4	0.50	0.006	0.007	0.093	0.016	1.1	1132
Peas, strained	1 oz[a]	28.0	24.80	11	1.00	0.10	2.30	6.0	0.27	4.0	12.0	32	1	1.90	0.023	0.017	0.289	0.020	7.4	160
Squash, strained	1 oz[a]	28.0	26.30	7	0.20	0.10	1.60	7.0	0.08	3.0	4.0	51	1	2.20	0.003	0.016	0.100	0.018	4.4	574
Zwieback	1 piece	7.0	0.30	30	0.70	0.70	5.20	1.0	0.04	1.0	4.0	21	16	0.40	0.015	0.017	0.092	0.006	nd	4

Beverages
(except milk or fruit & vegetable products)

Alcoholic

Food	Amount																			
Beer, 4.5% alcohol by volume	12 fl oz	360.0	332.00	151	1.10	0	13.70	18.0	trace	36.0	108.0	90	25	0	0	0.110	2.200	0.216	0	0
Gin, Rum, Whiskey, Vodka																				
80-proof	1 jigger (1.5 fl oz)	43.0	28.00	97	0	0	trace	3.0	trace	0	4.0	1	0	0	0	0	0	0	0	0
90-proof	1 jigger (1.5 fl oz)	43.0	26.00	110	0	0	trace	3.0	trace	0	4.0	1	0	0	0	0	0	0	0	0
100-proof	1 jigger (1.5 fl oz)	43.0	24.00	124	0	0	trace	3.0	trace	0	4.0	1	0	0	0	0	0	0	0	0
Wines, dessert 18.8% alcohol by volume	2 fl oz	60.0	46.00	82	0.10	0	4.60	5.0	0.20	3.0	6.0	45	2	0	0.010	0.010	0.100	0.024	0	0.010
Table 12.2% alcohol by volume	3.5 fl oz	100.0	86.00	85	0.10	0	4.20	9.0	0.40	8.0	10.0	92	5	0	0.010	0.010	0.100	0.040	0	0.040

Non Alcoholic

Carbonated

Food	Amount																			
Cola type	12 fl oz	339.0	305.00	132	0	0	33.90	27.0	1.40	3.0	51.0	0	20	0	0	0	0	0	0	0
Cream soda	12 fl oz	371.0	330.00	160	0	0	40.80	—	—	—	—	—	—	0	—	—	—	—	—	0
Fruit flavored	12 fl oz	372.0	327.00	171	0	0	44.60	—	—	—	—	—	—	0	—	—	—	—	—	0
Ginger ale	12 fl oz	339.0	312.00	105	0	0	27.10	27.0	1.40	3.0	51.0	0	20	0	0	0	0	0	0	0
Root beer	12 fl oz	370.0	331.00	152	0	0	38.90	—	—	—	—	—	—	0	—	—	—	—	—	0
Soda, club	12 fl oz	355.0	355.00	0	0	0	0	—	—	—	—	—	—	0	—	—	—	—	—	0
Soda, quinine	12 fl oz	366.0	337.00	113	0	0	29.30	—	—	—	—	—	—	0	—	—	—	—	—	0
Coffee, instant (2 oz powder in water)	1 cup=6 fl oz	180.0	176.00	2	trace	trace	trace	4.0	0.20	9.0	7.0	65	2	0	trace	trace	0.500	0.018	—	0
Tea, instant	1 cup=6 fl oz	180.0	179.00	3	0	0	0.70	0	0	4.0	0	45	0	0.02	0	0	0.500	0.011	6.0	0

Cereals and Grains

Food	Amount																			
Barley, uncooked, pearled, light	1/2 cup	100.0	11.00	349	8.20	1.00	78.80	16.0	2.00	37.0	189.0	160	3	0	0.120	0.050	3.100	—	—	0
Biscuits	1	28.0	21.00	103	2.10	4.80	12.80	34.0	0.40	6.0	49.0	33	175	trace	0.060	0.060	0.500	0.011	2.0	trace
Bran Flakes	1 cup	35.0	1.00	106	3.60	0.60	28.20	19.0	12.40	—	125.0	137	207	12.00	0.410	0.490	4.100	0.100	6.0	1650

Breads

Food	Amount																			
Boston Brown	1 slice	45.0	20.00	95	2.50	0.60	20.50	41.0	0.90	8.0	72.0	131	113	0	0.050	0.030	0.500	0.018	—	0
French	1 slice	35.0	11.00	102	3.20	1.10	19.40	15.0	0.80	—	30.0	32	203	trace	0.100	0.080	0.900	0.018	3.0	trace
Submarine Roll	1	135.0	41.00	392	12.30	4.10	74.80	58.0	3.00	8.0	115.0	122	783	trace	0.380	0.300	3.400	—	—	trace
Italian	1 slice	30.0	10.00	83	2.70	0.20	16.90	5.0	0.70	5.0	23.0	58	176	0	0.090	0.060	0.800	0.020	3.0	0
Raisin	1 slice	25.0	9.00	66	1.70	0.70	13.40	18.0	0.30	6.0	22.0	139	91	trace	0.010	0.020	0.200	0.009	—	trace
Rye, American	1 slice	25.0	9.00	61	2.30	0.30	13.00	13.0	0.40	6.0	37.0	36	139	0	0.050	0.020	0.400	0.023	4.0	0
White Enriched	1 slice	25.0	9.00	68	2.20	0.80	12.60	21.0	0.60	10.0	24.0	26	127	trace	0.060	0.050	0.600	0.009	9.0	trace
Whole Wheat	1 slice	25.0	9.00	61	2.60	0.80	11.90	25.0	0.80	6.0	57.0	68	132	trace	0.060	0.030	0.700	0.041	4.0	trace
Brownies w/nuts	1¾"x1¾"x7/8"	20.0	2.00	97	1.30	6.30	10.20	8.0	0.40	10.0	30.0	38	50	0	0.040	0.020	0.100	—	9.0	40
Buckwheat flour	1 cup	98.0	12.00	326	11.50	2.50	70.60	32.0	2.70	—	340.0	—	—	0	0.570	0.150	2.800	—	—	0
Bulghur, dry	1 cup	170.0	17.00	602	19.0	2.60	128.70	49.0	6.30	48.0	575.0	389	—	trace	0.480	0.240	7.700	—	—	trace

Cakes — made from mix

Food	Amount																			
Angel Food	1/12 cake	53.0	18.00	137	3.00	0.10	31.50	50.0	0.20	8.0	63.0	32	77	0	trace	0.060	0.100	0.006	1.0	0
Coffee	1/6 cake	72.0	22.00	232	4.50	6.90	37.70	44.0	1.20	11.0	125.0	78	310	trace	0.130	0.120	1.000	0.030	trace	120
Cupcake without icing	1	25.0	6.00	88	1.20	3.00	14.00	40.0	0.10	—	59.0	21	113	trace	0.010	0.030	0.100	0.010	trace	40
Cupcake w/choc. icing	1	36.0	8.00	129	1.60	4.50	21.30	47.0	0.30	—	71.0	42	121	trace	0.010	0.040	0.100	0.010	trace	60
Devil's Food w/choc. icing	1/12 cake	92.0	22.00	312	4.00	11.30	53.60	54.0	0.70	22.0	97.0	120	241	trace	0.030	0.070	0.300	0.045	30.0	140

• Approximately 1¾ = 2 tbsp.

*Sources and general notes for this table will be found at the end of the table.

Food	Amount	Weight g	Water g	Energy kcal	Protein g	Fat g	Total Carbo-hydrate g	Minerals: Cal-cium mg	Iron mg	Mag-nesium mg	Phos-phorus mg	Potas-sium mg	Sod-ium mg	Vitamins: Vitamin C mg	Thia-min mg	Ribo-flavin mg	Niacin mg	Vitamin B_6 mg	Folacin µg	Total Vitamin A I.U.
Gingerbread	1/9 cake	63.0	23.00	174	2.00	4.30	32.20	57.0	1.00	—	63.0	173	192	trace	0.020	0.060	0.500	—	—	trace
White w/choc. icing	1/12 cake	95.0	20.00	333	3.70	10.20	59.70	94.0	0.50	—	170.0	110	216	trace	0.020	0.080	0.200	—	—	60
Yellow w/choc. icing	1/12 cake	92.0	24.00	310	3.80	10.40	53.00	84.0	0.60	18	167.0	100	209	trace	0.020	0.070	0.200	0.036	7.5	130
Cakes—home recipe																				
Boston Cream Pie	1/12 cake	69.0	24.00	208	3.50	6.50	34.40	46.0	0.30	—	70.0	61	128	trace	0.020	0.080	0.100	—	—	140
Fruit, dark	1 slice	15.0	3.00	57	0.70	2.30	9.00	11.0	0.40	2.0	17.0	74	24	trace	0.020	0.020	0.100	0.012	trace	20
Pound	1 slice	30.0	5.00	142	1.70	8.90	14.10	6.0	0.20	4.0	24.0	18	33	0	0.010	0.030	0.100	0.012	2.0	80
Sponge	1/12 cake	66.0	21.00	196	5.00	3.80	35.70	20.0	0.80	—	74.0	57	110	trace	0.030	0.090	0.100	—	—	300
Cereals																				
Corn Flakes, plain	1 cup	25.0	1.00	97	2.00	0.10	21.30	1.7	0.60	4.0	9.0	30	251	9.00	0.290	0.350	2.900	0.020	1.0	1180
Corn, puffed	1 cup	20.0	0.70	80	1.60	0.80	16.20	4.0	2.30	—	18.0	—	233	7.00	0.230	0.280	2.300	—	—	940
Farina, quick cooking	1 cup	245.0	218.00	105	3.20	0.20	21.80	147.0	12.30	8.0	162.0	25	466	0	0.120	0.070	1.000	0.024	0	0
Oats, cooked oatmeal	1 cup	240.0	208.00	132	4.80	2.40	23.30	22.0	1.40	58.0	137.0	146	523	0	0.190	0.050	0.200	0.048	26.0	0
Rice, oven popped	1 cup	30.0	1.00	117	1.80	0.10	26.30	6.0	0.80	—	28.0	29	283	11.00	0.350	0.420	3.500	—	—	1410
Rice, puffed	1 cup	15.0	6.00	60	0.90	0.10	13.40	3.0	0.30	—	14.0	15	trace	0	0.070	0.010	0.700	0.010	1.0	0
Wheat & Barley	1 cup cooked	245.0	196.00	196	7.40	0.70	39.40	22.0	2.20	76.0	201.0	trace	250	0	0.170	0.050	—	0.200	16.0	0
Wheat Flakes, added sugar vitamins	1 cup	30.0	1.00	106	3.10	0.50	24.20	12.0	3.50	27.0	83.0	81	310	11.00	0.350	0.420	3.500	0.081	5.0	1410
Wheat, puffed	1 cup plain	15	0.50	54	2.30	0.20	11.8	4	0.60	—	48	51	1	0	0.080	0.030	1.200	—	—	0
Wheat, shredded	1 large biscuit	25	1.60	89	2.50	0.50	20.0	11	0.90	33.0	97	87	1	0	0.060	0.030	1.100	0.050	2.0	0
Cookies																				
Butter	5 cookies 2" diam.	25.0	1.10	115	1.60	4.20	18.00	32.0	0.20	—	24.0	15	105	0	0.010	0.020	0.100	—	—	115
Chocolate Chip	5 cookies 2¼" diam.	52.0	1.40	248	2.90	11.10	36.60	21.0	1.00	—	60.0	71	211	trace	0.020	0.040	0.200	—	—	65
Fig Bars	4 cookies 1½"x1¾"x½"	56.0	7.60	200	2.20	3.10	42.20	44.0	0.60	14.0	34.0	111	141	trace	0.020	0.040	0.200	0.052	6.0	60
Ginger Snaps	5 cookies 2" diam.	35.0	1.10	147	2.00	3.10	28.00	26.0	0.80	—	17.0	162	200	trace	0.020	0.020	0.200	—	—	25
Macaroons	2 cookies 2¾" diam.	38.0	1.70	181	2.00	8.80	25.10	10.0	0.30	—	32.0	176	13	0	0.020	0.060	0.200	—	—	0
Oatmeal with raisins	4 cookies 2-5/8" diam.	52.0	1.40	235	3.20	8.00	38.20	11.0	1.50	—	53.0	192	84	trace	0.060	0.040	0.300	—	—	30
Peanut (sandwich type)	4 cookies 1¾" diam.	49.0	1.10	232	4.90	9.40	32.80	21.0	0.40	—	57.0	86	85	trace	0.030	0.040	1.400	—	—	100
Sandwich	4 cookies 1¾" diam.	40.0	0.80	198	1.90	9.00	27.70	10.0	0.30	—	96.0	15	193	0	0.020	0.020	0.200	—	—	0
Sugar	5 cookies 2¼" diam.	40.0	3.20	178	2.40	6.70	27.20	31.0	0.60	—	41.0	31	127	trace	0.070	0.070	0.500	—	—	45
Corn Bread, southern style	1 piece 2½"x2½"x1½"	78.0	4.00	161	5.80	5.60	22.70	94.0	0.90	—	165.0	122	490	1.00	0.100	0.150	0.500	—	—	120
Cornmeal, whole ground	1 cup	122.0	15.00	433	11.20	4.80	89.90	24.0	2.90	129.0	312.0	346	1	0	0.460	0.130	2.400	—	—	620
Cornstarch	1 tbsp.	8.0	1.00	29	trace	trace	7	0	0	trace	0	trace	trace	0	0	0	0	—	—	0
Crackers																				
Animal	10	26.0	0.80	112	1.70	2.40	20.80	14.0	0.10	—	30.0	25	79	trace	0.010	0.030	0.100	—	—	30
Butter	5	16.0	0.70	75	1.20	3.00	11.10	25.0	0.10	—	43.0	19	180	0	trace	0.010	0.200	—	—	35
Cheese	5	17.2	0.70	83	2.00	3.70	10.40	58.0	0.20	—	53.0	19	178	0	trace	0.020	0.200	—	—	trace
Graham, Sugar/Honey	1 large	14.2	0.50	58	1.00	1.60	10.00	12.0	0.20	7.0	47.0	38	72	0	trace	0.020	0.100	0.010	3.0	—
Saltines	4	11.0	0.50	48	1.00	1.30	8.00	2.0	0.10	4.0	10.0	13	123	0	trace	trace	0.100	0.008	2.0	0
Peanut Butter & Cheese	4	28.0	0.70	139	4.30	6.80	15.90	16.0	0.20	—	51.0	64	281	0	0.010	0.020	1.000	—	—	10
Donut, Plain	1	42.0	10.00	164	1.90	7.80	21.60	17.0	0.60	7.0	80.0	38	210	trace	0.070	0.070	0.500	0.017	3.0	30
Macaroni																				
Cooked, plain	1 cup	130.0	83.00	192	6.50	0.70	39.10	14.0	1.40	25.0	55.0	103	1	0	0.230	0.130	1.800	0.030	5.0	0
and cheese	1 cup	200.0	116.00	430	16.80	22.20	40.20	362.0	1.80	58.0	322.0	240	1086	trace	0.200	0.400	1.800	0.090	13.0	860

Item	Serving																			
Muffins																				
Blueberry	1	40.0	16.00	112	2.90	3.70	16.80	34.0	0.60	10.0	53.0	46	253	trace	0.060	0.080	0.500	0.020	3.0	90
Bran	1	40.0	14.00	104	3.10	3.90	17.20	57.0	1.50	20.0	162.0	172	179	trace	0.060	0.100	1.600	—	—	90
Corn	1	40.0	13.00	126	2.80	4.00	19.20	42.0	0.70	—	68.0	54	192	trace	0.080	0.090	0.600	—	3.0	120
Plain	1	40.0	15.00	118	3.10	4.00	16.90	42.0	0.60	10.0	60.0	50	176	trace	0.070	0.090	0.600	0.020	—	40
Noodles																				
Egg, cooked	1 cup	160.0	113.00	200	6.60	2.40	37.30	16.0	1.40	36.0	94.0	70	3	0	0.220	0.130	1.900	0.032	4.0	110
Chow Mein, canned	½ cup	22.0	0.20	110	3.00	5.30	13.00	—	—	—	—	—	—	0	—	—	—	—	—	—
Pancakes																				
Home Recipe	4" diameter	27.0	13.00	62	1.90	1.90	9.20	27.0	0.40	4.0	38.0	33	115	trace	0.050	0.060	0.400	0.100	2.0	30
Mix, buckwheat	4" diameter	27.0	16.00	54	1.80	2.50	6.40	59.0	0.40	—	91.0	66	125	trace	0.030	0.040	0.200	—	—	60
mix, plain	4" diameter	27.0	14.00	61	1.90	2.00	8.70	58.0	0.30	4.0	70.0	42	152	trace	0.040	0.060	0.200	0.100	2.0	70
Pies, 9" diam.[a]																				
Apple	1/8 pie	118.0	56.00	302	2.60	13.10	45.00	9.0	0.40	5.0	26.0	94	355	1.00	0.020	0.020	0.500	0.047	5.0	40
Blueberry	1/8 pie	118.0	60.00	286	2.80	12.70	41.20	13.0	0.70	5.0	27.0	77	316	4.00	0.020	0.020	0.400	0.050	3.0	40
Cherry	1/8 pie	118.0	55.00	308	3.10	13.30	45.30	17.0	0.40	—	30.0	124	369	trace	0.020	0.020	0.600	—	—	520
Custard	1/8 pie	114.0	66.00	249	7.00	12.70	26.70	109.0	0.70	—	129.0	156	327	0	0.060	0.180	0.300	—	—	260
Lemon Meringue	1/8 pie	105.0	50.00	268	3.90	10.70	39.60	15.0	0.50	—	51.0	53	296	3.00	0.030	0.080	0.200	—	2.0	180
Mince	1/8 pie	118.0	51.00	320	3.00	13.60	48.60	33.0	1.20	—	45.0	210	529	1.00	0.080	0.050	0.500	—	—	trace
Pecan	1/8 pie	103.0	20.00	431	5.30	23.60	52.80	48.0	2.90	—	106.0	127	228	trace	0.160	0.070	0.300	—	—	160
Pumpkin	1/8 pie	114.0	67.00	241	4.60	12.80	27.90	58.0	0.60	7.0	79.0	182	244	trace	0.030	0.110	0.600	0.046	5.0	2819
Rhubarb	1/8 pie	118.0	56.00	299	3.00	12.60	45.10	76.0	0.80	—	31.0	188	319	4.00	0.020	0.050	0.400	—	—	60
Popovers	1	40.0	22.00	90	3.50	3.70	10.30	38.0	0.60	—	56.0	60	88	trace	0.060	0.100	0.400	—	—	130
Rice, added salt																				
brown, cooked	1 cup	195.0	137.00	232	4.90	1.20	49.70	23.0	1.00	58.0	142.0	137	550	0	0.180	0.040	2.700	0.300	15.0	0
White, cooked	1 cup	205.0	149.00	223	4.10	0.20	49.60	21.0	1.80	16.0	57.0	57	767	0	0.230	0.020	2.100	0.075	1.5	0
Parboiled	1 cup	175.0	128.00	186	3.70	0.20	40.80	33.0	1.40	—	100.0	75	627	0	0.190	0.020	2.100	—	—	0
Rolls and Buns																				
Danish Pastry	1	65.0	14.00	274	4.80	15.30	29.60	33.0	0.60	15.0	71.0	73	238	trace	0.040	0.100	0.500	—	5.0	200
Hard Roll	1 round	50.0	13.00	156	4.90	1.60	29.80	24.0	1.20	15.0	46.0	49	313	trace	0.130	0.120	0.140	—	6.0	trace
Frankfurter or Hamburger	1	40.0	13.00	119	3.30	2.20	21.20	30.0	0.80	10.0	34.0	38	202	trace	0.110	0.070	0.900	0.010	5.0	trace
Brown and Serve	1	26.0	7.00	84	2.20	1.90	14.20	20.0	0.50	10.0	23.0	25	136	trace	0.070	0.060	0.600	—	4.0	trace
Rye Flour	1 cup	88.0	10.00	308	10.00	1.50	65.80	24.0	2.30	64.0	231.0	179	1	0	0.260	0.110	2.200	—	—	0
Sesame Seeds	1 tbsp	8.0	0.40	47	1.50	4.30	1.40	9.0	0.20	1.0	47.0	—	—	0	0.010	0.010	0.400	—	5.0	—
Spaghetti																				
Plain, cooked	1 cup	130.0	83.00	192	6.50	0.70	39.10	14.0	1.40	17.0	85.0	103	1	0	0.230	0.130	1.800	0.026	3.0	0
Tomato sauce w/cheese	1 cup	250.0	192.00	260	8.80	8.80	37.00	80.0	2.30	30.0	135.0	408	955	13.00	0.250	0.180	2.300	0.100	2.0	1080
Meatballs w/tomato sauce	1 cup	248.0	174.00	332	18.60	11.70	38.70	124.0	3.70	42.0	236.0	665	1009	22.00	0.250	0.300	4.000	0.113	15.0	1590
Tortilla, corn, lime-treated	1 average 6" diam.	30.0	14.00	63	1.50	0.60	13.50	60.0	0.90	32.0	42.0	5	33	0	0.040	0.300	0.300	0.021	0	6
Waffles																				
Home-recipe	½ of whole	50.0	21.00	140	4.70	4.90	18.80	57.0	0.90	—	87.0	73	238	trace	0.090	0.130	0.700	—	—	170
Frozen	1 waffle	22.0	9.00	56	1.60	1.40	9.20	27.0	0.40	—	46.0	35	142	trace	0.040	0.040	0.300	—	—	30
From mix	½ of whole	50.0	21.00	138	4.40	5.30	18.10	120.0	0.70	13.0	172.0	98	343	trace	0.070	0.120	0.500	—	—	120
Wheat Flour																				
Whole	1 cup	120.0	14.00	400	16.00	2.40	85.20	49.0	4.00	136.0	446.0	444	4	0	0.660	0.140	5.200	0.400	35.0	0
White, all-purpose enriched	1 cup	137.0	16.00	499	14.40	1.40	104.30	22.0	4.00	34.0	119.0	130	3	0	0.600	0.360	4.800	0.080	22.0	0
Unenriched	1 cup	137.0	16.00	499	14.40	1.40	104.30	22.0	1.10	34.0	119.0	130	3	0	0.080	0.070	1.200	0.080	22.0	0
Wheat Germ, toasted	1 tbsp	6.0	0.20	23	1.80	0.70	3.00	3.0	0.50	20.0	70.0	57	trace	1.00	0.110	0.050	0.300	0.055	18.0	10
Dairy Products and Eggs																				
Cheeses																				
Blue	1 oz	28.0	12.02	100	6.07	8.15	0.66	150.0	0.09	7.0	110.0	73	396	0	0.008	0.108	0.2880	0.047	10.0	204
Brie	1 oz	28.0	13.73	95	5.88	7.85	0.13	52.0	0.14	—	53.0	43	178	0	0.020	0.147	0.108	0.067	18.0	189
Cheddar	1 oz	28.0	10.42	114	7.06	9.40	0.36	204.0	0.19	8.0	145.0	28	176	trace	0.008	0.106	0.023	0.021	5.0	300
Cottage, creamed	1/2 cup	105.0	82.91	108	13.12	4.74	2.82	63.0	0.15	6.0	138.0	88	425	—	0.022	0.171	0.130	0.070	13.0	171

[a] Unenriched flour used for crust.

Food	Amount	Weight g	Water g	Energy kcal	Protein g	Fat g	Total Carbohydrate g	Minerals						Vitamins						
								Calcium mg	Iron mg	Magnesium mg	Phosphorus mg	Potassium mg	Sodium mg	Vitamin C mg	Thiamin mg	Riboflavin mg	Niacin mg	Vitamin B6 mg	Folacin μg	Total Vitamin A I.U.
Cottage, dry curd	1/2 cup	72.0	57.84	62	12.52	0.31	1.34	23.0	0.16	3.0	76.0	24	10	0	0.018	0.103	0.112	0.060	11.0	22
Cottage, 2% fat	1/2 cup	113.0	89.62	102	15.53	2.18	4.10	77.0	0.18	7.0	170.0	109	459	trace	0.027	0.209	0.163	0.086	15.0	79
Cream	1 oz	28.0	15.24	99	2.14	9.89	0.75	23.0	0.34	2.0	30.0	34	84	0	0.005	0.056	0.029	0.013	4.0	405
Edam	1 oz	28.0	11.78	101	7.08	7.88	0.40	207.0	0.12	8.0	152.0	53	274	0	0.010	0.110	0.023	0.022	5.0	260
Feta	1 oz	28.0	15.66	75	4.03	6.03	1.16	140.0	0.18	5.0	96.0	18	316	0	—	—	—	—	—	—
Gouda	1 oz	28.0	11.75	101	7.07	7.78	0.63	198.0	0.07	8.0	155.0	34	232	0	0.009	0.095	0.018	0.023	6.0	183
Gruyère	1 oz	28.0	9.41	117	8.45	9.17	0.10	287.0	—	—	172.0	23	95	0	0.017	0.079	0.030	0.023	3.0	346
Mozzarella	1 oz	28.0	15.35	80	5.51	6.12	0.63	147.0	0.05	5.0	105.0	19	106	0	0.004	0.069	0.024	0.016	2.0	225
Mozzarella, part skim	1 oz	28.0	15.25	72	6.88	4.51	0.78	183.0	0.06	7.0	131.0	24	132	0	0.005	0.086	0.030	0.020	2.0	166
Parmesan, grated	1 tbsp	5.0	0.88	23	2.08	1.50	0.19	69.0	0.05	3.0	40.0	5	93	0	0.002	0.019	0.016	0.005	trace	35
Provolone	1 oz	28.0	11.61	100	7.25	7.55	0.61	214.0	0.15	8.0	141.0	39	248	0	0.005	0.091	0.044	0.021	3.0	231
Ricotta, whole milk	1/2 cup	124.0	88.91	216	13.96	16.10	3.77	257.0	0.47	14.0	196.0	257	104	0	0.016	0.242	0.129	0.053	—	608
Romano	1 oz	28.0	8.76	110	9.02	7.64	1.03	302.0	—	—	215.0	104	340	0	—	0.105	0.022	0.022	2.0	162
Roquefort	1 oz	28.0	11.16	105	6.11	8.69	0.57	188.0	0.16	8.0	111.0	26	513	0	0.011	0.166	0.208	0.035	14.0	297
Swiss	1 oz	28.0	10.55	107	8.06	7.78	0.96	272.0	0.05	10.0	171.0	31	74	0	0.006	0.103	0.026	0.024	2.0	240
American, pasteurized process	1 oz	28.0	11.10	106	6.28	8.86	0.45	174.0	0.11	6.0	211.0	46	406	0	0.008	0.100	0.020	0.020	2.0	343
Swiss, pasteurized process	1 oz	28.0	12.00	95	7.01	7.09	0.60	219.0	0.17	8.0	216.0	61	388	0	0.004	0.078	0.011	0.010	—	229
Cream																				
Half and Half	1 tbsp	15.0	12.08	20	0.44	1.72	0.64	16.0	0.01	2.0	14.0	19	6	0.13	0.005	0.022	0.012	0.006	trace	65
Light	1 tbsp	15.0	11.06	29	0.40	2.90	0.55	14.0	0.01	1.0	12.0	18	6	0.11	0.005	0.022	0.009	0.005	trace	108
Medium	1 tbsp	15.0	10.28	37	0.37	3.75	0.52	14.0	0.01	1.0	11.0	17	6	0.11	0.004	0.020	0.008	0.005	trace	141
Heavy	1 tbsp	15.0	8.66	52	0.31	5.55	0.42	10.0	trace	1.0	9.0	11	6	0.09	0.003	0.016	0.006	0.004	1.0	220
Whipped topping, pressurized	1 tbsp	3.0	1.84	8	0.10	0.67	0.38	3.0	trace	trace	3.0	4	4	0	0.001	0.002	0.002	0.001	—	27
Sour	1 tbsp	12.0	8.51	26	0.38	2.52	0.51	14.0	0.01	1.0	10.0	17	6	0.10	0.004	0.018	0.008	0.002	1.0	95
Eggnog	1 cup	254.0	188.90	342	9.68	19.00	34.39	330.0	0.51	47.0	278.0	420	138	3.81	0.086	0.483	0.267	0.127	2.0	894
Ice Cream																				
Vanilla, 10% fat	1/2 cup	66.0	40.43	135	2.40	7.16	15.86	88.0	0.06	9.0	67.0	128	58	0.35	0.026	0.164	0.067	0.031	1.5	272
Ice Milk, vanilla	1/2 cup	66.0	44.94	92	2.58	2.82	14.48	88.0	0.09	10.0	65.0	132	52	0.38	0.038	0.174	0.059	0.042	1.5	107
Sherbert, orange	1/2 cup	96.0	63.76	135	1.08	1.91	29.36	51.0	0.16	8.0	37.0	99	44	1.93	0.016	0.045	0.066	0.012	7.0	92
Coffee Whitener, liquid	1/2 fl oz	15.0	11.59	20	0.15	1.50	1.71	1.0	trace	trace	10.0	29	12	0	0	0	0	0	0	13
Whitener, powdered	1 tsp	2.0	0.04	11	0.10	0.71	1.10	trace	0.02	trace	8.0	16	4	0	0	0.003	0	0	0	4
Milk																				
Whole	1 cup	244.0	214.70	150	8.03	8.15	11.37	291.0	0.12	33.0	228.0	370	120	2.29	0.093	0.395	0.205	0.102	12.0	307
2% Fat	1 cup	244.0	217.67	121	8.12	4.68	11.71	297.0	0.12	33.0	232.0	377	122	2.32	0.095	0.403	0.210	0.105	12.0	500[a]
2% Fat, & milk solids	1 cup	245.0	217.71	125	8.53	4.70	12.18	313.0	0.12	35.0	245.0	397	128	2.45	0.098	0.424	0.220	0.110	13.0	500[a]
1% Fat	1 cup	244.0	219.80	102	8.03	2.59	11.66	300.0	0.12	34.0	235.0	381	123	2.37	0.095	0.407	0.212	0.105	13.0	500[a]
1% Fat & milk solids	1 cup	245.0	220.03	104	8.53	2.38	12.18	313.0	0.12	35.0	245.0	397	128	2.45	0.098	0.424	0.220	0.110	13.0	500[a]
Skim	1 cup	245.0	222.46	86	8.35	0.44	11.88	302.0	0.10	28.0	247.0	406	126	2.40	0.088	0.343	0.216	0.098	13.0	500[a]
Skim & milk solids	1 cup	245.0	221.43	90	8.75	0.61	12.30	316.0	0.12	36.0	255.0	418	130	2.47	0.100	0.429	0.223	0.113	13.0	500[a]
Buttermilk	1 cup	245.0	220.82	99	8.11	2.16	11.74	285.0	0.12	27.0	219.0	371	257	2.40	0.083	0.377	0.142	0.083	—	81
Dry, non-fat	1/4 cup	30.0	0.96	109	10.85	0.23	15.59	377.0	0.10	33.0	290.0	538	161	2.03	0.124	0.465	0.285	0.108	15.0	11
Condensed, sweetened	1 fl oz	38.2	10.38	123	3.02	3.32	20.78	108.0	0.07	10.0	97.0	142	49	0.99	0.034	0.159	0.080	0.019	4.0	125
Evaporated, whole	1 fl oz	31.5	23.32	42	2.14	2.38	3.16	82.0	0.06	8.0	64.0	95	33	0.59	0.015	0.100	0.061	0.016	2.0	77
Chocolate, whole	1 cup	250.0	205.75	208	7.92	8.48	25.85	280.0	0.60	33.0	251.0	417	149	2.28	0.092	0.405	0.313	0.100	12.0	302[a]
Chocolate, 2% fat	1 cup	250.0	208.95	179	8.02	5.00	26.00	284.0	0.60	33.0	254.0	422	150	2.30	0.092	0.410	0.315	0.102	12.0	500[a]
Goat, whole	1 cup	244.0	212.35	168	8.69	10.10	10.86	326.0	0.12	34.0	270.0	499	122	3.15	0.117	0.337	0.676	0.112	1.0	451
Shake																				
Chocolate, thick	11 oz	300.0	216.60	356	9.15	8.10	63.45	396.0	0.93	48.0	378.0	672	333	0	0.141	0.666	0.372	0.075	15.0	258
Vanilla, thick	11 oz	313.0	233.03	350	12.08	9.48	55.56	457.0	0.31	37.0	361.0	572	299	0	0.094	0.610	0.457	0.131	2.10	357
Yogurt																				
Plain	8 oz	227.0	199.53	139	7.88	7.38	10.58	274.0	0.11	26.0	215.0	351	105	1.20	0.066	0.322	0.170	0.073	17.0	279

Plain, lowfat & milk solids	8 oz	227.0	193.11	144	11.92	3.52	15.98	415.0	0.18	40.0	326.0	531	159	1.82	0.100	0.486	0.259	0.111	25.0	150
Plain, skim milk & milk solids	8 oz	227.0	193.47	127	13.01	0.41	17.43	452.0	0.20	43.0	355.0	579	174	1.98	0.109	0.531	0.281	0.120	28.0	16
Fruit, lowfat & milk solids	8 oz	227.0	170.93	225	9.04	2.61	42.31	314.0	0.14	30.0	247.0	402	121	1.36	0.077	0.368	0.195	0.084	19.0	111
Egg																				
Chicken, whole raw	1 egg	50.0	37.28	79	6.07	5.58	0.60	28.0	1.04	6.0	90.0	65	69	0	0.044	0.150	0.031	0.060	32.0	260
Chicken, white raw	1 egg	33.0	29.06	16	3.25	trace	0.41	4.0	0.01	3.0	4.0	45	50	0	0.002	0.094	0.029	0.001	5.0	0
Chicken, yolk, raw	1 egg	17.0	8.29	63	2.79	5.60	0.04	26.0	0.95	3.0	86.0	15	8	0	0.043	0.074	0.012	0.053	26.0	313
Chicken, fried w/butter	1 egg	46.0	33.06	83	5.37	6.41	0.53	26.0	0.92	5.0	80.0	58	144	0	0.033	0.126	0.026	0.050	22.0	286
Chicken, hard-cooked	1 egg	50.0	37.28	79	6.07	5.58	0.60	28.0	1.04	6.0	90.0	65	69	0	0.037	0.143	0.030	0.057	24.0	260
Chicken, omelet w/fat & milk	1 egg	64.0	48.83	95	5.96	7.08	1.37	47.0	0.93	8.0	97.0	85	155	0.13	0.039	0.156	0.042	0.058	22.0	311
Duck, whole raw	1 egg	70.0	49.58	130	8.97	9.64	1.02	45.0	2.70	12.0	154.0	156	102	0	0.109	0.283	0.140	0.175	56.0	930
Substitute, frozen	1/4 cup	60.0	43.86	96	6.77	6.67	1.92	44.0	1.19	—	43.0	128	120	—	0.072	0.232	—	0.080	—	810
Substitute, liquid	1.5 fl oz	47.0	38.89	40	5.64	1.56	0.30	25.0	0.99	—	57.0	155	83	0	0.052	0.141	0.052	—	—	1015
Substitute, powder	0.35 oz	10.0	0.38	44	5.49	1.29	2.16	32.0	0.31	—	47.0	74	79	0.07	0.022	0.174	0.057	—	—	122
Fast Foods																				
Burger Chef																				
Big Shef	1	186.0	nd	542	23.00	34.00	35.00	189.0	3.40	nd	278.0	384	622	2.00	0.340	0.350	5.400	nd	nd	282
Cheeseburger	1	104.0	nd	304	14.00	17.00	24.00	156.0	2.00	nd	198.0	220	535	1.00	0.220	0.230	3.200	nd	nd	266
French Fries	1 serving	68.0	nd	187	3.00	9.00	25.00	10.0	0.90	nd	76.0	581	4	14.00	0.090	0.050	2.100	nd	nd	trace
Rancher Platter	1	316.0	nd	640	30.00	38.00	44.00	57.0	5.10	nd	326.0	1370	444	24.00	0.300	0.370	8.700	nd	nd	367
Burger King																				
Cheeseburger	1	nd	nd	305	17.00	13.00	29.00	141.0	2.00	nd	229.0	219	562	0.50	0.010	0.020	2.200	nd	nd	195
Hamburger	1	nd	nd	252	14.00	9.00	29.00	45.0	2.00	nd	119.0	208	401	0.50	0.010	0.010	2.200	nd	nd	21
Whopper	1	nd	nd	606	29.00	32.00	51.00	37.0	6.00	nd	205.0	653	909	13.00	0.020	0.030	5.200	nd	nd	641
French Fries	1 serving	nd	nd	214	3.00	10.00	28.00	12.0	1.00	nd	87.0	666	5	16.00	0.010	0.010	2.420	nd	nd	0
Hot Dog	1	nd	nd	291	11.00	17.00	23.00	40.0	2.00	nd	117.0	170	841	0	0.040	0.020	2.000	nd	nd	0
Dairy Queen																				
Big Brazier Deluxe	1	213.0	nd	470	28.00	24.00	36.00	111.0	5.20	45.0	262.0	nd	920	2.50	0.340	0.370	9.600	0.380	nd	nd
Big Brazier Regular	1	184.0	nd	457	27.00	23.00	37.00	113.0	5.20	42.0	223.0	nd	910	2.00	0.370	0.390	9.600	0.340	nd	nd
Big Brazier w/cheese	1	213.0	nd	553	32.00	30.00	38.00	268.0	5.20	47.0	359.0	nd	1435	2.30	0.340	0.530	9.500	0.350	nd	495
Brazier Onion Rings	1 serving	85.0	nd	300	6.00	17.00	33.00	20.0	0.40	16.0	60.0	nd	nd	2.40	0.090	trace	0.400	0.080	nd	trace
Brazier Regular	1	106.0	nd	260	13.00	9.00	28.00	70.0	3.50	23.0	114.0	nd	576	1.00	0.280	0.260	5.000	0.130	nd	nd
Fish Sandwich	1	170.0	nd	400	20.00	17.00	41.00	60.0	1.10	24.0	200.0	nd	nd	trace	0.150	0.260	3.000	0.160	nd	trace
Fish Sandwich w/cheese	1	177.0	nd	440	24.00	21.00	39.00	150.0	0.40	24.0	250.0	nd	nd	trace	0.150	0.260	3.000	0.160	nd	100
Super Brazier Dog	1	182.0	nd	518	20.00	30.00	41.00	158.0	4.30	37.0	195.0	nd	1552	14.00	0.420	0.440	7.000	0.170	nd	trace
Super Brazier Chili Dog	1	210.0	nd	555	23.00	33.00	42.00	158.0	4.00	48.0	231.0	nd	1640	18.00	0.420	0.480	8.800	0.270	nd	nd
Buster Bar	1	149.0	nd	390	10.00	22.00	37.00	200.0	0.70	60.0	150.0	nd	nd	trace	0.090	0.340	1.600	0.120	nd	300
DQ Chocolate Dipped Cone, med.	1	156.0	nd	300	7.00	13.00	40.00	200.0	0.40	24.0	150.0	nd	nd	trace	0.090	0.340	trace	0.080	nd	300
DQ Chocolate Malt, med	1	418.0	nd	600	15.00	20.00	89.00	500.0	3.60	60.0	400.0	nd	nd	3.60	0.120	0.600	0.800	0.200	nd	750
DQ Chocolate Sundae, med	1	184.0	nd	300	6.00	7.00	53.00	200.0	1.10	32.0	150.0	nd	nd	trace	0.060	0.260	trace	0.080	nd	300
DQ Cone, med	1	142.0	nd	230	6.00	7.00	35.00	200.0	trace	24.0	150.0	nd	nd	trace	0.090	0.260	trace	0.080	nd	300
DQ Float	1	397.0	nd	330	6.00	8.00	59.00	200.0	trace	nd	200.0	nd	nd	trace	0.120	0.170	trace	nd	nd	100
DQ Freeze	1	397.0	nd	520	11.00	13.00	89.00	300.0	trace	nd	250.0	nd	nd	trace	0.150	0.340	trace	nd	nd	200
DQ Sandwich	1	60.0	nd	140	3.00	4.00	24.00	60.0	0.40	8.0	60.0	nd	nd	trace	0.030	0.140	0.400	trace	nd	100
Hot Fudge Brownie Delight	1	266.0	nd	570	11.00	22.00	83.00	300.0	1.10	40.0	250.0	nd	nd	trace	0.450	0.430	0.800	0.160	nd	500
Kentucky Fried Chicken																				
Original Recipe Dinner	1 dinner	425.0	nd	830	52.00	46.00	56.00	150.0	4.50	nd	nd	nd	2285	27.00	0.380	0.560	15.000	nd	nd	750
Extra Crispy Dinner	1 dinner	437.0	nd	950	52.00	54.00	63.00	150.0	3.60	nd	nd	nd	1915	27.00	0.380	0.560	14.000	nd	nd	750
Individual Pieces, Original Recipe, Drumstick	1	54.0	28.60	136	14.00	8.00	2.00	20.0	0.90	nd	nd	nd	nd	0.60	0.040	0.120	2.700	nd	nd	30
Keel	1	96.0	50.30	283	25.00	13.00	6.00	nd	0.90	nd	nd	nd	nd	1.20	0.070	0.130	nd	nd	nd	50
Rib	1	82.0	37.70	241	19.00	15.00	8.00	55.0	1.00	nd	nd	nd	nd	1.00	0.060	0.140	5.800	nd	nd	58
Thigh	1	97.0	48.30	276	20.00	19.00	12.00	39.0	1.40	nd	nd	nd	nd	1.00	0.080	0.240	4.900	nd	nd	74
Wing	1	45.0	19.10	151	11.00	10.00	4.00	nd	0.60	nd	nd	nd	nd	1.00	0.030	0.070	nd	nd	nd	nd
Long John Silver's																				
Breaded Clams	5 oz	nd	nd	465	13.00	25.00	46.00	nd	nd	nd	nd	nd	nd	nd	nd	nd	nd	nd	nd	nd
Cole Slaw	4 oz	nd	nd	138	1.00	8.00	16.00	nd	nd	nd	nd	nd	nd	nd	nd	nd	nd	nd	nd	nd
Corn on Cob	1 piece	nd	nd	174	5.00	4.00	29.00	nd	nd	nd	nd	nd	nd	nd	nd	nd	nd	nd	nd	nd

[a]Values based on addition of Vitamin A to level of 2,000 I.U. per quart.

Food	Amount	Weight g	Water g	Energy kcal	Protein g	Fat g	Total Carbohydrate g	Calcium mg	Iron mg	Magnesium mg	Phosphorus mg	Potassium mg	Sodium mg	Vitamin C mg	Thiamin mg	Riboflavin mg	Niacin mg	Vitamin B₆ mg	Folacin µg	Total Vitamin A I.U.
Long John Silver's																				
Fish with Batter	2 pieces	nd	nd	318	19.00	19.00	19.00	nd	nd	nd	nd	nd	nd	nd	nd	nd	nd	nd	nd	nd
Hush Puppies	3 pieces	nd	nd	153	1.00	7.00	20.00	nd	nd	nd	nd	nd	nd	nd	nd	nd	nd	nd	nd	nd
Ocean Scallops	6 pieces	nd	nd	257	10.00	12.00	27.00	nd	nd	nd	nd	nd	nd	nd	nd	nd	nd	nd	nd	nd
Shrimp with Batter	6 pieces	nd	nd	269	9.00	13.00	31.00	nd	nd	nd	nd	nd	nd	nd	nd	nd	nd	nd	nd	nd
Treasure Chest	2 pc fish / 2 peg legs	nd	nd	467	25.00	29.00	27.00	nd	nd	nd	nd	nd	nd	nd	nd	nd	nd	nd	nd	nd
Mc Donald's																				
Egg McMuffin	1	132.0	65.30	352	18.00	20.00	26.00	187.0	3.20	25.0	265.0	222	914	1.60	0.360	0.600	4.300	0.140	nd	361
Hot Cakes w/butter & syrup	1 serving	206.0	95.90	472	8.00	9.00	89.00	54.0	2.40	30.0	404.0	264	1071	2.10	0.310	0.430	4.000	0.060	nd	255
Big Mac	1	187.0	86.40	541	26.00	31.00	39.00	175.0	4.30	38.0	215.0	386	962	2.40	0.350	0.370	8.200	0.220	nd	327
Cheeseburger	1	114.0	51.40	306	16.00	13.00	31.00	158.0	2.90	24.0	134.0	244	725	1.60	0.240	0.300	5.500	0.100	nd	372
Filet O Fish	1 serving	131.0	55.90	402	15.00	23.00	34.00	105.0	1.80	29.0	158.0	293	709	4.20	0.280	0.280	3.900	0.080	nd	152
French Fries	1	69.0	27.80	211	3.00	11.00	26.00	10.0	0.50	23.0	49.0	570	113	11.00	0.150	0.030	2.900	0.010	nd	52
Hamburger	1 serving	99.0	44.60	257	13.00	9.00	30.00	63.0	3.00	21.0	88.0	234	526	1.80	0.230	0.230	5.100	0.110	nd	231
Quarter Pounder	1	164.0	81.20	418	26.00	21.00	33.00	79.0	5.10	38.0	179.0	442	711	2.30	0.310	0.410	9.800	0.250	nd	164
Quarter Pounder w/cheese	1	193.0	94.20	518	31.00	29.00	34.00	251.0	4.60	43.0	257.0	472	1209	2.90	0.350	0.590	15.100	0.250	nd	683
Apple Pie	1	91.0	38.30	300	2.00	19.00	31.00	12.0	0.60	7.0	23.0	39	414	2.70	0.020	0.030	1.300	0.080	nd	69
Cherry Pie	1	92.0	38.60	298	2.00	18.00	33.00	12.0	0.40	8.0	23.0	57	456	1.30	0.020	0.030	0.400	0.020	nd	213
McDonaldland Cookies	1 serving	63.0	1.90	294	4.00	11.00	45.00	10.0	1.40	10.0	51.0	58	330	1.40	0.280	0.230	0.800	0.020	nd	48
Chocolate Shake	1	289.0	207.00	364	11.00	9.00	60.00	338.0	1.00	51.0	292.0	656	329	2.90	0.120	0.890	0.800	0.120	nd	318
Vanilla Shake	1	289.0	216.00	323	10.00	8.00	52.00	346.0	0.20	35.0	266.0	499	250	2.90	0.120	0.660	0.600	0.120	nd	346
Pizza Hut																				
Thin'N Crispy																				
Beef	% of 10" pizza	nd	nd	490	29.00	19.00	51.00	350.0	6.30	nd	nd	nd	nd	1.20	0.300	0.600	7.000	nd	nd	750
Cheese	% of 10" pizza	nd	nd	450	25.00	15.00	54.00	450.0	4.50	nd	nd	nd	nd	1.20	0.300	0.510	5.000	nd	nd	750
Pepperoni	% of 10" pizza	nd	nd	430	23.00	17.00	45.00	300.0	4.50	nd	nd	nd	nd	1.20	0.300	0.510	6.000	nd	nd	1000
Supreme	% of 10" pizza	nd	nd	510	27.00	21.00	51.00	350.0	7.20	nd	nd	nd	nd	2.40	0.380	0.680	7.000	nd	nd	1250
Thick'N Chewy																				
Beef	% of 10" pizza	nd	nd	620	38.00	20.00	73.00	400.0	7.20	nd	nd	nd	nd	1.20	0.680	0.600	8.000	nd	nd	750
Cheese	% of 10" pizza	nd	nd	560	34.00	14.00	71.00	500.0	5.40	nd	nd	nd	nd	1.20	0.680	0.680	7.000	nd	nd	1000
Pepperoni	% of 10" pizza	nd	nd	560	31.00	18.00	68.00	400.0	5.40	nd	nd	nd	nd	3.60	0.680	0.680	8.000	nd	nd	1250
Supreme	% of 10" pizza	nd	nd	640	36.00	22.00	74.00	400.0	7.20	nd	nd	nd	nd	9.00	0.750	0.850	9.000	nd	nd	1000
Taco Bell																				
Bean Burrito	1 serving	166.0	nd	343	11.00	12.00	48.00	98.0	2.80	nd	173.0	235	272	15.20	0.370	0.220	2.200	nd	nr*	1657
Beef Burrito	1 serving	184.0	nd	466	30.00	21.00	37.00	83.0	4.60	nd	288.0	320	327	15.20	0.300	0.390	7.000	nd	nd	1675
Beef Tostado	1 serving	184.0	nd	291	19.00	15.00	21.00	208.0	3.40	nd	265.0	277	138	12.70	0.160	0.270	3.300	nd	nd	3450
Burrito Supreme	1 serving	225.0	nd	457	21.00	22.00	43.00	121.0	3.80	nd	245.0	350	367	16.00	0.330	0.350	4.700	nd	nd	3462
Combination Burrito	1 serving	175.0	nd	404	21.00	16.00	43.00	91.0	3.70	nd	230.0	278	300	15.20	0.340	0.310	4.600	nd	nd	1666
Pintos'N Cheese	1 serving	158.0	nd	168	11.00	5.00	21.00	150.0	2.30	nd	210.0	307	102	9.30	0.260	0.160	0.900	nd	nd	3123
Taco	1 serving	83.0	nd	186	15.00	8.00	14.00	120.0	2.50	nd	175.0	143	79	0.20	0.090	0.160	2.900	nd	nd	120
Tostada	1 serving	138.0	nd	179	9.00	6.00	25.00	191.0	2.30	nd	186.0	172	101	9.70	0.180	0.150	0.800	nd	nd	3152
Fruits																				
Apples																				
Fresh	1	180.0	152.00	96	0.30	1.00	24.00	12.0	0.50	9.0	17.0	182	2	7.00	0.050	0.030	0.200	0.054	4.0	150
Apple Juice	6 oz	186.0	163.00	87	0.20	trace	22.10	11.0	1.10	8.0	17.0	188	2	2.00	0.020	0.040	0.200	0.054	0	–
Apple Sauce (sweetened)	½ cup	128.0	97.00	116	0.20	0.20	30.40	5.0	0.60	5.0	7.0	83	2	2.00	0.020	0.020	0.050	0.039	3.0	50
Apricots																				
Canned in syrup	3 halves	85.0	65.00	73	0.50	0.10	18.70	9.0	0.30	6.0	13.0	199	1	3.00	0.020	0.020	0.300	0.043	—	1480
Dried sulfured	5 halves	18.0	4.00	46	0.90	0.10	11.60	11.0	1.00	11.0	19.0	172	trace	2.00	trace	0.030	1.200	0.030	2.0	3820
Nectar	6 oz	188.0	159.00	107	0.60	0.20	27.40	17.0	0.40	7.0	23.0	284	trace	6.00	0.020	0.020	0.400	0.060	—	1790
Avocado, raw	½	125.0	92.00	188	2.40	18.50	7.10	11.0	0.70	44.0	47.0	680	5	16.00	0.120	0.230	1.800	0.525	37.0	330
Bananas	1 med	175.0	132.00	101	1.30	0.20	26.40	10.0	0.80	37.0	31.0	440	1	12.00	0.060	0.070	0.800	0.380	32.0	230
Blackberries, fresh	1 cup	144.0	122.00	84	1.70	1.30	18.60	46.0	1.30	43.0	27.0	245	1	30.00	0.040	0.060	0.600	0.080	4.0	290

Food	Amount																		
Blueberries, fresh	1 cup	145.0	121.00	90	1.00	0.70	22.20	22.0	1.50	8.0	19.0	117	1	20.00	0.040	0.090	0.700	0.100	4.0	150
Cherries																				
Canned, in water, sweet	½ cup	135.0	117.00	60	1.10	0.30	14.80	19.0	0.40	12.0	16.0	162	1	4.00	0.030	0.030	0.200	0.020	4.0	75
Raw, sweet	10	75.0	60.00	47	0.90	0.20	11.70	15.0	0.30	10.0	13.0	129	1	7.00	0.030	0.040	0.300	—	—	70
Cranberries																				
Raw	1 cup	95.0	83.00	44	0.40	0.70	10.30	13.0	0.50	8.0	10.0	78	2	10.00	0.030	0.020	0.100	—	—	40
Juice	6 oz	190.0	158.00	124	0.20	0.20	31.40	10.0	0.60	—	6.0	19	2	30.00	0.020	0.020	0.100	—	—	trace
Sauce	1 cup	277.0	172.00	404	0.30	0.60	103.90	17.0	0.60	5.0	11.0	83	3	6.00	0.030	0.030	0.100	0.080	—	60
Dates, Pitted	5	40.0	9.00	110	0.90	0.20	29.20	24.0	1.20	23.0	25.0	259	1	0	0.050	0.040	0.900	0.050	5.0	20
Fruit Cocktail, canned in syrup	1 cup	255.0	203.00	194	1.00	0.30	50.20	23.0	1.00	18.0	31.0	411	13	5.00	0.050	0.030	1.000	0.020	—	360
Grapefruit																				
Canned, sweetened	1 cup	254.0	206.00	178	1.50	0.30	45.20	33.0	0.80	28.0	36.0	343	3	76.00	0.080	0.050	0.500	0.030	2.0	30
Fresh	½ of 3½" diam.	184.0	163.00	40	0.50	0.10	10.30	16.0	0.40	9.0	16.0	132	1	37.00	0.040	0.020	0.200	0.018	2.0	80
Juice, canned, unsweetened	6 oz	185.4	166.00	78	1.20	trace	18	12.0	0.60	12.0	24.0	300	trace	66.00	0.060	0.060	0.600	—	—	trace
Grapes																				
Concord	10	40.0	33.00	18	0.30	0.30	4.10	4.0	0.10	5.0	3.0	42	1	1.00	0.010	0.010	0.100	0.040	2.0	30
Grape Juice, canned	6 oz	190.0	158.00	125	0.40	trace	31.50	21.0	0.60	22.0	23.0	220	4	trace	0.080	0.040	0.400	0.040	4.0	—
Lemons																				
Fresh	½	40.0	36.00	7	0.30	0.10	2.20	7.0	0.20	1.0	4.0	38	trace	14.00	0.010	0.010	trace	—	0	10
Juice	1 tbsp	15.2	14.00	4	0.10	trace	1.20	1.0	trace	—	2.0	21	trace	7.00	trace	trace	trace	0.008	4	trace
Lemonade Concentrate, diluted	6 oz	185.0	164.00	81	0.10	trace	21.10	2.0	0.10	1.0	2.0	30	1	13.00	0.010	0.010	0.100	0.017	—	10
Limes	1	80.0	71.00	19	0.50	0.10	6.40	22.0	0.40	—	12.0	69	1	25.00	0.020	0.010	0.100	—	—	10
Limeade Concentrate, diluted	6 oz	185.0	164.00	76	0.10	trace	20.40	2.0	trace	—	2.0	24	trace	4.00	trace	trace	trace	—	—	trace
Mangos	1	300.0	261.00	152	1.60	0.90	38.80	23.0	0.90	54.0	30.0	437	16	81.00	0.120	0.120	2.500	—	—	11,090
Melons																				
Cantelope 5" diam.	½ melon	477.0	435.00	82	1.90	0.30	20.40	38.0	1.10	76.0	44.0	682	33	90.00	0.110	0.080	1.600	0.300	150.0	9240
Honeydew	1/10 melon	226.0	205.00	49	1.20	0.40	11.50	21.0	0.60	31.0	24.0	374	18	34.00	0.060	0.040	0.900	0.060	—	60
Watermelon	1/16 melon	926.0	857.00	111	2.10	0.90	27.30	30.0	2.10	70.0	43.0	426	4	30.00	0.130	0.130	0.900	0.600	16.0	2510
Nectarines	1	150.0	123.00	88	0.80	trace	23.60	6.0	0.70	19.0	33.0	406	8	18.00	—	—	—	—	—	2280
Oranges																				
Fresh	1	180.0	155.00	64	1.30	0.30	16.00	54.0	0.50	14.0	26.0	263	1	66.00	0.130	0.050	0.500	0.082	61.0	260
Juice, concentrate, diluted	6 oz	187.0	163.00	92	1.30	0.20	21.70	19.0	0.20	19.0	32.0	378	2	90.00	0.170	0.030	0.700	0.054	7.0	410
Juice, dehydrated, reconstituted	6 oz	186.0	164.00	86	1.10	0.40	20.10	19.0	0.40	—	30.0	388	1.5	82.00	0.150	0.050	0.800	—	—	375
Juice, fresh	6 oz	186.0	164.00	84	1.30	0.40	19.40	20.2	0.40	20.0	32.0	372	2	93.00	0.170	0.050	0.800	0.070	65.0	375
Papaya, raw	1 cup	140.0	124.00	55	0.80	0.10	14.00	28.0	0.40	—	22.0	328	4	78.00	0.060	0.060	0.400	—	—	2450
Peaches																				
Canned, sweetened	1 cup	256.0	202.00	200	1.00	0.30	51.50	10.0	0.80	16.0	31.0	333	5	8.00	0.030	0.050	1.500	0.050	28.0	1100
Dried, sulphured	5 halves	65.0	16.00	170	2.00	0.50	44.40	31.0	3.90	31.0	76.0	618	11	12.00	0.010	0.120	3.500	0.060	—	2535
Fresh	1½" diam	115.0	102.00	38	0.60	0.10	9.70	9.0	0.50	11.0	19.0	202	1	7.00	0.020	0.050	1.000	0.020	11.0	1330
Pears																				
Canned, sweetened	1 cup	255.0	203.00	194	0.50	0.50	50.00	13.0	0.50	12.0	18.0	214	3	3.00	0.030	0.050	0.300	0.034	15.0	10
Fresh, Bartlett	1½" diam	180.0	150.00	100	1.10	0.70	25.10	13.0	0.50	13.0	18.0	213	3	7.00	0.030	0.070	0.200	0.030	9.0	30
Pineapple																				
Canned, sweetened	1 slice, ¾" thick	255.0	204.00	189	0.80	0.30	49.50	28.0	0.80	19.0	13.0	245	3	18.00	0.200	0.050	0.500	0.175	5.0	130
Fresh	1 cup	84.0	72.00	44	0.30	0.20	11.50	14.0	0.40	10.0	7.0	123	1	14.00	0.080	0.030	0.200	0.072	1.0	60
Juice, canned unsweetened	6 oz	187.0	162.00	96	0.70	0.10	24.00	21.0	0.60	22.0	15.0	254	2	24.00	0.130	0.040	0.500	—	—	20
Plums																				
Canned, sweetened	1 cup	272.0	210.00	214	1.00	0.30	55.80	23.0	2.30	14.0	26.0	367	3	5.00	0.050	0.050	1.000	0.080	—	3130
Raw	1.1" diam	11.0	9.00	7	0.10	trace	1.80	1.8	0.10	1.0	1.7	30	trace	—	0.010	0.010	0.100	0.006	trace	30
Pomegranates	1, 3-3/8" diam	275.0	226.00	97	0.80	0.50	25.30	5.0	0.50	—	12.0	399	5	6.00	0.050	0.050	0.500	—	—	trace
Prunes																				
Dried, uncooked	10	75.0	21.00	164	1.40	0.40	43.50	33.0	2.50	30.0	51.0	448	5	2.0	0.060	0.110	1.000	—	—	1030
Juice	6 oz	192.0	154.00	148	0.80	0.20	36.50	27.0	7.90	19.0	38.0	451	4	4.0	0.020	0.020	0.800	—	—	

Food	Amount	Weight g	Water g	Energy kcal	Protein g	Fat g	Total Carbohydrate g	Calcium mg	Iron mg	Magnesium mg	Phosphorus mg	Potassium mg	Sodium mg	Vitamin C mg	Thiamin mg	Riboflavin mg	Niacin mg	Vitamin B6 mg	Folacin µg	Total Vitamin A I.U.
Raisins, seedless	⅔ oz	14.0	2.00	40	0.40	trace	10.80	9.0	0.50	4.0	14.0	107	4	trace	0.020	0.010	0.100	0.034	1.5	trace
Raspberries, black, fresh	1 cup	134.0	108.00	98	2.00	1.90	21.00	40.0	1.20	40.0	29.0	267	1	24.00	0.040	0.120	1.200	—	—	trace
Strawberries																				
Fresh	1 cup whole berries	149.0	134.00	55	1.00	0.70	12.50	31.0	1.50	18.0	31.0	244	1	88.00	0.040	0.100	0.900	0.090	22.0	90
Frozen, sweetened	1 cup sliced	255.0	182.00	278	1.30	0.50	70.90	36.0	1.80	23.0	43.0	286	3	135.00	0.050	0.150	1.300	0.105	22.0	80
Tangerines	1 med	116.0	100.90	39	0.70	0.20	10.00	34.0	0.30	—	15.0	108	2	27.00	0.050	0.020	0.100	—	—	360
Herbs and Spices																				
Allspice, ground	1 tsp	1.9	0.16	5	0.12	0.17	1.37	13.0	0.13	3.0	2.0	20	1	0.75	0.002	0.001	0.054	—	—	10
Anise Seed	1 tsp	2.1	0.20	7	0.37	0.33	1.05	14.0	0.78	4.0	9.0	30	trace	—	—	—	—	—	—	—
Basil, ground	1 tsp	1.4	0.09	4	0.20	0.06	0.85	30.0	0.59	6.0	7.0	48	trace	0.86	0.002	0.004	0.097	—	—	131
Bay Leaf	1 tsp	0.6	0.03	2	0.05	0.05	0.45	5.0	0.26	1.0	1.0	3	trace	0.28	trace	0.003	0.012	—	—	37
Caraway Seed	1 tsp	2.1	0.21	7	0.42	0.31	1.05	14.0	0.34	5.0	12.0	28	trace	0.34	0.008	0.008	0.076	—	—	8
Celery Seed	1 tsp	2.0	0.12	8	0.36	0.50	0.83	35.0	0.90	9.0	11.0	28	3	—	—	—	—	—	—	1
Chili Powder	1 tsp	2.6	0.20	8	0.32	0.44	1.42	7.0	0.37	4.0	8.0	50	26	1.67	0.009	0.021	0.205	—	—	908
Cinnamon, ground	1 tsp	2.3	0.22	6	0.09	0.07	1.84	28.0	0.88	1.0	1.0	11	1	0.65	0.002	0.003	0.030	—	—	6
Cloves, ground	1 tsp	2.1	0.14	7	0.13	0.42	1.29	14.0	0.18	6.0	2.0	23	5	1.70	0.002	0.006	0.031	—	—	11
Coriander Seed	1 tsp	1.8	0.16	5	0.22	0.32	0.99	13.0	0.29	6.0	7.0	23	1	—	0.004	0.005	0.038	—	—	27
Cumin Seed	1 tsp	2.1	0.17	8	0.37	0.47	0.93	20.0	1.39	8.0	10.0	38	4	0.16	0.013	0.007	0.096	—	—	20
Curry Powder	1 tsp	2.0	0.19	6	0.25	0.28	1.16	10.0	0.59	5.0	7.0	31	trace	0.23	0.005	0.006	0.069	—	—	1
Dill Seed	1 tsp	2.1	0.16	6	0.34	0.31	1.16	32.0	0.34	5.0	6.0	25	trace	—	0.009	0.006	0.059	—	—	1
Dill Weed, dried	1 tsp	1.0	0.07	3	0.20	trace	0.56	18.0	0.49	5.0	5.0	33	2	—	0.004	0.003	0.029	0.0150	—	3
Fennel Seed	1 tsp	2.0	0.18	7	0.32	0.30	1.05	24.0	0.37	8.0	10.0	34	2	—	0.008	0.007	0.121	—	—	—
Garlic Powder	1 tsp	2.8	0.18	9	0.47	0.02	2.04	2.0	0.08	2.0	12.0	31	1	—	0.013	0.004	0.019	—	—	3
Ginger, ground	1 tsp	1.8	0.17	6	0.16	0.11	1.27	2.0	0.21	3.0	3.0	24	1	—	0.001	0.003	0.093	—	—	3
Mace, ground	1 tsp	1.7	0.14	8	0.11	0.55	0.86	4.0	0.24	3.0	2.0	8	1	—	0.005	0.008	0.023	—	—	14
Marjoram, dried	1 tsp	0.6	0.05	2	0.08	0.04	0.36	12.0	0.50	2.0	2.0	9	trace	0.31	0.002	0.001	0.025	—	—	48
Nutmeg, ground	1 tsp	2.2	0.14	12	0.13	0.80	1.08	4.0	0.07	3.0	5.0	8	trace	—	0.008	0.001	0.029	—	—	2
Onion Powder	1 tsp	2.1	0.11	7	0.21	0.02	1.69	8.0	0.05	3.0	7.0	20	1	0.31	0.009	0.001	0.014	—	—	—
Oregano, ground	1 tsp	1.5	0.11	5	0.17	0.15	0.97	24.0	0.66	4.0	3.0	25	trace	1.49	0.005	—	0.093	—	—	104
Paprika	1 tsp	2.1	0.20	6	0.31	0.27	1.17	4.0	0.50	4.0	7.0	49	1	1.49	0.014	0.037	0.322	—	—	1273
Parsley, dried	1 tsp	0.3	0.03	1	0.07	0.01	0.15	4.0	0.29	1.0	1.0	11	1	0.37	0.001	0.004	0.024	0.003	—	70
Pepper																				
Black	1 tsp	2.1	0.22	5	0.23	0.07	1.36	9.0	0.61	4.0	4.0	26	1	—	0.002	0.005	0.024	—	—	4
Red or Cayenne	1 tsp	1.8	0.14	6	0.22	0.31	1.02	3.0	0.14	3.0	5.0	36	trace	1.38	0.006	0.017	0.157	—	—	749
White	1 tsp	2.4	0.27	7	0.25	0.05	1.65	6.0	0.34	2.0	4.0	2	trace	—	0.001	0.003	0.005	—	—	—
Poppy Seed	1 tsp	2.8	0.19	15	0.50	1.25	0.66	41.0	0.26	9.0	24.0	20	1	—	0.024	0.005	0.027	0.012	—	—
Poultry Seasoning	1 tsp	1.5	0.14	5	0.14	0.11	0.98	15.0	0.53	3.0	3.0	10	trace	0.18	0.004	0.003	0.045	—	—	39
Rosemary, dried	1 tsp	1.2	0.11	4	0.06	0.18	0.77	15.0	0.35	3.0	1.0	11	1	0.74	0.006	—	0.012	—	—	38
Saffron	1 tsp	0.7	0.08	2	0.08	0.04	0.46	1.0	0.08	—	2.0	12	1	—	—	—	—	—	—	—
Sage, ground	1 tsp	0.7	0.06	2	0.07	0.09	0.43	12.0	0.20	3.0	1.0	7	trace	0.23	0.005	0.002	0.040	—	—	41
Savory, ground	1 tsp	1.4	0.13	4	0.09	0.08	0.96	30.0	0.53	5.0	2.0	15	trace	—	0.005	—	0.057	—	—	72
Sesame Seed	1 tsp	2.7	0.13	16	0.71	1.48	0.25	4.0	0.21	9.0	21.0	11	1	—	0.019	0.002	0.126	0.004	—	2

Tarragon, ground	1 tsp	1.6	0.12	5	0.36	0.12	0.80	18.0	0.52	6.0	5.0	48	1	—	0.004	0.021	0.143	—	—	67
Thyme, ground	1 tsp	1.4	0.11	4	0.13	0.10	0.89	26.0	1.73	3.0	3.0	11	1	—	0.007	0.006	0.069	—	—	53
Turmeric, ground	1 tsp	2.2	0.25	8	0.17	0.22	1.43	4.0	0.91	4.0	6.0	56	1	0.57	0.003	0.005	0.113	—	—	—
Meat, Poultry and Seafood																				
Bacon																				
Cooked	2 med slices	15.0	1.00	86	3.80	7.80	0.50	2.0	0.50	4.0	34.0	35	153	—	0.080	0.05	0.8	.016	0	0
Canadian, cooked	1 slice 3-3/8'' diam	21.0	10.00	58	5.70	3.70	0.10	3.0	0.90	5.0	46.0	91	537	—	0.190	0.04	1.1	—	—	0
Bass																				
Striped, fried	1 fillet, ½ lb	200.0	122.00	392	43.00	17.00	13.40	—	—	—	—	—	—	—	—	—	—	—	—	—
Beef																				
Ground, 21% fat	1 Patty 3'' diam, ¼ lb	87.0	47.00	235	19.80	16.60	0	9.0	2.60	18.0	159.0	221	49	—	0.070	0.17	4.4	0.390	4.0	30
Round Steak, 19% fat	3 oz	85.0	46.00	222	24.30	13.10	0	10.0	3.00	25.0	213.0	272	60	—	0.070	0.19	4.8	0.300	3.0	20
Corn Beef, Hash, w/potato	1 cup	220.0	148.00	398	19.40	24.90	23.50	29.0	4.40	40.0	147.0	440	1188	—	0.020	0.20	4.6	0.160	—	—
Roast, chuck	3 oz	85.0	34.20	363	19.00	31.20	0	9.0	2.50	13.0	94.0	152	33	—	0.040	0.140	3.000	—	3.0	60
Roast, rib	3 oz	85.0	34.00	374	16.90	33.50	0	8.0	2.20	17.0	158.0	189	41	—	0.050	0.130	3.100	0.300	3.0	70
Steak, flank	¼ lb	113.0	69.70	222	34.60	8.30	0	16.0	4.30	—	170.0	276	60	—	0.060	0.260	5.200	—	—	12
Steak, sirloin	3 oz	85.0	49.90	176	27.40	6.50	0	11.0	3.30	18.0	222.0	307	67	—	0.070	0.210	5.400	—	3.0	10
Blue Fish, cooked	1 fillet, 1/3 lb	155.0	105.00	246	40.60	8.10	0	45.0	1.10	—	445.0	—	161	—	0.170	0.16	2.9	—	—	80
Chicken without skin																				
Light meat, Roasted	2 pieces 2½''x1-7/8''x ¼''	50.0	32.00	83	15.80	1.70	0	6.0	0.70	10.0	133.0	206	32	—	0.020	0.05	5.8	0.350	2.0	30
Dark meat, Roasted	4 pieces 1-7/8'' x 1'' x ¼''	40.0	26.00	70	11.20	2.50	0	5.0	0.70	6.0	92.0	128	34	—	0.030	0.09	2.2	0.250	2.0	60
Pot Pie	1/3 of a 9'' pie	232.0	131.00	545	23.40	31.30	42.50	70.0	3.00	—	232.0	343	594	5	0.260	0.26	4.2	—	—	3090
Chili Con Carne w/beans, canned	1 cup	255.0	185.00	339	19.10	15.60	31.10	82.0	4.30	66.0	321.0	594	1354	—	0.080	0.18	3.3	0.260	23.0	150
Clams																				
Canned, drained	1 cup minced	160.0	123.00	157	25.30	4.00	3.00	—	—	180.0	—	—	—	—	—	—	—	0.130	5.0	—
Raw	4–5	70.0	56.00	56	7.80	0.60	4.10	48.0	5.30	—	106.0	218	144	—	—	—	—	—	—	—
Cod, broiled	1 fillet, 1/6 lb	65.0	42.00	111	18.50	3.40	0	20.0	0.7	18.0	178.0	265	72	—	0.050	0.07	2.0	0.180	6.0	120
Crab																				
Canned, king	1 cup, drained	135.0	104.00	136	23.50	3.40	1.50	61.0	1.10	46.0	246.0	149	1350	—	0.110	0.11	2.6	0.400	trace	—
Cooked, flaked	1 cup	125.0	98.00	116	21.60	2.40	0.60	54.0	1.00	42.0	219.0	—	—	2	0.200	0.10	3.5	—	—	2710
Fish Cakes, fried	5 small 1¼'' diam	60.0	40.00	103	8.80	4.80	5.60	—	—	—	—	—	—	—	—	—	—	—	—	—
Fish Sticks																				
Breaded, cooked	4 sticks	112.0	74.00	200	18.80	10.00	7.20	12.0	0.40	20.0	188.0	—	—	—	0.040	0.08	2.0	0.060	18.0	0
Flounder, baked	1 fillet, 1/6 lb	57.0	33.00	115	17.00	4.70	0	13.0	0.80	17.0	196.0	335	135	1.00	0.040	0.05	1.4	0.097	—	—
Goose, roasted	3 oz	85.0	47.00	198	28.80	8.30	0	12.0	1.40	—	235.0	514	105	—	0.090	0.14	7.9	—	—	—
Haddock, fried	1 fillet, 1/3 lb	110.0	73.00	182	21.60	7.00	6.40	44.0	1.30	30.0	272.0	383	195	2.00	0.040	0.08	3.5	0.157	17.0	—
Halibut, broiled	1 fillet, 1/3 lb	125.0	83.00	214	31.50	8.80	0	20.0	1.00	29.0	310.0	656	168	—	0.060	0.090	10.400	0.425	20.0	850
Herring,																				
Pickled	1 piece 1¾''x7/8''x½''	15.0	8.9	33	3.10	2.30	0	—	—	—	—	—	—	—	—	—	—	—	—	—
Smoked	1 small fillet	20.0	12.00	42	4.40	2.60	0	13.0	0.30	—	51.0	—	—	—	—	0.060	0.700	0.040	—	10
Kidney																				
Beef, cooked	1 cup, slices ¼'' thick	140.0	74.00	353	46.20	16.80	1.10	25.0	18.30	25.0	342.0	454	354	trace	0.710	6.750	15.000	0.560	84.0	1610
Lamb, cooked																				
Chop, loin	2.3 oz	65.0	40.00	122	18.30	4.90	0	8.0	1.30	13.0	142.0	205	45	—	0.100	0.180	4.000	0.2	1.0	—
Chop, rib	2 oz	57.0	34.00	120	15.50	6.00	0	6.0	1.10	11.0	121.0	174	38	—	0.090	0.150	3.400	—	—	—
Leg	3 oz	85.0	53.00	158	24.40	6.00	0	11.0	1.90	19.0	202.0	273	60	—	0.140	0.260	5.300	0.272	3.0	—
Liver, cooked																				
Beef	3 oz	85.0	48.00	195	22.40	9.00	4.50	9.0	7.50	19.0	405.0	323	156	23	0.220	3.560	14.000	0.569	250.0	45,390
Calf	3 oz	85.0	44.00	222	25.10	11.20	3.40	11.0	12.10	6.0	456.0	385	100	31	0.200	3.540	14.000	0.570	—	27,800

Food	Amount	Weight g	Water g	Energy kcal	Protein g	Fat g	Total Carbo-hydrate g	Minerals						Vitamins						
								Cal-cium mg	Iron mg	Mag-nesium mg	Phos-phorus mg	Potas-sium mg	Sod-ium mg	Vitamin C mg	Thia-min mg	Ribo-flavin mg	Niacin mg	Vitamin B_6 mg	Folacin µg	Total Vitamin A I.U.
Liver, cooked																				
Chicken	1 liver	25.0	16.00	41	6.60	1.10	0.80	3.0	2.10	—	40.0	38	15	4	0.040	0.670	2.900	—	—	3080
Pork	3 oz	85.0	46.00	205	25.40	9.80	2.10	13.0	24.70	20.0	458.0	336	94	19	0.290	3.710	19.000	0.552	188.0	12,670
Lobster																				
Cooked	1 cup	145.0	111.00	138	27.10	2.20	0.40	94.0	1.20	32.0	278.0	261	305	—	0.150	0.100	—	—	—	—
Newburg	1 cup	250.0	160.00	485	46.30	26.50	12.80	218.0	2.30	—	480.0	428	573	—	0.180	0.280	—	—	—	—
Ocean Perch, fried	3 oz	84.0	50.00	192	16.20	11.40	5.70	27.0	1.20	—	192.0	243	129	—	0.090	0.090	1.500	—	—	—
Oysters																				
Eastern, raw	2–3	28.0	24.00	19	2.40	0.50	1.00	27.0	1.60	9.0	41.0	34	21	—	0.040	0.050	0.700	.014	3.0	90
Pork, cooked																				
Cured Baked Ham	3 oz	85.0	53.00	159	21.50	7.50	0	9.0	2.70	17.0	170.0	241	770	—	0.490	0.200	3.800	0.340	9.0	0
Fresh Baked Ham	3 oz	85.0	51.00	184	25.20	8.50	0	11.0	3.20	25.0	262.0	282	62	—	0.540	0.250	4.800	0.380	2.0	0
Loin	3 oz	85.0	47.00	216	25.00	12.10	0	11.0	3.20	—	264.0	280	61	—	0.92	0.260	5.500	—	—	0
Chops	1 chop[a]	56.0	29.00	151	17.10	8.60	0	7.0	2.20	14.0	181.0	192	42	—	0.630	0.180	3.800	—	—	0
Spareribs, Cooked	yield from ½ lb	90.0	35.70	396	18.70	35.00	0	8.0	2.40	—	109.0	150	33	—	0.390	0.190	3.100	—	—	0
Salmon																				
Canned Sockeye	½ can	110.0	74.00	188	22.40	10.20	0	285.0	1.30	32.0	378.0	378	574	—	0.040	0.180	8.100	0.300	10.0	255
Fresh, broiled	3 oz	85.0	54.00	156	23.10	6.30	0	—	0.90	35.0	351.0	378	99	—	0.150	0.060	8.400	0.255	6.0	150
Smoked	1 oz	28.0	16.00	50	6.10	2.60	0	4.0	—	9.0	69.0	—	—	—	—	—	—	0.198	2.0	—
Sardines Canned in oil	1 can	92.0	57.00	187	22.10	10.20	—	402.0	2.70	36.0	459.0	543	757	—	0.030	0.180	5.000	0.164	29.0	200
Sausage, Cold Cuts, & Luncheon Meats																				
Bologna	1 slice 4½" diam	28.0	16.00	86	3.40	7.80	0.30	2.0	0.50	—	36.0	65	369	—	0.050	0.060	0.700	0.030	1.0	—
Brown & Serve Sausage	1 patty 2-3/8"x1-7/8"x½"	23.0	9.00	97	3.80	8.70	0.60	—	—	—	—	—	—	—	—	—	—	—	—	—
	1 link 3-7/8"x5/8"	17.0	7.00	72	2.80	6.40	0.50	—	—	—	—	—	—	—	—	—	—	—	—	—
Deviled Ham, cooked	1 tbsp	13.0	6.00	46	1.80	4.20	0	1.0	0.30	—	12.0	—	—	—	0.020	0.010	0.200	—	—	0
Frankfurters	1 5"x¾" diam	45.0	25.00	139	5.60	12.40	0.80	3.0	0.90	4.0	60.0	99	495	—	0.070	0.090	1.200	0.049	2.0	—
Liverwurst	1 slice	28.0	15.00	87	4.60	7.30	0.50	3.0	1.50	7.0	68.0	—	—	—	0.060	0.370	1.600	0.279	2.0	1800
Salami	1 slice 3-1/8"x1/16"	10.0	3.00	45	2.40	3.80	0.10	1.0	0.40	—	28.0	—	—	—	0.040	0.030	0.500	0.013	0.3	—
Scrapple	1 slice 2¾"x2-1/8"x¼"	25.0	15.00	54	2.20	3.40	3.70	1.0	0.30	—	16.0	—	—	—	0.050	0.030	0.500	—	—	—
Scallops, steamed	¼ lb	114.0	83.00	127	26.30	1.60	—	130.0	3.40	—	383.0	540	300	—	—	—	—	—	22.0	—
Shrimp																				
Fried	¼ lb	113.0	64.00	255	23.00	12.20	11.40	82.0	2.30	69.0	216.0	260	211	—	0.050	0.090	3.000	0.068	2.0	—
Boiled	3 oz	85.0	66.00	80	17.80	0.70	0.40	66.0	1.40	36.0	177.0	173	107	9	0.020	0.030	2.800	0.042	2.0	34
Swordfish Broiled	1 piece 1/3 lb	145.0	93.70	237	38.20	8.20	0	37.0	1.80	—	375.0	—	—	—	0.050	0.070	14.900	—	—	2790
Tongue, beef	1 slice 3"x2"x1/8"	20.0	12.00	49	4.30	3.30	0.10	1.0	0.40	3.0	23.0	33	12	—	0.010	0.060	0.700	0.033	—	—
Tuna																				
Canned in oil	1 cup drained	160.0	97.00	315	46.10	13.10	0	13.0	3.00	43.0	374.0	—	—	—	0.080	0.190	19.000	0.688	3.0	130
Canned in water	3½ oz	99.0	69.00	126	27.70	0.80	0	16.0	1.60	25.0	188.0	276	41	—	—	0.090	12.200	0.400	8.0	—
Turkey, cooked	3 oz	85.0	53.00	150	28.00	3.30	0	—	1.00	20.0	—	349	70	—	0.040	0.120	9.400	0.300	3.0	—

Food	Measure																			
Light meat w/o skin	2 slices 4"x2"x¼"	85.0	56.00	173	25.50	7.10	0	—	2.00	20.0	—	—	84	—	0.030	0.200	3.600	0.300	7.0	—
Dark meat w/o skin	4 pieces 2½"x1-5/8"x¼"=3 oz	145.0	88.00	338	29.90	22.30	2.30	—	—	—	—	338	—	—	—	3.940	—	—	—	—
Turkey Giblets, Simmered	1 cup	—	—	—	—	—	—	—	—	—	—	—	—	—	—	—	—	—	—	—
Turkey Pot Pie	1/3 of 9" pie	232.0	130.00	550	24.10	31.30	42.90	63.0	3.20	—	234.0	459	633	5	0.260	0.300	5.800	0.300	—	3090
Veal, cooked																				
Cutlet	3 oz	85.0	51.00	184	23.00	9.40	0	9.0	2.70	20.0	196.0	258	56	—	0.060	0.210	4.600	0.300	15.0	—
Loin	3 oz	85.0	50.00	199	22.40	11.40	0	9.0	2.70	—	191.0	251	55	—	0.060	0.210	4.600	—	—	—
Stew meat	3 oz	85.0	50.00	200	23.70	10.90	0	10.0	3.00	16.0	128.0	190	41	—	0.080	0.250	5.400	—	—	—
Vegetables																				
Alfalfa Sprouts, raw	1 cup packed	100.0	90.00	40	5.00	0.6	5.00	30.0	1.40	—	—	—	—	15.00	0.1	0.2	1.5	—	—	—
Artichokes, cooked	1	300.0	260.00	10-53	3.40	0.20	11.90	61.0	1.30	12.0	83.0	361	36	10.00	0.080	0.050	0.800	0.300	—	180
Asparagus, fresh, cooked	4 spears	60.0	56.00	12	1.30	0.10	2.20	13.0	0.40	—	30.0	110	1	16.00	0.100	0.110	0.800	0.125	37.0	540
Bamboo Shoots	½ cup	76.0	69.00	20	2.00	0.20	3.90	13.0	0.40	—	45.0	403	—	3.00	0.110	0.050	0.400	—	—	15
Beans																				
Navy, cooked	½ cup	95.0	131.00	112	7.40	0.60	20.20	48.0	2.60	37.0	141.0	395	7	0	0.140	0.060	0.600	0.140	8.0	0
w/Pork & Tomato Sauce	1 cup	255.0	180.00	311	15.60	6.60	48.50	138.0	4.60	70.0	235.0	536	1181	5.00	0.200	0.080	1.500	0.950	24.0	330
Red Kidney, cooked	1 cup	185.0	128.00	218	14.40	0.90	39.60	70.0	4.40	70.0	259.0	629	6	—	0.200	0.110	1.300	0.800	20.0	10
Lima, cooked	½ cup	85.0	60.00	95	6.40	0.50	16.80	40.0	2.20	55.0	103.0	358	1	15.00	0.160	0.080	1.100	0.100	16.0	240
Mung, Sprouts	½ cup	52.0	46.00	19	2.00	0.10	3.50	32.0	0.70	—	34.0	117	3	10.00	0.070	0.070	0.400	—	—	10
Green, fresh, cooked	½ cup	62.0	58.00	16	1.00	0.20	3.40	32.0	0.40	14.0	23.0	95	3	8.00	0.050	0.050	0.300	0.039	3.0	340
Yellow, fresh, cooked	½ cup	62.0	58.00	14	0.90	0.20	2.90	32.0	0.40	—	23.0	95	4	8.00	0.050	0.050	0.300	—	—	145
Beets																				
Canned	½ cup sliced	85.0	76.00	32	0.90	0.10	7.50	16.0	0.60	12.0	16.0	142	200	3.00	0.010	0.030	0.100	0.040	16.0	15
Greens, cooked	½ cup	72.0	68.00	41	3.80	0.50	7.50	225.0	4.30	76.0	56.0	753	172	34.00	0.160	0.340	0.700	0.080	—	11,565
Broccoli, frozen, cooked	3 stalks	90.0	82.00	24	2.70	0.30	4.20	36.0	0.60	31.0	51.0	198	12	66.00	0.060	0.090	0.600	0.150	19.0	1710
Brussels Sprouts, cooked	1 cup	155.0	138.00	51	5.00	0.30	10.10	33.0	1.20	25.0	95.0	457	22	126.00	0.120	0.160	0.900	0.680	25.0	880
Cabbage																				
Chinese	1 cup	75.0	71.00	11	0.90	0.10	2.30	32.0	0.50	10.0	30.0	190	17	19.00	0.040	0.030	0.500	—	—	110
Cooked, shredded	1 cup	145.0	136.00	29	1.60	0.30	6.20	64.0	0.40	16.0	29.0	236	20	48.00	0.060	0.060	0.400	0.190	16.0	190
Raw, shredded	1 cup	90.0	83.00	22	1.20	0.20	4.90	44.0	0.40	12.0	26.0	210	18	42.00	0.050	0.050	0.300	0.140	48.0	120
Red, raw, shredded	1 cup	90.0	81.00	28	1.80	0.20	6.20	38.0	0.70	—	32.0	241	23	55.00	0.080	0.050	0.400	—	—	40
Spoon, pakchoy, cooked	1 cup	170.0	161.00	24	2.40	0.30	4.10	252.0	1.00	—	56.0	364	31	26.00	0.070	0.140	1.200	—	—	5270
Carrots																				
Cooked	½ cup diced	72.0	66.00	23	0.70	0.20	5.20	24.0	0.50	5.0	23.0	161	24	5.00	0.040	0.040	0.400	0.023	2.0	7615
Raw	1, 7½" long	81.0	71.00	30	0.80	0.10	7.00	27.0	0.50	13.0	26.0	246	34	6.00	0.040	0.040	0.400	0.112	12.0	7930
Cauliflower																				
Cooked	1 cup	125.0	116.00	28	2.90	0.30	5.10	26.0	0.90	16.0	53.0	258	11	69.00	0.110	0.100	0.800	0.200	4.0	80
Raw	1 cup	100.0	91.00	27	2.70	0.20	5.20	25.0	1.10	24.0	56.0	295	13	78.00	0.110	0.100	0.700	0.125	37.0	60
Celery, raw	1 stalk	40.0	38.00	7	0.40	trace	1.60	16.0	0.10	9.0	11.0	136	50	4.00	0.010	0.010	0.100	0.025	2.0	110
Chard, Swiss	1 cup	175.0	164.00	32	3.20	0.40	5.80	128.0	3.20	114.0	42.0	562	151	28.00	0.070	0.190	0.700	—	—	9450
Chick Peas (Garbanzos)	1 cup cooked	200.0	21.00	720	41.00	9.60	122.00	300.0	13.8	—	662.0	1594	52	—	0.620	0.300	4.000	0.250	11.0	100
Chicory	1 cup	90.0	86.00	14	0.90	0.10	2.90	16.0	0.50	12.0	19.0	164	6	—	—	—	—	—	—	trace
Collards, cooked	1 cup	190.0	170.00	63	6.80	1.30	9.70	357.0	1.50	72.0	99.0	498	—	144.00	0.210	0.380	2.300	0.340	40.0	14,820
Corn																				
Canned, cream style	1 cup	256.0	195.00	210	5.40	1.50	51.20	8.0	1.50	50.0	143.0	248	604	13.00	0.080	0.130	2.600	0.504	6.0	840
Canned, kernel	1 cup	210.0	158.00	174	5.30	1.10	43.10	6.0	1.10	43.0	153.0	204	496	11.00	0.060	0.130	2.300	0.425	5.0	740
Cob	1 ear	140.0	104.00	70	2.50	0.80	16.20	2.0	0.50	67.0	69.0	151	trace	7.00	0.090	0.080	1.100	—	—	310
Frozen, cooked	1 cup	165.0	127.00	130	5.00	0.80	31.00	5.0	1.30	36.0	120.0	304	2	8.00	0.150	0.100	2.500	—	—	580
Cow Peas, immature (Black-Eyed), cooked	½ cup	85.0	61.00	92	6.90	0.70	15.40	20.0	1.80	16.0	124.0	322	1	14.00	0.250	0.090	1.200	0.042	22.0	297

a Three chops to the pound.

Food	Amount	Weight g	Water g	Energy kcal	Protein g	Fat g	Total Carbohydrate g	Minerals						Vitamins						
								Calcium mg	Iron mg	Magnesium mg	Phosphorus mg	Potassium mg	Sodium mg	Vitamin C mg	Thiamin mg	Riboflavin mg	Niacin mg	Vitamin B6 mg	Folacin μg	Total Vitamin A I.U.
Cucumbers																				
Pared, 6-3/8" long	½	79.0	76.00	11	0.50	0.10	2.60	14.0	0.30	9.0	14.0	127	5	9.00	0.030	0.030	0.200	0.030	12.0	trace
Egg Plant, cooked, Drained	1 cup, diced	200.0	189.00	38	2.00	0.40	8.20	22.0	1.20	32.0	42.0	300	2	6.00	0.100	0.080	1.000	0.160	4.0	20
Kale, fresh, cooked	1 cup	110.0	96.00	43	5.00	0.80	6.70	206.0	1.80	41.0	64.0	243	47	102.00	0.110	0.200	1.800	0.400	50.0	9130
Lentils, cooked	½ cup	100.0	72.00	106	7.80	trace	19.30	25.0	2.10	20.0	119.0	498	—	0	0.140	0.120	1.200	—	5.0	40
Lettuce																				
Boston, shredded	1 cup	55.0	52.00	8	0.70	0.10	1.40	19.0	1.10	10.0	14.0	145	5	4.00	0.030	0.030	0.200	0.030	30.0	530
Iceberg, shredded	1 cup	55.0	52.00	7	0.50	0.10	1.60	11.0	0.30	6.0	12.0	96	5	3.00	0.030	0.030	0.200	0.033	111.0	180
Mushrooms																				
Fresh	1 cup	70.0	63.00	20	1.90	0.20	3.10	4.0	0.60	9.0	81.0	290	11	2.00	0.070	0.320	2.900	0.080	14.0	trace
Canned, solids & liquids	½ cup	100.0	93.00	17	1.90	0.10	2.40	6.0	0.50	8.0	68.0	197	400	2.00	0.020	0.250	2.000	0.060	8.0	0
Onions																				
Green	2 medium	30.0	26.00	14	0.30	0.10	3.20	12.0	0.20	3.0	12.0	69	2	8.00	0.020	0.010	0.100	—	12.0	trace
White, sliced	½ cup	58.0	52.00	22	0.90	0.10	5.00	16.0	0.30	7.0	21.0	90	6	6.00	0.020	0.030	0.100	0.071	6.0	25
Parsley, raw	10 sprigs 2½" long	10.0	8.5	4	0.4	0.1	0.9	20.0	0.60	4.0	6.0	73	5	17.00	0.010	0.030	0.100	0.020	4.0	850
Parsnips																				
Diced, cooked	1 cup	155.0	127.00	102	2.30	0.80	23.10	70.0	0.90	45.0	96.0	587	12	16.00	0.110	0.120	0.200	0.062	—	50
Peas, green, canned, cooked	½ cup	125.0	103.00	82	4.40	0.40	15.60	25.0	2.10	16.0	82.0	120	294	11.00	0.110	0.060	1.100	—	19.0	560
Fresh, cooked	½ cup	80.0	65.00	57	4.30	0.30	9.70	19.0	1.50	—	79.0	157	1	16.00	0.230	0.090	1.800	0.104	12.0	430
Frozen, cooked	½ cup	80.0	66.00	54	4.10	0.20	9.40	15.0	1.50	17.0	69.0	108	92	11.00	0.220	0.070	1.400	—	—	480
Peppers																				
Sweet, green	½ cup	40.0	37.00	9	0.50	0.10	1.90	4.0	0.30	7.0	9.0	85	5	51.00	0.030	0.030	0.400	0.10	2.0	170
Sweet, red	½ cup	40.0	36.00	13	0.60	0.10	2.90	5.0	0.20	—	12.0	—	—	82.00	0.030	0.030	0.200	—	10.0	1780
Potatoes																				
Baked	1 large	202.0	152.00	145	4.00	0.20	32.80	14.0	1.10	33.0	101.0	782	6	31.00	0.150	0.070	2.700	0.300	18.0	trace
French Fries	10 strips	50.0	22.00	137	2.20	6.60	18.00	8.0	0.70	9.0	56.0	427	3	11.00	0.070	0.040	1.600	0.090	5.0	trace
Mashed w/milk & fat	1 cup	210.0	168.00	197	4.40	9.00	25.80	50.0	0.80	28.0	101.0	525	695	19.00	0.170	0.110	2.100	0.180	24.0	360
Scalloped w/cheese	1 cup	245.0	174.00	355	13.00	19.40	33.30	311.0	1.20	—	299.0	750	1095	25.00	0.150	0.290	2.200	—	—	780
Sweet Potato, baked	1	146.0	93.00	161	2.40	0.60	37.00	46.0	1.00	17.0	66.0	342	14	25.00	0.100	0.080	0.800	0.238	27.0	9230
Canned	1 cup	200.0	144.00	216	4.00	0.40	49.80	50.0	1.60	36.0	82.0	400	96	28.00	0.100	0.080	1.200	0.140	38.0	15,600
Salad	1 cup	250.0	190.00	248	6.80	7.00	40.80	80.0	1.50	—	160.0	798	1320	28.00	0.200	0.180	2.800	0.015	5.0	350
Radishes	5	25.0	23.00	4	0.20	trace	0.80	7.0	0.20	1.5	7.0	72	4	6.00	0.010	0.010	0.100	0.400	—	trace
Sauerkraut, canned	1 cup	235.0	218.00	42	2.40	0.50	9.40	85.0	1.20	—	42.0	329	1755	33.00	0.070	0.090	0.500	—	—	120
Soy Beans																				
Cooked	1 cup	180.0	128.00	234	19.80	10.30	19.40	131.0	4.90	377.0	322.0	972	4	0.00	0.380	0.160	1.100	0.078	73.0	50
Curd (Tofu)	1 piece 2½"x2¾"x1"	120.0	102.00	86	9.40	5.00	2.90	154.0	2.30	133.0	151.0	50	8	0.00	0.070	0.040	0.100	—	—	0
Spinach																				
Raw	1 cup	55.0	50.00	14	1.80	0.20	2.40	51.0	1.70	30.0	28.0	259	39	28.00	0.060	0.110	0.3	0.152	40.0	4460
Fresh, cooked	1 cup	180.0	165.00	41	5.40	0.50	6.50	167.0	4.00	120.0	68.0	583	90	50.00	0.130	0.250	0.9	0.400	120.0	14,580
Frozen, cooked	1 cup	190.0	174.00	46	5.50	0.60	7.40	200.0	4.80	120.0	84.0	688	93	53.00	0.150	0.270	1.0	0.350	120.0	15,390
Squash																				
Summer, cooked[a]	1 cup, cubed	210.0	200.00	29	1.90	0.20	6.50	53.0	0.80	31.0	53.0	296	2	21.00	0.110	0.170	1.7	0.126	4.0	820
Winter, cooked[b]	1 cup, baked	205.0	166.00	129	3.70	0.80	31.60	57.0	1.60	34.0	98.0	945	2	27.00	0.100	0.270	1.4	0.200	—	8610
Winter, frozen	1 cup, cooked	240.0	213.00	91	2.90	0.70	22.10	60.0	2.40	28.0	77.0	497	2	19.00	0.070	0.170	1.2	—	—	9360
Succotash, frozen	1 cup, cooked	170.0	126.00	158	7.10	0.70	34.90	22.0	1.70	—	145.0	418	65	10.00	0.150	0.090	2.2	—	—	510
Tomatoes																				
Canned	1 cup	241.0	226.00	51	2.40	0.50	10.40	14.0	1.20	26.0	46.0	523	313	41.00	0.120	0.070	1.7	0.216	62.0	2170

Food	Measure																		
Fresh	1, 2-3/5" diam	135.0	126.00	27	1.40	0.20	5.80	16.0	0.60	17.0	33.0	300	4	28.00	0.070	0.050	0.9	0.126	23.0	1110
Juice	6 fl oz	182.0	170.00	35	1.60	0.20	7.80	13.0	1.60	18.0	33.0	413	364	29.00	0.090	0.050	1.5	0.300	18.0	1460
Paste	6 oz can	170.0	128.00	139	5.80	0.70	31.60	46.0	6.00	32.0	119.0	1510	65	83.00	0.340	0.200	5.3	0.650	32.0	5610
Paste	1 tbsp	14.0	11.00	12	0.50	0.10	2.60	4.0	0.50	3.0	10.0	126	5	7.00	0.030	0.020	0.4	0.050	3.0	468
Turnip, cooked	1 cup cubed	155.0	145.00	36	1.20	0.30	7.60	54.0	0.60	22.0	37.0	291	53	34.00	0.060	0.080	0.5	0.108	2.0	trace
Turnip, greens, cooked	1 cup	145.0	135.00	29	3.20	0.30	5.20	267.0	1.60	40.0	54.0	—	—	100.00	0.220	0.350	0.9	1.400	—	9140
Vegetable Juice Cocktail	6 fl oz	182.0	171.00	31	1.60	0.20	6.60	22.0	0.90	—	40.0	402	364	16.00	0.090	0.050	1.5	0.170	—	1270
Vegetables, mixed, Frozen	1 cup cooked	182.0	150.00	116	5.80	0.50	24.40	46.0	2.40	42.0	115.0	348	96	15.00	0.220	0.130	2.0	—	26.0	9010
Water chestnuts, raw	1 lb	454.0	355.00	276	4.90	0.70	66.40	14.0	2.10	54.0	227.0	1747	70	14.00	0.490	0.700	3.5	0.040	—	0
Watercress	1 cup, whole	35.0	33.00	7	0.80	0.10	1.10	53.0	0.60	7.0	19.0	99	18	28.00	0.030	0.060	0.3	—	70.0	1270
Miscellaneous																				
Condiments																				
Barbeque Sauce	1 cup	250.0	202.00	228	3.80	17.30	20.00	53.0	2.00	—	50.0	435	2038	13.00	0.030	0.030	0.8	—	—	900
Horseradish, prepared	1 tsp	5.0	4.00	2	0.10	trace	0.50	3.0	trace	—	2.0	15	5	—	—	—	trace	—	—	—
Mustard Brown	1 tsp	5.0	4.00	5	0.30	0.30	0.30	6.0	0.10	2.0	7.0	7	65	—	—	—	—	—	2.0	—
Mustard Yellow	1 tsp	5.0	4.00	4	0.20	0.20	0.30	4.0	0.10	2.0	4.0	7	63	—	—	—	—	—	2.0	—
Olives Green	10 large	46.0	36.00	45	0.50	4.90	0.50	24.0	0.60	7.0	7.0	21	926	trace	—	trace	—	0.011	7.0	120
Olives Ripe	10 giant	80.0	64.00	89	0.80	9.50	1.80	58.0	1.10	11.0	—	23	559	trace	—	trace	—	—	—	40
Pickles Dill	1 medium	65.0	61.00	7	0.50	0.10	1.40	17.0	0.70	14.0	—	130	928	4.00	trace	0.010	trace	0.006	2.0	70
Pickles Sour	1 medium	65.0	62.00	7	0.30	0.10	1.30	11.0	2.10	10.0	—	—	879	5.00	trace	0.010	trace	—	—	70
Pickles Sweet	1 small	15.0	9.00	22	0.10	0.10	5.50	2.0	0.20	2.0	—	—	—	1.00	trace	trace	trace	0.001	0.7	10
Pickles Relish	1 tbsp	15.0	9.00	21	0.10	0.10	5.10	3.0	0.10	2.0	—	—	107	2.00	—	—	—	—	—	—
Salt	1 tsp	5.5	0.01	0	0	0	0	14.0	6.0	—	—	trace	2132	0	0	0	trace	0	0	0
Soy Sauce	1 tbsp	18.0	11.00	12	1.00	0.20	1.70	15.0	0.90	19.0	—	66	1319	trace	0.010	0.050	0.1	—	trace	0
Tartar Sauce	1 tbsp	14.0	5.00	74	0.20	8.10	0.60	3.0	0.10	4.0	—	11	99	trace	trace	trace	trace	—	trace	30
Tomato Catsup	1 tbsp	15.0	10.00	16	0.30	0.10	3.80	3.0	0.10	8.0	—	54	156	2.00	0.010	0.010	0.2	0.019	2.0	210
Tomato Chili Sauce, bottled	1 tbsp	15.0	10.00	16	0.40	trace	3.70	3.0	trace	8.0	—	56	201	2.00	0.010	0.010	0.2	0.019	5.0	210
Vinegar Cider	1 tbsp	15.0	14.00	2	trace	0	0.90	1.0	0.10	1.0	—	15	trace	—	—	—	—	—	—	—
Vinegar White distilled	1 tbsp	15.0	14.00	2	—	—	0.80	—	—	—	—	2	trace	—	—	—	—	—	—	—
Fats and Oils																				
Butter Regular, salted	1 pat	5.0	0.80	36	0.040	4.10	trace	1.0	0.01	trace	—	1	41	0	trace	0.002	0.002	trace	trace	153
Butter Salted, whipped	1 pat	3.8	0.60	27	0.03	3.08	trace	1.0	0.01	trace	—	1	31	0	trace	0.001	0.002	trace	trace	116
Lard	1 tsp	13.0	0	117	0	13.00	0	0	0	—	—	0	0	0	0	0	0	0.003	0	0
Margarine	1 pat	5.0	0.80	36	trace	4.00	trace	1.0	trace	—	—	1	50	0	0	0	0	0	0	160
Oils Corn, Cotton-seed, Safflower, Sesame, Soy	1 tbsp	14.0	0	120	0	14.00	0	0	0	—	—	0	0	0	0	0	0	0	0	—
Oils Olive, Peanut	1 tbsp	14.0	0	119	0	13.50	0	0	0	—	—	0	0	0	0	0	0	0	0	—
Salad Dressing Blue Cheese Regular	1 tbsp	15.0	5.00	76	0.7	7.80	1.10	12.0	trace	—	11.0	6	164	trace	trace	0.020	trace	0.020	trace	30
Salad Dressing Blue Cheese Low Fat	1 tbsp	15.0	13.00	12	0.5	0.90	0.70	10.0	trace	—	8.0	5	177	trace	trace	0.010	trace	0.010	trace	30
French Regular	1 tbsp	16.0	6.00	66	0.1	6.20	2.80	2.0	—	—	2.0	13	219	—	—	—	—	—	—	—
French Low Fat	1 tbsp	16.0	12.00	15	0.1	0.70	2.50	2.0	—	—	2.0	13	126	—	—	—	—	—	—	—

[a] Crookneck, zucchini, scalloped varieties.

[b] Acorn, butternut, hubbard.

Food	Amount	Weight g	Water g	Energy kcal	Protein g	Fat g	Total Carbohydrate g	Minerals						Vitamins						
								Calcium mg	Iron mg	Magnesium mg	Phosphorus mg	Potassium mg	Sodium mg	Vitamin C mg	Thiamin mg	Riboflavin mg	Niacin mg	Vitamin B6 mg	Folacin µg	Total Vitamin A I.U.
Italian																				
Regular	1 tbsp	15.0	4.00	83	trace	9.00	1.00	2.0	trace	1.0	1.0	2	314	—	trace	trace	trace	0	0	trace
Low Fat	1 tbsp	16.0	14.00	8	trace	0.70	0.40	trace	trace	—	1.0	2	118	—	trace	trace	trace	0	0	trace
Mayonnaise	1 tbsp	14.0	2.00	101	0.2	11.20	0.30	3.0	0.10	0	4.0	5	84	—	trace	0.010	trace	0	0	40
Mayonnaise-type Salad Dressing	1 tbsp	15.0	6.00	65	0.2	6.30	2.20	2.0	trace	0	4.0	1	88	—	trace	trace	trace	0	0	30
Thousand Island																				
Regular	1 tbsp	16.0	5.00	80	0.1	8.00	2.50	2.0	0.10	—	3.0	18	112	trace	trace	trace	trace	—	—	50
Low Fat	1 tbsp	15.0	10.00	27	0.1	2.10	2.30	2.0	0.10	—	3.0	17	105	trace	trace	trace	trace	—	—	50
Nuts and Snacks																				
Almonds, roasted, salted	22	28.0	0.10	178	5.3	16.40	5.50	67.0	1.30	84.0	143.0	219	56	0	0.010	0.260	1.0	0.030	14.0	0
Brazil Nuts, shelled	6–8	28.0	1.30	185	4.1	19.00	3.10	53.0	1.00	65.0	196.0	203	trace	0	0.270	0.030	0.5	0.050	trace	trace
Cashews	18	28.0	1.50	159	4.9	13.00	8.30	11.0	1.10	80.0	106.0	132	4	0	0.120	0.070	0.5	0.120	8.0	30
Peanuts, roasted, salted	½ cup	72.0	1.00	421	18.7	35.80	13.60	54.0	1.50	120.0	288.0	486	301	0	0.230	0.100	12.4	0.288	19.0	—
Peanut Butter	1 tsp	16.0	0.30	94	4.0	8.10	3.00	9.0	0.30	28.0	61.0	100	97	0	0.020	0.020	2.4	0.005	2.0	—
Pecans, shelled	½ cup	54.0	2.00	371	5.0	38.40	7.90	40.0	1.30	77.0	156.0	325	trace	1.00	0.460	0.070	0.5	0.09	7.0	70
Pistachio Nuts	½ cup	76.0	4.00	449	14.6	40.60	14.40	99.0	5.50	120.0	378.0	735	—	—	0.500	—	1.1	—	—	173
Popcorn with oil, salt	1 cup	9.0	0.30	41	0.90	2.00	5.30	1.0	0.20	12.0	19.0	—	175	0	—	0.010	0.2	0.014	0	trace
Potato Chips	10	20.0	0.40	114	1.10	8.00	10.00	8.0	0.40	8.0	28.0	226	a	3.00	0.040	0.010	1.0	0.036	2.0	trace
Pretzels, 3-Ring	10	30.0	1.00	117	2.90	1.40	22.80	7.0	0.50	—	39.0	39	504	0	0.010	0.010	0.2	0.010	0	0
Walnuts, shelled																				
Black	½ cup	62.0	2.00	392	12.80	37.00	9.20	trace	3.80	118.0	356.0	288	2	—	0.140	0.070	0.4	—	—	190
English	½ cup	50.0	2.00	326	7.40	32.00	7.90	50.0	1.60	66.0	190.0	225	1	1.00	0.160	0.070	0.4	0.360	30.0	15
Soups[b]																				
Canned																				
Bean with pork	1 cup	250.0	211.00	168	8.00	5.80	21.80	63.0	2.30	—	128.0	395	1008	3.00	0.130	0.080	1.0	—	—	650
Beef Noodle	1 cup	240.0	224.00	67	3.80	2.60	7.00	7.0	1.00	—	48.0	77	917	trace	0.050	0.070	1.0	—	—	50
Chicken Noodle	1 cup	240.0	224.00	62	3.40	1.90	7.90	10.0	0.50	10.0	36.0	55	979	trace	0.020	0.020	0.7	0.071	0	50
Clam Chowder (Manhattan)	1 cup	245.0	225.00	81	2.20	2.50	12.30	34.0	1.00	—	47.0	184	938	trace	0.020	0.020	1.0	—	8.0	880
Cream of Mushroom	1 cup	240.0	215.00	134	2.40	9.60	10.10	41.0	0.50	—	50.0	98	955	trace	0.020	0.120	0.7	—	—	70
Split Pea	1 cup	245.0	209.00	145	8.60	3.20	20.60	29.0	1.50	14.0	149.0	270	941	1.00	0.250	0.150	1.5	0.120	2.0	440
Tomato	1 cup	245.0	223.00	88	2.00	2.50	16.70	15.0	0.70	17.0	34.0	230	970	12.00	0.050	0.050	1.2	0.048	9.0	1000
Vegetarian Vegetable	1 cup	245.0	225.00	78	2.20	2.00	13.20	20.0	1.00	—	39.0	172	838	—	0.050	0.050	1.0	—	—	2940
Dehydrated																				
Chicken Rice	1 cup	240.0	228.00	48	1.20	1.00	8.40	7.0	trace	—	10.0	10	622	0	trace	trace	0.2	—	—	trace
Onion	1 cup	240.0	230.00	36	1.40	1.20	5.50	10.0	0.20	—	12.0	58	689	2.00	trace	trace	trace	—	—	trace
Sugars and Sweets																				
Candy																				
Butterscotch	1 oz	28.0	0.40	113	trace	1.00	26.90	5.0	0.40	—	2.0	1	19	0	0	trace	trace	—	—	40
Caramels	1 oz	28.0	2.00	113	1.10	2.90	21.70	42.0	0.40	—	35.0	54	64	trace	0.010	0.050	0.1	trace	—	trace
Chocolate																				
Milk, plain	1 oz	28.0	0.20	147	2.20	9.20	16.10	65.0	0.30	16.0	65.0	109	27	trace	0.020	0.100	0.1	trace	1	80
Semi-sweet	1 oz	28.0	0.30	144	1.20	10.10	16.20	9.0	0.70	—	43.0	92	1	trace	trace	0.020	0.1	—	—	10
Sweet	1 oz	28.0	0.20	150	1.20	10.00	16.40	27.0	0.40	30.0	40.0	76	9	trace	0.010	0.040	0.1	—	—	trace
Fudge	1 oz	28.0	2.00	113	0.80	3.50	21.30	22.0	0.30	—	24.0	42	54	trace	0.010	0.030	0.1	—	—	trace

Food	Unit	Weight (g)															
Gum Drops	1 oz	28.0	3.00	98	trace	0.20	24.80	2.0	0.10	1	10	0	0	trace	trace	—	0
Jelly Beans	10	28.0	2.00	104	trace	0.10	26.40	3.0	0.30	trace	3	0	0	trace	trace	—	0
Marshmallows	1 large	7.0	1.00	23	0.10	trace	5.80	1.0	0.10	trace	3	0	0	trace	trace	0	0
Honey, strained	1 tbsp	21.0	4.00	64	0.10	0	17.30	1.0	0.10	11	1	1	trace	0.010	0.1	1.0	trace
Icings																	
Chocolate	1 cup[a]	275.0	39.00	1034	8.80	38.20	185.40	165.0	3.30	536	168	1	0.060	0.280	0.6	—	580
White, boiled	1 cup	94.0	17.00	297	1.30	0	75.50	2.0	trace	17	134	0	trace	0.030	trace	—	0
Jams and Preserves	1 tbsp	20.0	6.00	54	0.10	trace	14.00	4.0	0.20	18	2	trace	trace	0.010	trace	1.0	trace
Jellies	1 tbsp	18.0	5.00	49	trace	trace	12.70	4.0	0.30	14	3	1	trace	0.010	trace	0	trace
Marmalade, citrus	1 tbsp	20.0	6.00	51	0.10	trace	14.00	7.0	0.10	7	3	1	trace	trace	trace	—	—
Molasses																	
Light	1 tbsp	20.0	5.00	50	—	—	13.00	33.0	0.90	183	3	—	0.010	0.010	0.010	—	—
Medium	1 tbsp	20.0	5.00	46	—	—	12.00	58.0	1.20	213	7	—	trace	0.020	0.020	2.0	—
Blackstrap	1 tbsp	20.0	5.00	43	—	—	11.00	137.0	3.20	585	19	—	0.020	0.040	0.040	—	—
Sugar																	
Brown	⅓ cup, packed	110.0	2.00	410	0	0	106.00	94.0	3.80	378	33	0	0.010	0.040	0.2	0	0
	1 tsp	4.0	0.02	15	0	0	4.00	0	trace	0	trace	0	0	0	0	0	0
White, granulated	1 lump	5.0	0.03	19	0	0	5.00	0	0	0	trace	0	0	0	0	0	0
White, powdered	1 tbsp	8.0	0.04	31	0	0	8.00	0	trace	0	trace	0	0	0	0	0	0
Syrups																	
Maple	1 tbsp	20.0	6.00	50	—	—	12.80	20.0	0.20	35	2	0	—	—	—	—	—
Table blends Corn	1 tbsp	20.0	5.00	59	0	0	15.40	9.0	0.80	1	14	0	0	0	0	0	0
Cane and Maple	1 tbsp	20.0	6.00	50	0	0	12.80	3.0	trace	5	trace	0	0	0	0	0	0
Other																	
Baking Powder	1 tsp	3.0	0.05	4	trace	trace	0.90	58.0	—	5	329	0	0	0	0	0	0
Bouillon Cube	1	4.0	0.2	5	0.80	0.10	0.20	—	—	4	960	0	—	—	—	0	—
Chewing Gum, Candy coated piece	¾"x½"x½" piece	1.7	0.06	5	—	—	1.60	—	—	—	—	—	—	—	—	—	—
Cocoa, plain, dry	1 tbsp	5.0	0.10	15	0.90	1.00	3.00	5.0	0.60	80	trace	0	0.010	0.02	0.1	0	0
Cocoa Mix w/non fat dry milk	1 tbsp	7.0	0.20	27	0.70	0.70	5.20	19.0	0.10	42	27	0	0.010	0.03	0	0.001	1
Gelatin, dry	1 envelope	7.0	0.90	23	6.00	trace	0	2.0	—	—	—	—	—	—	—	—	—
Gelatin Dessert, plain	1 cup	240.0	202.00	142	3.60	0	33.80	4.0	—	—	122	0	—	—	—	0	—
Gravy, meat, brown	¼ cup	72.0	48.00	164	1.20	14.00	8.00	0	0.40	76	720	0	0.040	0.03	0.03	0.036	0
Puddings with milk	½ cup	130.0	91.00	161	4.40	3.90	29.60	133.0	0.40	177	168	0	0.030	0.19	0.1	0.065	169
Yeast																	
Bakers, compressed	1 pkg	18.0	13.00	15	2.20	0.10	2.00	2.0	0.90	110	3	trace	0.130	0.30	2.0	—	trace
Bakers, dry active	1 pkg	7.0	0.04	20	2.60	0.10	2.70	3.0	1.10	140	4	trace	0.160	0.38	2.6	0.10	trace
Brewers, debittered	1 tbsp	8.0	0.04	23	3.10	0.10	3.10	17.0	1.40	152	10	trace	1.250	0.34	3.0	0.10	trace

[a] Sodium content varies; may be 1000 mg per 100 g. [b] Prepared with water according to package directions. [a] Enough to frost 1 9'' diam cake layer.

Sources:
Adams, C. F. Nutritive Value of American Foods in Common Units. *Agriculture Handbook No. 456.* Agricultural Research Service, USDA. Washington, D.C. 1975.
Pennington, J.A. *Dietary Nutrient Guide.* Westport, Conn.: AVI Publishing Company, Inc., 1976.
Watt, B. K. and A. L. Merrill (with assistance of R. K. Pecot, C. F. Adams, M. L. Orr, and D. F. Miller). Composition of Foods—Raw, processed, prepared. *Agriculture Handbook No. 8.* Agricultural Research Service, USDA. Washington, D.C. 1963, reprinted 1975.
Young, E. A., E. H. Brennan, and G. L. Irving. Perspectives on fast foods. *Public Health Currents.* Ross Laboratories, Columbus, Ohio. Jan., Feb., 1979.
Church, C. F. and H. N. Church. Food values of portions commonly used, 12th edition. Philadelphia: J. B. Lippincott Co. 1975.
Posati, L. P. and M. L. Orr. Composition of Foods. Dairy and egg products; raw, processed, prepared. *Agriculture Handbook No. 8-1;* Agricultural Research Service, USDA. Washington, D.C. 1976.
Marsh, A. C., M. K. Moss, and E. W. Murphy. Composition of Foods. Spices and herbs. Raw, processed, prepared. *Agriculture Handbook No. 8-2;* Agricultural Research Service, USDA. Washington, D.C. 1977.
Gebhardt, S. E., R. Cutrufelli, and R. H. Matthews. Composition of Foods. Baby Foods. Raw, processed, prepared. *Agriculture Handbook No. 8-3;* Agricultural Research Service, USDA. Washington, D.C. 1978.

Notes:
Unless otherwise indicated, enriched flour is used in all products containing wheat flour.
— Indicates lack of reliable data for a nutrient believed to be present.
nd indicates no data.
Amino acid content of foods may be found in the article "Amino acid content of foods and biological data on proteins." FAO. No. 24, Rome, 1970.
Fatty acid content of foods may be found in the appropriate Handbooks No. 8 (revised editions), Handbook 456, and in the Journal of the American Dietetic Association series cited in Chapter 3.

APPENDIX I
Selected Nutrition Resources

American Council on Science
and Health
1995 Broadway
New York, NY 10023

American Dental Association
211 E. Chicago Avenue
Chicago, IL 60611

American Diabetes Association
2 Park Avenue
New York, NY 10016

American Dietetic Association
(ADA)
430 N. Michigan Avenue
Chicago, IL 60611

American Egg Board
1460 Renaissance Drive
Park Ridge, IL 60068

American Heart Association
(AHA)
7320 Greenville Ave.
Dallas, TX 75231

American Home Economics
Association (AHEA)
Division of Public Affairs
1010 Massachusetts Avenue,
N.W.
Washington, DC 20036

American Institute of Nutrition
9650 Rockville Pike
Bethesda, MD 20014

American Medical Association
Council on Foods and Nutrition
535 N. Dearborn Street
Chicago, IL 60610

American Public Health Association (APHA)
1015 Fifteenth St., NW
Washington, DC 20005

Anorexia Nervosa and Associated Disorders
Suite 2020
550 Frontage Road
Northfield, IL 60093

Community Nutrition Institute
(CNI)
1146 19th St., NW
Washington, DC 20036

Consumer Information Center
U.S. General Services Admin-
istration
Pueblo, CO 81009

Extension Service of State
Universities
County Extension Offices (see
local telephone listing)

Food and Agriculture
Organization of America, Inc.
Information Office
1776 F Street NW
Washington, DC 20437

Food and Agricultural Organi-
zation of the United Nations
UNIPUB Inc.
P.O. Box 433
New York, NY 10016

Director, Consumer Communi-
cations HFJ-10
Food and Drug Administration
(FDA)
5600 Fishers Lane
Rockville, MD 20852

Food and Nutrition Board
(FNB)
National Academy of Sciences
2101 Constitution Avenue
Washington, DC 20418

Food and Nutrition Information
and Educational Materials
Center
National Agricultural Library,
Rm. 304
Beltsville, MD 20705

Food and Nutrition Service
(federal programs including
Extension Service and
School Lunch)
U.S.D.A.
500 12th Street SW
Washington, DC 20250

Institute of Food Technologists
(IFT)
221 North LaSalle Street
Chicago, IL 60601

International Life Sciences
Institute-Nutrition Foundation (ILSI)
1126 16th Street, N.W.
Washington, DC 20036

La Leche League Interna-
tional, Inc. (LLLI)
9616 Minneapolis Ave.
Franklin Park, IL 60131

March of Dimes Birth Defects
Foundation (MOD)
1275 Mamaroneck Ave.
White Plains, NY 10605

Meals for Millions/Freedom
from Hunger Foundation
(MFM)
1800 Olympic Blvd.
P.O. Drawer 680
Santa Monica, CA 90406

National Dairy Council
6300 North River Road
Rosemont, IL 60018

National Institutes of Health
9000 Rockville Pike
Bethesda, MD 20205

National Food Processor's
Association
1401 New York Avenue, N.W.
Washington, DC 20005

National Livestock and Meat
Board
444 North Michigan Avenue
Chicago, IL 60611

Nutrition Today Society
P.O. Box 1829
703 Giddings Avenue
Annapolis, MD 21401

Public Affairs Committee, Inc.
381 Park Avenue South
New York, NY 10016

Society for Nutrition Education
(SNE)
1736 Franklin Street
Oakland, CA 94612

Superintendent of Documents
U.S. Government Printing Office
Washington, DC 20402

U.S. Department of Agriculture
Nutrition Program
Agricultural Research Service
Hyattsville, MD 20782

U.S. Department of Health and
Human Services
330 Independence Ave. SW
Washington, DC 20201

U.S. Department of Health and
Human Services
Maternal and Child Health
Services
Health Services Administration
Rockville, MD 20852

World Health Organization
777 United Nations Plaza
New York, NY 10017

*PERIODICALS AND MAGA-
ZINES*

CNI Weekly Report
Contemporary Nutrition
Dairy Council Digest
Food and Nutrition News
FDA Consumer
Nutrition Action
Nutrition and the M.D.
Nutrition Today
Professional Nutritionist

PROFESSIONAL JOURNALS

*American Journal of Clinical
Nutrition*
*American Journal of Public
Health*
Food Technology
Journal of the American Dental Association
Journal of the American Dietetic Association
Journal of the American Medical Association
Journal of Clinical Investigation
Journal of Food Science
Journal of Home Economics
Journal of Nutrition
The Lancet
Journal of Nutrition Education
*Medicine and Science in
Sports and Exercise*
Metabolism
*New England Journal of
Medicine*
Nutrition Research
Nutrition Reviews
Pediatrics
School Food Service Journal
Science

APPENDIX J
Basic Concepts of Chemistry and Biology

ATOMS AND MOLECULES

Chemistry is the study of the composition, structure, and properties of matter, the changes that matter undergoes, and the energy associated with these changes. **Matter** is anything that occupies space and has mass or weight. **Energy** is the capacity to do work; heat, electricity, and movement are familiar forms of energy.

The basic building blocks of all kinds of matter—liquid, solid, and gas—are called **atoms.** Although atoms are exceedingly small, they are nevertheless quite complex. Atoms have a central core, or **nucleus,** which contains particles with a positive electrical charge, **protons,** and neutral particles having no electrical charge, **neutrons.** Revolving around the nucleus like planets around the sun are negatively charged particles, **electrons.** Any atom—whether it is an atom of metal, such as iron, or of a gas, such as oxygen—contains the same number of protons as electrons, creating a balance between the positively charged protons and the negatively charged electrons.

The very smallest atom in existence consists of just one proton and one electron, with no neutrons. It is the hydrogen atom (Figure 1). Being the smallest, it is also the lightest, weighing only 1.67×10^{-24} grams. Complex numbers such as this are difficult to work with so scientists have devised a system of atomic weights in which hydrogen is assigned a weight of 1, for its single proton. Because an electron has a mass only $1/1,836$ as large as a proton, its extremely small contribution is disregarded in all calculations of atomic weight. Neutrons, however, have approximately the same mass as protons.

Atoms have a tendency to "lose" and "gain" electrons, thus disrupting their electrical balance or neutrality. When a hydrogen atom, for example, loses its single electron, we say it has an electrical charge of $+1$. Any charged atom is called an **ion.** A positively charged ion, one which has lost an electron or electrons, is a **cation.** A negatively charged atom, which has gained an electron or electrons, is an **anion.**

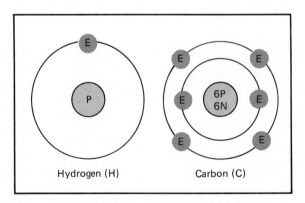

FIGURE 1

Hydrogen and Carbon Atoms.

The physical properties of matter, such as taste, odor, color, and weight depend on the composition and arrangement of atoms. Any physical change in matter, such as the melting of ice into liquid water, does not change the composition of its atoms. Other types of changes in matter, called chemical changes, involve rearrangement of atoms. Such rearrangements depend on the ability of atoms to share electrons. This sharing is known as covalent **bonding.**

A substance composed of only one kind of atom, such as oxygen, iron, and calcium, is called an **element.** When atoms of any one element bond together, the result is a **molecule** of that element. We speak of molecules of oxygen, for example. When atoms of two or more different elements combine, the resulting molecule is a **compound.** Some well-known examples are water, made up of hydrogen and oxygen atoms (see Figure 2) and sugar, made up of hydrogen, oxygen, and carbon atoms. A molecule is the smallest particle of any distinct substance, either an element or a compound.

Chemical Notation and Bonding

Only 103 elements have been identified on our planet. Their various combinations, however, produce hundreds of thousands of compounds. Table 1 lists the elements that are of greatest interest to the study of nutrition. Note that each element is represented by a **chemical symbol,** which chemists use in describing reactions between elements, molecules, and compounds.

A symbol or group of symbols which represents the composition of an element or compound is known as a **chemical formula.** For example, the chemical formula for common table salt is NaCl, representing the bonding of one *atom* of sodium and one *atom* of chlorine into one *molecule* of sodium chloride. This bonding is expressed by the **chemical equation:**

$$Na + Cl \rightarrow NaCl$$

To take another example:

$$4H + C \rightarrow CH_4$$

FIGURE 2   *Water Molecule.*
Two atoms of hydrogen combine with one atom of oxygen to form a water molecule.

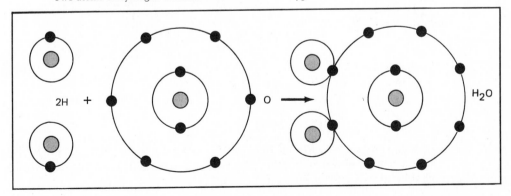

TABLE 1. *Elements Most Important to the Study of Nutrition*

Symbol	Element	Symbol	Element
H	Hydrogen	Mn	Manganese
C	Carbon	Fe	Iron
N	Nitrogen	Co	Cobalt
O	Oxygen	Ni	Nickel
Ca	Calcium	Cu	Copper
Na	Sodium	Zn	Zinc
Mg	Magnesium	I	Iodine
P	Phosphorus	F	Fluorine
S	Sulfur	Se	Selenium
Cl	Chlorine	Cr	Chromium
K	Potassium		

That is, four atoms of hydrogen plus one atom of carbon yields one molecule of methane.

By convention, chemical equations are written with the reactants (**substrates**) to the left of the arrow and the products to the right. Also by convention, no coefficient is indicated when only one atom or molecule of a substance is used or produced. However, when more than one atom or molecule is a reactant or a product, a coefficient is written in front of the appropriate symbol, as in the preceding four hydrogen atoms. Subscripts are used to indicate the number of atoms in any particular compound. As with coefficients, no subscript is used if only one atom is involved. Thus, one molecule of methane (CH_4) consists of one atom of carbon and four atoms of hydrogen.

Chemical reactions involve covalent bonding, which is a sharing of electrons. Chemists have developed yet another shorthand system to describe these bonds. It is based on pictorial diagrams representing the outermost ring of electrons in a particular atom. This outer ring, known as the **valence shell**, contains the electrons that are shared in chemical bonds. Carbon, for example, with four electrons in its outermost ring, can share four additional electrons and thus have a valence of 4. It is represented as:

$$\overset{\displaystyle |}{\underset{\displaystyle |}{C}}$$

Hydrogen has a valence of 1:

$$H$$

Oxygen has a valence of 2:

$$O$$

Nitrogen usually has a valence of 3:

$$\overset{\displaystyle |}{\underset{\displaystyle |}{N}}$$

In a *stable compound*, each of the available electrons is shared, or bonded. Thus, when carbon combines with other elements to form a stable compound, each carbon atom has four chemical bonds.

The bonding of carbon atoms is central to the study of nutrition. In fact, of all the 103 known elements, this one has proved so important that its compounds have been given a science of their own, **organic chemistry.** The number of carbon compounds known today exceeds the number of compounds prepared from all the other 102 elements.

Carbon compounds, usually called *organic compounds*, are composed of carbon atoms bonded to one another to form what are known as chains and rings. **Hydrocarbons** are the simplest organic compounds, containing only hydrogen and carbons. Methane is a simple example:

$$
\begin{array}{c}
\text{H} \\
| \\
\text{H} \quad \text{C} \quad \text{H} \\
| \\
\text{H}
\end{array}
$$

The bonding requirements for both carbon (valence 4) and hydrogen (valence 1) are met in this compound. In more complicated bonding, forms of hydrocarbons are produced through the replacement of one or more hydrogen atoms by **functional groups** of atoms. A grouping of atoms that imparts characteristic properties to a molecule and to the reactions in which it takes part is known as a functional group. Many organic compounds are classified according to their functional group or groups. The double lines connecting the carbon atoms with other atoms in these groups represent a double bond, which is the sharing of two electron pairs. Certain functional groups are particularly important in nutritional compounds, and they will become very familiar in the chapters that follow (see Table 2).

All the foods we eat contain carbon compounds. Although their chemical names may be unfamiliar, their everyday names are common household words:

- **Carbohydrates** (sugars and starches) are organic molecules containing C, H, and O, and occasionally N and S.
- **Proteins** are organic molecules containing C, H, O, N, sometimes S, and other elements.
- **Lipids** (or fats) are organic molecules containing C, H, O, and sometimes N or P.
- **Vitamins** are organic molecules containing C, H, O, and sometimes N, S, and Co.

Alcohol	$-\overset{\displaystyle |}{\underset{\displaystyle |}{\text{C}}}-\text{OH}$
Aldehyde	$-\overset{\displaystyle \text{O}}{\overset{\displaystyle \|}{\text{C}}}-\text{H}$
Ketone	$-\overset{\displaystyle \text{O}}{\overset{\displaystyle \|}{\text{C}}}-$
Acid	$-\overset{\displaystyle \text{O}}{\overset{\displaystyle \|}{\text{C}}}-\text{O}-\text{H}$

TABLE 2.
Some Nutritionally Important Functional Groups

These four classes of organic compounds present in foods are known as **nutrients**. Vitamins and minerals required in trace amounts are also known as **micronutrients**. Carbohydrates, proteins, and lipids are considered **macronutrients**. Also considered as nutrients are inorganic molecules, such as Na, K, P, S, Ca, Fe, and other elements, better known as the **minerals**, and **water**, which is a compound of H and O.

ORGANIZATION OF THE BODY

Your body and the foods you eat are made up of atoms and molecules. The process of nutrition involves the transformation of atoms and molecules present in food into the kind of atoms and molecules that make up the body. This transformation occurs inside the cells of all animal bodies.

Cells are the basic structural units ("building blocks") of any living organism. Each cell is like a miniature factory, which processes nutrients for energy, growth, and performance of its particular body-regulating function. Although there is no such thing as a "typical" cell, a representative one can be described, as shown in Figure 3.

The body is a highly organized system containing many types of cells, each specifically structured to fulfill a particular function. There are skin (epithelial) cells, blood cells (erythrocytes, or red cells, and leucocytes, or white cells), nerve cells (neurons), fat cells (adipocytes), bone cells (osteocytes), and muscle cells. (Note that the suffix *cyte* identifies many cells.) Cells are organized into **tissues**—muscle tissue, epithelial (skin) tissue, adipose (fat) tissue, bone tissue, nerve tissue—which, in turn, are organized into **organs**—the digestive organs—esophagus, stomach, small intestine, large intestine, pancreas, gall bladder, liver—and others such as the heart, brain, lungs, and reproductive organs. Organs may contain primarily one type of tissue, or they may be a functionally organized collection of several tissue types.

Several organs with related functions together make up larger **organ systems**, for example, the skeletal, respiratory, reproductive, nervous, circulatory, and digestive systems. The integrated product of all these functioning organ systems is, of course, the **organism**.

The organism, with all its component parts, consists entirely of atoms and molecules of chemical elements. Looking at the distribution of elements within the body (Table 3) we can see that carbon, oxygen, hydrogen, and nitrogen comprise about 96 percent of body weight. Other elements account for the rest, with the mineral calcium being by far the most abundant.

ANATOMY AND PHYSIOLOGY OF DIGESTION

Digestion is the mechanical and chemical process by which food is prepared for absorption. Obviously, chunks of meat, potatoes, and vegetables don't just float around in the body after a meal. Foods cannot be used without digestion and con-

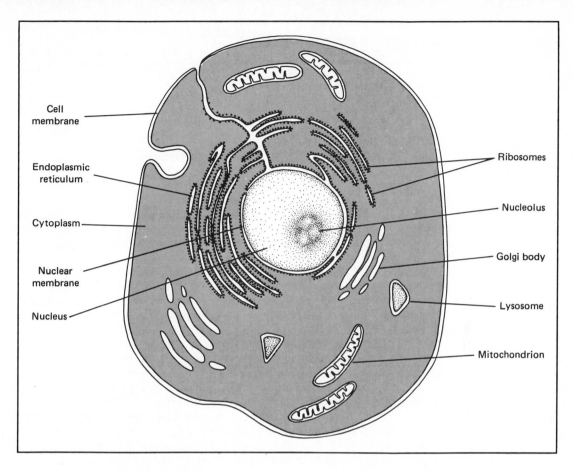

FIGURE 3   *A Cell.*

Most cells (with insignificant exceptions) contain the same components, or organelles.

The cell is enclosed by a double **plasma membrane**, a layered protein-lipid-protein sandwich that determines the shape of the cell and regulates the passage of materials into and out of it. The membrane is filled with a viscous fluid called **cytoplasm.** Cytoplasm provides an optimum environment for the organelles, in which the life functions of the cell are performed.

Within the cytoplasm is a cluster of material, the **nucleus**, which is the "brain" or control center of the cell. In the nucleus are **chromosomes** of deoxyribonucleic acid (DNA), the genetic material that carries the information necessary to create a complete new individual. DNA, which always remains in the nucleus of the cell, determines all cell activities by programming the synthesis of ribonucleic acids (RNA) that can move out of the nucleus to the cytoplasm, where they directly control cellular function. Other RNAs remain in the nucleus, located in a small body, the **nucleolus.**

Mitochondria (singular: *mitochondrion*) are the "powerhouses" of the cell. Mitochondria are responsible for the many chemical reactions related to energy production inside each cell. Some busy cells may contain thousands of mitochondria.

Endoplasmic reticulum is the name given to the system of membranous channels that transport materials throughout the cell. Endoplasmic reticulum (ER) with ribosomes (see below) around its outer surface is referred to as rough ER. Smooth ER has no ribosomes.

Ribosomes are small granules composed of protein and nucleic acid. Some ribosomes float free in the cytoplasm; others are bound to the endoplasmic reticulum. Protein synthesis occurs on the ribosomes.

Golgi bodies make up the system of intracellular membranes contiguous with the ER. Their function is the packaging and storage of various products that the cell will eventually secrete.

Lysosomes are membrane-bound vesicles that contain the enzymes that break down intracellular products and debris.

TABLE 3. *Distribution of Elements in the Human Body, Percent Body Weight*

Oxygen	65.00	Sulfur	0.25000	Iodine	0.0001
Carbon	18.00	Sodium	0.15000	Fluorine	0.0001
Hydrogen	10.00	Chlorine	0.15000	Silicon	0.0001
Nitrogen	3.00	Magnesium	0.05000	Copper	0.0001
Calcium	2.00	Iron	0.00400	Cobalt	0.0001
Phosphorus	1.10	Zinc	0.00020		
Potassium	0.35	Manganese	0.00013		

version into simpler substances that can pass through the cells of the small intestine (intestinal mucosa) and then into the blood or lymph.

The transformation of food requires both mechanical and enzymatic means. Both begin in the mouth, as food is chewed and mixed with saliva, meeting the first of many enzymes that facilitate its chemical breakdown. Enzymes are specialized protein molecules that catalyze chemical reactions; that is, enzymes speed up the rate of chemical reactions, although they themselves are not part of the product of the reaction. Enzymes increase the rate of chemical reactions by lowering the energy level required to drive these reactions. Enzymes are very specific: Each enzyme can catalyze only one type of reaction. Thus, each of the many chemical reactions occurring in the body employs a different, specialized enzyme. All enzymes can be reused. Some need to be replaced more quickly than others, however.

An enzyme can be visualized as a molecule having specific sites to accept a specific substrate, thereby making the substrate more chemically reactive. As illustrated in Figure 4, an enzyme can change compound X into compounds Y and Z, without being changed itself.

Some of the many enzymes of the digestive system are manufactured (synthesized) in the cells of the salivary glands (amylase), pancreas (lipase), stomach (pepsin), and small intestine (maltase). (Note that the suffix *ase* identifies many enzymes.) A complete explanation of the digestive enzymes and their reactions will follow in later chapters. For now, let us examine the digestive system diagrammed in Figure 5. The transformation of food begins with mechanical breakdown by the teeth. The mixture of chewed food and saliva (called a *bolus*) next moves to the **esophagus.** Rhythmic contractions of circular muscles in the wall of the esophagus

FIGURE 4   *Model of Enzyme.*

An enzyme combines with a substrate (the substance to undergo the reaction). A product is produced, after which the enzyme (unchanged) can be used again.

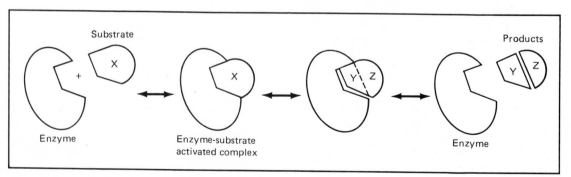

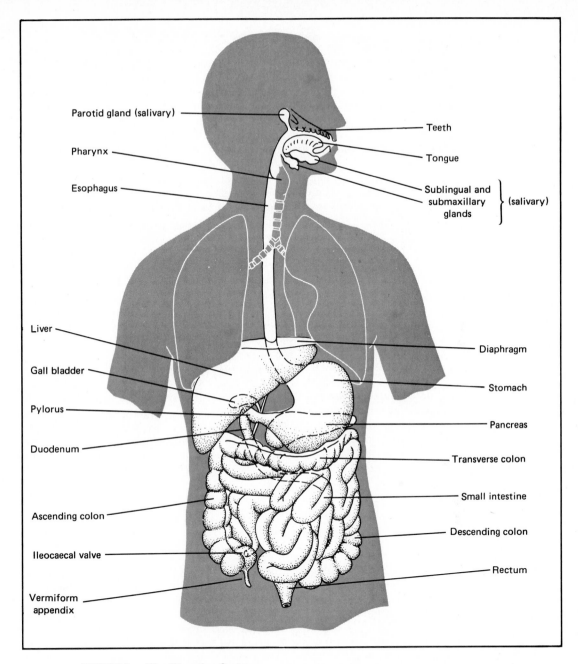

Parotid gland (salivary)

Pharynx

Esophagus

Teeth

Tongue

Sublingual and submaxillary glands $\}$ (salivary)

Liver

Gall bladder

Pylorus

Duodenum

Ascending colon

Ileocaecal valve

Vermiform appendix

Diaphragm

Stomach

Pancreas

Transverse colon

Small intestine

Descending colon

Rectum

FIGURE 5   *The Digestive System.*

move the bolus down the esophagus to the stomach by the process of **peristalsis.** In the stomach, powerful contractions churn the food and break up large pieces, maximizing their exposure to *gastric juices,* the mixture of hydrochloric acid and digestive enzymes secreted by glands in the stomach lining. Antacid advertising to the contrary, an acid stomach is quite necessary for digestion. Gastric juices work the food into a soupy fluid called **chyme.**

From the stomach, chyme passes through the pyloric valve into the small intestine for its final processing. Here the presence of chyme stimulates the release of many digestive enzymes from the pancreas and the intestinal glands. Each will act on different nutrients. Proteins are digested by a combination of several pancreatic and intestinal enzymes. Starch digestion is carried out by pancreatic amylase. Another pancreatic enzyme, lipase, acts to split molecules of fat into monoglycerides and fatty acids. The liver produces a fluid called **bile** that also aids in fat digestion. Bile is stored in the gall bladder and released into the small intestine as needed.

The entire small intestine of an adult is 7 or 8 meters (23 feet) long and 2.54 centimeters (1 inch) in diameter. This substantial length is made effectively even greater by numerous folds and ridges. In addition, the mucous lining of the small intestine is covered with small fingerlike projections called **villi** (singular: *villus*). The villi and their surrounding epithelial cells are, in turn, covered with numerous closely packed cylindrical outgrowths called **microvilli.** The microvilli make up the **brush border.** With all these folds, villi, and microvilli, the total surface area of the small intestine is about as large as half a basketball court. These intestinal cells are in a continuous state of turnover and renewal. In fact, the epithelium of the small intestine has the fastest turnover rate of any tissue in the body. Each villus loses one cell per hour from its tip. Calculating the extrusion from all the villi taken together yields a figure of 20 to 50 million cells per minute that are cast off into the lumen (inner space) of the small intestine. These cells may end up being digested and their contents absorbed or excreted from the body.

Large volumes of water are involved in the digestive process and must be recycled to prevent dehydration. In the large intestine, in the next stage of the absorptive process, water is reabsorbed. The large intestine is continuous with the small intestine at the lower right side of the body (as shown in Figure 5); then it ascends to the middle of the abdominal cavity, crosses to the left side, and then descends. This pathway forms three sections, called the *ascending, transverse,* and *descending* colons. From the large intestine, water travels back into the bloodstream, and waste matter passes into the rectum, ready for defecation through the anus.

Absorption

Digestion is only the beginning of the series of biological events that takes place as food is incorporated into the human body. Eventually, the nutrient materials in some form will reach every cell. Nutrients begin their travels by entering the bloodstream, or circulation, which will carry them to where they are needed. **Absorption** is the passage or transport of digested products into the bloodstream. It occurs in the small intestine and, to a much lesser extent, in the stomach.

Most absorption takes place at the mucosal membrane of the small intestine, where the extensive epithelial surface of the villi and microvilli provides a large area to which the nutrients passing through the intestinal lumen are exposed. As you can see in Figure 6, the villi are supported by a structure of connective tissue, interlaced with blood vessels and lymph ducts. During absorption, digested nutrients cross the intestinal epithelial layer into the blood vessels and lymph ducts. Because they occupy a central position between the lumen of the small intestine and the blood supply, these epithelial cells act as monitors of what is transported between the two compartments.

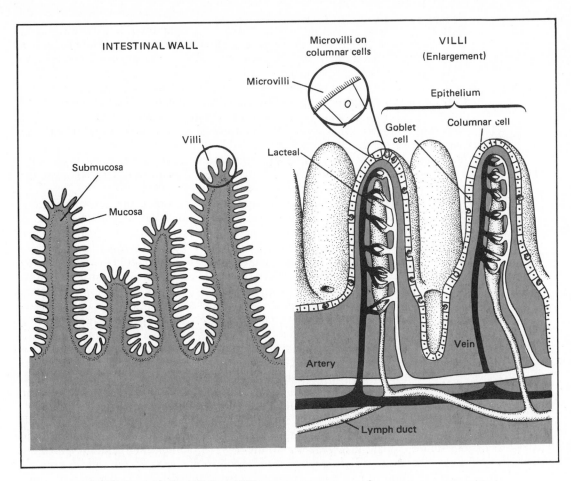

FIGURE 6 *Intestinal Wall and Villus.*
The primary site of nutrient absorption is in the mucosa, or interior surface membrane, of the small intestine, diagrammed at left. It is lined with thousands of projections or villa (singular villus), shown in detail at right. Each villus contains blood vessels and a special lymph vessel, the lacteal. The outer surface (epithelium) of each villus consists of columnar cells for absorption and goblet cells for production of mucus. From the columnar cells the microvilli extend, forming the brush border. All these structures vastly increase the surface area available for nutrient absorption.

A variety of transport mechanisms can be broadly classified into *passive* and *active* processes. In one type of **passive transport** thousands of tiny pores in the walls of the microvilli allow water and certain small water-soluble molecules to enter the intestinal cell. Molecules small enough to get through tend to cross the membrane until they are present in equal distribution (concentration) on both sides. In other words, molecules travel from an area of high concentration in the intestinal lumen to an area of lower concentration, until both areas come to have an equal concentration. This passive process is known as **diffusion** down a **concentration gradient**.

You can see diffusion at work if you drop some blue ink into a glass of water. It starts out as a dark, concentrated drop and then slowly diffuses until the water takes on an even, but lighter, blue color. In scientific terms, we say that the ink has diffused from an area of high concentration (the ink drop) to an area of low concentration (the whole glass of water).

The size and shape of epithelial pores are such that only certain molecules can fit through. Many nutrients are chemically unable to flow through these pores. To solve this problem, specific **carrier molecules** combine with these large molecules to permit diffusion through the cell. Transport carriers are proteins that constitute part of the membrane that must be crossed. They can bind themselves to a particular nutrient, help it through the membrane, and release it. Passive transport of this type is known as "carrier-mediated" or *facilitated* diffusion and is analogous to the use of graphite to ease a key into a lock.

Digestion results in a high concentration of nutrients in the intestinal lumen. Through passive diffusion, then, nutrient molecules are carried from their areas of high concentration in the lumen into the blood and lymph vessels. If the body were dependent only on diffusion, absorption would stop once the concentration gradient was equalized on both sides of the membrane. But that would deprive the body of the benefit of the nutrient molecules still remaining in the small intestine. Moreover, the concentration of some molecules is greater in the cell than in the lumen. To transport those molecules from an area of low concentration to high concentration is an **active transport** process requiring energy and a special transport carrier, as a result of which certain nutrients are "pumped" from the lumen into the intestinal cell. This active transport process is responsible for much of the absorption of calcium, iron, glucose, galactose, and amino acids in our bodies.

After the nutrients leave the small intestine, those that are fat soluble and those that are water soluble follow different routes. Water-soluble nutrients enter the bloodstream via nearby veins, which lead into the large portal vein (see Figure 7). The portal vein carries the nutrients to the liver, which monitors their passage into the general circulation. The nutrients not removed by the liver cells flow with the blood up through the hepatic vein to the heart. From here, the blood travels to the lungs, where it is oxygenated, and then returns to the heart. Blood, with its nutrient freight, is pumped into arteries that will carry it to small capillaries, present in tissues throughout the body. Nutrients move from the capillaries into the extracellular fluid that bathes all the cells of the body.

Fats and fat-soluble nutrients enter the lymphatic system, another circulatory system for transport of body fluids. The lymphatic system bypasses the liver, releasing its content into the general circulation through the thoracic duct and subclavian vein into the right atrium of the heart.

In digestion and absorption, foods are processed and their nutrients sent throughout the body. Most foods consist of combinations of nutrients. Despite all the different kinds of food humans eat and the different chemical reactions to which each is subjected, eventually all foods are digested and transformed into their component nutrients, and eventually all nutrients enter the general circulation for distribution throughout the body. In a sense, the gastrointestinal tract is a long, convoluted column or space enclosed by walls (sort of like a rubber hose) within the body cavity. Only after the end products of digestion have left the gastrointestinal tract and been absorbed into the blood stream can they really be considered as being "in" the body and accessible to the body's cells.

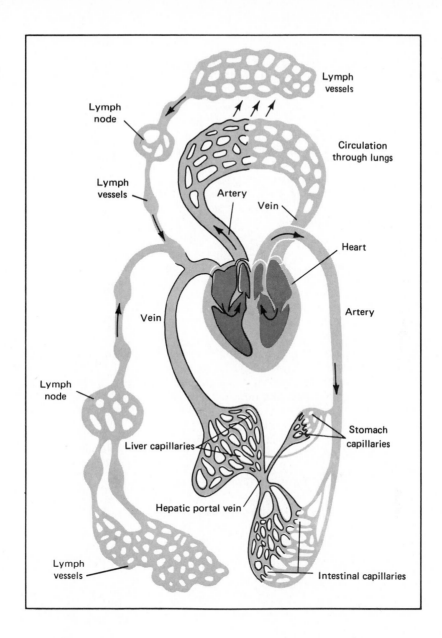

FIGURE 7

After absorption in the small intestine, nutrients (except for fats) enter the general circulation through veins which lead to the large portal vein, in which they are carried to the liver. The liver serves as a control system, selectively storing or releasing various metabolites, which enter the hepatic vein and are transported to the heart. Blood is pumped from the heart to the lungs for oxygenation and returns to the heart for circulation in the arteries. From the arteries blood goes into the capillary network that will carry it, with its nutrient contents, to all body tissues. Fats and fat soluble substances at first do not go through the liver but are carried by the lymphatic circulation, entering the general circulation through the thoracic duct and subclavian vein, which bring them to the heart.

Metabolism

Metabolism refers to all of the chemical processes that occur in the body from the time nutrients are absorbed until they are either made part of the body, used for energy, or excreted.

Metabolism occurs in two phases: anabolism, an *energy-using* process by which substances are built up (synthesized); and catabolism, an *energy-releasing* process by which body substances are broken down into simpler substances. Anabolism and catabolism are dynamic processes, both occurring at the same time but frequently proceeding at different rates. When anabolism exceeds catabolism, growth occurs. When catabolism predominates, the net effect on the body is deterioration, as in starvation, fever, and certain illnesses. In a healthy adult who is no longer growing, these processes reach an overall steady state in which cellular growth and cellular breakdown are balanced.

Metabolic processes occur in every cell of the body. They are regulated by chemicals produced inside the body (endogenous) and also by substances that are supplied from the diet, such as vitamins and minerals (exogenous). Enzymes are part of the metabolic machinery of the internal environment. In addition to the digestive enzymes, hundreds of other enzymes are necessary for anabolism and catabolism. The activity of enzymes, and thus their ability to catalyze reactions, is controlled and influenced by a variety of chemical regulators.

Hormones, for example, are also endogenously produced in body organs called glands. They are transported through the blood to *target* organs where they exert a controlling effect. Hormones act as messengers, ordering the increase or decrease of particular metabolic processes in the target organs. Other molecules that contribute to the control of metabolic processes are **coenzymes**, nonprotein substances that assist enzymes in their catalytic action. Coenzymes often contain vitamins, and we shall examine their role in Chapter 7.

The processes of anabolism and catabolism both produce waste products, all of which must be *excreted* from the body. The kidneys and the large intestine are the body's major waste-handling stations, producing urine and feces. The lungs and the skin are also organs for disposal of **metabolic wastes**. Feces consist mainly of materials that cannot be digested and are not, therefore, primarily metabolic wastes. The lungs serve as the main excretory passage for carbon dioxide and a small amount of water. Other waste products are lost through the skin by perspiration. Some nutrients are incorporated into the nails and hair, which are eventually lost. The kidneys, in addition to excreting wastes into the urine, also help the body to retain key nutrients. As needed, glucose, vitamins, minerals, amino acids, and water are reabsorbed into the blood, by way of the kidneys.

Metabolism, then, is vital to all body functions. The structural organization of all body systems and the processes of digestion, absorption, metabolism, and excretion constitute the internal environment that enables us to use the food we eat and eliminate that which is no longer useful.

GLOSSARY

Absorption The movement of digested food substances from the lumen of the intestine into intestinal cells, and from there into the bloodstream for distribution to other parts of the body.

Acetyl Coenzyme A (Acetyl COA) An important metabolic intermediate that provides energy for cellular function, and is used for the synthesis of cholesterol, fatty acids, and other biological compounds.

Acid Any substance that will release hydrogen ions in solution.

ACTH (Adrenocorticotropic Hormone) A pituitary hormone which regulates the secretion of hormones from the adrenal cortex.

Active Transport An energy-requiring process by which certain nutrients are "pumped" from one compartment to another against a concentration gradient.

Adenosine Triphosphate (ATP) A high-energy compound produced in metabolic pathways and the electron transport system; needed for cellular activity.

Adipocyte Cell that stores fat.

Aerobic Pathway See *Embden-Meyerhof pathway.*

Albumin A water-soluble protein that increases the solubility of fatty acids in the blood, and plays a role in maintaining blood volume.

Aldosterone An adrenal hormone that plays a major role in the regulation of sodium and potassium metabolism.

Amination The addition of an amino group (—NH_2) to a molecule.

Amino Acid Any one of a large group of organic acids characterized by an amino group (—NH_2). Structural unit of proteins.

Anabolism The energy-requiring metabolic processes in which body substances are synthesized from simpler substances.

Anaerobic Pathway See *Krebs cycle.*

Anecdotal Evidence See *Descriptive evidence.*

Animal Model An animal used as an experimental system in research. Rats are the animal model most widely used in nutritional studies.

Anion A negatively charged atom (an atom that has gained one or more electrons).

Anorexia Nervosa Self-imposed starvation, characterized by acute fear of becoming obese, disturbed body image, loss of at least 25 percent of original body weight, and several other criteria.

Antioxidant A substance that delays or prevents oxidation.

Appetite The desire for food; influenced by external (nonphysiological) stimuli.

Association A link between two or more variables; does not necessarily indicate a cause-effect relationship.

Atom The basic structural unit of all substances. All matter in the known universe consists of some 100 distinct types of atoms (elements). Atoms consist of protons, neutrons, and electrons.

Basal Metabolic Rate (BMR) The amount of energy expended for involuntary functions of the body per unit of time: measured under standard conditions; affected by age, sex, size, shape of the body, and physiological state.

Base Any substance that will release hydroxyl (—OH) ions.

Bile Digestive fluid produced by the liver and stored in the gall bladder. Aids in fat digestion and absorption.

Bioavailability The extent to which any nutrient in food is available for utilization by the body.

Biological Value An index of protein quality that reflects the percentage of absorbed dietary nitrogen utilized by the body.

Body Mass Index (BMI) Provides a basis for evaluating fatness or leanness. It is calculated as weight in kilograms divided by the square of the height in meters.

563

Bomb Calorimeter A device used to measure the amount of heat produced by a weighed sample of food, and thus the food's energy value.

Bonding Sharing of electrons by atoms.

Brush Border The collective term for the microvilli that cover the villi and epithelial cells of the small intestine.

Bulemia Characterized by alternate episodes of binging and purging, weight is usually maintained slightly below the normal range. According to some, may be part of anorexia nervosa, not a separate disease.

Calorie The amount of heat necessary to raise the temperature of one liter of water from 15° C to 16° C; a kilocalorie; 1 kilocalorie = 1 Calorie = 1000 calories = 4.184 kilojoules.

Calorimetry The measurement of heat change in an individual or system. As used in nutritional studies, the measurement of heat expenditure. (See *direct calorimetry; indirect calorimetry.*)

Carbohydrate An organic compound containing carbon, hydrogen, oxygen, and sometimes nitrogen and sulfur; a major nutrient class which provides a major source of energy in the human diet; sugars and starches.

Carrier Molecule Specialized protein molecule that enables large molecules to be transported across cell membranes.

Catabolism The energy-releasing metabolic processes in which body substances are broken down into simpler substances.

Catalyst Any substance that speeds up a chemical reaction. Although necessary for a reaction to occur, a catalyst (e.g., an enzyme) is the same in quantity and structure after the reaction as it was before.

Cation A positively charged atom (an atom that has lost one or more of its electrons).

Cell The basic structural and functional unit of living organisms.

Cellulose The most abundant of plant polysaccharides, and for humans, an indigestible carbohydrate; a component of dietary fiber.

Chemical Digestion Process in which biological catalysts or enzymes act on molecules in food to split them into smaller, different molecules.

Chemical Equation An equation that uses chemical formulas and other symbols to represent the changes of bonding that occur between atoms involved in a chemical reaction.

Chemical Formula The symbol or combination of symbols used by chemists to represent the composition of an element or compound (e.g., O_2, H_2O, NaCl).

Chemical Score An index of protein quality; compares the essential amino acid content of a test protein with that of a standard protein.

Chemical Structure In general terms, the arrangement of atoms in a molecule, or of molecules in a compound.

Chemical Symbol The letter or letters used by chemists to represent an element (e.g., H and Ca for hydrogen and calcium, respectively).

Cholesterol The chief sterol synthesized in the human body and present in all tissues; precursor of steroid hormones and vitamin D; dietary cholesterol is found primarily in egg yolks, liver, and organ meats.

Chromosome A giant molecule of DNA and protein located in the cell nucleus; it contains the genes and functions in heredity.

Chylomicrons The least dense type of lipoprotein; transport primarily triglycerides and also some cholesterol.

Chyme Semifluid thick mass consisting of food broken down by the digestive action of gastric juices in the stomach; passes into the small intestine.

Cis Form A term indicating that certain atoms or groups of atoms, relative to a double bond between two carbon atoms, are on the "same side" of a molecule.

Codon A three-nucleotide unit that represents the code for the production of a specific amino acid in the process of protein synthesis.

Coenzyme A nonprotein compound that functions to activate an enzyme.

Complete Protein A term for dietary protein that contains all the essential amino acids in amounts sufficient for growth and maintenance.

Complex Carbohydrate A general term for polysaccharides, molecules in which a number of monosaccharides are combined.

Compound A substance composed of two or more different elements (e.g., CO_2, H_2O).

Condensation Reaction A chemical reaction in which two or more molecules combine.

Controlled Experiment An experiment characterized by a test group and a control group. Experimental conditions are identical for both groups except for a single condition or factor (e.g., a food item). Comparison of results of the test group with those of the control group should reveal the effect (if any) of the test factor or condition.

Cretinism A serious form of thyroid hormone deficiency; symptoms include lethargy, mental retardation, stunted growth, enlarged tongue, and dry skin.

Crystalline Resembling a crystal (a solid body in which atoms are arranged in a symmetrical pattern).

Culture A patterned set of reactions, habits, customs, and ways of life characteristic of a particular group of people.

Cytoplasm The viscous fluid surrounding the cell nucleus and containing cellular organelles.

Deamination Removal of an amino group ($-NH_2$) from a molecule. Some amino acids can be converted to glucose in a process that begins with deamination.

Decarboxylation Removal of a single carbon (in the form of CO_2) from a molecule. Decarboxylation reactions play an important part in the metabolism of glucose.

Denaturation The disruption of the structural arrangement of the atoms in a protein molecule.

Deoxyribonucleic Acid (DNA) The hereditary material found in chromosomes.

Descriptive Evidence A set of facts that "describes" or summarizes a phenomenon. Also called *anecdotal evidence*, it consists essentially of casual impressions rather than recorded data. (Compare *epidemiological evidence; experimental evidence.*)

Diet The food and drink an individual usually consumes; A food regimen.

Dietary Recall A technique of dietary evaluation in which subjects are asked for specific details of their diet during the preceding 24 hours.

Diffusion The passive movement of substances from an area of high concentration to one of low concentration. Water and certain water-soluble nutrient molecules enter the cells of the intestinal lining via diffusion.

Digestion The process by which food substances are broken down into smaller units—mechanically and chemically—for absorption into the body.

Digestive System The specific group of organs responsible for the digestion and absorption of food substances. Major organs of this system include the esophagus, stomach, and intestine.

Digestive Tract A complex tube running through the body, through which food passes as it is absorbed, digested, and excreted.

Diglyceride A glycerol ester having two fatty acids; a lipid.

Direct Calorimetry Determination of the amount of heat released by the body.

Disaccharide A sugar molecule formed by a condensation reaction between two monosaccharides.

Disaccharidase One of a group of enzymes that hydrolyze disaccharides. Found in the cells of the brush border.

Disappearance Data The amount of a given food which leaves the marketplace, that is, disappears. No correction is made for losses.

Edema Tissue swelling caused by an excess of fluid in the interstitial space; seen in thiamin and protein deficiency, as well as some other medical conditions.

Electrolyte A substance that in solution is capable of conducting an electric current.

Electron Negatively charged particle that revolves about the nucleus of an atom. Its mass is negligible, but its negative charge exactly balances the single positive charge of one proton.

Element A substance consisting of only one kind of atom (e.g., oxygen, iron, carbon, hydrogen).

Embden-Meyerhof Pathway Simple glycolysis; a series of energy-producing reactions that can proceed in the absence of oxygen, unlike the Krebs cycle, which is aerobic (requires oxygen).

Emulsification Any process by which a water-insoluble substance is made more soluble. An emulsifier contains both water- and fat-soluble groups. It thus acts as a "bridge" between two substances that would not otherwise mix.

Endocrine System The system of organs (glands) that secrete hormones into the blood.

Endopeptidase One of a group of enzymes that hydrolyze dietary proteins by breaking internal peptide bonds.

Endoplasmic Reticulum (ER) An intracellular system of membranous channels that transport materials throughout the cell. Smooth ER has no ribosomes attached to it; rough ER does.

Energy The capacity to do work. Energy is measured in terms of kilocalories or kilojoules. 4.184 joules = 1 calorie; 4.184 kilojoules = 1 kilocalorie (1 Calorie).

Enterohepatic Circulation The return of bile components to the circulation and the liver from the intestine.

Enzyme A specialized protein molecule that catalyzes a biochemical reaction.

Epidemiological Evidence Evidence based on the occurrence and distribution of a factor or factors associated with a particular phenomenon in a population (e.g., the association of heart disease and obesity).

Epidemiology The study of the occurrence and distribution of factors associated with a particular phenomenon in a given population.

Esophagus The muscular canal through which food passes from the mouth to the stomach.

Essential As applied to nutrition, an essential substance is one that the body requires for growth and maintenance but cannot sythesize in adequate amounts.

Essential Amino Acids Those amino acids that must be supplied in the diet because the body cannot synthesize them.

Essential Fatty Acids Those fatty acids that must be supplied in the diet because the body cannot synthesize them.

Ester A compound resulting from the combination of an alcohol and an acid. Lipids are esters formed from alcohols and fatty acids.

Esterification The process of forming an ester from an alcohol and an acid.

Etiology The origins or causes of a disease.

Excretion The expelling of unused, unusable, and perhaps even detrimental materials back into the external environment.

Experimental Evidence Evidence derived from controlled experiments designed to test the validity of a scientific hypothesis.

Experimental Model A nonhuman system used in research studies. The most common such models in nutritional research are animals. See *animal model.*

External Environment The environment in which an organism exists (the environment outside an organism). See *internal environment.*

Extracellular Compartment The approximately 40 percent of total body water that is found outside cells. Consists of intravascular, interstitial, and transcellular fluids.

Fats Mixture of glycerides (esters of glycerol and fatty acids); commonly, lipids that are solid at room temperature, such as butter.

Fat-Soluble Vitamins Vitamins A, D, E, and K. Because of their chemical nature, they may accumulate in the body.

Fatty Acid An organic molecule; consists of a carbon and hydrogen chain with a carboxyl (acid) group at one end.

Fiber The indigestible remnant of dietary carbohydrate; dietary fiber.

Filtration (Hydrostatic Pressure) Fluid pressure in the blood vessels generated by the pumping action of the heart.

Food A collection of nutrients in a form which is eaten, digested, and metabolized to provide energy and materials that build and maintain the structure and regulate the function of the body.

Food Chain A scheme or sequence of feeding relationships that link member species of a biological community (e.g.: grass, zebra, lion).

Foodway A stylized food habit that has evolved as an adaptation to the physical and social environment.

Free Fatty Acid A fatty acid released from adipose tissue by hydrolysis of a triglyceride.

Fructose A 6-carbon monosaccharide found in many fruits. Also known as levulose, or fruit sugar.

Functional Group An atom or group of atoms that determine or greatly influence the chemical behavior of the molecule to which it is attached.

Galactose A 6-carbon monosaccharide; major component of lactose, or milk sugar.

Gerontology Field of study that explores the psychosocial, physiological, economic, and medical aspects of aging.

Gluconeogenesis Synthesis of glucose from a noncarbohydrate precursor.

Glucose A 6-carbon monosaccharide also known as dextrose, or corn sugar. Found in sweet fruits and certain vegetables.

Glyceride A glycerol ester formed from glycerol and a fatty acid. Mono-, di-, and triglycerides contain one, two, and three fatty acids, respectively. Glycerides constitute a major class of lipids.

Glycerol An important molecule (derived from glucose metabolism) from which glycerides are formed by combination with a fatty acid. See *ester*.

Glycogen The only polysaccharide of animal origin. Stored as an energy source in some tissues; manufactured during glucose metabolism in humans.

Glycogenic Amino acids that can be transformed into glucose.

Glycogenesis The production of glycogen in the body. Glycogen is the storage form of carbohydrate in animals.

Glycolysis The production of energy from the anaerobic breakdown of glucose. Also known as the *anaerobic pathway*.

Goiter Swelling of the thyroid gland, a consequence of iodine deficiency.

Golgi Body Cell organelle that functions in the "packaging" and storage of chemical substances before they are secreted.

Heme The iron-containing complex of the hemoglobin molecule.

Hexose A monosaccharide that contains six carbons (e.g., glucose).

Homeostasis The maintenance of a constant internal environment; the set of physiological mechanisms that maintains this environment as a constant.

Hormone A specialized chemical substance secreted into the blood by an organ or by specific cells of an organ which has a specific effect on "target" cells at some distance from the secreting organ.

Household Survey In nutritional studies, a method of dietary evaluation in which a trained interviewer visits the home to obtain information about household use of foods.

Hunger The sensation produced by the physiological need for food.

Hydrocarbon An organic compound that contains only the elements hydrogen and carbon.

Hydrogenation A process of adding hydrogen to polyunsaturated oils to solidify them. Margarine, for example, contains hydrogenated vegetable oils.

Hydrolysis A reaction in which a chemical bond is split by the addition of a molecule of water.

Hyperglycemia A higher-than-normal concentration of glucose in the blood.

Hyperthyroidism Overactive thyroid; occurs when regulatory mechanisms that control thyroid hormone synthesis do not function.

Hypervitaminosis Any condition resulting from the consumption (or administration) of excessive amounts of a vitamin.

Hypoglycemia A lower-than-normal concentration of glucose in the blood.

Hypothesis Explanation advanced to account for an observation. In scientific research a hypothesis must be confirmed by at least one controlled experiment before it can be accepted as a valid explanation.

Hypothyroidism Underactive thyroid; results in subnormal levels of thyroid hormones in the blood, from insufficient synthesis.

Incomplete Protein Dietary protein that contains less than the optimal amounts of essential amino acids.

Index of Nutritional Quality (INQ) A technique for identifying foods that have a beneficial nutrient:energy ratio. The formula is

$$INQ = \frac{\text{amount of nutrient in food/ddal of food}}{\text{allowance for nutrient/ddal allowance}}$$

Indirect Calorimetry Measurement of the amount of oxygen consumed (which is an index of the amount of energy liberated as heat).

Imino Acid Organic acid having an imino group ($-N^{|}H$). (Compare *amino acid*, NH_2.)

Inorganic Non-carbon-containing substance.

Insulin A pancreatic hormone that plays a crucial role in glucose metabolism. Any interference with the production or function of this hormone will produce symptoms of diabetes mellitus.

Internal Environment The set of conditions, processes, and substances found inside an organism. The nutritional health of an organism is largely a function of the interaction between the internal and the external environment.

International Units (IU) A standard unit that represents the biologic activity of a nutrient.

Interstitial Fluid Together with transcellular fluids accounts for 80 percent of all extracellular fluid in the body (e.g., fluids that bathe all cells, saliva).

Intestinal Lipase An enzyme that hydrolyzes medium- and short-chain triglycerides to glycerol plus short- and medium-chain fatty acids.

Intracellular Compartment The approximately 60 percent of body water that is contained in cells.

Intravascular Fluid The liquid component of the blood; constitutes 20 percent of the extracellular fluid in the body.

Ion Any atom that has lost one or more electrons (becoming a positively charged cation) or gained one or more electrons (becoming a negatively charged anion).

Isomer One of two or more compounds that are identical in chemical composition but differ in structure.

Joule A unit of energy measurement. 4.184 joules = 1 calorie; 4.184 kilojoules = 1 kilocalorie.

Ketone Bodies Fatty-acid derivatives that can function as energy sources.

Ketogenic Amino acids that cannot be converted to glucose.

Ketosis Excessive accumulation of ketone bodies caused by accelerated rate of tissue lipolysis.

Kilocalorie The basic unit of energy in nutrition. The amount of energy (heat) required to raise the temperature of 1 liter of water from 15 to 16 degrees Celsius.

Krebs Cycle The aerobic pathway for oxidation of carbohydrate, protein, and lipid to CO_2, H_2O, and energy.

Kwashiorkor Disease resulting from a deficit of protein relative to energy intake.

Lactase An enzyme required for the digestion of lactose (milk sugar).

Lacteal A specialized lymph vessel in a villus.

Lactose Milk sugar; a disaccharide produced from the condensation of glucose and galactose. It is the only significant dietary carbohydrate of animal origin.

Lean Body Mass A measure of body composition; fat-free body weight.

Lecithin Any of group of phospholipids; an important emulsifier.

Lipid One of a major class of nutrients; any one of a group of fats or fatlike substances.

Lipogenesis The process by which lipids are synthesized in the body.

Lipolysis The breakdown of triglycerides to glycerol and fatty acids.

Lipoprotein A molecule consisting of a lipid and a protein; involved in lipid transport in the blood.

Lysosome Cell organelle. A membrane-bound vesicle contai)ning digestive enzymes that break down intracellular products and debris.

Macronutrient A nutrient substance or element required in large quantity (100 milligrams or more per day).

Major (Macro-) Minerals Dietary minerals required in amounts of 100 milligrams or more per day. See *trace mineral.*

Maltose A disaccharide consisting of two glucose units. It is an intermediate product formed in the breakdown of starch in human digestion.

Marasmus Disease condition reflecting deficits of energy due to a generally inadequate food supply.

Matter Anything that occupies space and has mass (or weight).

Mechanical Digestion Process by which pieces of food are broken down into smaller bits that retain the same chemical identity. See also *chemical digestion.*

Metabolic Disturbance Any disruption of the normal processes of anabolism or catabolism.

Metabolic Wastes The unusable endproducts of anabolic and catabolic processes which are excreted from the body.

Metabolism All the chemical processes that occur in the body from the time nutrients are absorbed until they are utilized or excreted. See *anabolism; catabolism.*

Micelle A specialized aggregate of monoglycerides, fatty acids, cholesterol, phospholipids, and bile.

Micronutrient A vitamin or mineral required in trace amounts for health and growth.

Microvilli Cylindrical outgrowths from villi and surrounding epithelial cells. They constitute the brush border, and function in absorption.

Minerals A group of inorganic nutrients that includes Na, K, P, S, Ca, and Fe.

Mitochondrion (plural: mitochondria). Cell organelle that functions as the site of respiratory reactions involved in energy production.

Molecule A particle consisting of two or more atoms. The atoms may be the same element (as in O_2) or different elements (as in H_2O and CO_2).

Monoglyceride A glycerol ester containing one fatty acid.

Monosaccharide Any "simple sugar"—i.e., a sugar of the general formula $C_n(H_2O)_n$. Classes of monosaccharides are distinguished by the number of carbons they contain (e.g., hexoses all contain six carbons).

Monounsaturated Fatty Acid A fatty acid with one double bond.

Natural Food As defined by the Federal Trade Commission, any food that is minimally processed and contains no artificial ingredients.

Net Protein Utilization (NPU) Proportion of dietary nitrogen that is retained by the body; an index of protein quality.

Neutron Electrically neutral particle located in the nucleus of the atom.

Normoglycemia The condition of having normal levels of blood glucose.

Nucleic Acids DNA (deoxyribonucleic acid) and RNA (ribonucleic acid) found in the cell nucleus.

Nucleotide The basic structural unit of nucleic acid; consists of a purine or pyrimidine base combined with a sugar and phosphoric acid.

Nucleus, Atomic The central core of any atom, containing one or more protons and (except for hydrogen) one or more neutrons, contains almost all of the mass of the atom.

Nucleus, Cell A membrane-bound cluster of materials that functions to regulate the major activities of the cell; contains the chromosomes and the nucleolus.

Nutrients Nutritional substances found in food. These are: four classes of organic compounds (carbohydrates, proteins, lipids, and vitamins), minerals, and water.

Nutrition A term that has two meanings: (1) nutritional science, or the study of nutritional processes; (2) the overall process in which food substances are taken into the body and there transformed and utilized for the proper functioning of the body.

Nutritional Anthropology A discipline concerned with patterns of food acquisition and consumption.

Obesity An excess of body fat that can be estimated from skinfold measurements, underwater weighing, or other techniques.

Oil A lipid that is liquid at room temperature (e.g., corn oil).

Oligosaccharide A term sometimes used in referring to a carbohydrate consisting of two to ten monosaccharide units.

Organ A part of an organism, consisting of one or more tissues organized to perform a specific function.

Organ System Several organs with related functions, such as the respiratory, nervous, circulatory, and digestive systems.

Organelle Subcellular structure that performs a specialized function in a cell (e.g., ribosome).

Organic Substance in living matter that contains carbon.

Organic Chemistry The chemistry of carbon-containing compounds.

Organic Compound Carbon-containing compound. Four classes of such compounds are major nutrients: carbohydrates, proteins, lipids, and vitamins.

Organic Foods A general term for foods grown by methods that do not use pesticides or chemical fertilizers.

Organism A living thing capable of performing all life processes; may be unicellular (bacteria) or multicellular (plants and animals).

Osmosis The movement of water molecules through a membrane.

Osmotic Pressure The pressure that develops when two solutions with different concentrations of solute are separated by a membrane that is permeable only to the solvent.

Ossification The process of bone formation.

Osteoporosis A reduction of total bone mass, common among the elderly everywhere in the world.

Oxidation A chemical reaction that involves the addition of oxygen or the removal of hydrogen or electrons.

Passive Transport A process of diffusion by which substances move from one compartment to another down a concentration gradient; does not require energy.

Pentose A monosaccharide containing five carbon atoms.

Pepsin The primary digestive enzyme produced in the stomach; a proteolytic enzyme.

Peristalsis Rhythmic contraction of muscles of the gastrointestinal tract that aid in propelling material through the digestive system.

pH A chemical measure of relative acidity. A pH value of less than 7 is acidic; more than 7, basic. Physiological pH is 7.4.

Phospholipid A glyceride with fatty acids and a phosphate-containing group (e.g., lecithin).

Pica A craving for nonfood items (e.g., clay).

Plasma Membrane The membrane surrounding the cell. It functions to regulate the passage of substances into and out of the cell.

Polymer A general term for a large molecule consisting of many smaller molecules (or monomers) that are identical or may be of several different types. Polysaccharides are polymers, as are plastics.

Polypeptide A chain of amino acids linked by peptide bonds.

Polysaccharide A carbohydrate containing more than ten monosaccharides; also termed a "complex carbohydrate," in contrast to a simple sugar.

Polyunsaturated Fatty Acid (PUFA) A fatty acid with two or more double bonds.

Pregnancy-Induced Hypertension (PIH) Formerly called toxemia of pregnancy. A condition characterized by edema, high blood pressure, and protein in the urine (albuminuria).

Protein One of six major classes of nutrients; an organic compound consisting of amino acids linked by peptide bonds. Proteins perform a wide variety of structural and functional roles in the body.

Protein Efficiency Ratio (PER) Biologic method of estimating protein quality; defined as weight gain per amount of protein consumed.

Protein-Energy Malnutrition (PEM) A condition caused by insufficient protein and energy intake; characterized by retarded growth, weight loss, listlessness.

Protein Quality A measure of the biologic efficiency of dietary protein; depends on the kinds and amounts of amino acids contained in the protein.

Protein Turnover A term for the breakdown and replacement of protein.

Proton Positively charged particle located in the nucleus of the atom.

Ptyalin An enzyme, found in saliva, that breaks down starch to simple sugars. Also known as salivary amylase.

Pyruvate A metabolic intermediate formed from glucose in glycolysis, and from the deamination of alanine.

Rancid Having a rank smell or taste; spoiled food, especially fats and oils.

Respiratory Quotient (RQ) The ratio of the volume of CO_2 exhaled to the amount of O_2 inhaled.

Resting Metabolic Rate (RMR) Similar to BMR but measured under less rigorous conditions.

Retinol Equivalent (RE) The equivalent of one microgram of retinol; a unit of measure used for vitamin A.

Ribonucleic Acid (RNA) A nucleic acid which plays an important role in protein synthesis (messenger, ribosomal and transfer RNA).

Ribosome Small cellular organelle that functions as the site for protein synthesis. Ribosomes are found free in the cytoplasm and attached to the endoplasmic reticulum.

Ring Structure As used in this text, a diagram for conveniently representing certain large, complex molecules.

Saturated Fatty Acid A fatty acid all of whose carbon atoms are bound to four other atoms with single bonds (containing no double bonds).

Scientific Method A general term for the steps and procedures scientists follow in developing and testing an explanation (or hypothesis) of observed phenomena. Involves experimentation leading to evidence.

Simple Carbohydrate A general term for a monosaccharide or a disaccharide.

Skinfold Thickness A thickness of body fat accumulation, determined by measuring the thickness of a fold of skin.

Society A group with a distinctive culture; may be a tribe, village, ethnic group, or nation.

Solute A substance dissolved in another substance (known as the solvent).

Solvent A substance in which another substance (known as the solute) is dissolved.

Specific Dynamic Effect (SDE) The increase in metabolic rate observed after the digestion, absorption, and metabolism of food.

Starch Name given to most polysaccharides of plant origin.

Steatorrhea Excess lipid in the feces. May be caused by any of several factors which impair fat digestion and absorption.

Subclinical Signs Less obvious signs of a nutritional deficiency that would be overlooked in an ordinary physical examination.

Substance Matter that contains only one kind of atom or molecule.

Substrate Any substance on which an enzyme acts chemically.

Sucrose Table sugar; a disaccharide produced by condensation of glucose and fructose. A widely distributed plant sugar.

Tissue An aggregation of cells of the same type, such as muscle tissue, epithelial tissue, and nerve tissue.

Toxemia Any condition in which the blood contains toxic substances; toxemia of pregnancy is a condition characterized by edema, high blood pressure, and protein in the urine (albuminuria).

Trace Minerals Dietary minerals required in amounts no greater than a few milligrams per day.

Transamination In the synthesis of nonessential amino acids, the transfer of an amino group from an amino acid of one pair to the keto acid of another pair; requires the assistance of specific enzymes.

Transcellular Fluid Together with interstitial fluid accounts for 80 percent of all extracellular fluid in the body (e.g., fluids that bathe all cells, saliva).

Trans Form A term indicating that certain atoms or groups of atoms relative to a double bond between two carbon atoms, are on "opposite sides" of the molecule.

Triglyceride A glycerol ester containing three fatty acids.

Unsaturated Fatty Acid A fatty acid that contains one or more double bonds.

Urea The endproduct of protein metabolism that is excreted in urine.

Valence Shell The "shell" of an atom that contains those electrons involved in reactions with other atoms. The outermost electron shell.

Vegetarianism The practice of consuming a diet consisting exclusively or almost exclusively of plant foods and plant products.

Villi (Sing.: Villus) Small, fingerlike projections that line the small intestine. Function in absorption of nutrients into the body.

Vitamins A major class of nutrients, consisting of two types—fat-soluble and water-soluble.

Water An important nutrient containing hydrogen and oxygen.

Water Intoxication A potentially fatal condition caused by an intake of fluid that exceeds the maximum rate of urinary flow.

Wax A lipid with a high melting point; composed of esters of fatty acids with an alcohol other than glycerol.

INDEX

571

574

Morning sickness, 387
Mortality rates, maternal, 374
Muscles, life span and, 451
Mutant, 104
Myocardial infarction, 82
Myxedema, 295

National Center for Health Statistics, 400
National School Lunch Program, 499
Natural food, 567
Negative energy state, 131
Neomycin, 459
Nervous system, life span and, 451
Net protein utilization (NPU), 113, 567
Neutron, 550, 567
Niacin adenine dinucleotide (NAD), 381
Niacin (nicotinic acid, nicotinamide),
    219-24, 381
Nickel, 303
Nicotinamide, 219-24
Nicotinamide adenine dinucleotide
    (NAD), 220-21
Nicotinamide adenine dinucleotide
    phosphate (NADP), 220-21
Nicotinic acid, 219-24
Night blindness (nyctalopia), 178, 183
Nitrogen, 91
    balance studies, 112
    disposal of, 109
    loss, components of, 112
Nonheme iron, 281, 282
Non-insulin dependent diabetes mellitus
    (NIDDM), 36-37, 42
Normoglycemia, 567
Notation, chemical, 551-54
Nuclear membrane, 555
Nucleic acids, 38, 567
Nucleolus, 555
Nucleotide, 567
Nucleus, 555
    atomic, 568
    cell, 568
Nutrient composition of foods, 532
Nutrients, 495-97
    addition of, 492-93
    defined, 554, 568
Nutri-facts, 358
Nutrition, 1-21
    defined, 568
    ecology of, 9-19
    historical perspective on, 2-4
    information sources, 6-7, 548-49
    maternal, 374-75
    as science, 4-9
Nutritional anthropology, 514-15, 568
Nutritional status, basal metabolic rate
    and, 135
*Nutrition and Your Health, Dietary
    Guidelines for Americans*, 502-3, 504
Nutrition labeling, 355-58
Nutrition Program for older Americans,
    501
Nutrition surveys, 336-37
Nyctalopia, 178, 183

Obesity, 36, 42, 139-64, 280, 462, 466.
    See also Weight reduction
    childhood, 429-30
    concerns about, 142-44
    defined, 140-41, 568
    diagnosis of, 140-41
    hypothalmic, 144
    during infancy, 415-16
    etiology of, 144-49
    prevalence of, 141-42
    psychological costs of, 143
    teenage, 439-40
    treatment of, 149-50

Obligatory urinary nitrogen loss, 112
Observation, 4
Oil
    defined, 568
    mineral, 72-73, 459
Older Americans Act, 501
Oleic acid, 55, 56
Oligosaccharide, 26, 568
Omega-3 fatty acids, 56, 61
Omega-6 fatty acids, 56
Opsin, 178
Oral contraceptives, 460-61
Organ, 568
Organelle, 568
Organic chemistry, 553, 568
Organic compound, 568
Organic foods, 568
Organic matter, 17
Organic substance, 568
Organism, 554
Organ system, 568
Ornithine, 109
Orthomolecular medicine, 244
Osmosis, 314, 568
Osmotic pressure, 107, 568
Ossification (bone formation), 261, 568
Osteoblasts, 180
Osteoclasts, 180
Osteomalacia ("bone softening"), 192,
    466-67
Osteoporosis, 263, 266, 466, 568
Overeaters Anonymous, 164
Overweight, 462
Oxidation, 65
β-oxidation, 75-76
Oxidation, 568
Oxygen, 23
Oxygen transport, 283
Oxytetracycline, 228

Pancreatic juice, 69
Pancreatic lipase, 69
Pancreozymin, 100
Pangamic acid (pangamate; vitamin B_{15}),
    253
Pantothenic acid, 230-33
Para-aminobenzoic acid (PABA), 238,
    252-53
Parathyroid hormone (PTH), 188, 259,
    262, 267
Parents, childhood food behaviors and,
    422-25
Passive transport, 559-60, 568
Pasteurization, 251
Pectic substances, 34
Pellagra, 219, 223-24
Penicillamine, 384
Pentose, 23, 568
Pepsin, 100, 568
Pepsinogen, 100
Peptic ulcer, 463-64
Peptide bond, 92
Periodicals, 549
Peristalsis, 557, 568
Pernicious anemia, 241, 245
Persecution, hints of, 7
Personality types, 83, 280
Perspiration
    insensible, 310-11, 318
    sensible, 310-11
Pesticides, 485
pH, 107, 568
Phenylalanine, 91, 100, 104-5
Phenylketonuria (PKU), 45, 104-5
Phospholipase, 69
Phospholipid, 57, 65-66, 69, 568
    metabolism, 77-78
Phosphorus, 188-89, 266-68, 269, 382

Physical exercise, weight reduction and,
    156-58, 165
Physiology
    adult food patterns and, 467-69
    of digestion, 554-62
    lactation and, 390-91
    life span and, 451-53
Phytate, 260
Pica, 386, 568
Placenta (afterbirth), 366, 369-70
Plan, meal. *See* Meal planning
Planned survey, 5
Plaque, 431
Plasma membrane, 568
Policy, 497-504
Politics, food behavior and, 10
Polychlorinated biphenyls (PCBs), 393,
    409
Polydipsia, 36
Polymers, 26, 568
Polypeptide, 92-93, 104-6, 568
Polyribosome complex, 105
Polysaccharide, 26-27, 568
Polyunsaturated fatty acid (PUFA), 55-56,
    81, 568
Polyuria, 36
Portal vein, 35
Positive energy state, 131
Potassium, 274-76, 277, 322
Potential energy, 131
Poverty, 10, 484
Prader-Willi syndrome, 144
Preeclampsia, 386-87
Pregnancy, 365-89. *See also* Lactation
    adolescent, 372-73, 441
    alcohol and, 388-89
    anemia during, 386
    caffeine and, 388
    cravings and aversions during, 384-86
    energy demands of, 377-80
    food patterns during, 384-89
    gastrointestinal disturbances during, 387
    maternal hormones and tissues during,
        370-71
    maternal nutrition and, 374-75
    medication during, 388
    megaloblastic anemia of, 237, 239-40,
        244-45
    minerals and, 382-84
    nutritional supplementation during,
        375-76
    placenta, 369-70
    prenatal development, 366-69
    protein and, 116, 380-81
    psychoactive substances and, 388
    smoking and, 389
    toxemias, 386-87
    vitamins and, 381-82
Premenstrual edema, 324-25
Premenstrual syndrome (PMS), 237
Prenatal development, 366-69
Preservation of food, 487-88
Preservatives, 485
Pressure
    hydrostatic, 566
    osmotic, 568
Primary vitamin deficiency, 174
Procarboxypeptidase, 100
Production, food, 508, 509-11
Proelastase, 100
Professional resources, 6-7, 548-49
Progesterone, 324, 370-71
Proline, 91
Propionic acid, 75
Prostaglandins, 58, 79
Protein(s), 17, 89-128. *See also* Amino
    acid(s)
    adolescent requirement for, 437
    adult requirement for, 456
    for athletes, 326

577